Medical, Psychosocial and Vocational Aspects of Disability

Fourth Edition
2014

Edited by

Martin G. Brodwin, Ph.D., C.R.C.
California State University, Los Angeles

Frances W. Siu, Ph.D., C.R.C.
California State University, Los Angeles

John Howard, M.D., M.P.H.
George Washington University

Erin R. Brodwin, M.A.
City University of New York

Ashley T. Du, M.S.
California State University, Los Angeles

Elliott & Fitzpatrick, Inc.
Athens, GA

Medical, Psychosocial and
Vocational Aspects of Disability (4th ed.)

Edited by
Martin G. Brodwin, Ph.D., C.R.C.
Frances W. Siu, Ph.D., C.R.C.
John Howard, M.D., M.P.H.
Erin R. Brodwin, M.A.
Ashley T. Du, M.S.

All rights reserved. No portion of this book, in whole or in part, may be reproduced, copied, recorded, duplicated, transmitted, or stored in any form or medium without the written permission of the authors or the publisher.

© 2014 Martin Brodwin, Ph.D.

Hard Cover ISBN: 978-0-9855538-9-0

Published and distributed by: **Elliott & Fitzpatrick, Inc**.
1135 Cedar Shoals Drive
Athens, GA 30605
800-843-4977
email: myorder@elliottfitzpatrick.com

Table of Contents

Preface	**vii**

Part I - Introduction to Rehabilitation Medicine

Chapter 1 - A Case Study Approach, Rehabilitation Intervention, and the Medical Specialties — 1
Martin G. Brodwin, Ph.D., C.R.C. and Sandra K. Brodwin, M.S., C.R.C.

Chapter 2 - Human Body Systems — 17
Frances W. Siu, Ph.D., C.R.C. and Erin R. Brodwin, M.A.

Part II - Common Medical Conditions

Chapter 3 - Cancer — 37
Leo M. Orr, II, M.D. and Leo M. Orange, M.S.

Chapter 4 - Diabetes and Chronic Kidney Disease — 51
Martin G. Brodwin, Ph.D., C.R.C.

Chapter 5 - Cardiovascular Disease — 65
Harvey L. Alpern, M.D.

Chapter 6 - Chronic Obstructive Pulmonary Disease — 77
Hassan Bencheqroun, M.D.

Chapter 7 - HIV/AIDS — 87
John J. Howard, M.D., M.P.H.

Part III - Sensory Organ Conditions

Chapter 8 - Hearing Loss, Deafness, and Related Vestibular Disorders — 101
Shawn P. Saladin, Ph.D., C.R.C. and Sandra Hansmann, Ph.D.

Chapter 9 - Visual Disabilities — 117
Bill Takeshita, O.D., F.A.A.O., F.C.O.V.D., Robin Langman, M.S., C.R.C., and Rebekah Brod, M.A., M.F.T.

Chapter 10 - Chronic Pain Management — 131
Ashley T. Du, M.S., John Lindberg, M.D., and Brendon W. Bluestein, Ph.D.

Chapter 11 - Integrative Medicine — 143
Hua Gu, Ph.D., L.Ac. and Sandra Brodwin, M.S., C.R.C.

Part IV - Brain and Spinal Cord Conditions

Chapter 12 - Traumatic Brain Injury 155
Stacey Hunter Schwartz, Ph.D. and Michelle Ranae Wild, M.A.

Chapter 13 - Stroke 169
Andrew D. Barreto, M.D. and Frances Siu, Ph.D., C.R.C.

Chapter 14 - Epilepsy 181
*Robert T. Fraser, Ph.D., C.R.C., John W. Miller, M.D., Ph.D., and
Erica K. Johnson, Ph.D., C.R.C.*

Chapter 15 - Neurological Diagnoses 193
David B. Peterson, Ph.D., C.R.C. and Thomas VanVleet, Ph.D.

Chapter 16 - Spinal Cord Injury 205
*Gonzalo C. Centeno, M.S., Nancy M. Crewe, Ph.D., and
James S. Krause, Ph.D.*

Part V - Neuromuscular and Joint Conditions

Chapter 17 - Cerebral Palsy 219
Sherwood J. Best, Ph.D.

Chapter 18 - Muscular Dystrophy 233
Roy K. Chen, Ph.D., C.R.C.

Chapter 19 - Multiple Sclerosis 243
Barbara Barton, Ph.D., M.S.W. and Frances W. Siu, Ph.D., C.R.C.

Chapter 20 - Rheumatic Diseases 255
Thomas D. Beardmore, M.D. and Penny J. Chong, M.D.

Part VI – Psychosocial Conditions

Chapter 21 - Psychiatric Diagnoses 269
David B. Peterson, Ph.D., C.R.C. and George K. Hong, Ph.D.

Chapter 22 - Sexual Health and Disability 285
Leo M. Orange, M.S.

Chapter 23 - Addictions and Related Disorders 295
Frederick Payo, M.S. and Frances W. Siu, Ph.D., C.R.C.

Chapter 24 - Alcohol-Related Disorders 309
Roman Carlos, M.S., C.R.C.

Part VII - Developmental Conditions

Chapter 25 - Learning Disabilities 317
*Diane Haager, Ph.D., Christine C. Givner, Ph.D., and
Martin G. Brodwin, Ph.D., C.R.C.*

Chapter 26 - Intellectual Developmental Disorders 329
*Julie Ton, Ph.D., Mary A. Falvey, Ph.D., Kathryn D. Bishop, Ph.D., and
Susann Terry Gage, Ph.D.*

Chapter 27 - Autism Spectrum Disorder   **343**
*Frances W. Siu, Ph.D., C.R.C. and Jessica H. Franco, Ph.D.,
CCC-SLP, BCBA-D*

Part VIII - Assistive Technology and Reconstructive Repair

Chapter 28 - Orthotics, Amputation, and Prosthetics   **353**
Lance R. Clawson, B.S., C.P.O. and Martin G. Brodwin, Ph.D., C.R.C.

Chapter 29 – Societal Reintegration Following a Burn Injury   **367**
Cindy Rutter, R.N., B.S.N. and Ann Malo, R.N.

Chapter 30 - Evaluating Upper Extremity Function and Impairment   **377**
*George W. Balfour, M.D., Martin G. Brodwin, Ph.D., C.R.C.,
and Ashley T. Du, M.S.*

Chapter 31 - Assistive Technology and Universal Design   **389**
R. David Black, Ed.D., C.R.C. and Martin G. Brodwin, Ph.D., C.R.C.

Part IX – Genetics

Chapter 32 - Sickle Cell Disease and Hemophilia   **399**
John J. Howard, M.D., M.P.H.

Chapter 33 - Genetic Testing, Discrimination, and Counseling   **409**
John J. Howard, M.D., M.P.H.

Chapter 34 - Regenerative Medicine and Disability   **415**
John J. Howard, M.D., M.P.H.

Appendix   **423**

Index   **431**

PREFACE

Our sincere appreciation to the more than 90 universities and colleges in the United States and beyond that have selected *Medical, Psychosocial, and Vocational Aspects of Disability* as a textbook for rehabilitation education. It has also been used by continuing education programs, clinicians, and public and private rehabilitation agencies as a resource book. This fourth edition has three new chapters, including societal reintegration following a burn injury, assistive technology/universal design, and regenerative medicine and disability. Chapter One has a new section on medical specialties. There are ten new authors since the third edition. This edition, like the second and third editions, has major changes, modifications, additions, and updates.

Background

The enactment of the Americans with Disabilities Act (ADA) of 1990 signaled a new era in America for persons with disabilities. These individuals, often excluded from mainstream society, are participating in all phases of life to a far greater extent. Rehabilitation counselors, as well as educators, nurses, counselors in other settings, work evaluators, case managers, and family members participate in facilitating increasing progression into independent living, education, employment, and leisure activities for persons with disabilities. The ADA defined a person with a disability as someone who: "(1) has a physical or mental impairment that substantially limits one or more major life activities; (2) has a record of such an impairment; or (3) is regarded as having such an impairment."

Rehabilitation counseling involves assisting people with disabilities to acquire skills necessary for maximum functioning and independence. Professionals who have an understanding of medical and psychosocial aspects of disability and its relationship to employment are in demand within the counseling profession. Counselors need to read, understand, and interpret medical and psychological reports and other information regarding clients for whom they provide rehabilitation services. Knowledge of chronic illness and disability is crucial for counselors working with persons with disabilities. With comprehension of this information, counselors are better able to determine their clients' functional capabilities and limitations, including potential for rehabilitation.

Knowledge of functional capabilities and limitations allows the counselor and the individual with a disability to obtain information necessary for developing positive directions for rehabilitation. Rehabilitation services may include job modification, reasonable accommodation, educational pursuit, training or on-the-job training, supported employment, job placement, and independent living. The purpose of rehabilitation counseling is to empower the individual with a disability to successfully participate in all phases of life.

Overview

This is a textbook for students and a reference book for practicing counselors and other helping professionals. The intended audience includes rehabilitation counselors in public and private sectors, rehabilitation educators and students, vocational experts, work evaluators, counselors, and rehabilitation service providers. Allied health professionals in related disciplines also will benefit from the information within this text.

The reader is encouraged to have a medical dictionary available when reading this book. A glossary was not included, as the editors have found glossaries to be inadequate, both in providing sufficient explanations and in defining most of the required vocabulary. Various words throughout the text are provided with a short definition in parentheses.

The fourth edition of *Medical, Psychosocial, and Vocational Aspects of Disability* contains thirty-four chapters encompassing common disabilities encountered in the field of rehabilitation. Most of the chapters conclude with case studies to stimulate thinking and discussion about the topic. All case studies have a strong multicultural emphasis and are hypothetical scenarios. We believe the richness of cultural diversity adds an important dimension to the material.

We suggest the reader begin with Chapter 1, "A Case Study Approach: Rehabilitation, Intervention, and the Medical Specialties," as this chapter describes the case study analysis approach used throughout the book. Subsequent chapters can be reviewed in the order that best suites the needs of the reader.

Acknowledgments

The editors prepared the textbook to maintain the meaning and philosophy of each author, while conforming to a similar style within chapters. We sincerely appreciate each author's time and patience during the difficult writing and editing process. We believe that through their efforts, this text will provide readers with an excellent resource for medical and psychosocial aspects of chronic illness and disabling conditions, as well as the relationship to employment issues.

Martin G. Brodwin, Ph.D. C.R.C.
Professor
Rehabilitation Education Programs
California State University, Los Angeles

Chapter 1

A CASE STUDY APPROACH, REHABILITATION INTERVENTION, AND THE MEDICAL SPECIALTIES

Martin G. Brodwin, Ph.D., C.R.C.
Sandra K. Brodwin, M.S., C.R.C.

Introduction

Rehabilitation professionals need expertise concerning medical aspects of disabling conditions to work effectively with persons who have disabilities. Increasingly, rehabilitation counselors are expected to have greater knowledge and skills, and demonstrate case management expertise when working with employers to facilitate a return to work for individuals with chronic illnesses and disabilities. Counselors apply this expertise both when developing educational/vocational plans and determining functional limitations and rehabilitation potential. Knowledge of medical aspects of disability is a significant component when developing rehabilitation interventions. The *Vocational Profile* case study approach is one holistic method of evaluating a person's vocational potential using analysis of age, education, work history, occupationally significant characteristics of work, and transferable skills.

The basic criterion for acceptance for vocational rehabilitation is the existence of a disability which causes functional limitations and results in an impediment to employment. One of the attributes differentiating rehabilitation counselors from other counselors and mental health professionals is specialized knowledge and expertise related to disability. As no two people are alike, there are a variety of characteristics affecting each person's potential to benefit from rehabilitation services. Similar medical diagnoses have different effects, depending on a person's psychosocial circumstances, adaptation to functional limitations, vocational skills, education, and occupational history. Examples of components which affect rehabilitation potential for employment include (Brodwin, Parker, & DeLaGarza, 2010; Gilbride & Stensrud, 2012):

- Severity of disability (residual capacities and functional limitations)
- Age at onset of disability
- Current age
- Gender and ethnicity
- Psychological characteristics
- Pre-existing physical conditions
- Social functioning
- Educational and vocational training
- Employment
- Psychosocial adjustment to disability
- Use of assistive technology

Development of vocational and educational rehabilitation plans and programs relies heavily on the expertise of rehabilitation professionals. A realistic and practical objective for a vocational or educational plan must be formulated according to an individual's physical, intellectual, and emotional capacities. To establish a realistic and practical objective, the rehabilitation professional applies knowledge of the vocational profile, medical aspects of the disability, the individual's interaction with the environment, and the person's effort and persistence to accomplish goals.

This chapter addresses the functions of rehabilitation professionals when providing services in a variety of rehabilitation systems. The authors believe the use of the *vocational profile* approach will enhance a thorough case analysis and improve the opportunities for a person to become employed or reemployed. The chapter focuses on the importance of the holistic approach to enhance the potential for successful, meaningful, and satisfying rehabilitation. It discusses various aspects of functional limitations, rehabilitation potential, case intervention, a holistic approach, and the medical specialties.

Vocational Profile

The words, *Vocational Profile* are used specifically by Vocational Experts (VEs) for the Social Security Administration's (SSA) Office of Disability Adjudication and Review when testifying about disability-related issues. More broadly, however, the SSA vocational profile model is part of a nationally-mandated program that is uniform throughout the country. Vocational profiles are developed to include age, education, and work history categories as they relate to individuals, as well as occupationally significant characteristics and work skills transferability. The following categories – **age** (SSA Section # 404.1563), **education** (SSA Section # 404.1564), and **work experience** (SSA Section #s 404.1565, 404.1567, and 404.1568) – are taken from the guidelines of the Social Security Administration (Office of the Federal Register, 2001).

Age Category

Age is considered when evaluating the total person; as one ages, adaptation to new and unfamiliar situations becomes increasingly difficult. The magnitude of age as an evaluation factor varies with a person's work history. For example, if an individual has had only physically demanding jobs and developed few work skills, age can play a crucial role in rehabilitation.

Younger Person

An individual is considered to be within this category if under the age of 50. Generally, if in this category, the person's age will not impact the ability to adapt to new work.

Person Approaching Advanced Age

An individual between 50-54 years of age is considered a *person approaching advanced age*. A person in this age category who has a severe impairment and limited work experience may have major difficulty adjusting to many jobs within the labor market.

Person of Advanced Age

This category is appropriate if a person is between 55-59 years of age. With advancing age, it becomes more difficult to obtain employment, especially with an unskilled work background, a history of physically arduous work, and minimal education. Skills that can be transferred to similar jobs and work activity (often less physically demanding) become more relevant as the individual ages.

Close to Retirement Age

When individuals are 60 years of age or older, they are considered, by Social Security regulations to be *close to retirement age*. Skills at this age need to be highly transferable and are pivotal to success in the rehabilitation process.

Educational Level

Educational level is the amount of formal schooling a person has achieved. Grade level is only one means of assessment. When evaluating rehabilitation potential, the counselor needs to consider how long ago a person attended school, quality of the educational experience, additional informal or formal education, and other training that has occurred.

Illiteracy

Illiteracy means an inability to read or write. People are placed in this category if they cannot read or write simple messages, such as basic instructions, inventory lists, simple messages, and the like.

Marginal Education

Generally, *marginal education* indicates a formal education at the 6th grade level or less. The person who has a *marginal education* is limited to basic reasoning, arithmetic, and language skills.

Limited Education

A person of *limited education* has been formally educated between the 7th and 11th grades, without having attained a high school diploma or its equivalence.

High School Education and Above

High school education and above implies achieving a high school diploma or its equivalence. Attainment of a General Equivalency Diploma (GED) is at this level. Those with further education beyond high school are classified within this category. Individuals so classified have obtained reasoning, arithmetic, and language skills required for more complex work activity.

Work History

The following section of the vocational profile is subdivided into several categories. These include skill requirements, physical exertion, occupationally significant characteristics, vocational skills, and transferability of skills.

Skill Requirements

Unskilled Work

Work that requires little or no judgment for the completion of simple duties and is learned on the job in a short time is unskilled work. Unskilled jobs require 30 days or less to learn. While they are quickly learned, these jobs frequently require considerable strength. Primary work duties for an unskilled occupation could, for example, involve stock or material handling, machine feeding, sorting, simple assembling, or machine tending. Little specific vocational preparation or judgment are thus required. **A person does not gain work skills (transferable skills) by working in unskilled jobs.** When a worker develops skills, the work is considered to have changed to semiskilled work, as unskilled work never involves skills.

Semiskilled Work

Semiskilled work requires some skills but not complex work activity. This category consists of activities that are less complex than skilled work but more complex than unskilled work and can involve dexterity tasks such as working with tools, equipment, and measuring devices. These jobs may involve alertness and close attention to observing machine processes or inspecting, testing, or quality control. Such aspects also may include guarding equipment, materials, or persons against damage, loss, or injury. Typically, semiskilled work requires training from over 30 days to a maximum of two years.

Skilled Work

This category of work requires an individual to use judgment to determine fairly complex machine and manual operations performed to obtain the proper form, quality, and quantity of materials produced. Skilled work may require laying out work, estimating quality, determining suitability and needed quantities of material, making precise measurements, reading blueprints or other specifications, or making complex computations or mechanical adjustments to control or regulate the work. Other skilled jobs involve dealing with people, facts or figures, or abstract ideas at a high level of complexity. Skilled work typically requires more than two years of learning.

Physical Exertion Requirements

When reviewing a client's past relevant work experience, the counselor evaluates the level of physical exertion required at work. The individual's residual functional capacity (RFC) in conjunction with age, education, and work experience, are considered to determine whether the individual can engage in any other substantial gainful work which exists in the national economy. Physical exertion requirements are summarized in the following categories. Each functional level is defined (in accordance with terms used by the United States Department of Labor) by the extent of its requirements in the primary strength activities of sitting, standing, walking, lifting, carrying, pushing, and pulling. If medical reports regarding the client's disability indicate return to work at one exertional level, the counselor and client need to investigate work situations requiring equal or lesser physical exertion.

Occasionally means occurring from very little up to one-third of the work time. Typically, this is defined as ranging from 5 minutes up to 2½ hours per day. A *frequent* activity occurs one-third to two-thirds of the time (a total of 2½ to 5 hours). Since frequent lifting or carrying requires being on one's feet up to two-thirds of a workday, the full range of light work requires standing or walking, off and on, for a total of approximately 6 hours of an 8-hour workday. Sitting may occur intermittently during the remaining time. The lifting requirement for the majority of light jobs can be accomplished with occasional, rather than frequent, stooping. *Continuously* is defined as an activity which occurs for a total of more than 5 hours per day.

Sedentary Work

The regulations define sedentary work as involving lifting no more than 10 pounds at a time and occasionally lifting or carrying items weighing 5 pounds or less, such as files and small tools. Although sitting is involved, for some jobs a certain amount of walking and standing may be necessary in carrying out job duties. Jobs are sedentary if walking and standing are required less than occasionally and other sedentary criteria are met. By its very nature, work performed primarily in a seated position entails no significant stooping, kneeling, or bending.

Light Work

The regulations define light work as lifting no more than 20 pounds at a time with frequent lifting or carrying of objects weighing up to 10 pounds. Even though the weight lifted in a particular light job may be very little, a job is in this category when it requires a good deal of walking or standing – the primary difference between sedentary and most light jobs. A job is also in this category when it involves sitting most of the time but with some pushing and pulling of arm-hand or leg-foot controls, which require greater exertion than in sedentary work. Examples of these are a mattress sewing machine operator, motor-grader operator, and road-roller operator (skilled and semiskilled jobs in these particular instances). Relatively few unskilled light jobs are performed in a seated position.

Medium Work

The regulations define medium work as lifting no more than 50 pounds at a time with frequent lifting or carrying of objects weighing up to 25 pounds. A full range of medium work requires standing or walking, off and on, for a total of about 6 hours in an 8-hour workday to meet the requirements of frequent lifting or carrying objects weighing up to 25 pounds. As in light work, sitting may occur intermittently during the remaining time. Use of the arms and hands is necessary to grasp, hold, and turn objects, as opposed to the finer activities in most sedentary work, which require precision use of the fingers as well as use of the hands and arms. The lifting required for the full range of medium work usually requires bending-stooping at the frequent level or less. Stooping is a type of bending in which a person bends his or her body downward and forward by bending the spine at the waist. Crouching is bending both the legs and spine to bend the body downward and forward. In most medium jobs, being on one's feet for most of the workday is required.

Heavy Work

Lifting a maximum of 100 pounds occasionally with frequent lifting or carrying up to 50 pounds defines heavy work.

Very Heavy Work

Very heavy work involves lifting more than 100 pounds occasionally with frequent lifting or carrying of 50 pounds or more.

The following table summarizes the exertional categories of work.

TABLE 1
Exertional Categories of Work

Category	Lifting/Carrying	
	Frequent	Maximum (occasional)
Sedentary	2-5 pounds	10 pounds
Light	10 pounds	20 pounds
Medium	25 pounds	50 pounds
Heavy	50 pounds	100 pounds
Very Heavy	50 pounds or more	100 pounds or more

Occupationally Significant Characteristics

Occupationally significant characteristics are distinctive elements that contribute to the job, work environment, and work functions, but **do not involve skills or characteristics of a person**. Occupational characteristics exist independent of the worker and often can be modified, if necessary. Examples of occupationally significant characteristics include: eye-hand-foot coordination, visual perception, being around other people, exertional level of work (sedentary, light, medium, heavy, and very heavy), inside work, routine and repetitive job functions, activities requiring occasional bending and stooping, work involving fumes and irritants, among others.

An individual who has worked as a secretary, for example, may have some or all (depending on the particular job) of the following occupationally significant characteristics: indoor work, eye-hand coordination, sedentary work activity, work with other people, use of office equipment, clerical work, and work with information. In contrast, the work of a truck driver may include characteristics such as: manual dexterity, eye-hand-foot coordination, work within the transportation industry, medium exertion, working alone, and being in a variety of environmental conditions. Rehabilitation counselors need to be careful not to identify occupationally significant characteristics as skills. **As can be seen from these examples, occupationally significant characteristics do not involve the acquisition or use of skills**.

Vocational Skills and Transferability of Skills

Skills involve abilities that are learned during work, training, or educational programs. They are distinct from occupationally significant characteristics because they require work experience and the acquisition of abilities. Skills involve expertise or knowledge specific to work functions, such as the ability to use personal judgment, work with specific tools and equipment, operate complex machinery, and/or work with people or ideas at a high level of complexity.

The skills of a rehabilitation counselor include capability to communicate and organize, ability to counsel individuals regarding personal concerns, career development, and vocational pursuits; skills involved in helping persons secure employment; management and supervision capabilities; knowledge of medical aspects of chronic illness and disability, medical terminology, and medical treatments; and ability to work with troubled and distraught individuals with serious problems. In contrast, the skills of a secretary include: clerical skills; ability to operate various office machines; capability to use a computer and related equipment; compile, type, and file letters; aptitude to organize and maintain a record-keeping system; answer business telephones; communication capacities; and organizational skills required to maintain the clerical flow of an office.

The *Dictionary of Occupational Titles (D.O.T.)* (U. S. Department of Labor, 1991) and other resources can be used effectively when transferring skills from one job to another. Only skilled and semiskilled work provides transferable skills. Unskilled work, by definition, does not involve skills and, therefore, transferability of skills is not relevant to these positions. Skills, abilities, and knowledge found in skilled and semiskilled work can be transferred to a position requiring equal or lesser skills, but not to a position of greater skill requirements. An employee may be promoted to a more skilled position before acquiring the skills of that position and then learn the skills on the new job.

An example of transferability from a skilled position is illustrated by the occupation of rehabilitation counselor. Duties of this job can transfer to other skilled and semiskilled positions. Skilled positions include manager of a human resource department, college counselor, rehabilitation director, academic advisor, supervisor, teacher, mental health clinician, parole and probation officer, and vocational evaluator. The skills of a rehabilitation counselor also transfer to semiskilled work activities such as personnel interviewer, job analyst, job placement specialist, research assistant, and work evaluation technician. A semiskilled occupation, such as secretary, has transferable skills to other semiskilled work such as office clerk, receptionist, file clerk, general office worker, and word processor. Since the work is semiskilled, there is no transferability to skilled work.

When analyzing rehabilitation potential, all job possibilities need careful evaluation. Initial exploration includes determining the skill requirements of previous jobs held by the client to indicate potential transferable skills. The rehabilitation counselor can then identify other jobs within the same industry that use these skills. Next, the research process expands to jobs in related industries using transferability of skills. Finally, if no positions exist within the client's physical exertional (or emotional) restrictions using transferable skills, the counselor investigates alternative rehabilitation options. While determining transferability of skills, the counselor needs to assess how long ago the job was performed and whether the skills are outdated or forgotten, as well as the length of time the individual held the job.

If the client's skills are not immediately transferable to jobs within the current labor market (using direct job placement), the rehabilitation professional may consider on-the-job training, vocational training, and educational programs. The counselor and client use various criteria when selecting the type of plan best suited for the client.

The rehabilitation professional in a provider system applies expertise in medical aspects of chronic illness and disability to develop vocational and educational plans with practical, realistic, and obtainable objectives. The basis for the rehabilitation objective includes analysis of the client's age, education, work history, occupationally significant characteristics, transferable skills, capacities, and functional limitations (Brodwin, 2008). Roessler and Rumrill (1995), in a discussion of reasonable accommodations and job retention, discussed the need for postemployment services. These services reduce or remove barriers to successful employment outcomes. Three factors are crucial to successful job retention: (a) identification of barriers to employment and job accommodation strategies, (b) initiation of requests for accommodation, and (c) implementation of accommodations with cooperation of the employer.

Functional Limitations

A functional limitation is defined as "the inability to perform an action or set of actions because of a physical, mental, or emotional restriction" (Martin, Walls, Brodwin, Parker, Siu, & Kurata, 2012, p. 7). A clearly specified limitation of function helps the counselor understand the performance limitation(s) of the client. Restrictions can be analyzed with a clear understanding when medical conditions are stated in functional terms.

Examples

Client 1: An individual has a below the knee (BK) amputation of the left lower extremity. In functional terms, this person may be limited to maximum ambulation of one hour during an eight-hour workday, no ambulation on rough or uneven surfaces, no stair climbing, and no continuous standing.

Client 2: A person has a low back injury and a problem with lifting and carrying. Functionally, the individual is limited to lifting a maximum of 20 pounds on an occasional basis with repetitive lifting and carrying not to exceed 10 pounds (light work).

Client 3: This person has a psychiatric diagnosis involving moderate depression and anxiety. In functional terms, the individual needs low stress work with an understanding female supervisor (because of a problem with dominant male authority figures).

Client 4: The individual has a diagnosis of schizophrenia, chronic undifferentiated type. In functional terms, this person needs work that involves simple, routine, and repetitive activities with minimal personal interaction within a structured work environment.

Medical conditions described in functional terms enable the counselor to more readily understand the client's limitations. First, the rehabilitation professional assesses the client's vocational profile. The second step is to review the medical file and make sure the limitations are understood in functional terms. The rehabilitation counselor then determines the potential for vocational rehabilitation and return to work.

Rehabilitation Potential

For individuals to maximize their potential for rehabilitation, four factors need assessment: (a) the attainment of increased functioning in the areas of physical and emotional growth and development; (b) a sense of well being; (c) development of a personally satisfying level of independence; and (d) compatibility between the work and the person's capabilities and limitations. These four factors relate to employment and psychosocial adjustment. One's attitude and adaptation to disability also impact rehabilitation potential and success in a vocational or educational program.

Rehabilitation systems (e.g., disability management, long-term disability, Social Security, state vocational rehabilitation, and independent living) define a client's rehabilitation potential differently. A person may have rehabilitation potential within an independent living program but not with the state department of rehabilitation. Another individual may be considered to have rehabilitation potential within a public agency but not in certain private agency settings (such as long-term disability).

Counselors need an understanding of the distinct requirements of the particular rehabilitation system that is providing services (Brodwin, 2008). Each system has its own advantages and limitations. Once the counselor determines the client's rehabilitation potential within the specific system, a rationale is developed and presented to support the decision as to what rehabilitation services will be provided. The counselor needs to clarify if the medical conditions are temporary or permanent, and whether they may be expected to improve, remain the same, or deteriorate.

Additionally, one needs to assess whether the particular rehabilitation system providing services influenced this determination (e.g., eligibility criteria). The counselor should inform the client of the decision and the basis for that decision. If denying services, the counselor may be able to refer the client to another system where appropriate and applicable services or benefits are provided. If a client does not qualify for vocational rehabilitation services, the counselor may refer the person for Social Security benefits (SSDI, SSI). Each rehabilitation system evaluates rehabilitation potential, including length of time typically provided for rehabilitation services, medical expenses, rehabilitation costs, and the likelihood of return to gainful employment.

Rehabilitation Intervention

Through the provision of rehabilitation intervention, counselors may be able to modify environmental factors for clients with disabilities to empower them to succeed at productive activities. Modifications of the environment include accommodation, job modification, and restructuring of job sites.

Job Accommodation, Modification, and Restructuring

Reasonable accommodation is a logical adjustment made to a job or work environment that enables a qualified person with a disability to perform the duties of the position (Berkeley Planning Associates, 1982). Reasonable accommodation recommendations must be considered on an individual basis for each employee and employer. Cooperation on the part of the employer is essential to successful accommodation on the job.

Section 503 of the Federal Rehabilitation Act of 1973 and the Americans with Disabilities Act (ADA) of 1990 mandated reasonable accommodation. Employers have an obligation to make reasonable accommodation for physical and mental limitations, unless the accommodation imposes an *undue hardship* on the employer. Undue hardship depends upon several factors including cost, financial resources of the company, overall size of the employer, employer's operation (including composition and structure of the workplace), and the nature of the proposed accommodation.

The ADA stated that modifications necessary under the *reasonable accommodation* provisions include (Rubin & Roessler, 2008):

1. Restructuring a job to enable the person with a disability to perform the essential functions of the job.
2. Establishing a part-time or modified work schedule for employees with disabilities who are not capable of working a typical work day or work week.
3. Reassigning a person with a disability to a vacant position.
4. Acquiring or modifying equipment or devices (e.g., buying a hearing telephone amplifier for a person with a hearing impairment).
5. Adjusting or modifying examinations, training materials, or policies (e.g., giving an application examination orally to a person with dyslexia, or modifying a policy against dogs in the workplace for a person with a service dog).
6. Providing qualified readers or interpreters for people with vision or hearing impairments.
7. Giving an employee with a psychiatric illness a private place to work to alleviate stress.
8. Modifying the physical layout of a facility to make it accessible to employees who use wheelchairs or who have other impairments which make accessibility difficult.

Reasonable accommodation rarely involves considerable cost. Berkeley Planning Associates (1982) conducted a study for the U. S. Department of Labor on accommodation in private sector employment and noted the following results:

- About 50% of the reasonable accommodations surveyed cost less than $50
- Thirty percent cost between $50-$500
- Ten percent cost between $500-$2,000
- Ten percent cost in excess of $2,000

The Department of Labor study concluded that, based on the above figures, reasonable accommodation is *no big deal*. This study reported that the most expensive and extensive accommodations are usually provided to individuals with blindness and to persons who use wheelchairs. Frequently, reasonable accommodations that are expensive and extensive are provided by employers for current employees to maintain their ability to continue working. Assuming cooperation between employers and employees, most accommodations cost less than $100 (Muther, 1996).

Employers need to understand that accommodation efforts help persons with chronic illness and disabilities become employed or remain successful on the job. There appears to be no significant relationship between accommodation and upward mobility, either by providing an advantage to a specific employee or in limiting job potential. Highly skilled workers more often receive environmental adaptations of the workplace and special equipment, while lower skilled workers receive job redesign, retraining, and selective placement.

Large firms are most likely to hire and accommodate persons with disabilities for the following reasons (Berkeley Planning Associates, 1982; Gilbride & Stensrud, 2012):
1. The existence of affirmative action programs in larger firms.
2. The likelihood of encountering persons with disabilities because of the sheer numbers of workers employed.
3. The much greater diversity of job types in larger firms that lead to more possibilities of hiring and greater flexibility in job assignments.

Smaller firms are less likely to have (a) knowledge of and information about the ADA and (b) personnel who understand and can investigate potential accommodations.

Types of Reasonable Accommodation

I. **Physical access accommodation**
   A. A change or modification of the physical structure
   B. Examples - Accessibility/ambulation solutions
      1. Situate job on first floor
      2. Situate job near employee parking lot
      3. Situate job near restroom

II. **Resource accessibility accommodation**
   A. Providing an assistive person to enable the individual to do the job duties
   B. Examples
      1. Hearing impairment - Provide note taker or sign language interpreter
      2. Visual impairment - Provide reader or note taker
      3. Developmental disability (e.g., intellectual disability) - Provide a job coach

III. **Adaptive equipment accommodation**
   A. Provision of low tech and high tech assistive devices
   B. Examples
      1. Person with arthritis or carpal tunnel syndrome - Provide special pen/pencil holders
      2. Orthopedic problems
         a. Provide desk or chair modifications
         b. Provide speaker and earphone on telephone
      3. Reaching problems
         a. Provide a turntable on a desk
         b. Provide a special desk that has easy accessibility
      4. Neck problems - Provide a slant board on a desk
      5. Visual impairment - Provide a talking calculator or talking computer
      6. Hearing impairment
         a. Provide a telephone amplifier
         b. Provide a speaker telephone
      7. Quadriplegia - Provide a computer with specialized keyboard and an electronic wheelchair with assistive devices

IV. Job modification
A. Modifying the performance of job duties while maintaining the same job duties
B. Examples
1. Energy or ambulation problems - Salesperson can do more telephone sales and decrease field appointments
2. Energy problem - Design drafter can work part-time with an adjusted salary
3. Orthopedic problems
   a. Parking-lot attendant can use a chair for sitting instead of standing throughout the day
   b. Warehouse worker can lift and carry lesser weights by making more frequent trips with lighter weights
   c. Scheduling - Secretary can leave early *for physical therapy appointments by coming to work earlier*

V. Job restructuring
A. Changing some of the actual job duties performed (alter, eliminate, or replace job duties)
B. Examples
1. Ambulation problem - Rehabilitation counselor can be assigned more office work (labor market surveys, job development, job placement, initial interviews) and less field work (on-site job analysis, school visits, employer visits)
2. Emotional stress
   a. Social worker can be assigned more case file analysis and paperwork and less interviewing and field visits
   b. Attorney can be assigned more research, case preparation, and legal briefs and less time litigating in court
3. Lower extremity problems - Shipping and receiving clerk can be assigned more clerical work (typing reports, bills of lading, and expediting) and less lifting, carrying, standing, walking, and forklift driving

Job Accommodation Network (JAN) is a resource available for additional information about employer accommodations. They have an 800 toll-free telephone number. This telephone service is provided at no cost and allows the counselor, employer, and consumer access to information on restructuring possibilities and costs. Consultants are available Monday through Friday. Before calling JAN, one needs the specific medical restrictions of the client, job duties which are precluded as a result of the restrictions, and general information about the industry in which the job is located.

A Holistic Approach To Rehabilitation

Holistic rehabilitation stresses the importance of the person as a whole and the interdependence of the various facets of the individual. A person, with or without a disability, is not an isolated entity. There is continuous interaction between the person and the environment. Interventions in one area of the person's environment have an influence on other areas. Seven areas most pertinent to a holistic approach are the person's disability, psychological status, vocational experiences, educational background, social issues, spirituality/belief system, and culture (see Figure 1). Disability can be expressed in functional limitations. Psychological status involves emotional factors that impede rehabilitation planning (Vash & Crewe, 2004). The more extensive the person's vocational experiences and education, the greater the opportunities for success. Social functioning of the person involving interaction with family, friends, and associates is a factor to evaluate. Spirituality and one's belief system can enhance rehabilitation outcomes (Joseph E. Havranek, Ed.D., C.R.C., personal communication, March 2000). The counselor needs an understanding, careful consideration, and acceptance of the client's culture and ethnicity. Viewing rehabilitation from a holistic perspective enhances the probability of a successful outcome.

FIGURE 1
A Holistic View of the Individual

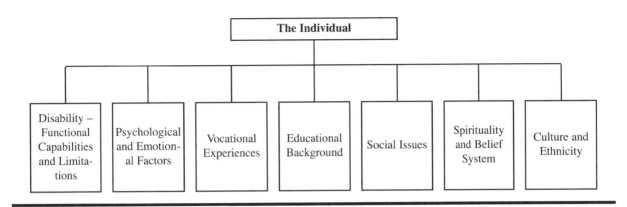

The Medical Specialties

This section includes ideas, concepts, and the writings of Jean Spencer Felton, M.D. He served as a physician and medical consultant to business and industry throughout southern California, and developed, organized, and taught the medical aspects of disability courses within the rehabilitation counselor education program at California State University, Los Angeles for many years. This section also uses information from the American Board of Medical Specialties (ABMS) (2013).

Rehabilitation counselors have frequent and explicit need to involve the services of a variety of medical specialists, and they should be thoroughly conversant with the scope of each of the recognized specialties. In the interests of general orientation to the medical profession, counselors need to be aware of the role of the family physician (general practitioner) in modern medicine.

Role of the Family Practitioner

Family physicians, formerly called general practitioners, have their own specialty board, the American Board of Family Medicine (ABFM), and a medical journal, the *Journal of the American Board of Family Medicine*. They are considered one of the 24 medical specialties by the ABMS. As stated by the president of the ABFM, in the Winter 2012 issue of their newsletter (The Phoenix), "Since its inception in 1969, the ABFM has been a leading innovator within the American Board of Medical Specialties."

Many people in urban communities tend to assume that all medicine today is practiced by specialists, but many families in this country receive all their medical care from family physicians (general practitioners), sometimes by choice and sometimes by necessity. In all probability, most of the clients who come to rehabilitation counselors' offices will have been seen by doctors in family practice; the medical records of those clients may open with reports from such physicians.

At their best, today's family practitioners are virtually as well rounded as internists (specialists in internal medicine). They are apt diagnosticians, and although of necessity they must be willing to assume an imposing amount of responsibility for independent action, they must also decide for their patients if and when a consultant in a specialized segment of medicine should be involved. Since there are many communities throughout the country where the specialties are conspicuously undermanned, it is by no means unusual for a doctor in family pracice to do obstetrics, anesthesiology, minor surgery, and even uncomplicated major surgery. Many family practitioners, without so labelling it, infuse their treatment of patients with supportive counseling.

The Specialty Boards

Within the medical specialties, the official organizations for certification, are the various specialty boards. There are currently 24 specialty boards in the following fields: aesthesiology, allergy and immunology, colon and rectal surgery, dermatology, emergency medicine, family medicine, internal medicine, medical genetics, neurological surgery, nuclear medicine, obstetrics and gynecology, ophthalmology, orthopedic surgery, otolaryngology, pathology, pediatrics, physical medicine and rehabilitation, plastic surgery, preventive medicine, psychiatry and neurology, radiology, surgery, thoracic surgery, and urology. Examples of the specialites include: American Board of Internal Medicine, American Board of Physical Medicine and Rehabilitation, American Board of Preventive Medicine, and American Board of Psychiatry and Neurology. There are multiple subspecialties under these specialty boards. For example, under the American Board of Physical Medicine and Rehabilitation are seven subspecialty areas: Brain Injury, Hospice and Palliative Care, Neuromuscular, Pain, Pediatric Rehabilitation, Spinal Cord Injury, and Sports Medicine.

From the point of view of the rehabilitation counselor, some of these specialties and the subspecialties within them are more relevant than others. Accordingly, the following discussion departs in some measure from the categories listed above.

Internal Medicine and Its Subspecialties

Internal Medicine is the specialty with the broadest scope, and the one whose jurisdiction is most difficult to define. The internist is sometimes identified as the physician who treats all disorders not requiring surgery. The range of the specialty of internal medicine can best be understood by identifying some of the major subspecialties which it includes:

Cardiology (heart) – The study of diseases of the heart. This usually includes disorders of the blood vessels, the two systems being termed jointly the cardiovascular system. It may also encompass evaluation of the lungs; often, the kidneys are involved.

Endocrinology (diabetes and other glandular disorders) – The study of the endocrine system, which secrete hormones. These glands include the pancreas, pituitary, pineal, thyroid, parathyroid, thymus, adrenals, ovaries, and testes.

Gastroenterology (colon and intestinal track) – The digestive system and its disorders, including the esophagus, stomach, intestinal track (gastrointestinal or GI system), pancreas, and liver.

Hematology (blood) – The study of disorders of the blood, bone marrow, and lymphatic systems.

Pulmonary (lungs) – Diseases of the lungs and bronchial tubes, which often involve evaluation of the upper respiratory tract (nose, pharynx, and throat), as well as the heart.

Geriatrics (care of the elderly) – Concerned with the health and well-being of older adults.

Rheumatology (arthritis) – Treatment of diseases involving the joints, muscles, and bones.

Oncology (cancer) – Focuses on treatment of cancer. The two types of clinical oncologists are surgical oncologists and radiation oncologists.

Other Medical Specialties

Anesthesiology – Physicians who administer local and general anesthesia before and during surgical procedures; they also participate in patient care before and after surgery. These physicians may be involved in the management of acute and chronic pain conditions.

Otolaryngology – The specialty which treats diseases of the ear, nose, and throat. The branch of medicine and surgery that specializes in diagnosis and treatment of diseases and disorders of the head and neck.

Ophthalmology – The specialty concerned with disorders of the eye; it is a surgical as well as a medical specialty.

Orthopedics – Involves conditions of the musculoskeletal system. Treats musculoskeletal trauma, sports injuries, degenerative diseases, infections, tumors, and congenital disorders.

Physical Medicine and Rehabilitation – A branch of medicine that aims to enhance and restore functional ability and quality of life to patients with physical impairments and disabilities.

Pediatrics – Medical care of infants, children, and adolescents. Includes treatement for physical, psychologic, and social problems which relate to growth and development.

Neurology – The study of diseases and disorders of the nervous system.

Psychiatry – The medical specialty devoted to the study, diagnosis, treatment, and prevention of mental disorders, including affective, behavioral, cognitive, and perceptual abnormalities. It is closely linked to the social sciences in its inquiry into human behavior.

Pathology – The science which deals wiith the nature of disease on the basis of the gross or microscopic examination of diseased tissue.

Preventive Medicine – The specialty concerned with measures taken to prevent diseases from occurring. The focus is on the environmental conditions conducive to good health and to diminish disease.

Occupational Medicine – The branch of clinical medicine most active in the field of Occupational Health. Occupational Medicine specialists work to ensure that the highest standards of health and safety at work can be achieved and maintained. Occupational Medicine serves as a link between medicine and the changing economic, social, and political trends.

Case Study – A Vocational Profile Approach

The following case study is an example of those found in the remaining chapters within this book. The case study describes a person with presenting disabilities. After the case study, there is a series of questions. Answers to the questions are provided to illustrate how to analyze case studies.

Case Study

Mr. Samuel Williams is 60 years of age and is currently married with three grown children. He has a Bachelor of Arts Degree in fine arts, completed a real estate course, and holds a current real estate license. For the past seven years, Mr. Williams has been active and successful in residential real estate sales. Previous to this, he was both a salesperson and an assistant manager in a men's specialty clothing store. The sales position lasted for five years, at which time Samuel was promoted to assistant manager.

This client has hypertension (high blood pressure) and a heart condition. Six months ago, he had a myocardial infarction (heart attack). The treating physician reported that Mr. Williams has coronary artery disease and has restricted him to a maximum of light work not involving excessive emotional stress. It was recommended he consider sedentary work, as it would be less physically demanding. No surgery is contemplated at this time.

The position of real estate sales agent, *Dictionary of Occupational Titles (D. O. T.)* #250.357-018 (U. S. Department of Labor, 1991), involves renting, buying, and selling real estate property for clients. An agent is paid on a commission basis and does not earn a salary. Real estate sales agents are familiar with all state and local regulations relating to the purchase and sale of property. They review trade journals and other publications to keep current in the field and to be informed about marketing conditions and property values. A real estate sales agent holds a current license issued by the state. Agents interview prospective clients to solicit listings. They accompany clients to property sites, show properties, quote purchase prices, and describe features and conditions of sale or terms of lease. Agents draw up real estate contracts, such as deeds, leases, and mortgages, and negotiate loans on properties. Real estate agents typically are paid on a commission-only basis.

In addition to these functions, Mr. Williams served as an office manager, supervising clerical personnel in the real estate office. This was on a part-time basis for which he was paid a salary.

Questions

1. Describe the client's vocational profile, including age, educational level, work history (skill and exertional levels), occupationally significant characteristics, and job skills.
2. How do the occupationally significant characteristics of the job impact Mr. Williams' disability?

3. What, if any, reasonable accommodations can you suggest for the client to return to his usual and customary occupation as a real estate sales agent or assistant manager?
4. What is this client's rehabilitation potential? Your rehabilitation supervisor is of the opinion this client may be too old for the provision of rehabilitation services. Comment on this issue.
5. What jobs can Mr. Williams perform using transferable skills?

References

American Board of Medical Specialties. (2013). *Specialties and subspecialties*. Chicago, IL: Author.

Americans with Disabilities Act of 1990 (ADA), PL 101-336, 42 U.S.C. §12101 et seq.

Berkeley Planning Associates. (1982). *A study of recommendations provided to handicapped employees by federal contractors* (Contract No. J-9-E-1-009). Berkeley, CA: Author.

Brodwin, M. G. (2008). Rehabilitation in the private-for-profit sector: Opportunities and challenges. In S. E. Rubin & R. T. Roessler, *Foundations of the vocational rehabilitation process* (6th ed., pp. 501–523). Austin, TX: Pro-ed.

Brodwin, M. G., Parker, R. M., & DeLaGarza, D. (2010). Disability and reasonable accommodation. In E. M. Szymanski & R. M. Parker (Eds.), *Work and disability: Contexts, issues, and strategies for enhancing employment outcomes for people with disabilities* (3rd ed., pp. 281–323). Austin, TX: Pro-ed.

Gilbride, D., & Stensrud, R. (2012). People with disabilities in the workplace. In R. M. Parker & J. B. Patterson (Eds.), *Rehabilitation counseling: Basics and beyond* (3rd ed., pp. 259–284). Austin, TX: Pro-ed.

Martin, F. H., Walls, R. T., Brodwin, M. G., Parker, R. M., Siu, F. W., & Kurata, E. (2012). Competitive employment outcomes of vocational rehabilitation. *Journal of Applied Rehabilitation Counseling, 43*, 3–10.

Muther, T. J. (1996). "Qualified" and "reasonable accommodations" under Title I of the ADA: Employer compliance. *Law Reporter, 15*(1), 18–20.

Office of the Federal Register. (2001). Code of federal regulations - 20 CFR. Washington, DC: United States Government Printing Office.

Rehabilitation Act of 1973, PL 93-112, 29 U.S.C. §701 et seq.

Roessler, R. T., & Rumrill, P. D., Jr. (1995). Promoting reasonable accommodations: An essential postemployment service. *Journal of Applied Rehabilitation Counseling, 26*, 3–7.

Rubin, S. E., & Roessler, R. T. (2008). *Foundations of the vocational rehabilitation process* (6th ed.). Austin, TX: Pro-ed.

U. S. Department of Labor. (1991). *Dictionary of Occupational Titles* (4th ed., revised). Washington, DC: Author.

Vash, C. l., & Crewe, N. M. (2004). *Psychology of disability* (2nd ed.). New York, NY: Springer.

About the Authors

Martin G. Brodwin, Ph.D., C.R.C., is Professor and Coordinator of the graduate Rehabilitation Counselor Education Program at California State University, Los Angeles. He is a vocational expert for the Office of Disability Adjudication and Review, Social Security Administration, providing testimony on disability-related issues. As a rehabilitation and vocational consultant, he provides assessment for long-term disability, case management, and reasonable accommodation. Dr. Brodwin has published over 100 refereed journal articles, book chapters, and books on the subjects of counseling, disability, rehabilitation, and accommodation in business and industry.

Sandra K. Brodwin, M.Ed., M.S., C.R.C., is a lecturer in the Rehabilitation Counselor Education Program at California State University, Los Angeles, and a vocational rehabilitation counselor for CIGNA Group Insurance in Glendale, California. In this role, Ms. Brodwin provides reasonable accommodation, job restructuring, employer consultation, and a full range of rehabilitation services for employees on long-term disability due to chronic illness, injury, and resultant disabilities. She has published book chapters and journal articles on the subjects of medical aspects of disabling conditions, counseling, disability, job analysis, and rehabilitation.

Chapter 2

HUMAN BODY SYSTEMS

Frances W. Siu, Ph.D., C.R.C.
Erin R. Brodwin, M.A.

Introduction

The human body is a complex network of some 63 trillion cells (McDowell & Windelspecht, 2004; Tortora & Derrickson, 2011). Cells are the body's building blocks—cells of the same origin comprise tissues; organs are composed of multiple tissue types. Organs that work together to carry out specific functions are known as body systems (Seeley, VanPutte, Regan, & Russo, 2011). These systems work together to meet the body's needs. Body systems can be broken down into two components: body functions, which include the physiological and psychological functions of body systems, and body structures, the anatomical components of the organs and limbs. Knowledge of the structure and function of the human body builds the foundation for understanding illnesses and disabilities (Martini & Nath, 2011). Preceded by an introduction to the chemical and cellular levels of the human body, this chapter provides readers with an overview of the skeletal system, muscular system, nervous system, cardiovascular and lymphatic systems, integumentary system, respiratory system, sensory system, digestive system, genitourinary system, and endocrine system. The visual and hearing systems are described in chapters in this book specific to those subjects.

Cellular and Chemical Levels

In the human body, building blocks of matter, called atoms, interact and combine to form molecules such as sugar, fat, water, and protein. These molecules in turn form organelles, such as the plasma membrane and nucleus, which make up cells (Seeley et al., 2011). Cells are the basic units of the human body; they carry out the functions of protection and support while providing the body systems with a means of communication. Cells additionally metabolize and release energy, provide the basic materials for genetic inheritance, and make movement possible. Each cell is encased by an outer layer known as the plasma membrane, which regulates what enters or leaves the cell. The hereditary material of the cell, Deoxyribonucleic Acid (DNA), is found inside the nucleus. DNA helps direct cell activities by utilizing Ribonucleic Acid (RNA) (Martini & Nath, 2011).

While the cellular level describes the physical structures that make up cells, the chemical level describes the chemical components within the cell. Oxygen, carbon dioxide, and water comprise the chemical levels of the cell. Oxygen fuels the chemical reactions that enable the cell to extract energy from food (Seeley et al., 2011). Carbon dioxide and energy are released during metabolism, the process by which organic molecules from an energy source are broken down. Water, another essential chemical, works in the cells to stabilize body temperature and protect against friction and trauma. Water directly participates in chemical reactions, such as dehydration and hydrolysis (Martini & Nath, 2011).

Tissue Level

Tissues are collections of similar cells and the substances surrounding them (Martini & Nath, 2011). There are four primary types of tissue:

- Epithelium forms the internal and external linings of various organs of the body. It is usually involved in activities such as diffusion, filtration, secretion, and absorption.
- Connective tissue connects and binds cells and other tissues together. Among the connective tissues, there are three types of specialized connective tissue (Seeley et al., 2011):
    - Cartilage is made up of collagen, proteoglycans, and water; its slightly elastic, gummy-like consistency allows body parts to spring back when compressed. The external parts of the ears and connecting tissues between the bones of the spine are examples.
    - Bone is a hard, calcified connective tissue composed of 35% organic substance, 45% inorganic substance, and 20% water that forms the internal framework of the body.
    - Blood contains cell fragments called platelets, which play a key role in blood clotting. The cells and platelets are suspended in plasma. There are two types of blood cells. *Red blood cells* transport oxygen through the arteries and waste through the veins, while *white blood cells* fight infections and cancer.
- Nervous tissue, which responds to stimuli and transmits impulses throughout the body, is composed of neurons (conductive cells) and neuralgia (support cells) (Moore, Dalley, & Agur, 2013). Neurons have cell processes called dendrites that receive electric impulses and axons that conduct them.
- Muscle tissue provides for bodily movement. Muscles are grouped according to the presence or absence of striations (microscopic bands) in the muscle cells (Adams, 2004). Types of muscle tissue include: skeletal, cardiac, and smooth muscle. Skeletal muscle is classified as striated voluntary (usually consciously controlled) while cardiac muscle is striated involuntary (not normally consciously controlled). Smooth muscle is characterized by nonstraited involuntary tissue (Seeley et al., 2011).

Organ Level

A body system is a group of organs that operate together to carry out a bodily function (Seeley et al., 2011). Some organs carry out a variety of functions. The hypothalamus, for example, interacts with the nervous system and endocrine system. Similarly, the kidneys act as the body's filtration system and secrete hormones.

The body systems which perform specific purposes in our daily lives also play a significant role in homeostasis, the process by which the body maintains its stability (Moore et al., 2013). Environmental factors that negatively affect the body systems can upset the body's internal constancy and state of homeostasis (Martini & Nath, 2011).

System Level

The Musculoskeletal System

As the name implies, the musculoskeletal system consists of the muscular system and skeletal system.

Skeletal Structure and Function

The human skeleton consists of 206 bones. Bones provide the body with its internal structural framework and protect its vital internal organs (Moore et al., 2013). For purposes of classification, bones are grouped into the axial and appendicular skeletons. The axial skeleton, formed by the bones of the head and trunk, is distinct from the appendicular skeleton, which includes the bones of the upper and lower limbs and the shoulder and hip bones.

The structure of the skeletal system permits movement, storage, and maintenance of chemical levels. Skeletal muscles attach at bone sites, allowing the body to move. Connective tissues in these areas house bone-forming cells responsible for repair. Bones also store important minerals like calcium and phosphate, and fats for cellular energy production (Martini & Nath, 2011).

FIGURE 1
Human Skeleton

Source: Health, Medicine, and Anatomy Reference Pictures. (2013). The human skeleton. Retrieved from http://healthfavo.com/detailed-human-skeleton-diagrams.html

Inside the compact outer shell of dense material encasing the bone marrow, a thriving environment exists. The inner mass, known as spongy bone, is less dense than compact bone and has numerous small cavities where red and white blood cells and platelets exist.

The skull is composed of two sets of bones: cranial bones and facial bones. Cranial bones, where the head muscles attach, protect and enclose the brain. Facial bones provide the framework for the face and mouth. Immovable joints connect all the bones in the skull—except for the mandible, which is attached to the skull via a freely movable joint. The cranium is made up of eight thin, eggshell-like bones that are self-bracing. The forehead is formed by the frontal bone, which also forms the upper half of the eye sockets. Two parietal bones make up the bulk of the cranium and comprise the sides of the skull. Temporal bones lie inferior to the parietal bones on both sides of the skull. The occipital bone, also named for the part of the brain it covers, shapes the posterior of the skull. The sphenoid bone encloses the cranial cavity (Tortora & Derrickson, 2011).

The spinal column, formed by 26 bones, connects the face and skull to the rest of the body. At the base of the flexible, curved spinal column is the sacrum, comprised of five fused vertebrae. Below the sacrum the coccyx is composed of four fused vertebrae. The entire spinal column is divided into three parts. Cervical vertebrae encompass the first seven vertebrae below the skull while thoracic vertebrae refer to the next 12, and lumbar to the last five vertebrae (Tortora & Derrickson, 2011).

Anterior to the spinal column is the sternum and rib cage. While 12 pairs of ribs exist, only the first seven are attached directly to the sternum. The rest are known as *false ribs*, meaning that they attach to the sternum indirectly or not at all. The seven attached ribs are connected to the sternum by cartilage. At the inferior end of the sternum, the xiphoid serves as an attachment point for the diaphragm.

On each side of the skeleton are the scapulae, posterior to the rib cage, connecting the upper arm to the rest of the skeleton by a bone called the clavicle which, together with the scapulae, comprises the shoulder girdles. The clavicle mainly acts as a brace holding the scapulae and the arms up and away from the ribs. It also enables people to raise their hands (Tortora & Derrickson, 2011).

The humerus is the only bone in the upper arm. At the end of the humerus are two bones: the radius and ulna. These long bones allow us to twist our hands from side to side. At the end of the radius and ulna Flie the carpals, collectively referred to as the wrist. The palm of the hand is supported by the metacarpals, while the three phalanges make up the fingers.

The rest of the body could not be connected to the lower extremities without the existence of one structure, the pelvis. The pelvis works to provide support for the body's internal organs. Its flaring sides are called the ilium. The two ring-shaped portions located inferior to the hip sockets are called ischium while the femur refers to the bone in the thigh (Goldman & Schafer, 2012). The patella (kneecap) guards the knee joint against injury and improves leverage of thigh muscles responsible for raising the lower leg. The tibia and fibula form the lower leg.

The foot is much like the hand in the way the bones are grouped. The first group of bones, the tarsals, form half the foot. The calcaneus forms the heel, while the talus connects the foot with the tibia and fibula. The rest of the foot, excluding the toes, is composed of metatarsals (Tortora & Derrickson, 2011).

Cartilage

Along with bone, cartilage helps give the skeletal system its shape. Cartilage is a dense connective tissue composed of cells called chondrocytes that are dispersed in a firm gel-like ground substance called the matrix. It is avascular (contains no blood vessels) and can be found in the joints, rib cage, ear, nose, throat, and between intervertebral disks (Tortora & Derrickson, 2011).

The Muscular System

The muscular system is the largest body system. The upper and lower extremities are almost entirely made up of muscles; over forty muscles are located in the skull alone. Muscles are distinct from all other tissues because of their unique ability to contract (Adams, 2004).

FIGURE 2
Muscular System

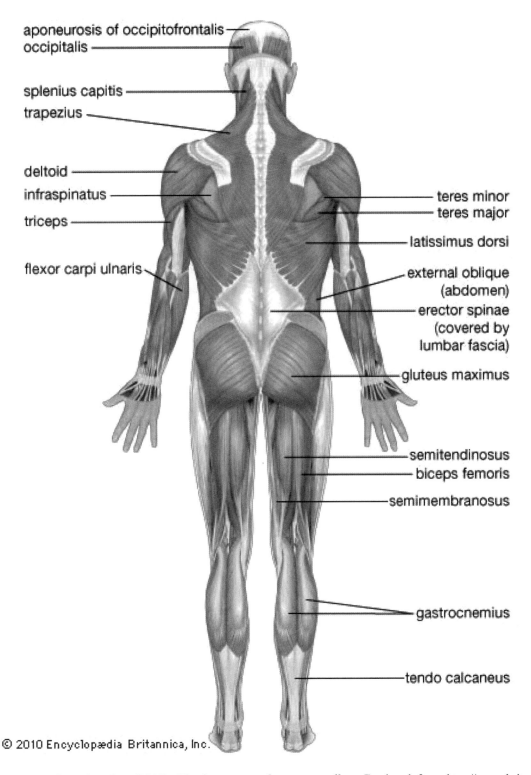

Source: Encyclopedia Britannica. (2010). *The human muscle system gallery*. Retrieved from http://www.britannica.com/EBchecked/media/147100/Posterior-view-of-human-muscular-system

One motor unit contains anywhere from two to as many as 2,000 muscle fibers. Blood vessels provide muscles with nutrients and oxygen and remove waste. Nerves deliver signals that cause muscles to contract and relax, resulting in movements as delicate as a blink of the eyelid or as powerful as a punch of the fist.

The three types of muscles include skeletal, smooth, and cardiac (Adams, 2004; Goldman & Schafer, 2012).

- Skeletal muscle is the strongest, lengthiest, and hardest working tissue in the body and is the longest form of muscle. Known as striated muscle tissue because of the way it criss-crosses over each fiber, skeletal muscle tissue owes part of its strength to its protective sheath-like covering. Skeletal muscle is also the only type of tissue that is voluntary.
- Smooth muscle is involuntary and is commonly found in hollow organs such as the stomach, bladder, and respiratory passages. Its main function is to propel objects. These tissue are spindle-shaped and arranged in sheets or layers.
- Cardiac muscle tissue is found only in the heart; it is striated, involuntary, and responsible for pumping blood throughout the heart. Cardiac muscle tissue is protected by connective tissue.

Joints, Tendons, and Ligaments

Besides muscles and bones, joints play a pivotal role in body movement. These connecting structures of bones are classified either according to degree of movement or type of connective tissue that joins them. Fibrous joints are those ends of bones connected by fibrous tissue without a joint cavity; they are capable of little or no movement. Cartilaginous joints are attached by hyaline cartilage and are slightly moveable. Synovial joints have joint cavities where the fibrous connective tissue holds the bones together. These joints are highly moveable, depending on their location. Synovial joints allow for various types of common movement such as gliding, angulations, rotation, and the combination of two or more movements. Elevation and depression, protraction and retraction, excursion, opposition and reposition, and inversion and eversion are some special movements also made possible by synovial joints (Tortora & Derrickson, 2011).

Both tendons and ligaments are soft collagenous tissues. While tendons connect muscles to bone and carry the tension forces between them, ligaments connect bone to bone. Both tendons and ligaments play a significant role in musculoskeletal biomechanics.

As the foundation of the body, the skeleton functions alongside the muscular system, which together provide the body with range of movement. The nervous system, integral to both the skeletal and muscular systems, provides the means by which all body systems function.

The Nervous System

The nervous system is the master controlling and communicating system of the body; it directs human thoughts, actions, and emotions. It is the most rapid-acting and complex system of the body, and functions via intra-cellular communication through electrical signals. The nervous system is typically discussed in two parts: the central nervous system (CNS) and the peripheral nervous system (PNS).

Central Nervous System

The CNS consists of the brain and spinal cord. As the command center of the nervous system, the CNS interprets incoming signals and responds to these signals based on past experiences, reflexes, and current conditions.

Peripheral Nervous System

The PNS is distinguished from the CNS, consisting of the nerves extending from the brain and spinal cord. These nerves, respectively called cranial nerves and spinal nerves serve as the communications link from the body to the CNS. The PNS is further divided into the following functional subdivisions:

- Sensory contains nerve fibers that carry impulses to the CNS from sensory receptors located throughout the body. There are two types of sensory fibers.

FIGURE 3
Neuron

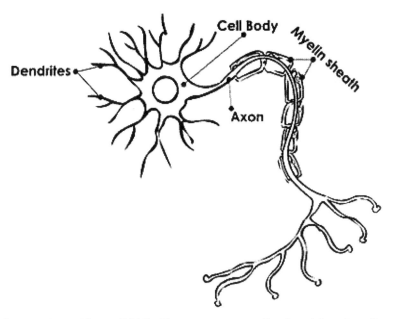

Source: National Institute on Drug Abuse. (2012). *Neurotransmission*. Retrieved from http://www.drugabuse.gov

- ○ Somatic afferents convey information from the skin, skeletal muscles, and joints.
- ○ Visceral afferents convey impulses from the visceral organs.
- Motor transports messages from the CNS to organs, muscles, and glands. The motor system is divided into two parts (Tortora & Derrickson, 2011).
  - ○ *Somatic nervous system*, composed of motor nerve fibers that connect the CNS to the skeletal muscles, is often referred to as the *voluntary nervous system*. These motor neurons respond mainly to external stimuli. Reflexes, automatic reactions to a stimulus, are usually controlled by the spinal cord and brain stem.
  - ○ *Autonomic nervous system*, consisting of nerve fibers that regulate the activity of smooth muscles, cardiac muscles, and glands, is not consciously controlled; therefore, it is generally referred to as the *involuntary nervous system*. The autonomic nervous system is subdivided into the sympathetic and parasympathetic nervous systems. These systems have opposing effects when they act upon the same organ. While the parasympathetic nervous system enhances activities and conserves energy, the sympathetic nervous system increases energy expenditures and prepares the body for action.

In the nervous system, there are two main types of cells – neurons and supporting cells. While neurons provide a pathway for messages traveling to and from the brain and spinal cord, supporting cells provide structural reinforcement, protection, insulation, and general assistance for neurons. As specialized cells, neurons provide for the transportation of signals. Although many different types of neurons exist, all neurons share common characteristics. For example, all neurons share large cell bodies and have fiber-like extensions called processes. Processes are further divided into dendrites and axons.

Dendrites convey signals toward the cell body. These short, numerous cells branch extensively around the nucleus. Perpendicular to the body of the neuron, the axon conducts signals away from the cell body. Along the length of the axon, the Schwann cells form an insulating layer called the myelin sheath. Branches of axons terminate in hundreds or thousands of telodendria branlets which, in turn, end in synaptic knobs.

Human Body Systems

FIGURE 4
Human Brain

Source: Health, Medicine, and Anatomy Reference Pictures. (2013). *Simple brain diagram labeled*. Retrieved from http://healthfavo.com/simple-brain-diagram-labeled.html

Synaptic knobs relay messages to other cells via neurotransmitters. Gaps in the synaptic knobs are called synapses.

Brain

The brain and body are linked by the spinal cord, a long bundle of white nerve matter residing in the middle of the spinal column. The spinal cord also serves as the center from which reflexes stem.

The brain has three divisions: brain stem, cerebellum, and cerebrum. The brain stem is the core for most life systems commands—vital functions that are not consciously controlled. The cerebellum, the next brain division, controls balance and muscle coordination. After the cerebellum, the most advanced part of the brain is the cerebral cortex—conscious thought takes place in this region. While the cerebellum can be divided into the left and right hemispheres, it can also be divided into functional parts. The right hemisphere, generally, is the artistic side of the brain. People who are *right brained* (the right hemisphere is dominate over the left) are thought to excel at activities involving abstract thinking, such as art and music. *Left brained* people are considered to be logical, allowing them to excel in math, physics, and other such logical thought processes. Although one sphere can be dominant, the two hemispheres are connected by the corpus callosum, which allows the two hemispheres to communicate (Fix, 2008).

FIGURE 5
Human Heart

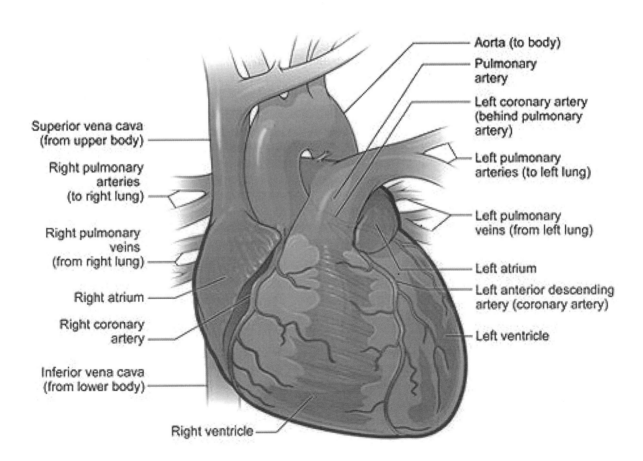

Source: National Heart Lung and Blood Institute. (2014). *Anatomy of the heart*. Retrieved from http://www.nhlbi.nih.gov/health//dci/Diseases/hhw/hhw_anatomy.html

The Cardiovascular System
(including the Lymphatic System)

The Cardiovascular System

The cardiovascular system controls a single vital function—blood circulation. Circulation is necessary for the growth and development of cells. The heart, the cardiovascular system's central organ, is responsible for moving blood throughout the body. Made of cardiac tissue, this vital fist-sized organ first pumps blood to the lungs, where it obtains oxygen. The heart then funnels the blood throughout the body via a series of arteries and veins. While the arteries carry oxygenated blood from the heart to the body, veins return the oxygen-depleted blood to the heart.

Centrally located in the upper body cavity, the heart can be divided into four chambers: left and right atria and left and right ventricle. The atria consist of the upper half of the heart, while the ventricles compose the lower portion. The left and right sides of the heart are divided by the septum. Four valves of the heart control circulation (Tortora & Derrickson, 2011).

Blood is composed of red and white blood cells, platelets, lymph, plasma, and water. Forty-five percent of blood consists of platelets (necessary for blood-clotting) and red and white blood cells. The remainder is liquid plasma, a mixture of glucose and water. Red blood cells, or erythrocytes, contain hemoglobin, the chemical compound that carries oxygen. White blood cells, or leukocytes, destroy and remove old cells and cellular debris and attack foreign or infectious agents (Collier, 2009).

FIGURE 6
Human Circulatory System

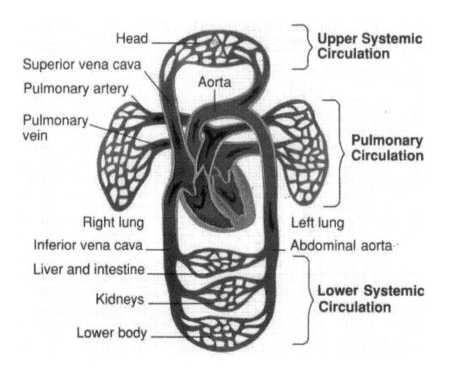

Source: Laas, M. (2009). *The circulatory system*. International School of Bremen. Retrieved from http://www.michael-laass.de/Circulatory%20System.htm

Blood enters the heart through the left atrium from the superior and inferior vena cava. The superior vena cava collects blood returning from the upper body. The inferior vena cava returns blood from the lower body. During the systolic phase of the heartbeat, deoxygenated blood from the superior and inferior vena cava enters the heart through the right atrium. In this phase of the heartbeat, the atria begin to fill while the ventricles contract to pump the blood. Additionally, the pulmonary and aortic valves open allowing blood to exit the ventricles. During the diastole phase, the atria contract, pumping blood into the ventricles, and the tricuspid and mitral valves open, allowing blood to enter.

New blood entering the right atrium is pumped by the tricuspid valve to the right ventricle. Once the pulmonary valve opens to the pulmonary artery, blood is carried to the lungs where it is oxygenated. The pulmonary artery is the only artery in the body that carries deoxygenated blood.

The oxygen in the lungs, first diffused through the alveoli sacs, is next pushed through the wall of the lungs into the bloodstream where the blood distributes oxygen throughout the body. To enable direct oxygenation of the cells, the arteries are branched into smaller arterioles. These separate further into capillaries, the smallest blood vessels, whose walls are thin and elastic. When oxygen is released from the hemoglobin, it is diffused across the capillary wall, traveling to a nearby cell and entering through its membrane.

The carbon dioxide that returns to the blood travels back to the lungs via the capillaries. The capillaries fork into smaller venules, which divide further into veins. Carbon dioxide and blood are carried back to the heart by the veins, completing the circulatory cycle (Moore et al., 2013).

The Lymphatic System

A specialized component of the circulatory system is the lymphatic system, consisting of moving fluid (lymph/interstitial fluid), vessels (lymphatics), lymph nodes, and organs (adenoid, tonsils, thymus, thoracic duct, small intestine, appendix, liver, and spleen). By moving blood in and out of arteries and into veins and through the lymph nodes and into the lymph, the body is able to eliminate the products of cellular breakdown and bacterial invasion (McDowell & Windelspecht, 2004). The lymphatic system functions 1) to absorb excess fluid, thus preventing tissues from swelling; 2) to defend the body against microorganisms and harmful foreign particles; and 3) to facilitate the absorption of fat. The lymph system is made up of T cells, B cells, antibodies, and platelets.

The skin plays a major role in preventing disease by protecting organs, blood vessels, and the lymph system. To combat bacteria, viruses, and disease, the skin contains lymph nodes. These nodes transport white blood cells (phagocytes) throughout the body via a network of vessels.

Mucous membranes, cells that line all openings of the body, provide a second line of defense against foreign bacteria. When dust particles enter the body, for example, they are trapped in the mucous membranes and then digested. Nose hair functions alongside the mucous membranes to protect the body; they act as an air filtration system.

Along with the lymph nodes, the lymphatic system includes lymph (interstitial fluid). Capillaries release excess water and plasma into intracellular spaces where they mix with lymph, a fluid containing proteins, fats, and a type of white blood cells called lymphocytes, the body's first-line defense in the immune system. Lymph flows from small lymph capillaries into lymph vessels that are similar to veins in having valves that prevent backflow. The contraction of skeletal muscle propels lymph fluid through the valves. Lymph vessels connect to lymph nodes, lymph organs (bone marrow, liver, spleen, thymus), and the cardiovascular system.

Besides functioning as a line of defense for the body, the lymphatic system functions as a separate circulatory system working parallel to the cardiovascular system. The lymphatic system absorbs fats, returns approximately three liters of fluid from our body tissues to the circulatory system on a daily basis, and transports selected nutrients from the digestive system to the circulatory system (Collier, 2009). The next line of body defense includes the integumentary system.

FIGURE 7
Human Skin Diagram

Source: Davis, F. A. (2009). *Taber's cyclopedia medical dictionary* (21st ed.). Philadelphia, PA: F. A. Davis

The Integumentary System

The integumentary system, commonly called the skin, encases the body. It functions as a protective barrier against the environment, and is involved in maintaining proper body temperature. The skin gathers sensory information from the environment and helps protect the body from disease. The skin's functioning is divided into three parts, representing three layers of skin: epidermis, dermis, and subcutaneous tissue (Martini & Nath, 2011; Goldman & Schafer, 2012).

The epidermis, the outer layer of skin, varies in thickness. It is thinnest on the eyelids and thickest on the palms of the hands and soles of the feet. When cells divide or multiply, they push other cells into higher layers, where they flatten and eventually die. Humans shed this surface layer every two weeks.

Dermis, which connects the skin to the tissue underneath, includes collagen, elastic tissue, and reticular fibers. It contains many specialized cells and structures such as hair follicles, sebaceous (oil) glands, and apocrine (scent) glands. This layer also contains eccrine (sweat) glands. Blood vessels and nerves course through this layer, transmitting sensations of pain, itching, and temperature. Specialized nerve cells in the dermis transmit sensations of touch and pressure (Martini & Nath, 2011).

Subcutaneous tissue is a layer of fat and connective tissue that houses larger blood vessels and nerves. This layer is vital in regulation of skin and body temperature; its size varies throughout the body and from person to person.

The Respiratory System

The respiratory system supplies the body with oxygen. After air is inhaled through the nose or mouth, it travels into the pharynx, passes through the larynx, and makes its way down the trachea. When air reaches the lungs, it is diffused into the blood via the alveoli (Martini & Nath, 2011).

Nasal Cavity

As people breathe, air enters the body through the nostrils. Inside the nose, the nasal cavity is divided by the septum and lined by the respiratory mucosa. In the roof of the nasal cavity, the mucosa house the olfactory receptors. The mucosa help warm and moisten air entering the body while trapping invading pathogens.

Sinuses

The nasal cavity is surrounded by the paranasal sinuses located in the maxillary, ethmoid, sphenoid, and frontal bones. The sinus chambers lighten the weight of the skull, act as resonance chambers for vocalization, and secrete mucous for the nasal cavity.

Pharynx

The pharynx (throat) is the muscular passageway that provides a means of transportation for air and food. Air enters the pharynx through its superior portion, the nasopharynx, and descends to the oropharynx and laryngopharynx. From the laryngopharynx, air moves into the larynx. Food mirrors the passage of air from the nasopharynx to the laryngopharynx. Instead of entering the larynx as air does, food enters the esophagus.

FIGURE 8
Respiratory System

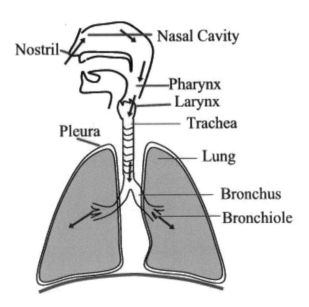

Source: Davis, F. A. (2009). *Taber's cyclopedia medical dictionary* (21st ed.). Philadelphia, PA: F. A. Davis.

Larynx

The larynx (voice box) routes food and air to the proper destination. The epiglottis prevents food from entering the superior opening of the larynx and traveling down the trachea, or windpipe. The epiglottis is opened by breathing, which allows air to pass freely to the lungs. Swallowing, conversely, causes the epiglottis to close. When the epiglottis is closed, food is forced down the esophagus. The mucous membranes of the larynx form the vocal folds. These folds are what give people the ability to speak; when expelled by air, the folds vibrate, resulting in vocal sound.

Trachea

The trachea, or windpipe, is a tube that connects the pharynx and larynx to the lungs, allowing for the passage of air. The trachea divides into the right and left bronchi, which enter the right and left lung. By the time air reaches the bronchi, it is warm, humidified, and cleansed of all pathogens. The tracheal walls, which beat constantly in the opposite direction of incoming air, are covered with ciliated mucous.

Lungs

Lungs are the primary organs of the respiratory system. Housed in the thoracic cavity, the lungs deliver oxygen to the bloodstream and release carbon dioxide. From the trachea, the bronchi enter the lungs, where they divide into smaller branches, or bronchioles, which divide further into respiratory zone structures. The respiratory zone is where the transfusion of air to blood takes place. These structures eventually divide into alveoli, which are responsible for the transfusion of oxygen into the blood.

The Sensory System

The sensory system is vital for survival, growth, development, and the experience of bodily pleasure. Sense perception depends on sensory receptors that respond to various stimuli. When a stimulus triggers an impulse in a receptor, the action potentials travel to the cerebral cortex where they are processed and interpreted as sensations. Some senses, such as pain, touch, pressure, and proprioception, are widely distributed in the body. These are called general senses. Other senses, such as taste, smell, hearing, and sight, are called special senses because their receptors are localized in particular areas (Tortora & Derrickson, 2011).

Sensory Components

The two components of sensory experience are reception and perception. Sensory reception is the process of receiving data from the internal and external environment through the senses and includes: visual (seeing); auditory (hearing); olfactory (smell); gustatory (taste); and tactile (touch).

Sensory perception is the conscious process of selecting, organizing, and interpreting data from the senses and transforming this data into meaningful information. This process is influenced by intensity, size, and shape, as well as by past experiences, knowledge, and attitudes. In some situations, the way in which a particular sensation is perceived depends on where it is interpreted in the brain. Nearly everyone is familiar with sensory adaptation in the sense of smell. A particular odor becomes unnoticed after a short time even though the odor molecules are still present in the air because the system quickly adapts to the continued stimulation (Moore et al., 2013).

General Senses

Visceral organs control general senses in the skin, muscles, and joints. General senses include touch, pressure, proprioception, temperature, and pain (Collier, 2009).

Touch and Pressure

As a group, the receptors for touch and pressure are widely distributed in the skin and are sensitive to forces that deform or displace tissues. Three of the receptors involved in touch and pressure are free nerve endings, Meissner's corpuscles, and Pacinian corpuscles. These receptors are important in sensing objects in continuous contact with the skin. While Meissner's corpuscles lie just beneath the epidermis and sense light touch stimuli, Pacinian corpuscles are deeper in the dermis and are sensitive to heavy pressure.

Temperature

Temperature receptors lie directly under the skin and are widely dispersed throughout the body. The sense of temperature is stimulated by cold receptors and heat receptors. Degree of stimulation depends on the number of each type of receptor stimulated. A person determines gradations in temperature by the degree of stimulation of each type of receptor. Extreme cold and extreme heat feel almost the same because the pain receptors are being stimulated.

The Digestive System

The digestive system, which prepares food for use, is one of the most complex systems of the body. When eaten, food cannot reach cells because it cannot pass through the intestinal walls to the bloodstream. The digestive system modifies food physically and chemically and disposes of unusable waste. Physical and chemical modification (digestion) depends on exocrine and endocrine secretions and the controlled movement of food through the digestive tract. It provides the body with the means of transforming food into energy. Food is transformed into enzymes, glucose, and other nutrients (Martini & Nath, 2011).

Mouth

Food enters the digestive system via the mucous membrane-lined oral cavity. The lips protect the mouth's outer opening, while the cheeks form its lateral walls. The hard and soft palates additionally form the anterior or posterior roof. The floor of the mouth is characterized by the muscular tongue. The breakdown of food requires mechanical and chemical processes. Taste buds, while making food enjoyable, also alert the body of potential hazards such as toxins.

Swallowing

Once food leaves the mouth, it crosses the respiratory tract. Swallowing empties the mouth and ensures that food does not enter the windpipe. This process involves coordinated activity of tongue, soft palate (pharynx), and esophagus. The first phase is voluntary, as food is forced into the pharynx by the tongue. After this phase, reflex controls swallowing. Food moves into the pharynx and onwards by peristalsis aided by gravity. The esophagus, the first part of the digestive tract, runs from the pharynx to the diaphragm and stomach (Goldman & Schafer, 2012).

Stomach

The stomach stores and digests food. Two sphincters, circular valve-like muscles placed outside organs, surround the two openings. Cardioesophageal sphincter guards the entrance from the esophagus while the pyloric sphincter guards the outlet. The stomach secretes acid (to continue the digestive process) and mucus (for self-protection). Food in the stomach is churned by three muscular layers to form chyme, a creamy substance voided via pyloric sphincter to the duodenum.

Small Intestine

The small intestine is the primary organ of the digestive tract. The first part of the small intestine, duodenum, curves around the pancreas, forming the entry of the common bile duct. Most food digestion occurs in the small intestine. In addition to digesting chyme, the small intestine is responsible for absorbing the processed food into the bloodstream so that energy can be derived from food.

Large Intestine

The large intestine stretches from a valve resting between the bottom of the small intestine and the top of the large intestine to the anus. The main job of the large intestine is to digest any undigested chyme and rid the body of unneeded wastes. The large intestine has many subdivisions including cecum, appendix, colon, rectum, and canal.

Accessory Organs

In addition to the main digestive organs, several accessory organs include the salivary glands, pancreas, liver, and gallbladder. Saliva, a mixture of mucus and serous fluids, is produced in various glands. The pancreas includes the endocrine and exocrine glands. Exocrine produces enzymes while endocrine produces insulin. Bile is produced by the liver and secreted via the hepatic duct and cystic duct to the gallbladder for storage. Bile salts and phospholipids emulsify fats. The liver is a multifunctional organ that receives fat and other nutrients from the small intestine via the hepatic portal system (Martini & Nath, 2011).

The Genitourinary System

The organs involved in production, formation, and release of urine and the sex organs make up the genitourinary system. This system includes the kidneys, ureters, bladder, urethra, and the organs of reproduction - ovaries, uterus, fallopian tubes, vagina and clitoris in women, and the testes, seminal vesicles, prostate, seminal ducts, and penis in men (Longo, Fauci, Kasper, Hauser, & Loscalzo, 2012*)*

Renal System

The kidneys are regulatory organs that maintain volume and composition of body fluid by filtering blood and secreting filtered solutes. Kidneys take blood from the aorta via the renal arteries and return it to the inferior vena cava via the renal veins. Urine, the filtered product containing waste materials and water, is excreted from the kidneys and passes down the ureters, collecting in the bladder. The bladder distends to accept urine, allowing large volumes to be collected without damaging the renal system. Urine is voided through the urethra (Martini & Nath, 2011).

Male Reproductive System

The organs of the male reproductive system are specialized for the following functions: production, maintenance, and transportation of sperm, protective fluid (semen), and male sex hormones. To best carry out these functions, the male reproductive anatomy includes internal and external structures. Most of the male reproductive system is located outside the body. These include the penis, scrotum, and testicles.

The penis, the male sex organ, is comprised of three parts: the root, which attaches to the wall of the abdomen; the body or shaft; and the glans, the cone-shaped end of the penis. The glans, which also is called the head, is covered with a loose layer of foreskin, sometimes removed through circumcision. The opening of the urethra, the tube that transports semen and urine, is at the tip of the glans penis. The body of the penis is cylindrical in shape and consists of three internal chambers made up of sponge-like erectile tissue. This tissue contains thousands of spaces that fill with blood during sexual arousal. As this process occurs, the penis becomes rigid and erect, allowing for penetration during sexual intercourse. Semen, which contains sperm, is expelled (ejaculated) through the end of the penis when the man reaches sexual climax (orgasm). When the penis is erect, the flow of urine is blocked from the urethra (Longo et al., 2012).

Scrotum is the loose pouch-like sac located behind the penis. It contains the testicles (also called testes), as well as many nerves and blood vessels. The scrotum functions as a climate control system to protect the testes; normal sperm development requires the testes to maintain a temperature slightly cooler than that of the body.

Testes, oval organs about the size of large olives, lie in the scrotum. The two testes are responsible for making testosterone (the primary male sex hormone) and for generating sperm. Within the testes, coiled masses of seminiferous tubules are responsible for producing sperm cells.

The internal organs of the male reproductive system, also called accessory organs, include the vas deferens, ejaculatory ducts, urethra, seminal vesicles, prostate, and Bulbourethral glands. The vas deferens, a long, muscular tube that travels from the epididymis into the pelvic cavity to just behind the bladder, transports mature sperm to the urethra in preparation for ejaculation. Ejaculatory ducts are formed by the fusion of the vas deferens and the seminal vesicles and empty into the urethra. Urethra, a tube that carries urine from the bladder to outside the body also controls ejaculation of semen.

The male reproductive system could not function without hormones, chemicals that stimulate or regulate the activity of cells or organs. The primary hormones involved in the functioning of the male reproductive system include the follicle-stimulating hormone, the luteinizing hormone, and testosterone.

Female Reproductive System

The female reproductive system is designed to carry out the following functions: 1) production of female egg cells necessary for reproduction, called the ova or oocytes, 2) transportation of the ova to the site of fertilization, and 3) production of female sex hormones. Conception, the fertilization of an egg by a sperm, normally occurs in the fallopian tubes. After conception, the uterus provides a safe environment for fetal development. In the absence of fertilization, the system carries out menstruation (monthly shedding of the uterine lining).

The female reproductive anatomy includes internal and external structures. The function of the external female reproductive structures (the genitals) is twofold: to enable sperm to enter the body and to protect the internal genital organs from infectious organisms. The main external structures of the female reproductive system include the labia majora, labina minora, Bartholin's glands, and the clitoris. The labina majora enclose and protect the other external reproductive organs. Labia minora lie just inside the labia majora and surround the openings to the vagina (the canal that joins the lower part of the uterus to the outside of the body) and urethra (the tube that carries urine from the bladder to outside the body). Bartholin's glands, located next to the vaginal opening, produce a fluid secretion. The two labia minora meet at the clitoris, a small, sensitive protrusion comparable to the penis in males. The clitoris is covered by a fold of skin called the prepuce, which is similar to the foreskin at the end of the penis.

The internal reproductive organs include the vagina, uterus, ovaries, and Fallopian tubes. The vaginal canal joins the cervix (the lower part of uterus) to the outside of the body. The uterus (womb), a hollow pear-shaped organ, is home for a developing fetus. The uterus is divided into two parts: the cervix, which is the lower part that opens into the vagina, and the main body of the uterus, called the corpus. The corpus can easily expand to hold a developing baby. A channel through the cervix allows sperm to enter and menstrual blood to exit. The small, oval-shaped glands located on either side of the uterus are called ovaries which produce eggs and hormones. The Fallopian tubes are attached to the upper part of the uterus and allow the ova (egg cells) to travel from the ovaries to the uterus. Conception, the fertilization of an egg by a sperm, normally occurs in the fallopian tubes. The fertilized egg then moves to the uterus, where it implants in the uterine wall.

Females of reproductive age experience cycles of hormonal activity that repeat at about one-month intervals. *Menstru*, meaning *monthly*, provides us with the term, menstrual cycle. Each such cycle prepares a woman's body for a potential pregnancy. The average menstrual cycle takes about 28 days and occurs in phases: the follicular phase, ovulatory phase (ovulation), and luteal phase. The term *menstruation* refers to the periodic shedding of the uterine lining.

The Follicular phase starts on the first day of the cycle. During this phase, the follicle stimulating hormone and luteinizing hormone are released from the brain and travel in the blood to the ovaries. These hormones stimulate the growth of about 15-20 eggs in the ovaries, each in its own *shell*, called a follicle. As the follicular phase progresses, one follicle in one ovary becomes dominant and continues to mature. This dominant follicle suppresses other follicles, which then stop growing and die. The dominant follicle continues to produce estrogen.

The Ovulatory phase, which begins about 14 days after the start of the follicular phase, is the midpoint of the menstrual cycle. During this phase, a rise in estrogen from the dominant follicle triggers a surge in the amount of luteinizing hormone produced by the brain, causing the dominant follicle to release its egg from the ovary.

The Luteal phase begins immediately after ovulation. Once it releases its egg, an empty follicle develops into a new structure called the corpus luteum. Progesterone prepares the uterus for a fertilized egg to implant. If intercourse has taken place and a man's sperm has fertilized the egg (a process called conception), the fertilized egg (embryo) will travel through the fallopian tube to implant in the uterus, resulting in pregnancy.

If the egg is not fertilized, it passes through the uterus, whose lining breaks down and sheds, starting the next menstrual period.

The Endocrine System

The endocrine system is an integrated system of small organs that controls the release of hormones. This system is instrumental in the regulation of metabolism, growth, development and puberty, tissue function, and mood (Longo et al., 2012; Martini & Nath, 2011).

The nervous system controls the sending of electrical messages that coordinate body movements. Conversely, the endocrine system uses chemicals, known as hormones, to communicate and coordinate functioning. Hormones, specific messenger molecules, are synthesized and secreted by a group of specialized cells called endocrine glands. These glands are ductless, meaning that their secretions (hormones) are released directly into the bloodstream to facilitate travel to target organs.

All hormones are characterized by specific shape, which is accordingly recognized by the corresponding target cells. The binding sites on the target cells are called hormone receptors. Many hormones come in antagonistic pairs that have opposite effects on the target organs. For example, insulin and glucagon have opposite effects on the liver's control of blood sugar level. Insulin lowers the blood sugar level by instructing the liver to take glucose out of circulation and store it, while glucagon instructs the liver to release some of its stored supply to raise the blood sugar level (Longo et al., 2012).

Hypothalamus and Pituitary

The major human endocrine glands include the hypothalamus and pituitary gland. The pituitary gland, called the *master gland*, is controlled by the hypothalamus. Together, these glands control many other endocrine functions and secrete a number of hormones, especially several important to female cycles (Moore et al., 2013).

A number of other hormones affect various target organs. One non-sex hormone secreted by the posterior pituitary is antidiuretic hormone or ADH. This hormone helps prevent excess water excretion by the kidneys. Another group of non-sex hormones include the endorphins which belong to a category of chemicals known as opiates and serve to deaden the pain receptors. Endorphins which are chemically related to morphine, are produced in response to pain.

Thyroid Gland

Thyroid hormones are responsible for the regulation of metabolism, body temperature, and weight. The thyroid gland requires iodine to manufacture hormones. If a person lacks dietary iodine, the thyroid cannot make its hormones, causing a deficiency.

Pancreas

The pancreas has two functions. First, it serves as a ducted gland, secreting digestive enzymes into the small intestine. Second, it functions using the islets of Langerhans to secrete insulin and glucagon to regulate blood sugar. By secreting glucagon, islets cells signal the liver to utilize carbohydrates and raise blood sugar level. These cells secrete insulin to command the liver to remove excess glucose from circulation.

Adrenal Glands

The adrenal glands sit on top of the kidneys and consist of the outer cortex and the inner medulla. While the medulla secretes epinephrine (adrenaline) and other similar hormones in response to stressors such as fright, anger, caffeine, or low blood sugar, the cortex secretes corticosteroids such as cortisone. Corticosteroids are anti-inflammatory regulators.

Gonads

In addition to producing gametes, the female ovaries and male testes secrete hormones. These hormones (sex hormones) are secreted by the gonads, which in turn are controlled by pituitary gland hormones. While both sexes make some of each hormone, male testes secrete primarily androgens, including testosterone. Female ovaries make estrogen and progesterone in varying amounts depending on menstrual timing.

Pineal Gland

The pineal gland is located near the center of the brain and is stimulated by nerves from the eyes. The pineal gland secretes melatonin at night when it is dark to promote sleep and depress activity of the gonads. Because melatonin production is affected by the amount of light to which a person is exposed, it additionally affects the circadian rhythm (having an activity cycle of about 24 hours), annual cycles, and biological clock functions (Martini & Nath, 2011).

Conclusion

By the time a human reaches adulthood, the body consists of approximately 100 trillion cells. Each is part of an organ system designed to perform essential life functions. The body's organ systems include: the skeletal system, muscular system, nervous system, cardiovascular and lymphatic systems, integumentary system, respiratory system, sensory system, digestive system, genitourinary system, and endocrine system. The human body is a fascinating and fantastic machine. No one understands all of its many mysteries, and no single source can do justice to its many parts. This chapter has provided an overview from the cellular level through ten body systems. The information learned in this chapter will be useful for the study of disabling conditions. As previous noted, the visual and hearing systems are discussed in chapters in this text specific to those areas.

References

Adams, A. (2004). The muscular system. In M. Windelspecht (Ed.), *Human body systems*. Westport, CT: Greenwood.

Collier, J. A. B. (2009). *Oxford handbook of clinical specialties* (8th ed). New York, NY: Oxford University.

Encyclopedia Britannica. (2010). *The human muscle system gallery*. Retrieved from http://www.britannica.com/EBchecked/media/147100/Posterior-view-of-human-muscular-system

Fix, J. (2008). *Atlas of the human brain and spinal cord* (2nd ed.). Sudbury, MA: Jones and Bartlett.

Goldman, L., & Schafer, A. I. (Eds.). (2012). *Goldman's Cecil medicine* (24th ed.). Philadelphia, PA: Elsevier Saunders.

Health, Medicine, and Anatomy Reference Pictures. (2013). *The human skeleton*. Retrieved from http://healthfavo.com/detailed-human-skeleton-diagrams.html

Health, Medicine, and Anatomy Reference Pictures. (2013). *Simple brain diagram labeled*. Retrieved from http://healthfavo.com/simple-brain-diagram-labeled.html

Laas, M. (2009). *The circulatory system*. International School of Bremen. Retrieved from http://www.michael-laass.de/Circulatory%20System.htm

Longo, D., Fauci, A., Kasper, D. L., Hauser, S., & Loscalzo, G. J. (2012). *Harrison's principles of internal medicine* (18th ed.). New York, NY: McGraw Hill.

Martini, F. H., & Nath, J. L. (2011). *Fundamentals of anatomy and physiology* (9th ed.). Upper Saddle River, NJ: Pearson.

McDowell, J., & Windelspecht, M. (2004). The lymphatic system. In M. Windelspecht (Ed.), *Human body systems*. Westport, CT: Greenwood.

Moore, K. L., Dalley, A. F., & Agur, A. M. R. (2013). *Clinically oriented anatomy* (7th ed.). Philadelphia, PA: Wolters Kluwer Health.

National Heart Lung and Blood Institute. (2014). *Anatomy of the heart*. Retrieved from http://www.nhlbi.nih.gov/health//dci/Diseases/hhw/hhw_anatomy.html

National Institute on Drug Abuse. (2012). *Neurotransmission*. Retrieved from http://www.drugabuse.gov/

Seeley, R. R., VanPutte, C., Regan, J., & Russo, A. (2011). *Anatomy and physiology* (9th ed.). New York, NY: McGraw-Hill.

Tortora, G. J., & Derrickson, B. H. (2011). *Principles of anatomy and physiology* (14th ed.). Hoboken, NJ: Wiley.

About the Authors

Frances W. Siu, Ph.D., C.R.C., is an assistant professor at California State University, Los Angeles (CSULA). She received her Ph.D. in Special Education and Counseling, option in Rehabilitation Counselor Education, from the University of Texas at Austin, her M.S. in Rehabilitation Counseling and B.S. in Psychology from CSULA. Research interests of Dr. Siu include psychosocial aspects of disability and violence against people with disabilities.

Erin R. Brodwin, M.A., received her Master of Arts degree in journalism from the City University of New York, and her B.A. in ethnic studies with a minor in environmental science from the University of California, San Diego. She is a recipient of the Malcolm R. Stacey Scholarship. While in college, Erin annually received Provost Honors for students with outstanding academic achievement.

Chapter 3

CANCER

Leo E. Orr, II, M.D.
Leo M. Orange, M.S.

Introduction

Cancer is a general term used to describe a group of tissues in which some cells in the human body grow uncontrollably, invade and destroy adjacent tissues, and, if malignant, spread from their organ of origin to other sites in the body. Additionally, cancer cells, unlike non-cancerous cells, are immortal and continue to grow and destroy normal tissue. Cancer can be malignant (spread from their organ of origin) or benign (grow only at their site of origin). Oncology is the branch of medicine concerned with the study, diagnosis, treatment, and prevention of cancer.

The human body contains billions of cells; each of these cells in turn contains 46 chromosomes that house DNA, the genetic blueprint of life. Approximately 22,000 protein coding genes within the chromosomes instruct the growth and function of each body organ (Tannock, Hill, Bristol, & Harrington, 2013). Chromosomes reproduce themselves by cell division, insuring that each daughter cell retains the same genetic information. However, cancer cells often show abnormally structured chromosomes and abnormal chromosome numbers. When these errors or mutations occur, genes send incorrect messages. When such an error is received, the cell begins to grow uncontrollably and rapidly, transmitting the new genetic characteristics to its progeny. If the growth proceeds to the point that a lump forms, it is called a malignant tumor or cancer.

The word *cancer* is derived from the Greek word *karkinos*, meaning crab. In the past, women who were found to have breast cancer often experienced large and highly visible veins surrounding the tumor with features resembling the claws of a crab. The earliest anthropological evidence of cancer was found in a million year-old skeleton of a man unearthed in Java, Indonesia. References to cancer are found in early Hindu and Egyptian writings; mummies from as early as the 3rd millennium BC showed signs of bone cancer. Though characterized by ancient roots, cancer has been interpreted with fear and stigma until recently (Raghavan et al., 2012).

For many years, the causes of transmission of cancer were unknown. At the beginning of the previous century, few methods existed to diagnose cancer at an early stage. The majority of individuals were diagnosed only after experiencing debilitation, pain, and oftentimes disfigurement. Surgery was the only treatment and was radical and only sporadically successful with patients who had advanced disease (Rossi, Cady, & Martin, 2000). The public thus learned to interpret the diagnosis of cancer as a severe and debilitating disability, ultimately causing death.

Cancer was often confused with findings of syphilis, another common but untreatable illness that often produced unsightly lesions. As a result of its common confusion with syphilis, individuals with cancer felt guilt and embarrassment of having a sexual connotation applied to the disease. Diagnosis of cancer came to be equated not only with physical effects such as severe pain, disfigurement, and disability, but with the emotional impact of dependence, isolation, and death. Even with modern methods of treatment and success rates, many fears and misconceptions continue to present challenges to physicians and counselors.

Incidence and Prevalence

Cancer currently affects one in four people in the United States. In 2012, over 1.64 million new cases were diagnosed; it is the second leading cause of death, following heart disease. Although cancer remains among the worst fears, it is becoming increasingly clear that cancer is no longer the *death sentence* which it had been called in the past. The most recent data on cancer incidence, mortality, and survival is based on incidence data from the National Cancer Institute (2012) and the SEER Cancer Statistics Review (Howlader et al., 2013). A total of 1,660,290 new cancer cases and 580,350 cancer deaths are projected to occur in the United States in 2013. Cancer death rates declined 20% from 1991 to 2009. They continue to decline in four major cancer sites (lung, colorectum, breast, and prostate). Between 2000 and 2009, the largest annual decline in death rates was for chronic myeloid leukemia (8.4%) and cancers of the stomach (3.1%). The reduction in overall cancer death rates since 1990 and 1991 in men and women translates to the survival of approximately one million individuals with cancer (American Cancer Society, 2012; Smith, Brooks, Cokkinides, Salsow, & Brawley, 2013).

The leading sites of new cancer cases are shown in Table 1.

TABLE 1
Leading Sites of New Cancer Cases - 2012 Estimates

Male	Female
Prostrate – 25%	Breast – 26%
Lung & bronchus – 14%	Lung & bronchus – 15%
Colon & rectum – 9%	Colon & rectum – 9%
Urinary bladder – 7%	Uterine corpus – 6%
Melanoma of the skin – 5%	Thyroid – 5%
Kidney & renal pelvis – 5%	Non-Hodgkin lymphoma – 4%
Non-Hodgkin lymphoma – 4%	Melanoma of the skin – 4%
Leukemia – 3%	Kidney & renal pelvis – 3%
Oral cavity & pharynx – 3%	Leukemia – 3%
Pancreas – 3%	Ovary – 3%
All other sites – 20%	All other sites – 20%

Source: American Cancer Society. (2012). *Cancer facts and figures.* Atlanta, GA: Author.

Although lung cancer incidence rates have recently stabilized, it still remains the leading cause of cancer death. This highlights the need for reduced smoking and avoidance of environmental tobacco smoke.

Among major racial/ethnic groups, African-Americans have the highest rate of new cancers. Rates are relatively low among American Indians/Alaska Natives with regionally higher rates of some cancers. These disparities are not likely due to genetic differences; rather, they are more likely caused by social, cultural, behavioral, and environmental factors (National Cancer Institute, 2012).

Etiology

Gene Transformation

A landmark scientific discovery was that normal genes may be altered and become cancer genes via oncogenes. Oncogenes, normally held in check by tumor suppressor genes, usually remain dormant. However, when a stimulus or chemical agent turns off the tumor suppressor genes, these oncogenes can be initiated to transform normal cells into cancer cells. Cancer is currently viewed as a multi-step process, with changes to the gene accumulating over time, leading to malignancy. When triggers for such growth derive from chemical or foreign sources, they are termed carcinogens (El-Deiry, 2003).

Environmental Factors

Major carcinogens associated with an increased risk of cancer include tobacco (30-32%), diet (30-35%), and viruses and infections (10%). There at least 45 known or suspected carcinogens present in tobacco and alcohol; these may be synergistic rather than additive in some cancer causation (Howlader et al., 2013). Tobacco use is linked to a number of malignancies, including those occurring in the lungs, larynx, pharynx, esophagus, bladder, pancreas, and cervix. Epidemiological studies have suggested that up to 37% of all cancers are due to the effects of smoking. Alcohol is associated with many cancers of the upper respiratory and digestive tracts; both alcohol and tobacco serve as initiators and promoters and are synergistic rather than additive in cancer causation (El-Deiry, 2003; Tannock et al., 2013). Other causes include gender factors (7%), unknown causes (5%), industrial occupations (4%), alcohol (3-4%), heredity (2%), environmental pollution (2%), radiation - environmental, medical, and diagnostic (1%), sunlight - ultraviolet (1%), and additives (1%).

Diet

Diet has a major effect on overall health, including the development of diseases, such as cancer. High fat intake appears closely related to an increased risk of cancer (Jacobsen et al., 2004; Kleinsmith, 2006). The evidence of the link between diet and cancer rates is undeniable. Migrant workers who take on the diet of a foreign country experience frequencies of cancer similar to those of natives of the country. Additionally, rates of cancer are correlated with changes in dietary practices. Striking examples include the decline in both fat consumption and cancer mortality in Europe during World Wars I and II, and the parallel increase in breast cancer rates and fat consumption in Japan.

Research has shown that poor diet and not being active are two key factors that increase a person's risk of cancer. Each year, more than 572,000 Americans die of cancer; about one-third of these deaths are linked to poor diet, physical inactivity, and obesity (American Cancer Society, 2012; Smith et al., 2013). Research studies have established that obesity correlates with a higher incidence of cancer. Recent studies suggest that people with a diet high in fat are more at risk of cancer of the colon, uterus, and prostate (Lichtman, 2010; Rossen & Rossen, 2012).

Occupational Causes

A minority of cancers are connected with occupational exposures (Cohen & Markman, 2008). Exposure to ultraviolet light (e.g., the sun) is known to increase the risk of skin cancer, while exposure to ionizing radiation is a rare but long recognized cause of cancer. Development of malignancy following exposure to atomic bomb blasts and intense nuclear radiation had been quantified. Viruses cause several different malignancies including cervical cancer, Burkitt's lymphoma, a variety of lymphocytic leukemias, and AIDS-related neoplasms.

Genetics

Genetic factors are powerful but uncommon determinants of cancer. Many families demonstrate increased risk of breast, ovary, colon, lung, and malignant melanomas. When identifiable abnormal oncogenes are found in family clusters with breast and ovarian cancer, family members have up to a 50% higher risk of developing that type of tumor. Although controversial, the discovery of a genetic predisposition in an unaffected individual may allow for increased cancer surveillance, possible early destruction of a new neoplasm, and other preventive treatment modalities (Kleinsmith, 2006).

Symptoms of Cancer

Tumor presence can usually be found in several ways: (a) the tumor presses on nearby tissues producing pain; (b) the tumor becomes so large that it is seen or felt; (c) the malignancy grows into nearby blood vessels and produces bleeding; and (d) the tumor causes a change in the way some organs work, resulting in symptoms (Smith et al., 2013). For example, persistent dysphagia (trouble swallowing) may indicate a tumor involving the esophagus. The symptoms of pressure, bleeding, a mass, unusual appearance, or interference with function, are reflected in the American Cancer Society's (2012) list of *seven early warning signs* (noted by the letters C-A-U-T-I-O-N):

Change in bowel or bladder habits.

A sore that does not heal.

Unusual bleeding or discharge.

Thickening or lump in the breast or elsewhere.

Indigestion or difficulty swallowing.

Obvious change in mole or skin nodule.

Nagging cough or hoarseness.

Diagnosis

Physical Examination

If a person identifies any of the early signs of cancer, an appointment with a physician for cancer screening is warranted. During cancer screening, the physician examines the body, emphasizing the parts of the body most prone to malignancy. Salient regions include the nose and throat, breasts in women, and prostate in men. Pelvic examinations in women, including Pap smears, are essential to aid in detecting cancer of the cervix, uterus, and ovaries. The examination also includes questions about abnormal bodily functions and information about a family history of cancer.

Laboratory Testing

Nonspecific Tests

Blood tests that reveal abnormalities in the blood and indicate the presence of illness are analyzed. These tests provide clues used to determine whether more definitive testing is needed. Anemia or abnormalities in white blood cells or platelets suggests the need for more specific tests. Likewise, screening of serum chemistries is standard; this laboratory test highlights function of the kidneys, liver, pancreas, and other internal organs. A chest x-ray may be conducted during screening.

Specific Tests

Specific tests are ordered if a physician suspects the presence of a malignancy. Serologic tumor markers are the most important blood tests indicating the presence of cancer. Blood serology confirms a physician's diagnosis, and is useful in monitoring a neoplasm following treatment to confirm that a remission has occurred.

Imaging Studies

Imaging studies include the use of x-ray, computerized tomography (CT) scans, magnetic resonance imaging (MRI), position emission tomography (PET) scans, radionucleide scans, and selective angiography (Cohen & Markman, 2008). These studies identify the tumor location, tumor size, and involvement of surrounding tissue. An ultrasound can detect cancer and be used to guide tissue biopsies.

Interventional Treatments

At times, physical examinations are insufficient and modern medical instruments are used for direct visualization inside body cavities. Thin, flexible telescopes are introduced into the lungs, bladder, rectum and colon, esophagus and stomach, and the nasopharynix. Instruments which allow for examination of the abdominal cavity are referred to as laparoscopic instruments. A thoroscopy involves the introduction of a visualizing scope into the thoracic (Raghavan et al., 2012).

Biopsy

A definitive diagnosis of cancer depends on a microscopic evaluation of a small amount of tissue analyzed by a pathologist. Special histochemical stains or immunologic markers help identify a neoplasm. Biopsies are obtained with special needles used to sample tissue, fluid from body cavities (through aspiration), or from tissue removed during a surgical procedure. Pathologic examination is usually the final step in diagnosis prior to the formulation of a treatment plan. The pathologist's evaluation is crucial in determining the origin of the cancer. The four broad cancer classifications are as follows (American Cancer Society, 2012).

1. Sarcomas – cancer of the bones, muscles, and connective tissue.
2. Carcinomas – cancer of epithelial cells which line the lungs, colon, breasts, and prostate.
3. Leukemias – cancer of the blood and bone marrow.
4. Lymphomas – cancer of the infection-fighting organs.

Staging Classifications

Once cancer is diagnosed, the physician must determine the extent to which it has spread (metastasized). Staging is a method used to describe if the cancer is localized or has spread to other organs. The most modern staging classification includes the *TNM* system with subscript numbers 0 - 4 (0 = least; 4 = most) by the American Joint Commission on Cancer (American Cancer Society, 2012):

T = Tumor size, location, and adjacent tissue involvement (T_1 through T_4).

N = Regional lymph node involvement with tumor (N_0 = no tumor involvement with lymph nodes; $N_1 - N_4$ = increasing degrees of tumor involvement with lymph nodes).

M = Absence (M_0) or degree of spread (metastases) to distant organs ($M_1 - M_4$).

Thus, a tumor staged $T_2N_1M_0$ is less extensive and potentially more curable than one staged $T_1N_1M_1$ (Rossi et al., 2000; Tannock et al., 2013).

An older staging system is still used to a limited extent. In this system, Stage I refers to a state in which the tumor is confined to a single area, usually the tissue of origin. With involvement of adjacent or regional lymph nodes, the cancer is considered to be in Stage II. Stage III involves the local spread of cancer beyond the confines of the tissue or organ initially involved. In Stage IV, cancer has metastasized to distant sites of the body.

Functional Capacity Categories

The patient's functional capacity is categorized using either the Eastern Cooperative Oncology Group (ECOG) or the Karnofsky scale. Because the ECOG is the most commonly used categorization method, the Karnofsy Scale is not described here.

ECOG performance scale:

O Normal activity without physical limitations.
I Symptomatic, but able to complete daily activities.
II Assistance needed at times, but can be out of bed more than 50% of the time.
III Needs skilled care; in bed more than 50% of the time.
IV In bed 100% of the time.

When determining the modality and extent of treatment possibilities, the patient's age, degree of tumor-associated weight loss, nutritional level, and presence of comorbid conditions (i.e., heart disease, lung disease) need to be considered (Kleinsmith, 2006). These factors will help in development of an individualized treatment plan.

Treatment

Once a definitive diagnosis is obtained, the physician develops and recommends a treatment plan. Major modalities for cancer treatment are surgery, radiation, chemotherapy, and biologic therapy. These methods are employed alone or in combination, depending on the nature of the malignancy and stage of the tumor. Bone marrow and stem cell transplantation are used in selected circumstances. The treatment modality chosen depends primarily on the stage of the neoplasm, the degree to which the neoplasm impacts the patient's health and ability to function, overall health of the patient, and feasibility for surgical intervention.

Surgery

Surgery is the oldest form and the most effective cancer treatment. More cancers are cured with surgical interventions than with any other treatment modalities. Surgery is often curative and is the primary treatment approach for several types of cancer. These include stomach, colon, head and neck, prostate, sarcoma, skin, thyroid, and certain lung cancers. Surgical procedures occur during the diagnosis, treatment, and post-treatment phases of cancer management to (Tannock et al., 2013):

- Diagnose or stage the disease, either with a biopsy or an open operation to remove nonessential organ parts.
- Remove the primary tumor which may be curative or used to improve the effectiveness of other treatments by reducing tumor volume. It may also relieve pain and improve quality of life.
- Remove other tumors that escaped prior treatment or are due to recurrent disease.
- Relieve symptoms. Used when the tumor blocks or compresses vital organ structures and functions.
- Reconstruct or rehabilitate. Examples include reconstructive surgery following mastectomy, removal of cancer of the head and neck, and extensive limb surgery.
- Support radiation and chemotherapy. Catheters filled with radiation implants are surgically placed in body cavities or organs to access deep-seated cancers when curative treatment with external beam radiation alone is inadequate. Treatment includes implantation of a venous access port to facilitate delivery of concentrated chemotherapy.

Radiation Therapy

About half of all cancer patients require radiation during treatment. This modality is used alone or in combination with chemotherapy, surgery, or both. The main goal is cure or relief of major symptoms. Radiation therapy employs high-energy x-rays, electron beams, and radioactive isotopes to destroy cancer cells. Malignant cells are destroyed through a process called ionization, which damages the DNA in the nuclei of cells so that cell division is stopped. There are several methods of delivering radiation, including external beam radiation, internal radiation, and hyperthermia.

External Beam Radiation

This treatment involves delivery of electrons, x-rays, or gamma rays. Generally, the equipment emits either low energy (orthovoltage) or high energy (megavoltage) beams. The *gamma knife* is a very high energy apparatus capable of brief, focused, and intense treatment to the target area using stereotactic techniques.

Internal Radiation

Internal radiation involves use of interstitial radiation, radiation implants, and brachytherapy. Radioactive seeds are placed temporarily or permanently into the cancer area. Intracavity radiation is used primarily for tumors of the cervix, uterus, and esophagus. Special hollow applicators are implanted within the body (where the applicator usually remains for two to three days), followed by insertion of a radioactive isotope.

Hyperthermia

Hyperthermia is based on the knowledge that malignant tumors are more susceptible to destruction by heat than normal tissues. This therapy is rarely used.

Side Effects

Common side effects of radiation therapy include nausea, fatigue, skin inflammation, and temporary lowering of blood counts. Specific side effects characterize different cancer types. If radiation is given to the brain, for example, hair loss occurs. After treatment to the head and neck, the patient may experience dry mouth. Diarrhea is a side effect of rectal and bladder therapy, while frequent urination often occurs after prostate radiation. Neoplasms that are treated by radiation with a curative intent include prostate, head and neck, rectum, Hodgkin's lymphoma, and certain lung cancers (Tannock et al., 2013).

Chemotherapy

Chemotherapy is another form of treatment that involves use of medications to interrupt cancer cell growth by attacking specific stages of cell division. These drugs are often administered in combination with other treatments. A major drawback of chemotherapy is the eventual development of drug resistance. Many cancers acquire the ability to overcome or evade the toxic effects of pharmaceuticals.

Delivery routes and methods for administration of chemotherapy include (a) oral administration; (b) intravenous (the most common route); (c) ambulatory infusion pump (employed for long-duration chemotherapy); (d) intra-arterial infusions (used for deep-seated localized tumors, found in liver cancer); and (e) intracavitary (used for some neoplasms of the chest cavity lining and ovaries). Since chemotherapeutic agents destroy rapid growing abnormal tissues, other rapid growing tissue such as hair follicles, gut mucosae, and bone morrow are often temporarily affected (Tannock et al., 2013). Common effects of chemotherapy include fatigue, nausea, diarrhea, hair loss, sore mouth, loss of sensation or tingling in fingers, diminished appetite or taste, and compromised blood count.

Chemotherapy is a curative treatment for some malignancies and is also used for palliative causes. Adjuvant treatment involves the use of drugs to eradicate microscopic or subclinical areas of cancer that may remain following surgery (Armitage & Antman, 2008).

Biologic Therapy

Biologic therapies are used to treat cancer by helping the functioning of the immune system. They are also referred to as biologic agents, biological response modifier therapy, and immunotherapy. Biologic therapy works with the immune system helping to fight cancer or control side effects of the disease or its treatments (Raghavan et al., 2012; Tannock et al., 2013).

While biologic therapy and chemotherapy may seem alike, treatments work in different ways. Biologic therapy helps the body's immune system fight cancer while chemotherapy attacks cancer cells. Biologic therapy aids the immune system in its fight against cancer in the following three ways:
- Stops or slows the growth of cancer cells.
- Helps the immune system destroy or eliminate cancer cells.
- Keeps cancer from spreading to other parts of the body.

Transplantation

Bone marrow transplants are performed to treat illnesses in which the stem cells are defective or preclude the production of normal cells. Bone marrow contains immature (stem) cells capable of continuously producing blood cells. Bone marrow transplantation is recommended when bone marrow or the immune system is defective. Many cancers are combated with high doses of radiation which irreversibly damages bone marrow, the most sensitive of all tissues to chemotherapy and radiation.

Types of Transplants

Allogenic. Allogenic transplants involve the transfer of marrow from one individual to another. Donors are matched immunologically as close as possible using a process known as human leukocyte antigen typing. The closer the match of a transplant, the less likely of immune incompatibility and *graft versus host disease*.

Autologous. This technique harvests cryopreserves from the patient's own marrow and stem cells. Marrow or stem cells are then reintroduced after high-dose radiation or chemotherapy has ablated the old marrow. There is no risk of marrow rejection with this technique.

Syngeneic. Syngeneic transplantation is when bone marrow is obtained from a person's identical twin. There is no risk of rejection.

Complications

After receiving a bone marrow transplant, individuals are at high risk for infection (Kleinsmith, 2006). The greatest window of susceptibility occurs between marrow ablation and repopulation of the bone marrow spaces by the transplanted marrow. Some people experience excessive bleeding after a transplant, while others develop pneumonia, usually caused by cytomegalovirus infection. Complications associated with marrow grafts occur when new marrow recognizes the host as foreign and begins attacking various tissues including the liver, skin, and intestines. Heart damage is an additional potential obstacle (Rossi et al., 2000).

Current Treatment Rates

Twenty-five years ago, only one in ten children survived cancer. Today, seven out of ten children (70%) who develop cancer are living five years after diagnosis, and one of every 1,000 Americans between the ages of 20 and 40 is a survivor of childhood cancer (Mariotto et al., 2009).

In the past, testicular cancer (the leading cause of death due to cancer among men 15 to 35 years of age) usually constituted a fatal diagnosis. Today, 90% of men who are diagnosed with testicular cancer are cured (Huddart et al., 2005). Likewise, the breast cancer death rate of women in the United States fell 6.3% between 1991 and 1995 and 9.3% in women under age 65. This drop in death rate is attributed to improvements in consumer awareness, modern testing methods, mammography, and modern treatments (National Cancer Institute, 2012).

Negative Effects of Cancer Treatment

Negative effects of cancer treatment vary for each individual; everyone experiences symptoms of varying intensity (El-Deiry, 2003). The most common physical changes and negative effects experienced from cancer treatment include: hair loss, weight loss or gain, appetite loss or increase, fatigue, disfigurement from surgery, difficulty concentrating, nausea and vomiting, diarrhea, pale skin and changes in skin tone, sleep disruption, and sexual dysfunction.

For many people diagnosed with cancer, the most prominent and challenging negative effect is fatigue, an effect of chemotherapy that can be overwhelming and persistent. Chemotherapy can involve months of strong medications that cause fatigue and weakness as the body tries to negotiate the healing process and regenerate affected tissue. Family, friends, and co-workers of the individual may experience stress and emotional involvement as a result of the individual's concerns and emotional changes, which in turn further impacts the person experiencing these changes (Raghavan et al., 2012).

Psychosocial Implications – Stress and Adjustment Reactions

The diagnosis and treatment of cancer is a stressful event, followed by a range of distressing symptoms, including anxiety and depression. While these symptoms are likely to be transient, the experience of cancer is not a single, undifferentiated event. Rather, people with cancer encounter a series of stressful events and challenges over time that poses different demands and difficulties. A person's distress may become heightened at particular times, such as at the time of diagnosis or disease recurrence, before surgery, at the commencement of adjuvant therapy, during the advanced disease stage, or when presenting for medical surveillance (Mystakidou, 2006).

Severe Emotional Distress

Stress and adjustment problems may include negative feelings lasting for one or more weeks. If such problems are not acknowledged, they may develop into more serious emotional states. Major psychological disorders resulting from emotional distress include major depressive episodes, anxiety disorders, PTSD, and negative emotional, behavioral, or cognitive states that are overwhelming and persistent (lasting more than two weeks) (Oeffinger & McCabe, 2006).

Anxiety

Some anxiety in response to a stressful life event is normal; however, severe anxiety can interfere with relationships, social or occupational functioning, and disrupt personal health. Symptoms associated with anxiety include heightened physical arousal, sleep disturbance, impaired concentration and decision-making, agitation, and anger. Severe anxiety problems include panic attacks, pervasive and generalized worrying, treatment phobias, social anxiety, and post-traumatic stress reactions.

Depression

Depression undermines the capacity of the person to cope with illness, and is associated with increased medical symptoms and impairment in social, educational, and vocational functioning (Livneh, 2000). Patients with depression are three times more likely to be non-compliant with medical treatment recommendations. Depressed patients with breast cancer, for example, have been found to be less likely to accept adjuvant chemotherapy (Wimberly, Carver, & Laurenceau, 2005). Depression is a major risk factor for potential suicide.

Diagnosis of a major depressive episode is best evaluated by the severity of the depressed mood, loss of interest and pleasure, the degree of feelings of hopelessness, guilt, and worthlessness, and the presence of suicidal thoughts (Mystakidou, 2006). Recurrent tearfulness is often accompanied by social withdrawal and loss of motivation. Patients with depression may feel they are unable to control their negative feelings; as a result, these feelings begin to dominate one's life.

Suicide

Accurate figures of the incidence of suicide in patients with cancer are difficult to obtain. Studies undertaken in Sweden and Denmark suggested that the incidence of suicide is higher in people with cancer than in the general population, and that suicide is more likely to occur during the first year after diagnosis (Jacobsen et al., 2004).

Risk factors for suicide include severe depression, a family history of suicide, past history of self-harm, alcohol or other substance abuse issues, poor social support, and a negative outlook for the future (Mystakidou, 2006). Assessment and exploration of an individual's suicidal thoughts is crucial to early recognition and treatment of psychological distress (Jacobsen et al., 2004).

Post-Traumatic Stress Disorder (PTSD)

Classifications of mental disorders have been revised to include diagnosis of a potentially life-threatening illness as a sufficient stressor for the precipitation of PTSD. There is limited but increasing research on traumatic symptomatology in patients with cancer. Most of this research has focused on patients with breast cancer (Oeffinger & McCabe, 2006). The stressor criteria for PTSD have recently been modified to include life-threatening illnesses, such as cancer, as precipitating traumatic events (American Cancer Society, 2012; Smith et al., 2013).

Sexuality Issues

Sexuality encompasses body image, self-esteem, mood, support, intimacy, and a sense of emotional connection. The role of body image in sexuality is illustrated by the number of patients reporting sexual problems whose cancers do not directly affect sexual organs (Livneh, 2000). This finding suggests the need to address patients' issues of sexuality regardless of the cancer site. Psychological factors such as emotional stress, depression, and grief may diminish interest in sex and create performance anxiety. Pressures of not working or feelings of being a burden affect one's sexuality (Orange, 2009).

As a topic in counseling, sexuality has received little scholarly attention. Professional training in sexual health is equally limited. Although literature demonstrates the integral role sexuality plays in the life of patients, physicians rarely introduce the subject during clinical encounters (Wimberly et al., 2005). Patients who have chronic diseases find that because of the complexity of their illnesses and medical treatments, concerns regarding sexuality are often ignored. Without prompting on the part of the counselor or physician, patients are reluctant to voice sexual concerns (Huddart et al., 2005). Yet, it is often these patients with chronic illnesses who have difficulties with sexual functioning (Brodwin, Orange, & Chen, 2004). By understanding the impact of chronic illness on sexual functioning, health care professionals can more readily screen for and help the person manage sexual dysfunction, thereby enhancing quality of life.

Emotional Adjustment

The psychosocial aspects of cancer including dependence, stigma, discrimination, and self-concept, can have negative effects equal to the physical components of the disease. To achieve physical, mental, and emotional health, individuals need time to adjust to the diagnosis. The acute stress of illness and treatment can result in distress and dysfunction in all areas of life. Due to the stigmatizing effects of disability in society, people with disabilities tend to develop negative feelings about their own and other types of disabilities and limitations (Brodwin, Orange, & Brodwin, 1994).

The recurrence of physical symptoms signals the reactivation of those psychological associations that accompanied initial diagnosis and treatment. As a form of negative information, these symptoms constitute the resurgence of feelings of stress, helplessness, fear, and pain, at times leading to depression and withdrawal. This can cause serious adjustment problems when left untreated. Depression is a reaction to the experience of loss, chronic frustration, and radical changes in lifestyle. Psychological and social supports function as stress buffers, helping a person modulate the somatic effects of stress (Livneh, 2000).

Rehabilitation researchers and counselors have long recognized the benefits of identifying and addressing the psychosocial needs of the client who currently has or is recovering from cancer (Alfano and Roland, 2006; Mystakidou, 2006). Cancer is unpredictable and symptoms can vary daily. To address and adapt to this unpredictability, individuals and healthcare professionals should focus on the following psychosocial issues during the rehabilitation process: (a) feelings of loss of control during treatment; (b) difficulty coping with physical changes; (c) need for social support within the family and community; (d) impact and consequences of role changes and need for internal and external resources to aid in adjustment; (e) interpersonal issues associated with stress; and (f) psychosocial factors related to both unemployment and potential return to work (Livneh, 2000).

Rehabilitation Potential and Employment Issues

Challenges

Work is a vital aspect of self-worth and identity. While many persons who have had cancer view return to work as the apex of achievement, those resuming employment face many challenges including discrimination, avoidance, financial concerns, reduced opportunities for advancement, and changes in physical and emotional capacity.

Many people return to employment during or after experiencing illness and medical treatment. Cancer survivors benefit from making contributions within the workplace and society, as well as financially contributing to their families. An essential component of rehabilitation is support and collaboration from the employer (McDonough, 1992). Unfortunately, cancer survivors face problems when employers have misconceptions about the consequences of cancer, medical treatment, and survival.

Together, survivors of cancer and vocational rehabilitation counselors can dispel the following societal myths about the disease: (a) health insurance rates for employee coverage increase when individuals who have cancer are hired; (b) attendance by these workers is substandard and job turnover is high; (c) employees who have cancer are less flexible; and (d) cancer survivors are less able to perform essential job functions, thereby imposing more duties on other employees and entailing added costs to employers (Slivon, Hicken, & Marini, 1994). These myths continue to have a negative impact (Brodwin & Orange, 2014).

To Disclose or Not to Disclose

Whether or not to disclose a disability or functional limitations to a potential employer is a difficult decision. Negative attitudes, stereotypes, and fears about people with cancer form major hurdles for cancer survivors who wish full participation in the work place. Even with federal legislation incorporated within the Americans with Disabilities Act (ADA) of 1990, it is not always clear if the individual should disclose the presence of a disability. The most appropriate response depends on personal choice and functional limitations. If a disability affects a worker's performance on the job, or if accommodation is necessary to perform the duties of the position, disclosure is potentially beneficial. The ADA states that an employer is not entitled to information about a disability unless it directly relates to (a) ability to perform the job, and (b) a request for reasonable accommodation.

Reasonable Accommodation and the Americans with Disabilities Act

The ADA provides protection for individuals with a history of cancer, regardless of whether the cancer is cured, in remission, or being treated. According to the ADA, people with limitations due to past or current disabilities are to be given the same opportunities as everyone else. Reasonable accommodations for individuals with disabilities under the statute include: modifications or adjustments to a job or work to participate in the application process, perform essential job functions, and enjoy the rights and privileges available to other employees. An employer is not required to provide accommodations under ADA unless the employee discloses that a disability exists.

Empowerment and Employment

Employment is a significant component of building one's identity and conception of self-worth. Individuals who have been diagnosed with a disease like cancer may place increased emphasis on work because it focuses on capabilities, rather than on illness and limitations. Work thus becomes a haven away from medical intervention, providing routine as well as psychosocial stability. It also provides familiarity, potential for reward, and a source of companionship. Being around people who are supportive is not only a source of comfort, but acts as an alternative to the isolating effects of cancer, and helps the individual surviving cancer maintain a sense of autonomy and control (Simon, 1999).

Counselors facilitate empowerment by encouraging and supporting a person's efforts to take an active role in the rehabilitation process. Determining the client's knowledge and awareness with respect to the disease and prognosis helps clarify directions for inquiry. People who survive cancer and understand their disability and its implications are better able to actively participate in decision making during medical treatment and rehabilitation (Brodwin & Orange, 2014).

Multicultural Perspectives

Americans with disabilities face varying societal beliefs, feelings, and behaviors from society. As noted by McDonough (1992), "Americans in society have a negative attitude about the disabled in general and those in the workplace in particular" (p. 58). Persons who possess attributes that are viewed negatively by the prevailing group in a society tend to be devalued by that society; individuals with disabilities often are evaluated and judged by the disability. Rehabilitation literature emphasizes the maintenance of positive regard and advocacy for people who have disabilities (Brodwin et al., 1994).

Rehabilitation serves to empower individuals with disabilities, allowing them to maximize their capabilities while minimizing limitations. As a strategy, rehabilitation works to maximize the potential for independent living. Rehabilitation philosophy emphasizes a multidisciplinary approach to guide people with disabilities to their pre-injury potentials of physical, mental, social, educational, vocational, and recreational status.

Counselors must be aware and understand the complexities of the multicultural society in which they live. If quality counseling services are to be provided to ethnic minority persons with disabilities, rehabilitation counselors and other human service professionals must be sensitive in interactions with culturally diverse individuals.

To be effective, rehabilitation counselors must be able to address the issues, needs, and beliefs of a culturally diverse population, while maintaining respect and positive attitudes toward cultural and gender differences. Counselors rehabilitate the *whole person* and dedicate their efforts to increasing the quality of life for all individuals, including survivors of cancer.

Case Study

Steve McPherson is married, 22 years of age, and the father of one child. Although Steve dropped out of high school, he attended adult education and successfully completed his G.E.D. He is a partner in a small but highly successful company involved with telephone and communication systems installation. By trade, he is an electrician and a member of the local electricians' trade union.

The *Dictionary of Occupational Titles* (U. S. Department of Labor, 1991) classifies Mr. McPherson's job as telephone electrician (telephone and telegraph) (*D.O.T.* # 822.281-018). Steve and his business partner install, test, and repair telephone and communication systems. They update and expand old equipment, install new computerized systems, and wire burglar alarm devices and related equipment. The work involves the use of hand tools and testing devices, an ability to read schematics, and knowledge of electrical and electronic principles. Lifting and carrying on the job involves a maximum of 50 pounds, with repetitive lifting up to 25 pounds.

Mr. McPherson felt in good physical and emotional health when he noticed a non-tender lump on his right scrotum. Two months later, he was diagnosed with embryonic cell carcinoma of testicular origin, well-differentiated, stage $T_2N_0M_0$. Steve underwent a right orchiectomy (testicle removal) and lymph node dissection and received a complete course of chemotherapy. Three months postoperatively, he was assessed as being disease-free with an excellent prognosis. Steve returned to work, continued to have an active family life, and maintained sexual function.

Approximately one year later, a routine cancer follow-up visit (including a chest x-ray) revealed a solitary metastatic right lower lobe pulmonary lesion. His oncologist initiated chemotherapy using a combination of agents and the lesion disappeared. Again, the oncologist believed him disease-free or *in remission*. After completion of chemotherapy, Steve returned to work and was fully independent.

Two years hence, Mr. McPherson was diagnosed with lung cancer. Within one month of open chest surgery to remove the cancer, Steve developed left-sided brain seizures. After a new diagnosis which identified metastatic testicular disease of the brain, he underwent neurosurgery for removal of the brain tumor.

After undergoing the craniotomy procedure, Steve again developed left-sided weakness in the form of significant loss of strength in his left arm and leg. He not only required crutches for ambulation, but had poor balance, and was required to be in bed or in a chair most of the day.

Following radiation therapy, Steve received physical and occupational therapy. He maintained a 25% residual deficit in his left, nondominant upper extremity and could walk for short distances with a cane. The symptoms gradually subsided and he was able to return to work part-time at a functional capacity of sedentary work. His major responsibilities became administrative, including work site analysis, writing bids, and service contract negotiations. Mr. McPherson remained asymptomatic and was able to gradually increase his work effort to full time at the sedentary level of exertion.

Questions

1. Discuss the various forms of cancer treatment.
2. Identify psychosocial implications of cancer.
3. Why was radiation therapy not given to his lung nodules?
4. Was the diagnosis of $T_2N_0M_0$ accurate? Please explain.
5. What were some precautions for Steve to take in returning to work?
6. Provide a vocational profile for Mr. McPherson including age, educational level, exertional and skill level of work activity, occupationally significant characteristics, and transferable skills (if any).
7. Was the return to modified work realistic? How were transferable skills used in this return to work?
8. What other vocational possibilities are there using transferable skills or additional training?

References

Alfano, C. M., & Rowland, J. H. (2006). Recovery issues in cancer survivorship: A new challenge for supportive care. *Cancer Journal, 12*(5), 432–443.

American Cancer Society. (2012). *Cancer facts and figures.* Atlanta, GA: Author.

Americans with Disabilities Act of 1990 (ADA), PL 101-336, 42 U.S.C. §12101 *et seq.*

Armitage, J. O., & Antman, K. H. (Eds.). (2008). *High-dose cancer therapy: Pharmacology, hematopoietins, and stem cells* (3rd ed.). Philadelphia, PA: Lippincott Williams and Wilkins.

Brodwin, M. G., & Orange, L. M. (2014). Attitudes toward disability. In J. D. Andrew & C. W. Faubion (Eds.), *Rehabilitation services: An introduction for the human services professional* (3rd ed., pp. 164–185). Linn Creek, MO: Aspen.

Brodwin, M. G., Orange, L. M., and Chen, R. K. (2004). Societal attitudes toward sexuality regarding people with disabilities. *Directions in Rehabilitation Counseling, 15*, 45–53.

Brodwin, S. K., Orange, L. M., & Brodwin, M. G. (1994). Disabled clients: What every therapist needs to know. In L. Vandecreek, S. Knapp, & T. L. Jackson (Eds.), *Innovations in clinical practice: A source book:* Vol. 13 (pp. 419–430). Sarasota, FL: Professional Resource.

Cohen, L., & Markman, M. (2008). *Integration oncology.* Totowa, NJ: Humana.

El-Deiry, W. S. (2003). *Tumor suppressor genes.* Totowa, NJ: Humana.

Howlader, N., Noone A. M., Krapcho, M., Garshell J., Neyman, N., Altekruse, S. F., . . . Cronin, K. A. (Eds), (2013). *SEER Cancer Statistics Review, 1975-2010.* Bethesda, MD: National Cancer Institute.

Huddart, R., Norman, A., Moynihan, C., Horwich, A., Parker, C., Nicholls, E., & Dearnaley, D. (2005). Fertility, gonadal, and sexual function in survivors of testicular cancer. *British Journal of Cancer, 93*(2), 5–9.

Jacobsen, P. H., Holmich, L. R., McLaughlin, J. K., Johansen, C., Olsen, J. H., Kjoller, K., & Friis, S. (2004). Mortality and suicide among Danish women with cosmetic breast implants. *Archives of Internal Medicine, 164*, 2450–2455.

Kleinsmith, L. J. (2006). *Principles of cancer biology* (2nd ed.). San Francisco, CA: Pearson Benjamin Cummings.

Lichtman M. A. (2010). Obesity and the risk for a hematological malignancy: Leukemia, lymphoma, or myeloma. *Oncologist, 15*, 1083–1101.

Livneh, H. (2000). Psychosocial adaptation to cancer: The role of coping strategies. *Journal of Rehabilitation, 66*(2), 40–49.

Mariotto, A. B., Julia, H., Rowland, K.,Yabroff, R., Scoppa, S., Hachey, A., & Feuer, E. J. (2009). Long-term survivors of childhood cancers in the United States. *Cancer Epidemiological Biomarkers Preview, 18*(4), 1033.

McDonough, H. (1992). You and the ADA. *Graduating Engineer*, 56–58.

Mystakidou, K. (2006). Psychological distress of patients with advanced cancer. *Cancer Nursing, 29*(5), 38–42.

National Cancer Institute. (2012). *Cancer trends progress report*. U. S. Department of Health and Human Services, National Institutes of Health (NIH Publication No. 05-5498). Retrieved from http://www.cancer.gov

Oeffinger, K. C., & McCabe, M. S. (2006). Models for delivering survivorship care. *Journal of Clinical Oncology, 24*, 5117–5124.

Orange, L. M. (2009). Sexuality and disability. In M. G. Brodwin, F. W. Siu, J. Howard, & E. R. Brodwin (Eds.), *Medical, psychosocial, and vocational aspects of disability* (3rd ed., pp. 263–272). Athens, GA: Elliott and Fitzpatrick.

Raghavan, D, Blanke, D. R., Johnson, D. H., Moots, P. L., Reaman, G. H., Rose, P. G., & Sekeres, M. H. (Eds.). (2012). *Textbook of uncommon cancer* (3rd ed.). Hoboken, NJ: Wiley.

Rossen L. M., & Rossen E. A. (2012). *Obesity 101*. New York, NY: Springer.

Rossi, R. L., Cady, B., & Martin, R. F. (Eds.). (2000). *Multidisciplinary approach to cancer*. Philadelphia, PA: W. B. Saunders.

Simon, D. (1999). *Return to wholeness: Embracing body, mind, and spirit in the face of cancer*. New York, NY: Wiley.

Slivon, D., Hicken, N., & Marini, I. (1994). Employer attitudes towards hiring persons with visible disabilities. *Journal of Job Placement, 10*(2), 23–26.

Smith R. A., Brooks D., Cokkinides V., Salsow D., & Brawley, O. W. (2013). Cancer screening in the United States: A review of current American Cancer Society guidelines, current issues in cancer screening, and new guidance on cervical cancer screening and lung cancer screening. *Cancer Journal for Clinicians, 63*, 87–105.

Tannock, I. F., Hill, R. P., Bristow, R., & Harrington, L. (Eds). (2013). *The basic science of oncology* (5th ed.). New York, NY: McGraw-Hill.

U. S. Department of Labor. (1991). *Dictionary of occupational titles* (4th ed., text rev.). Washington, DC: Author.

Wimberly, S. R., Carver, C. S., & Laurenceau, J. P. (2005). Perceived partner reactions to diagnosis and treatment of breast cancer: Impact on psychosocial and psychosexual adjustment. *Journal of Consultation and Clinical Psychology, 73*(2), 300–311.

About the Authors

Leo E. Orr, II, M.D., is in private practice in Los Angeles, California. At the Don P. Loker Cancer Center and Good Samaritan Hospital, he is involved in clinical research with primary interests in the development of tumor markers for early detection of cancer and biopharmacology research. Dr. Orr is Co-founder and Co-director of the Transfusion-free Center at Good Samaritan Hospital, and Assistant Clinical Professor at the University of Southern California Medical School.

Leo M. Orange, M.S., is Director of Disabled Students Programs and Services at Oxnard College in Oxnard, California, and a part-time assistant professor in the rehabilitation education program at California State University, Los Angeles. Mr. Orange is a cancer survivor who was successfully treated by his co-author, Dr. Orr, in 1985. He has written many book chapters and articles in rehabilitation and counseling journals addressing reasonable accommodation, multicultural counseling, psychosocial aspects of disabilities, and sexuality.

Chapter 4

DIABETES AND CHRONIC KIDNEY DISEASE

Martin G. Brodwin, Ph.D., C.R.C.

Introduction

Persons with diabetes mellitus (commonly called diabetes) account for nearly half of the cases of renal disease. It is for this reason we have combined the material on diabetes and renal failure. Individuals who do not have diabetes but have renal disease are also included within the section on kidney disease. The first part of the chapter discusses diabetes, while the second part includes chronic kidney disease and renal failure.

Diabetes Mellitus

Diabetes is recognized as the 6th leading cause of death in the United States. A chronic disorder, diabetes is characterized by abnormal elevations in blood glucose (blood sugar) resulting from defects in insulin secretion, insulin action, or both (American Diabetes Association, 2010, 2013a). Along with abnormal blood glucose, diabetes is associated with a set of physical abnormalities collectively referred to as diabetes complications. It is these complications that are responsible for the mortality and morbidity associated with diabetes. Diabetes is the leading cause of such conditions as blindness, end-stage kidney disease, and lower extremity amputation. Additionally, diabetes is also a risk factor for high blood pressure (hypertension), stroke, heart disease, and peripheral neuropathy (Andreoli, Benjamin, Griggs, Wing, & Fitz, 2010).

Prevalence

Diabetes mellitus (diabetes), popularly referred to as *sugar diabetes*, is a health concern of worldwide proportion. It is estimated that there are 25.8 million children and adults in the United States who have diabetes; 18.8 million are diagnosed, while 7.0 million are undiagnosed. This disease is one of the most common in the world. By the year 2030, it is estimated that 366 million people worldwide will be diagnosed with diabetes. The countries with the largest number of confirmed cases of diabetes worldwide are India, China, and the United States, respectively. In 2010, there were 1.9 million new cases of diagnosed diabetes in the United States in people aged 20 years and older (American Diabetes Association, 2011). One in 400 children has diabetes. In people 65 years and older, 10.9 million have diabetes, which is 27% of all people within that age group (American Diabetes Association, 2013b).

As projected by the American Diabetes Association (2013b), the number of people who will have diabetes in this country will double or triple by the year 2050. As many as one in every three to five people will have diagnosed or undiagnosed diabetes.

Risk Factors

The four major risk factors for diabetes development are genetics, age, obesity, and race. A positive family history of the disease increases the potential risk of developing diabetes (American Diabetes Association, 2010, 2013a). Aging also increases one's risk, as glucose tolerance and the ability of the body to metabolize sugar deteriorates with the aging process. Obesity induces insulin resistance; therefore, overweight individuals are more likely to develop diabetes. Diabetes is more common among Hispanics, while prevalence ranks second among African American; third among Asian Americans, and Caucasians have the least risk.

Costs

As noted by the American Diabetes Association (2013b), the total cost of diagnosed diabetes in 2012 was $245 billion, an increase of 41% since 2007. Of this amount, $176 billion was spent for direct medical costs and $69 billion in reduced productivity.

Diagnosis

Blood glucose values are a vital determining factor in the current American Diabetes Association criteria for diagnosis of diabetes (American Diabetes Association, 2013a). A fasting blood glucose greater than 126 mg/dl (milligrams per deciliter) is considered abnormal. When blood glucose is greater than 200mg/dl and is concurrent with symptoms of diabetes, such as polyuria (increased urination), polydipsia (increased thirst), and unexplained weight loss, a physician may diagnose an individual with diabetes.

Type I And Type II Diabetes

There are two major forms of diabetes. Type I diabetes (Insulin-Dependent Diabetes Mellitus) results from autoimmune destruction of the insulin-producing cells of the pancreas (â-cells). This type is characterized by absolute insulin insufficiency. This was formerly referred to as juvenile-onset diabetes, brittle diabetes, or ketosis-prone diabetes. Type I diabetes accounts for 5-10% of the cases of diabetes, and most patients manifest severe symptoms resulting from little or no insulin secretion. Even though primarily a disease with onset in childhood or adolescence, it can occur at any age.

Type II diabetes (Non-Insulin-Dependent Diabetes Mellitus) is the most common form of the disease (90-95% of the cases of diabetes) and is associated with defects in insulin secretion and/or insulin resistance at the tissue level. Type II diabetes, formerly referred to as maturity-onset diabetes or non-ketosis prone diabetes, is found especially in overweight individuals as obesity itself causes some degree of insulin resistance. Type II diabetes can remain undiagnosed over many years because insulin resistance and elevated blood sugar occur gradually. Over time, Type II patients may require oral agents to lower their elevated blood sugar and ultimately insulin supplementation therapy.

Gestational diabetes (GDM) occurs when glucose intolerance occurs during pregnancy. This term is applied regardless of whether insulin or only dietary modification is used for treatment. GDM complicates about 4% of all pregnancies in the United States. Subsequent to delivery, in most cases blood glucose levels return to normal (American Diabetes Association, 2010, 2013a).

Complications

Both types of diabetes develop similar complications. These are discussed below.

Peripheral Neuropathy

Patients with diabetes frequently exhibit abnormal nerve function, especially in the lower extremities. Common symptoms of this complication are painful sensations in the feet such as burning or tingling, known as parasthesias. The individual also may experience a loss of sensation. Because of decreased feeling in the lower extremities, these areas of the body are more susceptible to trauma. Such trauma may lead to foot ulcers, infection, and ultimately lower extremity amputation. The cause of diabetic neuropathy is unknown; theories include decreased blood supply and abnormal chemical metabolism of the involved nerves (Marrero, 2011; Skyler, 2012).

Peripheral Vascular Insufficiency (PVI)

PVI involves narrowing and/or occlusions of arteries, especially in the lower extremities. When larger blood vessels are involved, the disorder is referred to as macro-vascular disease, while occlusion of the smaller blood vessels at the tissue level is called micro-vascular disease. In PVI, the patient experiences a significant decrease in blood flow, precluding the delivery of nutrients and oxygen beyond the areas of occlusion. Peripheral vascular insufficiency is a major contributing factor in development of foot ulcers, infection, gangrene, and subsequent amputation (Unger, 2012).

Combined Peripheral Vascular Insufficiency and Peripheral Neuropathy

In combined peripheral vascular insufficiency and peripheral neuropathy, the lower extremities of the individual with diabetes are affected by both conditions. This potentially lethal coexistence causes the involved lower extremity to be particularly vulnerable to further problems (Izumi, Satterfield, Lee, & Harkless, 2006). The loss of protective sensations in a limb leads to trauma, resulting in foot ulcers and subsequent infection. Peripheral vascular insufficiency slows healing of such lesions and makes therapy a difficult process. Frequently, the end result is amputation. In the United States, diabetes is the leading cause of lower extremity amputation.

Diabetic Retinopathy

Diabetic retinopathy is the major cause of new cases of blindness in adults annually (American Diabetes Association, 2013a). In diabetic retinopathy, the small arteries in the retina of the eye develop lesions known as micro-aneurysms which become weak and are subject to bleeding. These lesions often lead to hemorrhaging, which can severely interfere with vision.

Diabetic Nephropathy/Renal Failure

This is the main cause of kidney disease, renal failure, and the need for dialysis. Diabetic nephropathy is a progressive kidney disease, usually occurring about 15 years after the onset of diabetes. It is caused by diabetes-induced abnormalities within the capillaries in the kidney glomeruli. This abnormality interferes with normal kidney function and causes abnormal loss of protein in the urine and buildup of metabolic waste products in the blood. Diabetic nephropathy is usually progressive and may ultimately result in end-stage kidney disease and renal failure. About 44% of new cases of renal disease are linked to diabetes (Rennke & Denker, 2012).

Arteriosclerosis

Arteriosclerosis, also known as atherosclerosis, or *hardening of the arteries*, is not a specific complication of diabetes, but is often seen at an early age in patients with diabetes. This condition may develop throughout the vascular system while, in some cases, it may manifest only in specific areas, such as the lower extremities or heart.

Cardiovascular Disease

In addition to arteriosclerosis, the heart is subject to many complications in patients with diabetes. Although not a specific complication of diabetes, the strong association between diabetes and development of cardiovascular disease is evident. The risk of cerebral vascular accidents (stroke) also is much greater. Cardiovascular events, such as myocardial infarction (heart attack) and strokes are recognized as the leading causes of death among patients with diabetes (Skyler, 2012).

Lower Extremity Amputation

Lower extremity amputation is a frequent occurrence. Approximately half of all nontraumatic amputations in this country occur to people who have diabetes (Ali et al., 2013). Risk of amputation is twice as likely in individuals with diabetes. The frequent co-existence of peripheral neuropathy and peripheral vascular insufficiency increase vulnerability to trauma as numbness makes it difficult to feel pain. If the skin is broken during a trauma and not treated, severe infection may follow. Peripheral vascular insufficiency makes therapy of foot infections slow and difficult. Local spread of infection may occur in the soft tissue. Osteomyelitis, infection in the underlying bone, may occur. Spread of infection via the blood, known as septicemia, can be life threatening. In such a scenario, amputation may be the only viable solution. Before serious infection develops, medical treatment is essential to prevent possible amputation (Skyler, 2012).

Blood Glucose Control and Development of Complications of Diabetes

Prior to the discovery of insulin in 1922, patients with insulin-dependent diabetes had limited life spans. With the advent of insulin therapy, patients with diabetes enjoyed longer lives but now had to address the complications associated with diabetes. Medical research has proven that blood sugar control and complication development are inter-related for both Type I and Type II diabetes. Improved blood glucose control is associated with a significant reduction in complication development. Education is clearly the most worthwhile method with which to treat, manage, and prevent or delay complications (American Diabetes Association, 2013a).

Therapy of Diabetes

Modern therapy offers various management strategies designed to control blood glucose levels and thus minimize development of long-term complications. Simple in theory but difficult in practice, diabetes requires four variables to be carefully balanced. These variables are diet, exercise, medication, and careful management of blood sugar levels through blood sugar testing (Falvo, 2014). The patient with diabetes is committed to continuous involvement in daily management of his or her condition. Patient education and knowledge is crucial; aside from contact with a physician or other health care practitioner, health care of diabetes is primarily self-care (Marrero, 2011).

Diet

Adherence to a healthy food plan is mandatory for all patients with diabetes and is a cornerstone of therapy. Yet, diet is also the single most difficult aspect of therapy to teach and learn. Dietary regulation may be all that is required for some Type II diabetes patients to control their diabetes, especially those who are significantly overweight. Each patient with diabetes should have a specific dietary program prescribed by a knowledgeable professional. The total number of calories and the proportions of carbohydrate, protein, and fat that make up those calories are all crucial factors. Flexibility is key to maintaining a prescribed diet. Emphasis needs to placed on an individualized healthy diet which the person is more likely to follow and maintain, taking into account cultural factors.

Exercise

Exercise can help lower blood glucose levels and may be of benefit in maintaining peripheral arterial circulation. However, variability of physical exercise when it is not maintained on a daily basis, may contribute to development of labile blood glucose and hypoglycemic episodes, especially in patients using insulin. Patients with Type II diabetes, who tend to be older, may be limited in their exercise tolerance due to cardiovascular disease, peripheral vascular problems, or other medical conditions. All patients with diabetes, despite age or physical shape, should engage in regular physical activity.

Insulin

Insulin, a necessary component of diabetes treatment, necessitates daily injections. Insulin is required therapy for Type I diabetes and for some Type II patients. Insulin, now manufactured by recombinant DNA technology, is identical to human insulin in chemical structure and has completely replaced animal source insulin. Biochemists have been able to alter the structure of the basic insulin molecule and produce insulin analogs with differing properties, onset, and duration of action.

The four types of insulin are rapid acting, short acting, intermediate acting, and long acting (Falvo, 2014). Currently, the majority of insulin-dependent patients require mixtures of different insulin types. Most patients use rapid acting insulin in conjunction with an intermediate or longer acting insulin, administered in multiple daily injections. Continuous subcutaneous insulin infusion is available for use via an insulin pump.

Oral Hypoglycemic Agents

There are several different classes of oral medications, with varying modes of action, available for therapy of Type II diabetes patients who are unable to maintain adequate blood glucose control using diet and exercise alone. The major mechanism of action of such drugs is stimulation of the pancreas to release stored insulin. These medications are not indicated for Type I diabetes since this form is characterized by absolute insulin insufficiency.

Patients with diabetes using insulin therapy are at risk of *insulin* reactions, referred to as hypoglycemia (low blood sugar). Such reactions may occur when the individual misses a meal, increases physical exercise, or inadvertently takes too much insulin. Insulin-dependent patients are educated to recognize and treat the symptoms of this common situation. If appropriately recognized, treatment is relatively easy, and includes immediate ingestion of carbohydrate (sugar) in a readily available form, such as eating candy or fruit. This ingestion will usually raise the blood sugar level and relieve a hypoglycemic situation in a few minutes. Oral hypoglycemic agents, like insulin, may also cause low blood glucose under certain conditions. These medications help the person avoid hyperglycemia (high blood sugar) which, if untreated for several days, can cause *diabetic coma*, a medical emergency.

Blood Sugar Testing

The introduction of small, inexpensive, and accurate blood glucose sensors for home use makes the self-monitoring of blood glucose easily accessible. It is necessary for patients with diabetes to perform self-monitoring of blood glucose daily to gauge and maintain their levels of blood sugar. The procedure is simple and fast; a drop of blood, obtained from a finger or forearm via a small lancing device, is placed on a test strip, which is read by a blood glucose meter in a few seconds. The result is displayed visually. Type II patients with diabetes should perform self-monitoring 1-4 times daily, while Type I patients should monitor blood glucose 4-6 times daily for ideal control. Self monitoring of blood glucose is an effective self-management technique to manage and maintain blood glucose control.

Many individuals are on insulin pump therapy. This offers the person flexibility and better blood glucose control. The insulin pump is a small device, about the size of a cell phone, which the person wears externally. It delivers precise doses of rapid-acting insulin to closely match the body's needs. Small amounts of insulin are delivered continuously for normal body functions. Additional insulin is delivered *on demand* by the person pushing a button on the meter before he or she eats or to correct a high blood sugar level.

First available in 2013, a continuous glucose monitoring system enables a patient to check his or her blood glucose level at any time, by simply pushing a button on a meter. A sensor is worn on the body which reads the blood glucose level and sends the reading continuously to the meter which is carried by the person like a cell phone. The meter alerts the individual when blood glucose is abnormally high or low, and indicates whether blood sugar is trending up, down, or remaining the same.

Functional Limitations

A person who maintains good blood glucose control and lacks complications will have few, if any, work restrictions. Persons taking insulin or oral hypoglycemic agents should try to avoid working irregular hours or rotating work shifts. It is desirable to have a work schedule that remains consistent for optimum control of blood glucose. Fluctuations in exercise cause variations in blood glucose levels. An occupation that requires consistent amounts of physical activity throughout the workday is preferred to one in which physical demands vary greatly. Of course, jobs often require a variety of work duties with differing physical demands. A knowledgeable person with good fundamental diabetes control can adjust medication and diet to compensate for varying physical activity (Brodwin, Parker, & De La Garza, 2010).

People taking insulin need a readily available source of sugar to combat potential insulin reactions. All individuals who are insulin-dependent should carry candy or another source of sugar to alleviate insulin reactions immediately when they occur. Persons who are in good metabolic control manage occasional minor hypoglycemic episodes so that they go unnoticed by others at the workplace.

An individual with diminished vision may require job accommodation. The degree of visual loss and prognosis for further loss are vital factors. The greater the amount of visual loss, the more the counselor needs to evaluate occupations requiring less reliance on vision for primary work functions. Secondary job duties may be modified or eliminated through provision of reasonable accommodation (Brodwin et al., 2010).

Lower extremity complications require job modification involving less ambulating, lifting, carrying, and standing (Unger, 2012). The degree of lower extremity involvement determines the amount of work restrictions required. If a lower extremity amputation has occurred, sedentary work is realistic. The level of amputation and the individual's adaptation are considered before restricting him or her to sedentary work. Fortunately, above-the-knee amputations are rarely necessary for persons with diabetes.

Mild to moderate neuropathy of the lower extremities does not preclude heavier types of work, whereas moderately severe to severe neuropathy may preclude all but sedentary work activity (Falvo, 2014). The worker, treating physician, and counselor can offer advice on the appropriateness of certain physical activities at the workplace and at home. Additional limitations of function may occur when there are skin problems at an amputation site. Minor skin problems can quickly develop into ulcerations, which impede proper fit of a prosthesis, limit ambulation, and require medical care.

Complications involving the circulatory system significantly limit physical activity. The counselor can be guided by the restriction of physical activity noted by the treating physician. Persons with renal failure usually have multiple complications. Depending on the multiplicity of complications and degree of renal failure, work activity may be restricted to part-time, at best. The counselor needs to evaluate the possibility of working at home for certain individuals.

Emotional factors play a role in control of diabetes from a physiological and psychological perspective; emotional instability complicates treatment. A stressful event may result in a temporary rise in blood glucose levels. If an occupation is stressful and affects good blood glucose control, intervention by a rehabilitation counselor is appropriate. When providing rehabilitation services, the counselor needs to assess the stressful components of work. Some people handle emotional stress well and almost *thrive on stress*. For some, occupational stress is not a significant factor.

The longer diabetes has been present, the greater the potential complications. Yet, complications are at least partially dependent on the degree of control of blood glucose a person has maintained over the long term, how quickly a physician is consulted for treatment, and adherence to medical recommendations. Although some people remain relatively free of complications, rehabilitation professionals see those persons who have complications interfering with work functions.

Rehabilitation Potential

People with diabetes under good control and with no complications will not be referred for vocational rehabilitation. Attitude is important in this and other disabilities. The person with diabetes who has a positive attitude and outlook has much greater potential for successful rehabilitation.

For individuals with diabetes using insulin, proper therapy, and adaptation to medical recommendations increase the chances of successful rehabilitation planning. Poor control and failure to adhere to medical advice impedes chances for a successful outcome.

Visual loss impacts the ability to perform many job functions. This is dependent on the amount and type of visual acuity required to conduct various job duties. It may be possible to redefine work responsibilities through the provision of reasonable accommodation. Visual loss affects rehabilitation potential to a variable extent (Brodwin et al., 2010).

Many persons of working age with lower extremity amputation are good candidates for fitting and use of prostheses. The purpose of prosthesis is to restore mobility and increase independence. Most amputations due to complications of diabetes are below the knee. If the prosthesis fits well and is used properly and regularly, rehabilitation potential remains positive. In most cases, a person with a bilateral lower extremity amputation requires a wheelchair for mobility.

Rehabilitation potential must be evaluated on an individualized basis. Factors include physical limitations, control of daily blood sugar levels, motivation, attitude, psychosocial functioning, and coping strategies. Ninety-seven percent of 300 physicians surveyed by the Integrated Benefits Institute (2002) stated that "return-to-work is good medicine." The American College of Occupational and Environmental Medicine Guidelines (2006) noted that safe, early return-to-work programs are in patients' best interests and promote recovery. Prolonged absence from work makes adjustment to the job more challenging and decreases the probability of the individual returning to work. Counselors knowledgeable in medical aspects of diabetes, ways to provide reasonable accommodation in business and industry, and a caring attitude can do much to assist clients with diabetes maximize their work potential and independent functioning.

Chronic Kidney Disease and Renal Failure

Persons with diabetes mellitus account for nearly half of these cases. In the following section, the reader will find information on chronic kidney disease and its connection to diabetes. Individuals who do not have diabetes but have kidney disease are also included within this section.

Most adults go about their daily activities unaware of the various body systems continuously functioning to keep their bodies healthy. The urological system is one of these. When in good health, the average person maintains only the cognizance to relieve the pressure resulting from urinary bladder distension through urination. Because of the general lack of public knowledge about body systems, internal malfunctions often require professional intervention. Despite advances in health care, some people are affected by disorders that permanently disrupt kidney function. This condition, known as end-stage renal (kidney) disease is incompatible with normal life functioning, causing serious health problems and potentially resulting in early death.

Prevalence and Costs

In this country, it is estimated that 26 million people have chronic kidney disease while millions of others are at increased risk. An estimated 527,000 people have irreversible kidney failure or end-stage renal disease, and require dialysis or a kidney transplant to survive. Each year, about 90,000 people die of kidney failure; it is the 8th leading cause of death in this country. Approximately 2% of the United States population has kidney disease; African Americans and Hispanics are at increased risk. The annual cost for end-stage renal disease is over $50 billion. Twenty-eight percent of all Medicare spending is for kidney disease (Centers for Disease Control and Prevention, 2012).

Kidney Functioning

The role of the kidneys exemplifies the interdependence of various body systems. The urine excretory function of the kidneys plays a major role in maintaining a chemical balance within the body, and comprises one of the most effective filtering systems known to humankind (Andreoli et al., 2010). The two kidneys in the body function separately; to sustain life, only one healthy kidney is needed.

Physiology

When filtering the blood, the kidneys have a remarkable ability to retain blood cells and certain proteins while passing on unwanted waste products. As the filtrate continues by way of the tubules within the kidneys, the process of re-absorption takes place. In this process, the tubules take back certain substances that have been filtered out and return them to the bloodstream, while allowing other products to be eliminated through the urine. This helps maintain the chemical composition and balance of the blood (McAninch & Lue, 2012).

Malfunctioning of the Kidneys

When the kidneys begin to fail, they lose their ability to perform the functions of absorption and excretion; this disruption leads to a chemical imbalance with abnormal clinical consequences. In some diseases, for example, the kidneys retain sodium. When this happens, the body retains water, causing generalized edema swelling. The person gains weight and appears to be bloated. As the severity of edema increases, the volume of fluid within the body increases. As a consequence, there is a rise in blood pressure; this places a strain on the heart as it must pump harder to circulate the blood.

During renal failure, unwanted by-products are retained within the body. When toxic chemicals build up, they cause uremia, which can be life threatening. Failing kidneys not only retain but also excrete abnormal amounts of certain proteins, which are essential in maintaining the delicate fluid balance of the body (Neelakantappa & Lowenstein, 2011).

Other Essential Kidney Functions

Additionally, the kidneys produce hormones. Hormones are chemicals produced in an organ and released into the bloodstream, affecting the cells of other organs and altering their functioning processes. Erythropoietin, a hormone produced by the kidneys, stimulates the production of red blood cells in the bone marrow. In failing kidneys, the decreased production of this hormone results in anemia (a deficiency of red blood cells).

Activated Vitamin D, produced within the kidneys, affects the absorption of calcium required for normal bone formation. Renin is also synthesized by the kidneys and plays a significant role in the regulation of blood pressure. It activates the hormone, angiotensin, which triggers the release of aldosterone from the adrenal glands. Aldosterone causes the kidneys to retain sodium, expanding blood volume and increasing blood pressure (McAninch & Lue, 2012).

Renal Failure

The term *renal failure* refers to the malfunctioning of both kidneys to such an extent that kidney function is below the level required to sustain life. The functional progress of acute or chronic renal failure is most often monitored by repeated laboratory measurement of urea and creatinine blood levels over time.

Loss of Kidney Function

Common causes of permanent loss of kidney functioning include (El Nahas & Levin, 2009; McAninch & Lue, 2012):

- Diabetes mellitus with nephropathy
- Hypertension
- Congenital defects
- Trauma due to accidents; in these cases, the individual usually does well with one kidney
- Autoimmune reactions that damage the glomerulus
- Infection due to various types of bacteria that ascend from the bladder and infect the kidneys
- Restricted circulation in the glomerular tuft, such as in arteriosclerosis (hardening of the arteries), thrombosis (blood clot), and hypertension (high blood pressure)

Acute and Chronic Kidney Failure

Kidney failure can be acute or chronic. Acute kidney failure has a sudden onset and is characterized by a rapid decline in normal kidney function due to trauma, bleeding, shock, burns, and other causes. Symptoms are related to the severity of failure and extent of involvement of other body systems (Rennke & Denker, 2012). Immediate management of acute kidney failure is needed to prevent possible permanent damage of the kidneys and the entire renal system. Though many symptoms of acute kidney failure are treated successfully, some cases result in chronic renal failure.

The number of people with end-stage kidney disease is increasing because people are living longer, along with the increased prevalence of diabetes in the aging population. Chronic renal failure begins as a slow, progressive decline in kidney function that results in the build-up of metabolic waste products within the body. At the outset, chronic renal failure prevents the kidneys from adequately regulating the body's water content. As the disease progresses, the individual begins to have back pain, increased frequency of and burning with urination, the presence of blood in the urine, and frequent urination at night. As toxic substances continue to build up, the person becomes less alert and loses the ability to concentrate. Nausea and vomiting occur which can lead to malnutrition, coma, and death (Thomas, 2004).

End-stage renal failure progresses gradually. It is categorized into three stages:

- Renal Impairment – Early-stage renal disease involving a 40%-70% loss of function
- Renal Insufficiency – Second stage renal disease involves a 75%-85% loss of function
- Renal Failure – End-stage renal disease where less than 15% of function remains

Dialysis

Human kidneys, like many other organs of the body, have a reserve capacity meaning that they are able to perform their normal work load with as little as 10% remaining function. Beyond this point, life is not sustainable. In cases where less than 10% of function remains, one must seek alternative or substitute kidney functioning. Two alternatives are dialysis and kidney transplantation.

Dialysis serves to support and rehabilitate an increasing number of persons with end-stage irreversible renal failure. Greater than 350,000 people in this country are receiving dialysis. Most of these individuals are on hemodialysis rather than peritoneal dialysis (Neelakantappa & Lowenstein, 2011). The process of dialysis makes use of the physical properties of a semi-permeable membrane. When two solutions, one more concentrated with small particles or molecules than the other, are separated in a container by a semi-permeable membrane, the concentrated substances move across the membrane until the two solutions become equal in concentration. Microscopic holes in the semi-permeable membrane allow for diffusion of waste products but prevent the passage of proteins or cells, such as red and white blood cells, which would otherwise be lost (Lerma, Berns, & Nissenson, 2012). Dialysis removes excess fluids and impurities from the body and serves as a substitute for functioning kidneys. Two principal forms of dialysis are (a) hemodialysis and (b) peritoneal dialysis.

Hemodialysis

This is a circular process wherein the person's arterial blood is transported outside the body to a dialysis machine where it is cleansed of waste products and returned to the circulatory system. In contrast to the transitory use of hemodialysis during acute kidney failure where the condition is temporary, hemodialysis for chronic renal failure is a lifetime requirement. As a consequence of repeated and life-long needle puncture of the involved blood vessels, thick scar tissue eventually develops which makes the procedure difficult and painful. To avoid this complication, a surgical procedure known as an arteriovenous fistula is performed. It produces a large vein that can be entered safely and easily with large needles for the three times a week procedure (Thomas, 2004).

While dialysis is a life-saving procedure, it is not as efficient as normal kidney functioning. The patient with end-stage renal disease undergoes dialysis for three to five hours a day three days per week. In contrast to human kidneys that function 24 hours a day, dialysis results in the gradual build-up of waste products from one treatment to the next. Depending on the extent of this accumulation, the person may experience fatigue, loss of appetite, and have lapses in concentration.

There are newer regimens of hemodialysis. These include short daily hemodialysis, daily nocturnal hemodialysis, and long overnight hemodialysis three times weekly at home. These new techniques are intended to improve the efficiency of dialysis and thereby increase life expectancy, as 20% of people with end-stage renal disease die annually (Neelakantappa & Lowenstein, 2011).

Peritoneal Dialysis

Peritoneum is the lining of the abdominal cavity. This tissue has the properties of a semi-permeable membrane, allowing the process of diffusion to take place in the abdominal cavity. An incision is made through the anterior abdominal muscle wall; through this opening, a tube (catheter) is inserted into the abdominal space. Sterile dialysate (solution used to clear waste products) is introduced and allowed to remain in the cavity four to six hours, or overnight. During this time, through the process of diffusion, impurities pass through the peritoneum into the dialysate. The dialysate and its collected impurities are then eliminated from the body (Lerma & Nissenson, 2011).

Kidney Transplantation

Over 150,000 individuals in the United States have undergone a kidney transplant (Neelakantappa & Lowenstein, 2011). When possible, kidney transplantation is the best alternative for end-stage renal disease. A major complication of this procedure, however, is the negative reaction of the immune system to a foreign organ. In this scenario, a new donor kidney is not recognized as the body's own, but rather is rejected as an invader threatening the body. To overcome this reaction to kidney transplantation, the recipient must undergo a medication regimen to suppress the immune system.

A national computerized kidney-harvesting program serves to locate donor kidneys and eligible recipients. Donor kidneys, however, are ideally obtained from living relatives to avoid the recipient's immune system rejection of a new kidney. Potential donors are carefully evaluated for compatibility (El Nahas & Levin, 2009).

Cadaveric donor kidneys come from individuals who have recently died as a result of fatal brain trauma. In these cases, the compatibility procedures undergone mirror those performed for transplants from living donors. Surgical procedures for kidney transplantation are usually successful. In these procedures, a donor kidney is implanted in the front groin area of the body and the recipient's non-functioning kidneys are left intact as long as they do not seriously impact the patient's overall health.

To suppress the immune system and avoid donor kidney rejection, medications are prescribed. Careful laboratory monitoring is essential as too low a concentration in the bloodstream exposes the kidney to rejection and high doses inhibit the body's capability to protect itself against infection. People who have had transplants remain on immune suppressors throughout their lives (Morris & Knechtle, 2008). As there are a great deal more people needing kidneys than those that become available, an individual may have to wait for several years before a donor kidney is obtainable.

In comparison with dialysis, kidney transplantation has advantages that positively affect the person's medical and vocational rehabilitation potential. The person with a kidney transplant does not spend three to five hours a day three times a week on a dialysis machine experiencing, in some cases, wide fluctuations in body chemistry. Furthermore, the individual is not exposed to the hazards of bleeding, clotting, and infection associated with constant use of needles and fluid exchanges.

Emotional Issues

Kidney failure causes severe emotional stress for both the individual undergoing treatment and his or her family members. Uncertainty of the future is a major stressor in all chronic conditions, including end-stage renal failure. Even after a successful kidney transplant uncertainty remains as the new kidney may be rejected at any time. People on dialysis experience a drastic shift in lifestyle, as the tri-weekly dialysis procedures take precedence over all other life activities. With effective treatment, however, improvements in quality of life occur. If a person receives a transplant, overall health and outlook on life improves substantially as one regains control over life. Some transplant recipients who are not employed return to work and function effectively. A return to work is more feasible for those who have undergone successful kidney transplantation than when receiving dialysis. Sedentary and light work activities are recommended for both transplant and dialysis patients to facilitate a return to the vocational environment. Emotional counseling and support groups further aid in the process of coping with the psychosocial aspects of this condition.

Complicating Factors Affecting Employment

Anemia

When kidneys severely malfunction, such as in end-stage renal disease, they do not produce erythropoietin, resulting in the development of anemia. The body responds to the paucity of red blood cells by increasing the breathing and heart rates to circulate fewer cells more rapidly and serve the same function (Andreoli et al., 2010). To help prevent anemia from occurring, human erythropoietin is prescribed, which is available by means of recombinant DNA.

Infection

For people on hemodialysis, the frequent introduction of needles into blood vessels and the repeated need to control blood leaks lowers resistance to infection. To avoid complications, individuals and paramedical team members must adhere rigidly to appropriate aseptic techniques.

Rigid Treatment Requirements

When undergoing hemodialysis, most people require three to five hours of treatment each day three days a week. As a result, individuals must plan their home and work activities around treatment times, giving dialysis precedence over work and other life activities (El Nahas & Levin, 2009). Many dialysis centers operate 24 hours a day, allowing recipients of dialysis to work regular daytime hours.

Rehabilitation Potential

Many persons who have left their jobs because of declining kidney function may be able to successfully return to work once they are on a consistent treatment regimen, such as a dialysis program, or after receiving a kidney transplant. Dialysis and kidney transplant recipients should avoid jobs involving physically strenuous work activities. Maintenance of optimal health is essential for persons on dialysis since they are predisposed to anemia, have lowered resistance to infection, and experience fatigue. To help maintain a life-long program of well being, including a well-balanced diet and an appropriate exercise program, hospitals employ a team of professionals consisting of the treating physician, dietician, medical social worker, clinical psychologist, and vocational rehabilitation counselor to encourage, counsel, and assist the person (Lerma & Nissenson, 2011). Ideally, the counselor coordinates the services of all participants on the client's behalf in such a way as to bring about a successful return to independence, daily activities, and employment.

Despite passage of the Americans with Disabilities Act (ADA) (1990), job placement remains challenging for those who have had kidney transplantation or are currently undergoing dialysis. Employers have the perception that their overall medical insurance costs will increase and the individual may have too many days off work due to illness. The rehabilitation counselor can help the person overcome obstacles like these by being persistent in following up with employers and medical insurance companies to assure the medical and employment stability of the client and, if needed, to explain the client's rights under the ADA (Brodwin et al., 2010).

Case Study

Ms. Consuelo Mendoza is 44 years old and immigrated to the United States from Puerto Rico. Currently, she lives with her sister and her sister's 13 year-old son. While in her native country, she worked as a flight attendant, received a college education, and subsequently became employed as a language arts middle school teacher. Since arriving in this country, Ms. Mendoza has worked as a secretary, home health aide, and salesperson in a women's dress shop. On a part-time basis for many years, Consuelo taught ESL (English as a second language [English Language Learners]) classes and tutored Spanish-speaking individuals wanting to learn or become proficient in English.

Since late adolescence, Consuelo has had Type II diabetes. At age 40, she was diagnosed with kidney disease. As a result, she is restricted to a maximum of light work, although her treating physician would prefer that she work in a sedentary capacity. In end-stage renal failure for the past year, she has been put on a list to receive a kidney transplant. Ms. Mendoza requires dialysis three times a week for approximately four hours each time, which she receives in the evenings and on weekends. For the year she has been on dialysis, she has worked only part-time as an ESL teacher and tutor.

Recently, Consuelo has sought vocational rehabilitation services because her part-time work does not provide her with sufficient income. There have been some months when she earns enough income to meet all her expenses and other times when she does not.

Questions

1. Identify factors significant in assessing rehabilitation potential of this client.
2. Discuss Type I and II diabetes and complications that can occur. Relate this to the case study. What may have caused this client to have renal failure?
3. Describe the two types of dialysis and kidney transplantation. Identify advantages of a transplant over dialysis.

4. Considering that Ms. Mendoza is on dialysis and may be receiving a kidney transplant within the year, what kinds of rehabilitation services will you provide at the present time and in the future? Are there any considerations needed for Consuelo's diabetes?
5. What issues related to dialysis and kidney transplant need to be considered in vocational planning?
6. Describe issues of reasonable accommodation for clients on dialysis.
7. Because of strong religious beliefs and her own fears concerning surgery, Ms. Mendoza is conflicted about receiving a transplant. As her rehabilitation counselor, how would you handle these mixed feelings she has shared with you?

References

Ali, M., Bullard, K. M., Saaddin, J. B., Cowie, C. C., Imperatore, G., & Gregg, E. W. (2013). Achievement of goals in U. S. diabetes care, 1990-2010. *New England Journal of Medicine, 368*, 1613–1624.

American College of Occupational and Environmental Medicine Guidelines. (2006). Preventing needless work disability by helping people stay employed. *Journal of Occupational and Environmental Medicine, 48*(9), 972–987.

American Diabetes Association. (2010). Diagnosis and classification of diabetes mellitus. *Diabetes Care, 35*(Supplement 1), S64-S71. www.diabetes.org.

American Diabetes Association. (2011). *2011 national diabetes facts sheet.* www.diabetes.org.

American Diabetes Association. (2013a). *Diabetes information – "All about diabetes."* www.diabetes.org.

American Diabetes Association. (2013b). *Diabetes fact sheet.* www.diabetes.org.

Americans with Disabilities Act. (1990). 42 U.S.C. § 12101 et seq.

Andreoli, T. E., Benjamin, I., Griggs, R. C., Wing, E. J., & Fitz, J. G. (2010). *Andreoli and Carpenter's Cecil essentials of medicine* (8th ed.). Philadelphia, PA: Saunders Elsevier.

Brodwin, M. G., Parker, R. M., & DeLaGarza, D. (2010). Disability and reasonable accommodation. In E. M. Szymanski & R. M. Parker (Eds.), *Work and disability: Contexts, issues, and strategies for enhancing employment outcomes for people with disabilities* (3rd ed., pp. 281–323). Austin, TX: Pro-ed.

Centers for Disease Control and Prevention. (2012). *Vital and health statistics.* Hyattsville, MD: Author.

El Nahas, M. E., & Levin, A. (Eds.). (2009). *Chronic kidney disease: A practical guide to understanding and management.* New York, NY: Oxford University.

Falvo, D. R. (2014). *Medical and psychosocial aspects of chronic illness and disability* (5th ed.). Burlington, MA: Jones and Bartlett Learning.

Integrated Benefits Institute. (2002). *Physicians managing disability: Identifying opportunities and constraints.* http://ibiweb.org

Izumi, Y., Satterfield, K., Lee, S., & Harkless, L. B. (2006). Risk of reamputation in patients with diabetes stratified by limb and level of amputation: A ten-year observation. *Diabetes Care, 29*, 566–570.

Lerma, E., Berns, J., & Nissenson, A. (2012). *Current essentials of nephrology and hypertension.* New York, NY: McGraw Hill Lange.

Lerma, E. V., & Nissenson, A. (2011). *Nephrology secrets* (3rd ed.). Philadelphia, PA: Elsevier.

Marrero, D. G. (2011). Diabetes mellitus. In S. Flanagan, H. H. Zaretsky, & A. Moroz (Eds.), *Medical aspects of disability: A handbook for the rehabilitation professional* (4th ed., pp. 159–175). New York, NY: Springer.

McAninch, J. W., & Lue, T. F. (Eds.). (2012). *Smith and Tanagho's general urology* (18th ed.). New York, NY: Lange Medical Books/McGraw-Hill.

Morris, P. J., & Knechtle, S. J. (2008). *Kidney transplantation: Principles and practices.* Philadelphia, PA: Saunders Elsevier.

Neelakantappa, K., & Lowenstein, J. (2011). Chronic kidney disease. In S. Flanagan, H. H. Zaretsky, & A. Moroz (Eds.), *Medical aspects of disability: A handbook for the rehabilitation professional* (4th ed., pp. 491–507). New York, NY: Springer.

Rennke, H. G.. & Denker, B. M. (2012). *Renal pathophysiology: The essentials.* Philadelphia, PA: Lippincott Williams & Wilkins.

Skyler, J. S. (Ed.). (2012). *Atlas of diabetes* (4th ed.). New York, NY: Springer.

Thomas, N. (2004). *Advanced renal care.* Malden, MA: Blackwell.

Unger, J. (Ed.). (2012). *Diabetes management in primary care* (2nd ed.). Philadelphia, PA: Lippincott Williams & Wilkins.

About the Author

Martin G. Brodwin, Ph.D, C.R.C., is Professor and Coordinator of the graduate Rehabilitation Counselor Education Program at California State University, Los Angeles. As a vocational expert for the Office of Disability Adjudication and Review, Social Security Administration, he provides testimony on disability-related issues. Dr. Brodwin has published over 100 refereed journal articles, book chapters, and books on the subjects of medical aspects of disability, counseling, disability, rehabilitation, and reasonable accommodation in business and industry.

Acknowledgment

The author would like to acknowledge Drs. Richard D. Hornichter and Fernando A. Tellez for their contributions to earlier versions of this chapter.

Chapter 5

CARDIOVASCULAR DISEASE

Harvey L. Alpern, M.D.

Introduction

Heart disease is the leading cause of death in the United States in both men and women. About 600,000 people die of heart disease every year (Centers for Disease Control and Prevention [CDC], 2013). This accounts for one in every four deaths. Additionally, heart conditions are the third leading cause of incapacitation and often affect physical, emotional, and vocational functioning (Klag, 2012).

The purpose of this chapter is to help rehabilitation counselors comprehend medical evaluations that identify cardiovascular impairments so they can use this understanding to help an individual restore independent functionality in the workplace. This chapter describes the New York Heart Association's (NYHA) classification system of heart disease, the different kinds of heart disease, diagnosis and treatment, therapeutic and diagnostic procedures, disability rating, functional limitations, and rehabilitation potential for individuals with cardiovascular impairment. The author concludes with a case study of an individual who has several disabilities, including coronary artery disease.

This chapter discusses the causes, symptoms, pathology, and evaluation of physical capabilities of persons with cardiovascular disease. Increasingly, the direction of medical research and treatment is on determining the principle course of heart disease in the employed population. Modern research is directed toward preventing and decreasing the progression of this disease, with the goal of increasing longevity and improving quality of life and productivity. There is also an emphasis on less invasive procedures. The rehabilitation counselor's challenge is to assist this growing population to remain vocationally competitive and productive.

The following seven major types of heart conditions are discussed within this chapter: (1) congenital heart disease in adult life; (2) valvular heart disease; (3) mitral valve prolapse; (4) cardiomyopathy; (5) hypertension and hypertensive heart disease; (6) coronary artery disease; and (7) congestive heart failure. These are the major types of cardiovascular conditions that rehabilitation counselors will encounter.

In the first five categories, heart strain or progressive heart muscle failure may eventually develop into congestive heart failure. In all groups, employability is dependent on a timely diagnosis, the potential for correcting or improving the disease process, anatomical abnormalities, and provision of rehabilitation services. In coronary artery disease, which represents the largest category, there is progressive inability of the heart muscle to function properly, primarily as a result of decreased blood flow to the heart muscle due to occluded coronary arteries (Nabel & Braunwald, 2012). After a given quantity of muscle mass has been damaged or destroyed, pump failure or congestive heart failure, can result in the inability of the heart to pump sufficient blood to the rest of the body.

Functional and Therapeutic Classifications of Heart Disease

The following discussion refers to the functional capacity of the heart and is adapted from criteria from the NYHA. Physicians and researchers accept this protocol as a standard of classification for cardiac conditions. The two classifications are evaluated to derive a cardiac status determination (Criteria Committee of the New York Heart Association, 1984).

Functional Classification – NYHA

Functional Classification is an estimate of a person's symptoms. It is described in four classes, I through IV (see Figure 1). Class I represents a person with no symptoms, while Class IV is an individual who develops discomfort with any physical activity and has symptoms even at rest. Classes II and III describe symptoms between these extremes, and are individuals most likely to be seen by rehabilitation counselors.

Therapeutic Classification – NYHA

Therapeutic Classification reflects the amount of physical activity recommended by the treating cardiologist considering all factors. There are five classes from Class A representing those individuals with no physical activity restriction to those in Class E whose physical activity is almost totally restricted. Counselors will most likely see persons in Classes B through D.

It must be noted that the NYHA classification is dependent on the subjective reporting of the patient. Impairment ratings should preferably be done using objective guidelines, such as described in the section Disability Rating of this chapter.

TABLE 1
Classifications of Patients with Heart Disease

	Functional Classes
Class I	Patients with heart disease who have no symptoms of any kind. Ordinary physical activity does not cause fatigue, palpitation, dyspnea, or angina pain.
Class II	Patients who are comfortable at rest but have symptoms with ordinary physical activity.
Class III	Patients who are comfortable at rest but have symptoms with less than ordinary effort.
Class IV	Patients who have symptoms at rest.
	Therapeutic Classes
Class A	Patients whose physical activity need not be restricted.
Class B	Patients whose ordinary activity need not be restricted, but who should be advised against severe activity.
Class C	Patients whose ordinary activity should be restricted.
Class D	Patients whose ordinary activity should be markedly restricted.
Class E	Patients who should be at complete rest in bed or a chair.

Source: Criteria Committee of the New York Heart Association. (1984). *The diseases of the heart and blood vessels: Nomenclature and criteria for diagnosis* (6th ed.). New York, NY: Little, Brown.

Congenital Heart Disease in Adult Life

Congenital heart disease is a condition caused by various malformations of the heart, which develop during gestation and become apparent in infancy or childhood. Many congenital heart problems require surgical or manipulative procedures early in life to improve cardiovascular function. Not all untreated individuals have residual problems; however, those who live into adulthood develop serious problems that require intervention to improve or correct abnormalities (Lange & Hillis, 2012). Early adult heart failure is a major problem necessitating aggressive treatment and evaluation to determine functional limitations and work restrictions (Skala, Freeland, & Carney, 2005). Rehabilitation counselors must obtain medical information describing these limitations before attempting to reemploy an individual with cardiovascular limitations.

Valvular Heart Disease

For adults under 65 years of age, valvular heart disease is usually a result of childhood rheumatic fever. It is an inflammatory condition that may damage the heart valves. Impairment of the heart valves can lead to dysfunction in the ventricles, heart failure, and possible death (Carabello, 2012). Inadequate closure of the mitral value occurs so that blood flows backward into the atria during ventricular contraction (Jacobson & Rahko, 2012). If the damage affects the performance of the heart, it is called rheumatic heart disease. In the United States, rheumatic fever was once a devastating disease common in the early part of the twentieth century. Improved understanding of prevention and antibiotic treatment has reduced not only the incidence and recurrence rate of rheumatic fever, but its severity and frequency as well (Bonow, Mann, Zipes, & Libby, 2011). Rheumatic heart disease as a cause of permanent disability has markedly diminished over the years.

Rheumatic valvular disease, however, is still a major source of concern. One chief complication of this disease is that depending on the severity of the original acute process, a person may become symptomatic during his or her middle teens through the mid-30s. Acute rheumatic fever leads to acute cardiomyopathy (abnormal changes in the heart muscle). The disease causes damage to the heart valves, including the mitral valve, aortic valve, and tricuspid valve, respectively. The mitral and aortic valves may become stenotic (i.e., constricted or narrowed), insufficient (i.e., the valve leafs do not come together, thus allowing leakage), or both. Although not subject to stenosis, the tricuspid valve can become insufficient. The greater the number of valves affected, the sooner the person develops heart failure, and the more severe the failure. Severe damage of a valve requires surgical intervention to correct the damage or replace the valve with an artificial one (Carabello, 2012).

Benefiting from emerging technology of prosthetic heart valve replacement, a growing number of people with rheumatic valvular disease can hold jobs that do not require heavy lifting or exposure to trauma. Individuals with valve replacement require medication to prevent abnormal blood clotting. A commonly prescribed preparation for this condition is Coumadin (warfarin sodium). People on this and similar medications bruise easily and should not work in areas where physical trauma could occur (Moser & Riegel, 2008). Today, there are an increasing variety of valve prostheses available. Surgery, when combined with medication and performed early in the disease process, can enable a person with valvular disease to lead a normal life. Cardiac testing helps determine one's work potential, both before and subsequent to surgery.

Mitral Valve Prolapse

Mitral valve prolapse (mitral stenosis) is one of the most common valvular abnormalities; the most common cause is rheumatic fever in childhood. It involves a narrowing of the heart valve, or an incompetent valve which does not close completely. In recent years, there has been an increase in the diagnosis of mitral valve prolapse (MVP). The exact cause of the condition is unknown. Possible causes include an undetected congenital defect, viral infection, or most likely, a degeneration of the heart valve. The most common symptoms experienced are anxiety, fatigue, palpitations, and chest pain. Frequently, the discovery of an asymptomatic extra heartbeat can alert a physician to a possible diagnosis of mitral valve prolapse. MVP may be accompanied by a degeneration of the valve musculature. In some cases, this mucous degeneration affects the tricuspid valve. When both mitral and tricuspid valves are diseased, the person develops valvular insufficiency due to severe mitral regurgitation (Carabello, 2012). This condition, if left untreated, may progress to heart failure.

A test commonly known as an echocardiogram (ECG, EKG) confirms a diagnosis of MVP, generally a benign condition. Although progression to a severe condition is rare, when such progression does occur, it may lead to severe mitral regurgitation associated with heart failure. If this is the case, surgery is compulsory. If a Holter monitor (a device worn by a person during normal activity as an ECG) reveals significant arrhythmia and the person is symptomatic, beta-blocker medication is used for treatment (Klag, 2012; Moser & Riegel, 2008).

Cardiomyopathy

Medical Implications

This group of diseases, also known as myocardiopathies (cardiac muscle weakness), involves inflammation, resulting in weakness within the heart muscle. Cardiomyopathy is a disease of the heart muscle making it weak and unable to function effectively. It may be secondary to infectious processes, usually viral or chemical toxic exposure, as well as part of the disease process of diabetes mellitus and alcohol abuse (Topol, Califf, Prystowsky, Thomas, & Thompson, 2007). Virus cardiomyopathies are more frequently found in younger people. The virus causes inflammation and weakness of the heart muscle and sometimes interferes with normal nerve conduction throughout the heart. During the acute phase, individuals may require hospitalization and possible intensive care to become medically stabilized. People with cardiomyopathies may additionally require short-term medication, or in more serious cases, a pacemaker for cardiac irregularities and life-long medication.

Some people experience arrhythmias in the form of extra heartbeats even after the acute phase, and require medication for control. Additional symptoms include weakness, fatigue, fluid accumulation in the extremities (sometimes in the lungs), difficulties in breathing, fainting, and nausea. Others need medication to support the myocardium (the muscle layer of the heart). In most cases, after the acute stage has passed, the person can continue in customary work requirements, with the exception of heavy lifting and arduous labor. A physician may recommend surgical correction of associated valve abnormalities (Mola, Whiteson, & Rey, 2011).

Diabetes Mellitus

When it is not optimally controlled, diabetes may cause complications resulting in poor function of one or more organs or systems of the body. Although an infrequent occurrence, poorly controlled diabetes may cause cardiac muscle disease and renal disease, resulting in progressive, congestive heart failure. Thus, individuals with diabetes must maintain normal blood glucose, body weight, and appropriate diet to lessen such possible complications. The probability and severity of diabetic cardiomyopathy is diminished when proper medical care is attained. If a diagnosis of cardiomyopathy is given, however, a patient is usually restricted to light or sedentary work (Moser & Riegel, 2008).

Alcoholic Cardiomyopathy

Toxic effects of alcohol and poor nutrition bring about alcoholic cardiomyopathy. Proper medical care for the person with alcoholism and complete abstinence from alcohol (and tobacco) reduces the severity of the myocarditis (inflammation of the myocardium). General improvement in health and overall functioning are the goals of alcohol rehabilitation programs, requiring total abstinence from alcohol and illicit drugs, good nutrition, and treatment of complications. Every effort is made to provide and maintain an ongoing therapeutic prevention program, such as Alcoholics Anonymous (AA).

Hypertension and Hypertensive Heart Disease

Hypertension (high blood pressure) occurs when the pressure of the blood against the walls of the vessels exceeds normal limits for a sustained period of time (Mola et al., 2011). About 50 million people in this country have hypertension, many with no recognizable symptoms. An additional 45 million people have pre-hypertension and are more susceptible to develop hypertension. Although hypertension in and of itself is not incapacitating, if prolonged and untreated, it may become a major risk for heart attack, heart failure, stroke, peripheral vascular disease, and kidney failure (Victor, 2012). The major goal of treatment is to lower a person's blood pressure, which will reduce possible complications. Once the pressure is lowered, it is essential that the patient do everything possible to maintain good blood pressure control and have regular medical visits (Bashore, Granger, Hronitzky, & Patel, 2013).

During the normal heart cycle, action of the heart can be compared to a hydraulic pump. When the heart muscle contracts, it propels blood out of the heart chambers. This forceful action is called systole. Pressure is high during this expulsive phase. The phase immediately following, when the heart muscle is at rest, is called the diastole. Blood pressure, as expressed as a fraction, is written with the systolic pressure on top and diastolic pressure on the bottom (e.g., 120/80 = systolic/diastolic). Diastolic pressure thus represents blood pressure when the heart is at rest; elevated diastolic blood pressure is a serious condition. Systolic pressure greater than 140 mm Hg (mercury), and diastolic pressure greater than 90 mm Hg is considered hypertension.

Causes of Hypertension

Ninety-five percent of hypertension cases are of unknown causes. The remaining five percent are related to kidney disease, endocrine abnormalities, increased cardiac output, and vascular abnormalities (Bonow et al., 2011). Heredity is a factor in hypertension; therefore, there is a genetic predisposition to heart disease. Surgical intervention or specific medical regimens benefit many secondary cases of hypertension.

Detection of Hypertension

Symptoms of hypertension may surface suddenly without warning. Commonly encountered nonspecific complaints such as fatigue, headache, nosebleed, change in vision, or muscle weakness are typical. Complications include coronary artery disease, renal failure, stroke, and peripheral vascular disease. Since most individuals do not have symptoms, hypertension has been called the *silent killer*.

When hypertension is suspected, physical examination includes assessment for any abnormalities of the hypertensive person's kidneys, heart, and cerebrovascular system. Additionally, chest x-ray, electrocardiogram, and echocardiogram are used to assess cardiac status. If hypertension is thought to be associated with coronary artery disease, a physician may conduct cardiac stress testing to clarify the diagnosis (Bonow et al., 2011).

Complications

Hypertension may cause significant renal damage leading to kidney failure; this damage contributes to further perpetuation of hypertensive problems. Frequently associated with hypertension, peripheral vascular disease is a major cause of disability. Unlike hypertension, this complication causes pain in the lower extremities brought on by exercise, and due to diminished blood flow in the legs. With a diagnosis of hypertension, the physician evaluates physical activity levels and suggests modifications, depending on the presence of complications (Mola et al., 2011). Physical limitations experienced with hypertension primarily result from coronary artery disease, heart failure, stroke, and renal failure. Each of these conditions has specific guidelines as to physical disability and resulting levels of activity (Alpern, 1996). Through consultation with the treating physician to identify functional limitations, the rehabilitation counselor is able to assist the individual through the vocational rehabilitation process.

Levels of disability for individuals with hypertension are related to the occurrence and severity of complications and presence of end-organ damage (Mola et al., 2011). Persons responsive to treatment may be able to continue their customary work activities. Individuals with hypertension who do not have major systemic complications but are unable to perform their current jobs may turn to vocational retraining for support and future success. Despite a diagnosis of hypertension, most people continue leading productive lives without serious limitations in work activity, recreation, and life style. Learning to control emotional stress is a significant factor in overall management of hypertension.

Coronary Artery Disease

Coronary artery disease (also known as coronary heart disease) is a broad term describing many heart-related conditions, all involving narrowed coronary arteries affecting blood flow to the heart. In this country, more than 12 million people have this condition (CDC, 2013). Symptoms usually occur only when the disease is advanced, making it a particularly dangerous condition. Individuals reporting symptoms generally have one or more of the following: discomfort, dull ache or sharp chest pain, especially with strenuous physical activities; discomfort in the shoulder, throat, or left arm; and shortness of breath (Bashore et al., 2013). These symptoms are referred to as angina pectoris. Extreme narrowing of the coronary arteries (arteriosclerosis) can result in heart attack or heart failure.

Coronary artery disease is the leading cause of death in the United States; approximately 715,000 Americans suffer from heart attacks each year. More than 385,000 of these people die. Of those who experience heart attacks each year, 525,000 are experiencing one for the first time; 190,000 occur in individuals who have already had at least one before. Many people have coronary artery disease not associated with myocardial infarction (heart attack). Overall, the disease costs $109 billion annually, including total payments for health care services, medications, and lost productivity (CDC, 2013). The various medical conditions associated with coronary artery disease also can lead to major problems and disability (Mola et al., 2011).

Etiology

Risk factors for coronary artery disease include high cholesterol levels, hypertension, diabetes, emotional stress, a poor diet (rich in fats), overweight and obesity, physical inactivity (e.g., lack of exercise), excessive alcohol use, and cigarette smoking. Of the risk factors mentioned, the most significant are high cholesterol, blood pressure elevation, and cigarette smoking, especially when these factors are combined. High cholesterol leads to accumulation of plaque in the coronary vessels and restricted blood flow. Nicotine from cigarette smoking diminishes blood flow by constricting vessel walls during smoking.

Manifestations of Coronary Artery Disease

Coronary artery disease leads to myocardial anoxia (insufficient oxygen to the heart muscle), due to diminished or absent blood flow. When this occurs, the person experiences chest pain (angina pectoris) and pressure that radiates from the left shoulder and arm, or sometimes from the heart to the abdomen. Other symptoms include a feeling of high anxiety or impending doom, sweating, pale (cyanotic) face, labored breathing, and rapid pulse (Bashore et al., 2013). This disease affects the myocardium and nerve conducting pathways, causing abnormal nerve conduction. Irregular heartbeats (arrhythmias) or ventricular fibrillation (rapid, ineffective pulsations of the heart) occur. During this time, the heart muscle receives insufficient oxygen; if this condition persists, the affected myocardium dies (myocardial infarction). Persistent arrhythmias result in an inefficient pumping action of the heart.

Heart arrhythmias are heart rhythms that deviate from the normal pattern and pace of the heart. People are often unaware of the condition. Those who report having symptoms typically have one or more of the following: weakness, fatigue, dizziness, lightheadedness, and an irregular pulse due to changes in blood flow to vital organs (Nabel & Braunwald, 2012).

Four major clinical signs of coronary artery disease are angina pectoris, myocardial infarction, arrhythmias, and congestive heart failure. Angina pectoris is precipitated by physical exertion and relieved by rest or cessation of the specific physical activity. Discomfort may last from a few seconds to several minutes, but can be a forerunner of a myocardial infarction (Reeder & Prasad, 2012). Shortness of breath, a feeling of the need to sit up in bed, and leg edema (swelling) are experienced during or as a precursor to congestive heart failure.

Myocardial Infarction

A heart attack occurs when a coronary artery becomes partially or completely occluded by plaque. This clot can develop suddenly at a narrow space in the artery. When the plaque ruptures, it cuts off the heart's oxygen supply, permanently damaging heart tissue.

Warning signs and symptoms usually begin with chest discomfort, similar to angina pectoris. This pain is more severe, however, and longer lasting than in the case of angina. Associated symptoms include upper body pain or discomfort in the arms, back, neck, jaw, or upper stomach; shortness of breath; nausea; and light-headedness or cold sweats (CDC, 2013). A physician may use blood testing and catheterization of the heart vessel to assess possible blockage. In some cases, however, there are no warning signs. In these unfortunate cases, sudden death may occur.

Diagnosis and Treatment

Ideally, an individual with symptoms of myocardial infarction is immediately hospitalized. Paramedics initiate treatment by administering pain relievers and oxygen. In the emergency room, a physician may administer a clot-dissolving medication called a thrombolytic agent to improve blood flow in the affected artery (Reeder & Prasad, 2012). Alternatively, the patient may be referred to a catheterization laboratory for immediate evaluation and possible angioplasty and stent placement (Topol et al., 2007).

After stabilization of the acute event and observation of the patient in a critical care hospital unit, symptoms and medical findings dictate ongoing treatment, which may involve a medical regimen and possible surgery. Medications are prescribed to control angina and arrhythmias. Nitroglycerine, for example, is a short-acting serum that dilates the coronary arteries to relieve angina. The treating physician may prescribe other medications to relieve arrhythmias and help the body eliminate excess fluid (Massie, 2012; McMurray & Pfeffer, 2012).

For most individuals, the physician recommends a rehabilitation program involving gradual increases in physical activity. This program begins in the hospital and is continued on an outpatient basis, often in a cardiac rehabilitation program. The program provides information on coronary artery disease including dietary and weight management, proper exercise programs, information on medications, assistance with stress reduction, and cessation of smoking. Cardiac rehabilitation involves a comprehensive and multidisciplinary program individualized for each person, with the goal of improving and maximizing both physical and psychosocial functioning.

If damage to the heart is severe, resulting in end-stage heart disease, the cardiologist may recommend a heart transplant. However for a transplant, the patient must be in sufficiently adequate health to withstand this extensive medical procedure.

Diagnosis

Echocardiogram (EKG, ECG)

An echocardiogram is a non-invasive procedure involving the use of high frequency ultrasound to show a functioning heart and its moving parts. An EKG displays the muscle activity measured from various directions. This display indicates overall rhythm of the heart and weaknesses in different parts of the heart muscle to measure and diagnose abnormal rhythms of the heart. EKG can identify damaged heart muscle for an individual who has had a heart attack.

Holter Monitor

A Holter monitor is a small, battery-powered device that is carried like a cell phone and records a continuous electrocardiogram for up to 24 hours. The individual is asked to keep a written record of the time of any special symptoms and physical exertion. Results are compared with the corresponding time on the EKG to denote abnormalities. If longer periods of time are required to monitor a rare event, an event monitor is attached to the skin that only runs when triggered by the patient with onset of the event.

Cardiac Radionuclide Imaging

Cardiac radionuclide imaging involves a procedure wherein a liquid radioactive substance (tracer) with an affinity to heart muscle is injected into a vein. A gamma camera scans the heart to detect that portion of heart muscle that has poor circulation and does not take up tracer material.

Treatment

Cardiac Catheterization

In cardiac catheterization, a thin catheter tube is inserted into an artery or vein and guided into the heart. Different types of catheters are designed to instill medications or dyes that appear on x-ray, allowing physicians to view abnormalities in heart structure, function, and circulation.

Surgical Procedures

Several surgical procedures are used to correct the narrowing or blockage of coronary arteries associated with cardiovascular problems. Coronary angioplasty involves the surgical insertion of a balloon-type device (catheter) into a narrowed artery to flatten the occlusion and allow blood to flow more freely. Laser angioplasty uses lasers to clear plaque; catheters also can be used to install stents, tube-shaped metal devices that remain in place at the problem site to hold the artery open (Mola et al., 2011).

Medical evaluation of coronary artery disease includes radioactive tracers or coronary arteriogram. Using a catheter (introduced in another body area and guided into the heart), the cardiologist injects the substance by means of the catheter directly into coronary vessels. The cardiologist is able to visualize blood flow restrictions, called stenosis, brought about by an accumulation of cholesterol plaques within coronary vessel walls. This condition is treatable through angioplasty or coronary bypass surgery. While angioplasty is effective when the person has only one or two narrowed arteries, it is not practical when more arteries are obstructed. When this occurs or when angioplasty proves unsuccessful, the physician may recommend coronary artery bypass surgery. Instead of repairing the affected region, this procedure reroutes blood around that particular region. Physicians may use robotic and endoscopic techniques to resolve the problem (Bashore et al., 2013).

Congestive Heart Failure

Congestive heart failure is the end stage of deteriorated heart function. An impaired heart must work harder to deliver a sufficient supply of blood to the body. Eventually, it becomes unable to pump the amount of blood needed by the various body systems. The heart chambers gradually enlarge (cardiac hypertrophy); the muscle walls become thicker. Symptoms include dyspnea (shortness of breath), edema in the lower extremities, fatigue, weakness, and abdominal discomfort. This disorder occurs either suddenly (due to a heart attack) or over a period of years. If the underlying problem is treated, however, the condition can be improved.

Cardiac Transplantation

When a person's heart is damaged to the point of end-stage heart disease, a heart transplant may be the only option. Over the years, the success of cardiac transplantation surgery has gradually improved (Jessup, 2012). To become eligible for a heart transplant, a patient needs to be in adequate general health; he or she must be able to withstand the surgical procedure itself, a prolonged recovery time, and a strict medical regimen. In addition to the operation, even being placed on a transplant list is emotionally stressful (McMurray & Pfeffer, 2012). The individual does not know when the surgery will occur or even if it will happen, and must respond immediately when a donor heart is ready. The person's health may deteriorate while on the waiting list for a donor heart. Similar to the patient, his or her family will experience emotional stress, anxiety, and possible depression.

When successful surgery is accomplished, the person is given immunosuppressants to prevent the body from rejecting the donor heart. Long-term exercise training after transplantation in a cardiac rehabilitation program increases exercise capacity. Three to six months is necessary to become sufficiently functional for work. However, emotional factors often impede a successful return to work (Jessup, 2012). Negative employer attitudes toward people with chronic, medical conditions also make it more difficult to secure gainful employment.

Functional Limitations

Functional limitations of people with cardiovascular disorders depend on the severity of the condition and whether medical treatment alleviates the symptoms. Individuals with mild congestive heart failure controlled by medication may be able to continue their usual work with minimal modifications. Workers performing physically arduous jobs need changes in employment. People with moderate heart failure who are limited to light or sedentary work may seek rehabilitation counseling services. Persons with severe conditions have extremely limited capacities for physical exertion and employment; some require cardiac transplantation, for which there is a lengthy waiting list. Exercise testing provides the level in METs where a patient becomes symptomatic with dyspnea; a poor heart rate response at that point suggests a negative prognosis.

Disability Rating

The treating physician determines the extent of disability resulting from coronary artery disease after carefully evaluating data obtained from a medical history, objective testing documentation, and response to treatment. Historical information is correlated with the NYHA classifications (see Figure 1) to determine symptomatic as well as therapeutic classification of the person's status, and in assessing ability to perform various activities (Alpern, 1996).

The NYHA classification system is one of the most helpful clinical determinants in establishing levels of cardiac disability. Physicians utilize these guidelines to classify patients on both functional and therapeutic levels. Factors relating to disability are compared with objective evaluations, which are then correlated with the results of exercise testing on a treadmill. The cardiologist performing an exercise test estimates the energy expenditure of physical activity in terms of oxygen consumption required to accomplish certain tasks.

The basic metabolic unit for this estimation is the MET (metabolic equivalent). Studies have established MET requirements for various activities, both occupational and recreational. Workload is expressed in METs, which corresponds to the amount of oxygen required to perform a given activity. For example, a patient performs a Bruce Protocol exercise level of nine minutes (on a treadmill). This individual could be expected to perform up to ten METs activity, indicating ability to perform mid-heavy to heavy activity by the NYHA, Functional Class 1 and Therapeutic Class A. The Bruce and Naughton treadmill tests are used to determine functional classification of disabilities. Performance test levels have been correlated with levels of physical activity that relate to a variety of job activities (Alpern, 1996; Bonow et al., 2011).

Information obtained from the patient's history and objective data from stress treadmill testing and other laboratory and physical findings are used to establish a classification of impairment and determine an optimal level of physical activity (Alpern, 1996). Goals of treatment are to decrease existing impairment and improve functional capacity to help the person establish a meaningful and productive life.

Physical Limitations

Most individuals, depending on the extent of cardiovascular disease, can perform at least light work. Some can engage in medium level work activity. Heavy lifting and carrying is usually discouraged, while moderate activities, such as standing and walking, are considered beneficial. The physician recommends physical exercise as part of the recovery process. Exercise testing reveals the exertion limit in METs so that a decision may be made as to the possibility of employment and type of work. Undue emotional stress is contraindicated.

Chest pain (angina pectoris) occurs in some people with cardiac disease. This involves severe pain and a feeling of constriction around the heart area, including radiation of pain down the left arm. Angina is caused by an insufficient supply of blood to a portion of the heart and may occur with physical overexertion. Pain is usually transitory and relieved by oral medication (nitroglycerine), which dilates the arteries. After angina pectoris, the person may resume work activity, usually in a few minutes, but is cautioned to avoid the activity that precipitated the event. A rehabilitation counselor needs to provide vocational guidance in accordance with the person's physical capacity. If angina is not relieved with medication, angioplasty or coronary bypass surgery may be recommended (Skala et al., 2005).

Some people experience arrhythmias and heart palpitations (throbbing sensations) in the chest area. These sensations may occur because of excessive physical activity. In all cases, the counselor needs to inquire about client compliance with prescribed medications. The cardiovascular system is affected by environmental extremes of temperature. Poor air quality must be avoided by many with cardiovascular disease. A counselor's awareness of this and other factors in the work environment helps promote successful rehabilitation.

Psychosocial Limitations

The experience of hospitalization and separation from home and family produces emotional stress. Early intervention can decrease this stress by helping the person cope in a more realistic manner. Fear, anxiety, and depression are common emotions felt by persons with any chronic condition, including cardiovascular disease (Livneh & Bishop, 2012). The impact these emotions produce on one's life can range from minimal to devastating. Emotional support and counseling can help individuals cope with anxiety and depression and adjust to daily life with a disability. Denial, a normal psychological defense, is often part of the adjustment to life with a disability. If this denial causes a person to ignore symptoms, it may be dysfunctional and lead to selection of an inappropriate rehabilitation plan.

Today, treatment emphasizes early ambulation and involvement in a cardiac rehabilitation program as preventive measures to help avoid immobilizing reactions (McMurray & Pfeffer, 2012). With modern advances in technology and medical treatment along with rehabilitation intervention, one minimizes symptoms of psychological distress. As a result of modern treatment, most people regain strength and functional capacity to return to being productive and gainfully employed.

Rehabilitation Potential

Multidisciplinary cardiac rehabilitation programs have assisted persons with cardiovascular problems in increasing performance during work, recreation, and leisure (Mola et al., 2011; Bashore et al., 2013). Improved physical functioning and enhanced mental and social capacities aid in facilitating an active and productive life. A comprehensive and multidisciplinary treatment approach allows persons with cardiovascular problems to achieve increased awareness of their underlying conditions, and participate in exercise as a preventive and therapeutic measure. With the cardiac rehabilitation programs, individuals are able to increase strength, endurance, and improve overall functioning and psychological outlook. By educating the patient in the various manifestations of cardiovascular disease, the counselor can improve rehabilitation potential. Many persons with cardiac problems do not understand their condition, its severity, or their functional limitations. Some refuse to regularly and consistently take prescribed medications. Denial may play a part in this, along with the misconception that a lack of symptoms means medications are no longer necessary.

Rehabilitation potential for persons with Functional Class I and Therapeutic Class A (see Figure 1) is excellent; these individuals have only slight restrictions in overall activities. Most do not require rehabilitation counseling services. Counselors see persons with Functional Classes II and III and Therapeutic Classes B through D, who need to modify their work activity to become reemployed. The amount of work adjustment necessary depends on the extent of cardiovascular disease and the physical and emotional components of the person's work activity. Individuals with Functional Class IV and Therapeutic Class E display such severe symptoms that their potential for rehabilitation is minimal.

Factors that may negatively influence return to work include: (a) duration of temporary disability, (b) perception of an inability to work, and (c) availability of disability income benefits. Rehabilitation potential is best for an individual who completes a cardiac rehabilitation program and feels positive about the results of therapy and the future (Paris et al., 1997). Development of appropriate educational and vocational goals consistent with physical and emotional restrictions is essential. Vocational rehabilitation ranges from returning to a former job with the same employer and minimal modifications, to establishing entirely new vocational objectives including a new occupation and occupational setting.

Investigation of job modification through reasonable accommodation helps both employee and employer maintain a productive work situation. One must consider both physical and emotional stress factors present in the employment environment, especially because emotional components are more difficult to define. Each person perceives emotional stress differently. Negative attitudes of employers may complicate and interfere with a successful return to work.

A final dimension in the rehabilitation of persons with cardiovascular disease is employer discrimination (Brodwin, Parker, & DeLaGarza, 2010). Rehabilitation counselors can help educate employers and dispel negative stereotypes they may possess toward persons with chronic disease. As stated by Yuker (1992), "employers value employees who have job skills, social skills, and dependability" (p. 17). Employers who have had past experiences with employees who have disabilities usually develop positive attitudes toward them. As more people with disabilities return to or enter the labor force and prove to be motivated and productive employees, we can expect further positive attitude change. Counselors play a crucial role in initiating and continuing this process.

Case Study

Joyce Albert is a 52 year-old married Korean American woman with multiple disabilities, including coronary artery disease, hypertension, and diabetes. One year ago, after being diagnosed with coronary artery disease, she had successful heart bypass surgery, and does not currently require medication for her condition. Ms. Albert has never participated in a cardiac rehabilitation program. In addition to coronary disease, she has been successfully controlling diabetes with insulin for the past ten years, and she keeps her hypertension under control with medication. Additionally, Joyce has mild to moderate anxiety and depression.

For nine years before attending graduate school in social work, Ms. Albert worked as a self-employed photographer. This involved lifting and carrying up to 40 pounds of equipment, long hours, and frequent traveling. Before becoming self-employed, Ms. Albert worked for various photographic studios, starting out as a photography assistant and working her way up to photographer. Joyce left each job within one year because she felt that none of her managers were satisfied with her work, although the managers noted satisfaction with her work on several occasions.

Joyce's first position following receipt of her M.S.W. was a children's social worker. After two years, she left this position because she believed her clients were never satisfied with her services. Her supervisors, however, consistently rated Joyce's work as excellent. She next obtained employment as an eligibility worker, but resigned after one year due to complaints from a client. The supervisor attempted to keep Ms. Albert as an employee by reassuring her that complaints were common among all eligibility workers; nevertheless, she left the job. Following these social work positions, Joyce decided to leave the field to secure employment as a photography assistant.

Ms. Albert was evaluated using an exercise study. She successfully accomplished five METS. There was no evidence of ischemia on a perfusion nuclear study at each exertional level. Her physician restricted Ms. Albert to a maximum of medium work with no undue emotional stress.

Questions

1. Provide a vocational profile for Ms. Albert.
2. Mr. Alpert feels his wife should be seeing a Korean, female counselor. You are neither Korean nor female, and have been assigned the case. Although there is a Korean, female counselor in your agency, your supervisor wants you to keep the case. Discuss whether you will work with this client and the cultural and interpersonal implications involved with this situation.
3. What are Joyce's functional limitations, both physical and emotional, that may effect employment?
4. Outline three possible rehabilitation plans for this client.
5. Are there any additional services that may help this individual return to work? Explain.

References

Alpern, H. L. (1996). Cardiac disability. In S. L. Demeter, G. B. J. Anderson, & G. M. Smith (Eds.), *Disability evaluation* (pp. 385–395). St. Louis, MO: Mosby.

Bashore, T. M., Granger, C. B., Hronitzky, P., & Patel, M. R. (2013). Heart disease. In S. J. Papadakis, S. J. McPhee, & M. W. Rabow (Eds.), *Current medical diagnosis and treatment* (pp. 324–431)). New York, NY: McGraw Hill-Lange.

Bonow, R. O., Mann, D. L., Zipes, D. P., & Libby, P. (2011). *Braunwald's heart disease: A textbook of cardiovascular medicine* (9th ed.). Philadelphia, PA: Elsevier Saunders.

Brodwin, M. G., Parker, R. M., & DeLaGarza, D. (2010). Disability and reasonable accommodation. In E. M. Szymanski & R. M. Parker (Eds.), *Work and disability: Contexts, issues, and strategies for enhancing employment for people with disabilities* (3rd ed., pp. 281–323). Austin, TX: Pro-ed.

Carabello, B. A. (2012). Valvular heart disease. In L. Goldman & A. I. Schafer (Eds.), *Goldman's Cecil medicine* (24th ed., pp. 334–337). Philadelphia, PA: Elsevier Saunders.

Centers for Disease Control and Prevention (CDC). (2013). *Heart disease: Facts*. Atlanta, GA: Author.

Criteria Committee of the New York Heart Association. (1984). *The diseases of the heart and blood vessels: Nomenclature and criteria for diagnosis* (6th ed.). New York, NY: Little, Brown.

Jacobson, K. M., & Rahko, P. S. (2012). Mitral valve prolapse. In E. T. Bope & R. D. Kellerman (Eds.), *Conn's current therapy* (pp. 454–457). Philadelphia, PA: Elsevier Saunders.

Jessup, M. (2012). Cardiac transplantation. In L. Goldman & A. I. Schafer (Eds.), *Goldman's Cecil medicine* (24th ed., pp. 482–486). Philadelphia, PA: Elsevier Saunders.

Klag, M. J. (2012). Epidemiology of cardiovascular disease. In L. Goldman & A. I. Schafer (Eds.), *Goldman's Cecil medicine* (24th ed., pp. 256–260). Philadelphia, PA: Elsevier Saunders.

Lange, R. S., & Hillis, L. D. (2012). Congenital heart disease. In E. T. Bope & R. D. Kellerman (Eds.), *Conn's current therapy* (pp. 422–427). Philadelphia, PA: Elsevier Saunders.

Livneh, H., & Bishop, M. L. (2012). Psychosocial impact of chronic illness and disability. In R. M. Parker, E. M. Szymanski, & J. B. Patterson (Eds.), *Rehabilitation counseling: Basics and beyond* (5th ed., pp. 167–197). Austin, TX: Pro-ed.

Massie, B. M. (2012). Heart failure: Pathophysiology and diagnosis. In L. Goldman & A. I. Schafer (Eds.), *Goldman's Cecil medicine* (24th ed., pp. 295–302). Philadelphia, PA: Elsevier Saunders.

McMurray, J. J. V., & Pfeffer, M. A. (2012). Heart failure: Management and prognosis. In L. Goldman & A. I. Schafer (Eds.), *Goldman's Cecil medicine* (24th ed., pp. 303–318). Philadelphia, PA: Elsevier Saunders.

Mola, A., Whiteson, J., & Rey, M. J. (2011). Cardiovascular disorders. In S. R. Flanagan, H. H. Zaretsky, & A. Moroz (Eds.), *Medical aspects of disability: A handbook for the rehabilitation professional* (4th ed., pp. 119–145). New York, NY: Springer.

Moser, D., & Riegel, B. (2008). *Cardiac nursing: A companion to Braunwald's heart disease*. St. Louis, MO: Saunders/Elsevier.

Nabel, E. G., & Braunwald, E. (2012). A tale of coronary disease and myocardial infarction. *New England Journal of Medicine, 366*(1), 54–63.

Paris, W., Calahoun-Wilson, G., Stentz, B., Dahr, A. S., Tebow, S., Hart, J., & Harrison, J. (1997). Employment and the transplant patient. *Journal of Rehabilitation, 63*, 10–14.

Reeder, G. S., & Prasad, A. (2012). Acute myocardial infarction. In E. T. Bope & R. D. Kellerman (Eds.), L. Goldman & A. I. Schafer (Eds.), *Conn's current therapy* (pp. 399–406). Philadelphia, PA: Elsevier Saunders.

Skala, J. A., Freeland, K. E., & Carney, R. M. (2005). *Heart disease*. Toronto, Canada: Hogrefe and Huber.

Topol, E. J., Califf, R. M., Prystowsky, N., Thomas, J. D., & Thompson, P. D. (Eds.). (2007). *Textbook of cardiovascular medicine* (3rd ed.). Philadelphia, PA: Lippincott-Raven.

Victor, R. G. (2012). Arterial hypertension. In L. Goldman & A. I. Schafer (Eds.), *Goldman's Cecil medicine* (24th ed., pp. 373–389). Philadelphia, PA: Elsevier Saunders.

Yuker, H. E. (1992). Attitudes toward persons with disabilities: Conclusions from the data. *Rehabilitation Psychology News, 19*(2), 17–18.

About the Author

Harvey L. Alpern, M. D., is in private practice with an emphasis on cardiac disability. Formerly, he was Clinical Chief of Cardiac Rehabilitation at Cedars-Sinai Medical Center in Los Angeles, California, and currently is Assistant Clinical Professor of Medicine at the University of California, Los Angeles. Dr. Alpern is a Fellow of the American College of Cardiology and Past-President of American College of Disability Evaluating Physicians. For many years, Dr. Alpern has been serving as a medical expert for the Office of Disability Adjudication and Review of the Social Security Administration.

Chapter 6

CHRONIC OBSTRUCTIVE PULMONARY DISEASE

Hassan Bencheqroun, M.D.

Introduction

An obstructive lung disease is defined as a limitation of air flow into the lungs. Lung damage due to various factors can make patients take longer to exhale. This impairment is called obstruction or airflow limitation. The two major obstructive lung diseases encountered are asthma and chronic obstructive pulmonary disease (COPD). This chapter discusses COPD.

COPD is defined as a preventable and treatable disease state, in which the airflow limitation is not fully reversed when treated with inhaled medicines called bronchodilators (in contrast to asthma which is fully reversible). In addition, COPD is usually progressive, and associated with an abnormal inflammatory response of the lungs to noxious particles or gases, primarily caused by cigarette smoking. In the past decade, research has established that although COPD affects the lungs, it also produces significant physical consequences to the overall inflammation it generates (Celli et al., 2004; Decramer, Janssens, & Mirevitlles, 2012; Fabbri, Luppi, Beghé, & Rabe, 2008).

Incidence and Prevalence

Chronic lower respiratory disease, primarily COPD, is the third leading cause of death in the United States, with mortality rates still rising (Rabe, 2007). Although COPD has been traditionally associated with men, the numbers of men and women who died from COPD-related causes leveled around the year 2000.

Globally, about 24% of people over the age of 40 with a history of smoking have airflow limitations, compared to 12% for individuals who have never smoked (Lamprecht et al., 2011). Prevalence of COPD rises with age. In addition, up to 60-85% of people with COPD (mostly mild/moderate severity) appear to be undiagnosed (Hoyert & Xu, 2012; Hvidsten, Storesund, & Wentzel-Larsen, 2010). Besides tobacco smoking, secondhand smoke, air pollution, biomass exposure, and work exposure to fumes and dust can cause COPD in susceptible individuals.

Pathology

At the lung tissue level, COPD is characterized both by destruction of the lung tissue with loss of its elasticity (called emphysema), and by infiltration of the walls of the small airways by inflammatory cells (causing chronic bronchitis). These two broad COPD types are usually presented as distinct entities, when in reality they coexist and overlap to varying degrees in virtually everyone with COPD. Researchers are just starting to understand the reasons for these variable phenotypes and their clinical importance.

Not everyone who smokes develops COPD. Several pathophysiological and pathobiological processes must interact for the disease to develop. These include a complex interplay of genetic determinants, lung growth, and environmental stimuli. The disease is further aggravated by exacerbations, particularly in patients with severe or untreated disease. While studies have not isolated specific microorganisms during exacerbations, it is now known that exacerbations treated with antibiotics have a better response than those not treated, suggesting that infections may be responsible in the pathogenesis of COPD exacerbations

(Stefan, Rothberg, Shieh, Pekow, & Lindenauer, 2013). Moreover, due to the nature of the disease and its direct link to cigarette smoking, it often coexists with other disease states, which are likewise related to smoking. These comorbidities include ischemic heart disease, stroke, diabetes, and lung cancer.

Symptoms

A patient with COPD often first experiences shortness of breath (dyspnea). This occurs primarily during physical exertion ranging from vigorous exercise, chores around the house, laundry, cleaning, pushing a cart at the supermarket, to more mundane activities such as taking a shower, making a bed, putting on shoes, or walking up stairs. In the advanced stages of COPD, dyspnea can become so distressing that it occurs during rest and is constantly present. Other symptoms of COPD include a persistent cough, mucus production, chest tightness, and on occasion, weight loss.

Symptoms often become temporarily more pronounced and severe and are referred to as exacerbations. They are usually preceded by a common *cold*, acute bronchitis, or both. Exacerbations are not random, but clustered around each other, often making the progression of the disease worse. During exacerbations, the patient may appear to be breathing faster and shallower, or through pursed lips. There is active use of the muscles in the neck to help with breathing, and longer exhalation time due to the airflow limitation (Bourbeau, 2010; Wedzicha & Seemungal, 2007).

In extreme circumstances, people with advanced COPD may develop respiratory failure. The body becomes unable to meet the demands for oxygen, and the person requires assistance of a ventilator until the precipitating factor is treated. Advanced COPD may overburden the heart, which is working against rising pressure in the chest to channel blood flow. This causes a complication of advanced COPD called *cor pulmonale*, a form of heart failure exerted mainly on the right side of the heart, and presents with swelling of the ankles and shortness of breath.

Diagnosis

Obstruction or airflow limitation is diagnosed using Pulmonary Function Testing, a test which measures forced airflow exhaled in one second (called Forced Expiratory Volume or FEV1) and the total forced exhaled volume (called Forced Vital Capacity or FVC). A diagnosis of COPD occurs if the ratio of FEV1/FVC is less than 70%. The patient is then given a bronchodilator medicine to inhale before a second test is given. If the FEV1 improves by 12% or more, it suggests the obstruction is reversible (i.e., asthma). If it shows less than 12% improvement, then the obstruction is only partially or not at all reversible (i.e., COPD).

In certain situations, arterial blood gas, or a blood sample taken from an artery, may show low oxygen (hypoxemia) and/or high carbon dioxide. The inability to exchange oxygen for carbon dioxide is a symptom of patients with COPD. Once the diagnosis of COPD is made, the physician has to determine the severity of the disease. The Global Initiative for Chronic Obstructive Lung Disease (GOLD) classification is the main method used to describe the different severities of COPD (Rabe, 2007).

GOLD is a collaboration between the National Institutes of Health (NIH) and the World Health Organization (WHO) for the advancement of knowledge, prevention, and treatment of COPD worldwide. In the GOLD classification, the worse a person's airflow limitation is, the lower their FEV1. As COPD progresses, FEV1 tends to decline. Based on the value of FEV1, GOLD staging uses mild, moderate, severe, and very severe categories to classify COPD (Rabe, 2007).

Associated Diseases

The most common comorbidities of COPD are ischemic heart disease, diabetes, sarcopenia (muscle wasting), cachexia (loss of weight), osteoporosis (decrease in bone mass), depression, and lung cancer (Decramer & Rennard, 2008). These comorbidities influence the course of COPD, increasing the risk for admission to a hospital or causing death. Comorbidities of COPD are responsible for over 50% of expenditures for the disease (Fabbri et al., 2008).

The BODE Index was developed to include more meaningful clinical data with the FEV1 and enhance the predictability of prognosis and mortality. The BODE Index stands for: the body-mass index, airflow obstruction (FEV1), dyspnea, and exercise capacity index (Cote & Celli, 2005).

Management of COPD

Inhalers constitute the mainstay of treatment. They encompass bronchodilator and anti-inflammatory medications. The airways are made of smooth muscles and airway mucosa (the lining inside the airways). Research has found several molecules called receptors embedded in the smooth muscle of the airways. Activation of these receptors leads to dilation and partial reversal of the airflow limitation, in turn alleviating some shortness of breath associated with the disease. Those receptors are called â2 receptors; they lead to bronchodilation when turned on (activated), hence the discovery of â2 agonist bronchodilators. Cholinergic receptors, in contrast, lead to bronchodilation when turned off (blocked). Therefore, anticholinergic inhalers lead to bronchodilation, helpful for people with COPD.

Physicians frequently prescribe both â2 agonists and anticholinergic agents. Development of fast acting and long acting inhalers has widened the types of medications used for treatment, with the fast acting inhalers being the *rescue* medicine, and the long acting inhalers being the *maintenance* medicine.

Additionally, since a certain degree of inflammation accompanies the disease, anti-inflammatory inhalers (corticosteroids) are prescribed to combine with bronchodilators in order to treat symptoms, both during exacerbations and on a maintenance basis (Decramer et al., 2012). Besides improving symptoms, these treatments are thought to lead to some positive disease modifications.

Medical Limitations

Muscle Dysfunction

Patients with COPD often complain of shortness of breath during activity, reduced exercise capacity, and a progressive decline in lung function with increasing age. However, aside from decline of lung function, muscle weakness seems to be a central component that contributes to reduced exercise capacity and poor quality of life, and is a separate predictor of morbidity and mortality.

Limb and respiratory skeletal muscle dysfunction in patients with COPD have been attributed to several factors. These include the presence of low grade inflammation throughout the body, poor nutrition, long term inactivity due to difficulty breathing, advancing age, intermittent or long term reduced oxygen, oxidative stresses along with protein degradation, and poor vascular circulation. Weakness in muscles is often generalized to all muscle groups tested, impacting mostly lower extremity function, and resulting in patients becoming less physically active.

Nutritional Status

The Obesity Paradox concept emerged in studying various COPD populations. COPD patients who are overweight or obese were found to survive longer than their counterparts with lower Body Mass Index. This suggests that nutritional status has an impact on the functional status of patients (Celli et al., 2004; Sabino, Silva, & Brunetto, 2010).

Dynamic Hyperinflation

In COPD, pressure in the chest during exhalation compresses rather than expands the airways. In theory, breathing more forcefully increases airflow. However, in COPD, there is often a limit to how much this can actually increase airflow, a condition called expiratory flow limitation.

Consequently, the patient is unable to exhale completely before taking the next breath. This is particularly common during exercise, when breathing must be faster and exhalation is shorter. When the lungs do not deflate completely, some volume of air from the previous breath still remains in the lungs before the next breath is started. This result is a process called dynamic hyperinflation, characterized by stacking of breaths and trapping of air inside the lungs. The lungs become inflated to a point where patients feel they can no longer inhale and need to stop the activity or exercise because they are constantly out of breath (Kim, Mofarrahi, & Hussain, 2009).

Pulmonary Rehabilitation

Rehabilitation Potential and Methods

The benefits of pulmonary rehabilitation have been shown to be effective, long lasting, reproducible, and cost saving (Mota et al., 2007). These benefits translate into improved ventilatory efficiency, longer walking distances, enhanced ventilatory muscle function, and less breathlessness (Cooper, 2009).

Pulmonary rehabilitation does not directly improve lung mechanics or oxygen and carbon dioxide exchange. Instead, it improves the function of other body systems, minimizing the effects of lung dysfunction. High-intensity rehabilitative exercise programs improve function by reconditioning the muscles to tolerate higher work rates.

If lower limb muscle function is the primary limitation, delaying fatigue directly enhances exercise tolerance. More specifically, rehabilitation targets endurance capability of the leg muscles with walking, using a stationary bicycle, and exercising on a treadmill. If respiratory muscle function seems to be the primary limitation, increasing the efficiency of breathing, and decreasing the level of hyperinflation will be the focus. This in turn decreases demand on respiratory muscles and breathlessness during physical exertion.

It is important to optimize the clinical status of each individual with regards to medical therapy while undergoing the rehabilitation program. Bronchodilation, oxygen supplementation, and antibiotic maintenance are treatments to reduce the potential for exacerbations and allow for completion of the prescribed rehabilitation program.

Composition of a Rehabilitation Program

The most commonly encountered type of program for pulmonary rehabilitation in the United States is multidisciplinary, hospital-based, outpatient, with incorporated education classes. The education component may include smoking cessation advice, translation of the exercises performed in the home setting, demonstration of proper use of inhaled therapy and oxygen use, promotion of adherence to therapy, and development of an action plan for earlier detection and treatment of COPD exacerbations (Fuld et al., 2005). Some other programs may also be provided at home, in the community, or as an in-patient. Usually, each patient will undergo 6 to 12 weeks of rehabilitation. A specially trained coordinator (nurse, physical therapist, or respiratory therapist) is responsible for designing the day exercise plan and delivering the therapy, while a pulmonologist oversees the overall program.

Adverse Effects of Rehabilitation

Safety measures are part of all rehabilitation programs for COPD patients. Given the co-existence of cardiovascular disease with COPD, vigilance towards cardiovascular events should be undertaken before a patient starts an exercise program evaluation. Use of fast-acting bronchodilators is recommended for patients with exercise-induced bronchospasm (Casaburi & ZuWallack, 2009). Precautionary measures should be taken to provide a safe environment for individuals with COPD.

Contraindications to Rehabilitation

Pulmonary rehabilitation is not recommended for patients with functional impairment due to orthopedic or neurologic disorders, or those with unstable cardiac disease (unstable angina or recent myocardial infarction [heart attack]). Other relative contraindications include the inability to comprehend or cooperate with treatment plans.

Outcomes of Rehabilitation in COPD

For three outcomes, the benefit is unequivocal: exercise capacity (in increasing type of exertion, steady exertion, and walking tests), severity of shortness of breath, and health-related quality of life. For these three outcomes, the magnitude of benefit is generally superior to any other COPD therapy (Ries et al., 2007).

Psychosocial outcomes can be achieved through classes that provide action plans on how to cope with exacerbations, while promoting self-sufficiency among patients with COPD. Social interaction with individuals with the same disease helps build support systems and decreases depression related to the disability. This has been demonstrated to optimize the effectiveness of the rehabilitation program regarding quality of life (Wittmann, Spohn, Schultz, Pfeifer, & Petro, 2007).

Unfortunately, access to pulmonary rehabilitation is minimal, due to such factors as geographic considerations, socioeconomic situation, and so forth. Home-based rehabilitation programs have been presented as an alternative to expand the benefit to larger populations (Vieira, Maltais, & Bourbeau, 2010). Maintenance of benefits gained in a pulmonary rehabilitation program is essential to continued success.

Rehabilitation After a COPD Exacerbation

Pulmonary rehabilitation is recommended as part of long-term management of COPD. A push toward incorporating it following a recent exacerbation or hospitalization follows the rationale that patients may be more likely to adhere to the lifestyle change, smoking cessation, and other medical recommendations. A recent review suggested that pulmonary rehabilitation is effective in reducing the chance of hospitalization and mortality following an acute exacerbation of COPD. In addition, pulmonary rehabilitation following acute COPD exacerbation also results in improvements in health-related quality of life, as well as exercise capacity (Jette, Bourgeois, & Buchbinder, 2010).

Vocational Aspects

With respect to COPD, return to work can be considered the best measure of health outcomes. As such, it is aligned with the goals of pulmonary rehabilitation, aimed at helping individuals improve daily living and restoring the ability to function independently. In addition, proper evaluation of the patient's capacities is essential to vocational rehabilitation. After completion of pulmonary rehabilitation, the potential to return to work depends upon the degree of functional and respiratory impairment, as well as adherence to lifestyle modifications recommended to the patient.

Recommendations for Return to Work

Individuals with COPD should avoid inhaling irritants at the workplace (ie., gases, fumes, dust), and sudden and wide changes in ambient temperatures. Work in high altitudes may be discouraged for patients with moderate or severe COPD. Tolerance for physical exertion may also be limited. This could be improved with supplemental oxygen and bronchodilation. Some patients may be advised for home employment, or work in facilities that can accommodate respiratory equipment and flexible rest schedules.

Pulmonary Disability

Disability is a broad term that encompasses impairment, limitations in activity, and restrictions in participation. The Americans with Disabilities Act (ADA) of 1990 has a three-part definition of disability. Under ADA, an individual with a disability is a person who: (1) has a physical or mental impairment that substantially limits one or more major life activities; or (2) has a record of such an impairment; or (3) is regarded as having such an impairment (Americans with Disabilities Act [ADA], 2012).

Many individuals with COPD are considered to have disabilities under the ADA. They can request reasonable accommodations from current or perspective employers under the ADA, and can ask for assistance from the state department of rehabilitation.

A disability may be multifactorial, representing the interplay of a person's own hindrances, as well as adverse environmental factors. Individuals with COPD may have a respiratory impairment with such level of severity that they are unable to engage in substantial gainful activity. This can be due to advanced irreversible lung obstruction or various hospitalizations because of exacerbations. A COPD patient may qualify for Social Security disability if he or she is unable to work due to severe limitations in one or more of the following areas (Social Security Disability Representation, 2013):

- Walking, standing, sitting, lifting, pushing, pulling, reaching, carrying, or handling

- Seeing, hearing, and speaking
- Understanding/carrying out and remembering simple instructions
- Responding appropriately to supervision, co-workers, and usual work situations
- Adjusting to changes in work routines

Role of the Rehabilitation Counselor

Employment provides individuals with COPD with a sense of purpose and a role beyond that of being a patient. A daily routine and time spent away from home helps improve financial, emotional, and physical health. The counselor and healthcare professionals play pivotal roles in helping persons with COPD in recovery and return to work (Marini & Stebnicki, 2009). The patient's vocational potential should be assessed from various aspects including personal-social background, family support, financial resources, prior job satisfaction, recent life changes, psychological and social dysfunction, substance abuse, and transferable skills (Brodwin, Parker, & DeLaGarza, 2010).

Vocational and Rehabilitation Aspects of COPD

Team Approach

Successful vocational rehabilitation of patients with COPD can be achieved through effective participation of all members of a rehabilitation team. The team includes the rehabilitation program physician whose primary goal is to optimize the activity level of the patient. Working alongside the medical team members are the occupational therapist, social worker, rehabilitation counselor, and job placement specialist. The ideal time to begin vocational counseling is during the psychosocial interview when the patient may still be able to return to prior employment, with or without reasonable accommodation.

Unfortunately, some patients are subject to severe respiratory infections frequently requiring hospitalization. This may result in a patient's inability to cope with regular employment, causing a disruption of socioeconomic status that imposes significant psychological impact on the individual and family, often leading to feelings of despair and uselessness (Mahler, 1998; Ries et al., 2007).

Vocational Factors

Information is obtained from the patient regarding personal-social background and educational-vocational history. The history needs to include all prior work, job duties, dates of employment, salaries, job duties, job satisfaction, reasons for termination of employment, and a transferable skills analysis. Information about present means of financial support, educational background, as well as social and psychological factors is taken into consideration in vocational counseling. Rehabilitation counselors, the other multidisciplinary team professionals, and liaisons with community agencies, make a significant impact on the psychosocial and vocational aspects of pulmonary rehabilitation (Baydur, 2009).

Persons with COPD may be classified into four clinical and vocational rehabilitation groups (Hodgkin, Celli, & Connors, 2008):

1. Individuals who can return to their previous work activities.
2. Individuals who should be retrained for more suitable work.
3. Individuals who are capable of work only in sheltered employment.
4. Individuals who can be trained for self-care only.

Proper evaluation and categorization of the patient's capacities are essential to successful educational and vocational rehabilitation. When selecting patients for vocational rehabilitation, counselors need to consider such factors as recent changes in lifestyle and evidence of rapid clinical deterioration, personality change, substance abuse, and psychological or social dysfunction (Brodwin et al., 2010). Counselors must additionally assess whether a person's cardiorespiratory reserve will enable a return to a previous job on a full or part-time basis. If the individual's tolerance to work requires job modification, the rehabilitation counselor can help facilitate this process. Once the patient is physically rehabilitated, training in new vocational areas commensurate with educational level and decreased respiratory capacity may be needed.

Sheltered or Home Employment

Some people who have COPD can only function in locations where special respiratory equipment is available, such as in sheltered employment or at home. Occupational therapists, rehabilitation counselors, and job placement specialists work together to help locate settings for employment. The occupational therapist provides training in energy-saving methods for those who have a difficult time with self-care. This helps the individual perform tasks including housekeeping, shopping, and other activities of daily living with less dependence on others. An occupational therapist may recommend the following to the person to help conserve needed energy (Baydur, 2009; Hodgkin et al., 2008):

1. Perform activities slowly.
2. Avoid noxious fumes.
3. Avoid areas of excessive heat, cold, and humidity.
4. Plan ahead to decrease ambulation and minimize body movement.
5. Change activities frequently.
6. Spread activities that promote fatigue or dyspnea throughout the day.
7. Transport heavy objects using carts or tables with wheels.
8. Perform most work activities while standing with the work surface (table) at hip level to minimize flexion and abduction.
9. Perform most work activities while standing with the work surface at a body level that minimizes trunk flexion and hyperextension.
10. Store utensils, tools, and similar devices in cabinets where height minimizes active trunk flexion, hyperextension, and active flexion of the shoulder girdle.
11. Use electric appliances (can opener, mixer, electric knife) to eliminate or minimize manual performance of daily activities.

Several factors impede vocational rehabilitation. These include psychosocial problems, severity of respiratory impairment, progression of disease, advancing age, limitation in skills and capabilities, and poor labor markets in certain fields.

Conclusion

In the past, COPD was considered solely a pulmonary disease, but now it has taken its place among systemic diseases, which have consequences for more than one organ, and require interventions beyond medical therapy alone. Pulmonary rehabilitation coupled with adequate patient-centered education, optimization of therapy, and psychosocial support, results in significant improvement of health status, improves patients' quality of life, and reduces the socioeconomic impact on society.

Case Study

Mr. Leroy Smith is a 57-year-old white male, who completed high school but has no further education. He is divorced and takes care of his two teenage boys on his own. This client shared that it has been a struggle to spend time with his sons because of his work schedule. Furthermore, he often finds himself short tempered from stress at work and occasionally "blows up" at his boys. As stated by the client, he is increasingly becoming more concerned about his career in construction because of his aging body. Since graduating high school, Leroy has been in the construction industry.

Because of a persistent cough with phlegm production for over six months, Mr. Smith sought medical attention. Three months ago, he first visited a doctor, who prescribed antibiotics; this medication did not fully resolve the problem. Leroy smokes one pack of cigarettes a day, and has done so since he was 20 years old. On several occasions, he attempted to quit but was unsuccessful.

Leroy noted that he was having trouble lifting heavy equipment, which was not a problem before. He has shortness of breath when walking up stairs and often has to stop to rest. His physical examination shows "rattling and wheezing" on auscultation of his lungs on both sides. He is able to speak comfortably when well rested. His pulmonary function tests indicated a severe obstruction, which showed some response to the inhaler he was given for the test. Chest imaging indicated he has emphysema.

Questions

1. Provide a vocational profile for Leroy. Using a multidisciplinary approach, identify additional information you need to best help this client and discuss how you will obtain the information.
2. What is the patient's medical condition? Discuss.
3. Identify factors that can be modified in the patient's life (triggers and medical therapy).
4. What recommendations can be made for the patient to keep his job?
5. Describe rehabilitation potential for Mr. Smith based on his condition.

References

Americans with Disabilities Act (ADA) of 1990, P.L. 101-336, U.S.C. § 12101 et seq.

Americans with Disabilities Act (ADA). (2012). *A guide to disability rights laws*. Retrieved on January 24, 2013 from http://www.ada.gov/cguide.htm

Baydur, A. (2009). Chronic obstructive pulmonary disease and neuromuscular disorders affecting the respiratory system. In M. G. Brodwin, F. W. Siu, J. Howard, and E. R. Brodwin (Eds.), *Medical, psychosocial, and vocational aspects of disability* (3rd ed., pp. 97–109). Athens, GA: Elliott & Fitzpatrick.

Bourbeau, J. (2010). Preventing hospitalization for COPD exacerbations. *Seminars in Respiratory and Critical Care Medicine, 31*(3), 313–320.

Brodwin, M. G., Parker, R. M., & DeLaGarza, D. (2010). Disability and reasonable accommodation. In E. M. Szymanski & R. M. Parker (Eds.), *Work and disability: Contexts, issues, and strategies for enhancing employment outcomes for people with disabilities* (3rd ed., pp. 281–323). Austin, TX: Pro-ed.

Casaburi, R., & ZuWallack, R. (2009). Pulmonary rehabilitation for management of chronic obstructive pulmonary disease. *New England Journal of Medicine, 360*(13), 1329–1335.

Celli, B. R., Cote, C. G., Marin, J. M., Casanova, C., Montes de Oca, M., Mendez, R. A., . . . Cabral, H. J. (2004). The body-mass index, airflow obstruction, dyspnea, and exercise capacity index in chronic obstructive pulmonary disease. *New England Journal of Medicine, 350*(10), 1005–1012.

Cooper, C. B. (2009). Desensitization to dyspnea in COPD with specificity for exercise training mode. *International Journal of Chronic Obstructive Pulmonary Disease, 4*(4), 33–43.

Cote, C. G., & Celli, B. R. (2005). Pulmonary rehabilitation and the BODE index in COPD. *European Respiratory Journal, 26*(4), 630–636.

Decramer, M., Janssens, M., & Miravitlles, M. (2012). Chronic obstructive pulmonary disease. *Lancet, 379* (9823), 1341–1351.

Decramer, M., & Rennard, S. (2008). COPD as a lung diease with systemic consequences, clinical impact, mechanisms, and potential for early intervention. *Journal of Chronic Obstructive Pulmonary Disease, 5*, 235–356.

Fabbri, L., Luppi, F., Beghé, B., & Rabe, K. F. (2008). Complex chronic comorbidities of COPD. *European Respiratory Journal, 31*(1), 204–212.

Fuld, J. P., Kilduff, L. P., Neder, J. A., Pitsiladis, Y., Lean, M. E., Ward, S. A., & Cotton, M. M. (2005). Creatine supplementation during pulmonary rehabilitation in chronic obstructive pulmonary disease. *Thorax, 60*(7), 531–537.

Hodgkin, J. E., Celli, B. R., & Connors, G. L. (2008). *Pulmonary rehabilitation: Guidelines to success* (4th ed.). Philadelphia, PA: Mosby Elsevier.

Hoyert, D. L., & Xu, J. (2012). Deaths: Preliminary data for 2011. *National Vital Statistics Reports, 61*(6), 1–52.

Hvidsten, S. C., Storesund, L., & Wentzel-Larsen, T. (2010). Prevalence and predictors of undiagnosed chronic obstructive pulmonary disease in a Norwegian adult general population. *Clinical Respiratory Journal, 4*(1), 13–21.

Jette, D. U., Bourgeois, M.C., & Buchbinder, R. (2010). Pulmonary rehabilitation following acute exacerbation of chronic obstructive pulmonary disease. *Physical Therapy, 90*(1), 9–12.

Kim, H. C., Mofarrahi, M., & Hussain, S. N. (2009). Skeletal muscle dysfunction in patients with chronic obstructive pulmonary disease. *International Journal of Chronic Obstructive Pulmonary Disease, 3*(4), 637–658.

Lamprecht, B., McBurnie, M. A., Vollmer, W. M., Gudmundsson, G., Welte, T., Nizankowska-Mogilnicka, E., . . . Buist, S. A. (2011). COPD in never smokers: Results from the population-based burden of obstructive lung disease study. *Chest, 139*(4), 752–763.

Marini, I., & Stebnicki, M. (2009). *The professional counselor's desk reference*. New York, NY: Springer.

Mahler, D. A. (1998). Pulmonary rehabilitation. *Chest, 113*, 263S–268S.

Mota, S., Güell, R., Barreiro, E., Solanes, I., Ramírez-Sarmiento, A., Orozco-Levi, M., . . . Sanchis, J. (2007). Clinical outcomes of expiratory muscle training in severe COPD patients. *Respiratory Medicine, 101*(3), 516–524.

Rabe, K. F., Hurd, S., Anzueto, A., Barnes, P. J., Buist, S. A., Calverley, P., . . . Zielinski, J. (2007). Global strategy for the diagnosis, management, and prevention of chronic obstructive pulmonary disease: GOLD executive summary. *American Journal of Respiratory Critical Care Medicine, 176*(6), 532–555.

Ries, A. L., Bauldoff, G. S., Carlin, B. W., Casaburi, R., Emery, C. F., Mahler, D. A., . . . Herrerias, C. (2007). Pulmonary rehabilitation: Joint ACCP/AACVPR evidence-based clinical practice guidelines. *Chest, 131*(5 Suppl), 4S–42S.

Sabino, P. G. Silva, B. M., & Brunetto, A. F. (2010). Nutritional status is related to fat-free mass, exercise capacity, and inspiratory strength in severe chronic obstructive pulmonary disease patients. *Clinics* (Sao Paulo), *65*(6), 599–605.

Social Security Disability Representation. (2013*). Chronic obstructive pulmonary disease (COPD) and Social Security Disability Insurance*. Retrieved on February 1, 2013 from http://www.allsup.com/about-ssdi/ssdi-guidelines-by-disability/chronic-obstructive-pulmonary-disease-(copd).aspx

Stefan, M. S., Rothberg, M. D., Shieh, M. S., Pekow, P. S., & Lindenauer, P. K. (2013). Association between antibiotic treatment and outcomes in patients hospitalized with acute exacerbation of COPD treated with systemic steroids. *Chest, 143*(1), 82–90.

Vieira, D. S., Maltais, F., & Bourbeau, J. (2010). Home-based pulmonary rehabilitation in chronic obstructive pulmonary disease patients. *Current Opinion in Pulmonary Medicine, 16*(2), 134–143.

Wedzicha, J. A., & Seemungal, T. A. (2007). COPD exacerbations: Defining their cause and prevention. *Lancet, 370* (9589), 786–796.

Wittmann, M., Spohn, S., Schultz, K., Pfeifer, M., & Petro, W. (2007). Patient education in COPD during inpatient rehabilitation improves quality of life and morbidity. *Pneumologie, 61*(10), 636–642.

About the Author

Dr. Hassan Bencheqroun is a Pulmonary and Critical Care Specialist with a medical practice at Eisenhower Medical Center in Rancho Mirage, California. Board certified in Internal Medicine and Pulmonary Disease, he was presented with the Patients' Choice Award for two consecutive years, and is on the 2010 list of Top Physicians of America. Additionally, he received a Compassionate Doctor Recognition Award in 2011-2012. Dr. Bencheqroun's specialties are in internal medicine, lung diseases, and critical care.

Chapter 7

HIV/AIDS

John J. Howard, M.D., M.P.H.

Introduction

In 1981, the first four cases of a new immunodeficiency syndrome in young gay men were reported in the United States (Gottlieb et al., 1981). Since then, the causative agent—the human immunodeficiency virus (HIV)—has infected tens of millions of people worldwide. By the end of 2011, an estimated 34 million people were living with HIV worldwide and 1.7 million died from diseases and cancers associated with the acquired immunodeficiency syndrome (AIDS) (Joint United Nations Programme on HIV/AIDS, 2012).

HIV/AIDS has not only had a profound impact on the medical world, but problems caused by HIV/AIDS have touched families, schools, communities, business, industry, courts, religious institutions, and government—throughout the world (Piot & Quinn, 2013). AIDS has brought many controversial issues to the forefront of public discussion, including discrimination against HIV-infected persons in housing, employment, and health care, the duty of government to protect its citizens from communicable diseases like HIV/AIDS, and the obligation of physicians and nurses to provide care for persons with HIV/AIDS despite a fear of contagion.

When HIV/AIDS was first recognized in 1981, few thought that persons with HIV/AIDS would ever have rehabilitation potential. At that time, AIDS was medically diagnosed only after HIV had completely destroyed the immune system. Medical progress has transformed HIV/AIDS from a severely activity-limiting condition with a very short survival time, into a condition with significant rehabilitation potential. The important medical advances which have occurred over the past 30 years have improved both the quantity and quality of life for persons with HIV/AIDS. Many HIV-affected persons can now benefit from early recognition of rehabilitation potential, establishment of therapeutic goals, and prompt referral to a rehabilitation counselor.

This chapter presents a comprehensive overview of the medical aspects of HIV/AIDS. First, the chapter discusses the modes of HIV transmission, prevention of HIV infection, and the natural history of HIV infection. Second, the chapter presents the clinical manifestations of HIV/AIDS. The chapter then describes treatment strategies against HIV itself (primary treatment) and against the different types of HIV-related infections and tumors (secondary treatment). Lastly, the chapter focuses on the functional and vocational limitations associated with HIV/AIDS, and on the rehabilitation potential for persons affected by this disease.

Modes of HIV Transmission

HIV infection occurs through the introduction of HIV-containing blood cells or bodily fluids from an infected individual into the bloodstream of an uninfected person. This occurs either through sexual or blood-related contact.

Sexual Contact

Sexual transmission is the most common mode of HIV transmission. Penetrative sexual intercourse involving the passage of HIV-containing white blood cells and bodily fluids, such as semen or vaginal secretions, can result in HIV transmission. The efficiency with which sexual contact transmits HIV varies with the particular type of sexual practice and gender of the sexual partners involved. Epidemiologic data points to anal intercourse between two males, especially for the receptive partner, as the most efficient means of sexual transmission.

Blood Contact

HIV transmission can occur through blood-related contact in different ways. Whole blood from an HIV-infected blood donor can be transfused to an uninfected person, or a blood-clotting factor isolated from the blood of an HIV-infected blood donor can be transfused into an uninfected person with a blood-clotting disorder. HIV transmission through blood contact has markedly decreased in the United States due to mandatory screening of all blood donations and heat inactivation of blood-clotting products.

Shared needle behavior through intravenous drug use accounts for most blood-related HIV transmissions. Intravenous drug users often share their *equipment* (e.g., needles or syringes) with other drug users. This equipment can contain minute amounts of HIV-infected blood, and when shared with an uninfected person, HIV transmission may occur. HIV can also be transmitted from an infected pregnant woman to her fetus. This route of HIV transmission, called maternal-fetal transmission or *vertical transmission*, accounts for most of the cases of pediatric HIV/AIDS globally. Before the advent of anti-HIV therapies, approximately half the infants born to HIV-infected mothers developed clinical HIV/AIDS. The use of medications have dramatically decreased the proportion of babies infected from HIV-infected mothers.

HIV can also be transmitted inadvertently in a health care setting. The routes of transmission that occur in these occupational settings are needlestick (sharp object injuries) and direct skin or mucous membrane contact with blood or other potentially infectious materials. For example, HIV can be transmitted when an uninfected health care worker is stuck with a needle or cut with a scalpel which contains blood from an HIV-infected patient (Marcus & Centers for Disease Control [CDC], 1988). The greatest risk in occupational exposure occurs when a healthcare worker sustains a needlestick injury with a large volume of blood from a patient whose blood contains a high HIV concentration (Daily, 1997).

Prevention of HIV Transmission

General Measures

Public health education is directed at interrupting the sexual transmission of HIV among high risk individuals by encouraging people to engage in safe sex practices (using condoms during sexual intercourse), and by avoiding shared needle behaviors through intravenous drug use.

HIV Vaccine

Development of an effective HIV vaccine has faced immense challenges (Baden & Dolin, 2012). For instance, the natural immune response against HIV is inadequate and this process fails to eradicate the virus. Furthermore, HIV quickly integrates itself into the DNA of the host cell, where it can hide, remain latent, and essentially be invisible to the immune system. Finally, the extraordinary ability of HIV to mutate makes it substantially more complex than any other human virus, potentially making any vaccine obsolete very quickly (Johnston & Fauci, 2008). Despite these formidable obstacles, numerous HIV/AIDS vaccine formulations have been tested since 1988, but none have, as yet, proven successful.

Natural History of HIV Infection

Acute Retroviral Syndrome

Most people infected with HIV are initially unaware of the infection, although a few individuals experience symptoms of a condition called *acute retroviral syndrome*. Acute HIV infection is called *retroviral syndrome* because HIV is a member of the family of viruses called *retrovirus*.

The natural history of acute HIV infection is characterized by a very high level of HIV viremia (the presence of virus in the blood) and a vigorous immune response (Rosenberg, 1997). During the peak of HIV viremia, the CD4+ helper T-lymphocyte cell count (major target of HIV) declines precipitously and the CD8 cytotoxic T-lymphocyte cell count increases to fight the invading HIV. Within 5 to 30 days of initial HIV infection, during the peak of HIV viremia and CD4+ and CD8 immunological activity, some individuals become acutely ill with symptoms of acute retroviral syndrome (Cohen, Shaw, McMichael, & Haynes, 2011a). Acute retroviral syndrome manifests itself as a flu-like illness characterized by fever, swollen lymph nodes, sore throat, rash, fatigue, weight loss, and myalgias (muscle aches) and lasts about 14 days.

HIV Antibody Formation

A prolonged period of well-being follows recovery from acute retroviral syndrome, during which time the HIV viral load in the blood decreases, the number of CD4+ T-lymphocytes increases, and HIV antibodies become detectable. Most individuals do not realize they are infected with HIV until they undergo a blood test for the presence of HIV antibodies and are told they are *HIV positive*. HIV antibody testing is usually performed in an outpatient clinic setting, but *home test collection systems* (where the individual collects the blood at home, sends the sample to a laboratory, and then telephones an information line for the result) and *true home tests* (where the individual actually performs the test at home) are increasingly being utilized. In late 2006, the CDC issued recommendations that urged all health care providers in the United States to include HIV testing as a routine part of their patients' healthcare. In this way, more people can learn whether they are HIV-infected, allowing them to benefit from earlier access to treatment and reducing the risk of infecting their partners (CDC, 2006b). The presence of detectable HIV antibodies in the blood is the most common way a person is diagnosed as HIV positive (CDC, 1992).

Progressive Immunodeficiency

Even though a person can remain asymptomatic for long periods after being infected with HIV, the virus begins to destroy the body's immune system almost immediately after HIV infection occurs. The virus spreads throughout the body, infecting the entire immune system (including circulating blood cells, like CD4+ T-lymphocytes, and stationary tissues such as the lymph nodes) as well as many other cells of the body (Stebbing, Gazzard, & Douek, 2004).

The immunological destructive process begins at the cellular level when the virus attaches itself to a particular white blood cell, the CD4+ T-lymphocyte. Once inside the white blood cell, HIV replicates into tens of thousands of new HIV particles, a process which eventually kills the CD4+ T-lymphocyte. Since this cell is responsible for coordinating the body's immune response to certain invading microorganisms, the relentless destruction of CD4+ cells is the major cause of the progressive immunodeficiency, the hallmark of HIV/AIDS.

The destruction of CD4+ T-lymphocytes due to continuous low level viral replication is a constant feature of the *untreated*, infected state. At the time of initial HIV infection, there is a short but intense burst of HIV replication. The body responds by forming HIV antibodies and producing a surge in the number of CD8 lymphocytes. As a result, viral replication partially subsides. In fact, the laboratory discovery that HIV replication is very rapid during the clinical latent period (average daily production of 10^{10} HIV copies) was the impetus for development of a new approach to anti-HIV or antiretroviral treatment, called highly active retroviral treatment or *HAART* (Dybul et al., 2002). Earlier and more aggressive antiretroviral treatment of HIV with multiple antiviral medications has become the standard of primary treatment for HIV/AIDS.

Throughout the period of time while infected individuals are without symptoms, HIV continues to replicate, damaging an increasing amount of CD4+ cells. The pace of this destructive process against the immune system varies. Even though the vast majority of HIV-infected individuals experience several years of relative immunological and clinical stability (median time period is about ten years), a small percentage experience rapid immunological progression to advanced HIV disease despite adequate antiretroviral therapy (rapid progressors). Approximately 5% of HIV-infected persons maintain a normal CD4+ T-lymphocyte cell count and an undetectable viral load for long periods of time (*long-term nonprogressors*). During this long latent period when an individual is without symptoms, infected individuals may unknowingly transmit HIV to others by sexual transmission or through blood contact.

Clinical Manifestations

Early HIV Disease

When the AIDS epidemic was initially identified, the CDC defined AIDS to facilitate tracking the number of persons who manifested the syndrome. According to the original 1981 CDC surveillance case definition, AIDS existed under two conditions. First, the individual had to be diagnosed with one of the qualifying types of infections or tumors, which were moderately indicative of the presence of a cellular immunodeficiency. Second, the individual could *not* have any known medical reason to have such an infection or tumor, such as receiving chemotherapy for cancer or receiving medications associated with the development of immunosuppression (CDC, 1981). In 1986, the AIDS surveillance case definition was refined to take into account the development (in 1984) of the HIV antibody test (CDC, 1987). In 1992, the CDC recognized that HIV infection resulted in a spectrum of levels of HIV-generated disease: asymptomatic, early, and late or advanced disease (AIDS).

The criteria for HIV infection for persons over 13 years of age include: (1) a positive HIV antibody screening and confirmatory test; and (2) direct identification of the virus in host tissues by isolation, HIV antigen detection, or a positive result by any other highly specific licensed test for HIV. In their 1992 revision, the CDC emphasized the importance of measuring the number or percentage of CD4+ T-lymphocytes and provided three categories based on such measurements: (1) Category 1, which means a count of greater or equal to 500 CD4+ lymphocytes per microliter; (2) Category 2, which indicates 200 to 499 CD4+ cells per microliter; and (3) Category 3, which means a count of less than 200 CD4+ cells per microliter. Currently, an individual is said to have *AIDS* when they have laboratory confirmation of HIV infection (e.g., a positive HIV antibody test) and a CD4+ T-lymphocyte count of less than 200 CD4+ cells or a CD4+ T-lymphocyte percentage of total lymphocytes less than 14% (CDC, 1992; Social Security Administration [SSA], 2005).

In addition to laboratory testing, CDC has defined three clinical categories of HIV infection (CDC, 1992). Category A consists of asymptomatic HIV infection, persistent generalized swelling of the lymph nodes, or acute retroviral infection. Category B consists of a variety of symptomatic conditions that meet at least one of the following criteria: (a) the condition is attributed to HIV infection or is indicative of a defect in cell-mediated immunity; or (b) the condition is considered by a physician to have a clinical course, or to require management that is complicated by HIV infection. Examples of Category B conditions include: oral candidiasis (thrush), persistent vulvovaginal candidiasis, oral hairy leukoplakia, herpes zoster (shingles), and peripheral neuropathy.

In general, early symptomatic HIV disease (Category B) is characterized by relatively non-specific signs (what the physician notices) and symptoms (what the patient notices). These include swollen glands or lymph nodes, mild intermittent fever, and fatigue or low energy. In people with early symptomatic HIV disease, these signs and symptoms worsen while new symptoms appear. Left untreated, HIV-infected individuals begin to manifest daily fever, night sweats, fatigue and weakness, weight loss, intermittent diarrhea, oral thrush or candidiasis (yeast growing on the tongue and along the sides of the mouth), and experience various immunodeficiency-related skin conditions or rashes.

Advanced HIV Disease

The CDC's Clinical Category C includes qualifying infectious diseases and types of cancer. When present, any of these conditions result in a diagnosis of advanced HIV disease or AIDS. Qualifying conditions for a diagnosis of AIDS under CDC's Clinical Category C include: candidiasis of the lungs or esophagus; invasive cervical cancer; disseminated or extrapulmonary coccidiodomycosis; extrapulmonary cryptococcosis; cytomegalovirus eye disease with loss of vision; encephalopathy; herpes simplex ulcers over one month in duration or involving the lungs or esophagus; disseminated or extrapulmonary histoplasmosis; chronic intestinal isosporiasis; Kaposi's sarcoma; Burkitt's, immunoblastic or brain lymphoma; tuberculosis; disseminated or extrapulmonary *Mycobacterium avium* complex; *Pneumocystis carinii* pneumonia (PCP); recurrent pneumonia; progressive multifocal leukoencephalopathy; salmonella septicemia; toxoplasmosis of the brain; and wasting syndrome. Once a Category C infectious disease or type of cancer has occurred, the person remains in Category C whether or not the disease or cancer condition improves or is cured with treatment.

The infections included in Category C are caused by different bacterial, viral, fungal, or protozoal organisms. These organisms share in common an inherently low level of virulence or ability to harm individuals with competent immune systems. Since these microorganisms rarely cause disease in immunocompetent individuals, they are called *opportunistic infections.* Opportunistic infections take advantage of the *opportunity* of the body's defenseless posture caused by HIV to produce infection. Before the introduction of HAART in 1996, the most common opportunistic infectious disease seen in advanced HIV disease was *Pneumocystis carinii* pneumonia or *PCP* (Thomas & Limper, 2004). The number of patients with advanced HIV disease and AIDS who present with PCP has declined significantly; the most frequent complications of advanced HIV or AIDS involving the chest have become acute bronchitis, bacterial pneumonia, and, increasingly, hospitalizations for cardiac conditions (Grubb et al., 2006).

Treatment Strategies

Due to medical advances in the treatment of HIV/AIDS, deaths from HIV/AIDS decreased 75%, and the occurrence of AIDS-defining diseases decreased by 73% between 1994 and 1997 (Palella et al., 1998). Persons with HIV/AIDS now function at higher levels for longer periods of time (Dybul et al., 2002) due to advances in antiretroviral therapy (primary treatment) and advances in treating the infections and tumors that make up AIDS (secondary treatment).

Primary Treatment

Primary treatment can be directed either at interrupting the life cycle of the virus itself (antiretroviral therapy) or aimed at positively modulating the body's immune response to the virus (immunomodulator therapy). Both types of primary treatment are designed to contain HIV growth, one by suppressing viral growth, the other by boosting the body's protective immune response against HIV. Both antiretroviral therapy and immunomodulator therapy have the goal of preventing the development of secondary infections and tumors associated with advanced HIV disease or AIDS (see Category C, infectious diseases and types of cancer listed above).

Several classes of antiretroviral medications have been discovered to be effective against HIV. The first class of antiretroviral medications developed were nucleoside analogs that inhibited a vital enzyme HIV used to reproduce itself called reverse-transcriptase. This class of anti-HIV drugs are called nucleoside reverse transcriptase inhibitors (NNTIs). In 1986, a nucleoside analog called zidovudine (AZT) was the first antiretroviral medication shown to prolong the lives of persons with AIDS.

In the 1990s, significant knowledge about the life cycle of HIV was discovered, making it possible to design drugs that interrupt different phases of HIV's life cycle. Two additional classes of antiretroviral drugs—non-nucleoside reverse transcriptase inhibitors (NNRTIs) and protease inhibitors (PIs)—were introduced in the 1990s. Protease inhibitors block HIV replication in the late phase by binding to HIV protease which stops maturation of newly formed HIV virus, and as a result the capsid of the virus does not form properly (Stix, 2006). By 1996, the widespread use of these newer medications—especially protease inhibitors—markedly reduced the mortality rate associated with HIV/AIDS.

Antiretroviral medications of these major classes are now used in simultaneous combination—HAART. *HAART* is the simultaneous administration of three to four or more antiretroviral medications. The therapeutic aim of combination therapy is complete suppression of HIV growth as measured by the viral load early in the course of HIV infection (Friedland, 1990). An *undetectable* viral load serves as laboratory confirmation that HIV growth has been suppressed. HAART therapy has been credited for prolonging the life of persons living with advanced HIV disease or AIDS by an estimated 13 years (Walensky et al., 2006).

Two newer classes of antiretroviral drugs include: (1) fusion or entry inhibitors which interfere with HIV's ability to fuse with the cellular membrane, thereby blocking entry of HIV into the CD4+ T-lymphocyte and interfering with an essential early step in viral replication (Poveda, Briz, Quinones-Mateu, & Soriano, 2006); and (2) integrase inhibitors which inhibit the complex, multi-step process of integration of HIV provirus into the host genome (Havlir, 2008; Walmsley et al., 2013). Another class of antiretroviral medication, maturation inhibitors, is still in development (Nguyen et al., 2011). If successful, they could potentially prevent HIV from properly assembling and maturing. For example, these treatments could block HIV from forming a protective outer coat or from emerging from human cells.

Drug Resistance

HIV's inherent mutability can make it resistant to even the newest anti-retroviral medication or an entire class of medications. The phenomenon of viral resistance was demonstrated shortly after the introduction of the first antiretroviral, AZT (Larder, Darby, & Richman, 1989). As many as half of HIV infected persons under treatment have been found to be infected with viruses that are resistant to at least one drug in their current combination therapy regime (Richman et al., 2004). When resistance is identified, patients must have their drug regiment changed to continue viral suppression. Even under current HAART regimens, patients must continue taking medications, and change them frequently, because of residual replication-competent HIV hiding in viral reservoirs throughout the body. However, innovative approaches are being tried to purge HIV from these latent viral reservoirs which would greatly aid in long-term suppression of the virus (Marsden & Zack, 2009).

Side Effects

Even when viral suppression is achieved, antiretroviral medications can produce serious side effects which often necessitate discontinuation of a medication. The most common side effects include lowered red cell count (anemia), fatigue, headaches, sore tongue, nausea, vomiting, muscle aches, hepatitis and pancreatitis, numbness and pain in the arms and legs (peripheral neuropathy), elevated blood sugar (diabetes mellitus), elevated fats in the blood (hypertriglyceridemia), and fat wasting of face and limbs with central obesity (peripheral lipodystrophy) (Dube & Sattler, 1998; Lenhard et al. 2000). As each new antiretroviral medication is introduced into practice, new side effects emerge. Even for people living with HIV/AIDS and employed, management of side effects can pose a challenge for them and their rehabilitation counselor.

Immunomodulation Therapy

Primary treatment also can be directed at *boosting* the function of the body's immune system (immunomodulation). Several drugs are available that do not interrupt the life cycle of HIV within the body, but improve the immune system's ability to defend itself. For example, chemicals that are naturally produced by the cells of the body's immune system to fight infections, such as interferons and interleukins, are now synthesized in the laboratory. They can be given to HIV-infected individuals to help their immune system overcome HIV infection. Another form of immunomodulation that shows promise in augmenting the body's immune defenses against HIV involves the use of *therapeutic vaccines*. The goal of vaccine therapy in already infected individuals is to induce the immune system to better recognize, and more effectively fight HIV than it does in response to natural HIV infection.

HIV Eradication

Success in the treatment of HIV/AIDS has given rise to the hope that HIV can be completely eradicated after the administration of a sufficiently lengthy period of antiretroviral suppressive therapy. Two obstacles, however, lie in the path of achieving complete HIV eradication. First, there are various HIV-infected tissue compartments, such as the germinal centers of lymph nodes, which cannot be reached by antiretroviral drugs. Unless HIV can be destroyed in these so-called *sanctuary sites*, complete eradication of the disease is difficult. Second, even after an undetectable level of HIV is attained following a lengthy period of antiretroviral suppressive therapy, HIV is still capable of regrowth. This is possible because of the prolonged life span of some *latently infected cells*, which after undergoing cell division, can serve as a source of infectious HIV (Wong et al., 1997a, 1997b). However, there has been one well documented case of an HIV-infected adult who experienced complete eradication of replication-competent HIV-1 after a hematopoietic stem cell transplant (Hutter et al., 2009). Even though the goal of complete viral eradication of HIV remains elusive, it has become the subject of considerable research (Hammer, 2013).

Antiretroviral Treatment as Prevention

Until an effective HIV treatment is a reality, public health efforts are directed in identifying HIV-infected individuals and treating them early in the course of infection with antiretroviral therapy (Hammer, 2011). During the past 20 years, the use of antiretroviral therapy for the prevention of HIV has been carefully studied. Evidence that antiretroviral treatment of a HIV-infected partner reduces the rate of infection in the HIV negative partner and that immediate therapy slows progression in a newly-infected person now is strong (Cohen et al., 2011b). These findings have led to the *test and treat* approach to prevent the spread of HIV. The premise of *test and treat* is that HIV/AIDS can be eliminated from society if all adults are tested for the presence of HIV and treated with antiretroviral medications regardless of their level of immunodeficiency (Health Resources and Services Administration [HRSA], 2012).

Secondary Treatment

Secondary treatment is directed not against HIV itself, but against the specific infections and tumors that are indirectly caused by HIV infection. Secondary therapies are aimed at curing or controlling the HIV/AIDS infections and tumors.

Functional Limitations

Energy-restricting disorders are the most common functional impairments resulting from HIV/AIDS infection. Fatigue often occurs, especially in individuals who have a low CD4+ T-lymphocyte cell count. As HIV-related immunodeficiency progresses, persons infected with HIV begin to experience decreased states of energy that restrict activities of daily living. Employed individuals with HIV not well controlled on medications experience frequent exhaustion, and often require midday rest periods.

Respiratory and Cardiac Disorders

A major contributor to energy restriction in advanced HIV disease is the presence of a respiratory infection. The single most common AIDS-defining disease is PCP which causes shortness of breath and fatigue during an acute episode and persists for weeks after recovery. Other potentially disabling respiratory conditions include respiratory tuberculosis, bacterial pneumonias, cytomegalovirus (CMV) pneumonia, and respiratory Kaposi's sarcoma. HIV can also affect the heart, causing an inflammation of the heart muscle itself (myocarditis) or the thin lining around the heart (pericarditis). Both conditions restrict energy by causing shortness of breath, chest pain, and fatigue.

Gastrointestinal Disorders

Individuals infected with HIV often have functional impairments caused by gastrointestinal disorders. Chief among these are infectious and non-infectious diarrheal diseases that cause prolonged bouts of profuse diarrhea, impairing a person's ability to absorb vital nutrients from food. This malabsorption causes progressive weight loss, profound fatigue, and an aversion to food out of fear of triggering diarrhea. In addition, painful oral lesions are common in HIV infection and include recurrent and painful aphthous ulcers (canker sores) and fungal and viral conditions like candidiasis and herpes simplex, which may impair the ability to chew.

Liver Disorders

Hepatitis C virus (HCV) and hepatitis B virus (HBV) infections are common in HIV-infected individuals because of shared routes of viral transmission. Liver disease due to chronic HBV and HCV infection is becoming a leading cause of death among persons with HIV infection worldwide; risk of death related to liver disease is inversely related to the CD4+ cell count (Koziel & Peters, 2007). An increase in the incidence of hepatocellular carcinoma and hepatotoxic effects associated with antiretroviral drugs in patients with HCV and HBV co-infection has been observed (Weber & the Data Collection on Adverse Events of Anti-HIV Drugs Study Group, 2006).

Musculoskeletal Disorders

In addition to internal organs, HIV affects joint, muscle, and bone tissues. Prevalence of musculoskeletal disorders in individuals affected with HIV is high (up to 50%) and increases with disease progression. Arthralgias (painful joints) and frank arthritis (inflammation of the joints) are the most common forms of musculoskeletal disorders. The following three conditions involve the muscles: (1) AZT myopathy (found in patients on AZT and manifested by proximal muscle weakness, myalgias, and muscle wasting); (b) HIV-related polymyositis (muscle weakness in patients not on AZT); and (c) infectious myositis (tenderness and swelling of a muscle caused by staphylococcal bacteria) (Rodriguez, 1998). Management of musculoskeletal pain includes the use of analgesic medications (some of which produce drowsiness and impaired judgment). The physician may prescribe physiotherapy, hypnosis, acupressure, or acupuncture. Musculoskeletal disorders associated with HIV can partially or totally impair ambulation because of pain or muscle weakness in one or both legs.

Neurological and Sensory Disorders

Nearly 20% of patients with HIV/AIDS experience some neurological dysfunction. Neurological disorders related to HIV include: (1) those that affect the central nervous system (brain and spinal cord); (2) those affecting the peripheral nervous system (nerves to the arms and legs); and (3) those affecting sensory organs, such as the eyes.

Disorders affecting the peripheral nervous system include painful sensory neuropathies of the arms and legs that result in pain and weakness, both of which restrict an individual's activities. Impairment of the brain causes limitations ranging from serious (such as recurrent seizures due to an opportunistic infection or a tumor) to mild (such as mild dementia or mental slowness due to an HIV-related cognitive impairment). Opportunistic infections and tumors, which can affect the central nervous system, include toxoplasmosis (a protozoan infection causing seizures), cryptococcal meningitis (a fungal infection causing inflammation of the lining of the brain), and various types of brain tumors, such as lymphoma. In addition, sub-acute encephalitis (AIDS encephalopathy or *AIDS dementia complex*) is the most insidious neurological problem. Symptoms such as poor memory, inability to concentrate, verbal and motor slowing, affective and behavioral changes, and social apathy are the chief manifestations of AIDS dementia (CDC, 2006a). Individuals with AIDS dementia complex manifest a myriad of cognitive impairments, such as short-term memory deficits and a decrease in concentration ability, as well as affective and behavioral disorders ranging from impatience, irritability and mania, to apathy, social withdrawal, and even psychosis. Finally, sensory organs like the eye can be affected by HIV. Most commonly, visual loss due to infection of the retina either by HIV itself or by cytomegalovirus (CMV) can occur. A person who loses any degree of vision faces physical challenges, such as loss of reading and writing, mobility impairments, and other daily living limitations.

Metabolic Disorders

The most debilitating metabolic complication is called *HIV wasting syndrome* and its severity correlates with the level of immunodeficiency. The HIV wasting syndrome is manifested by weight loss (in excess of 10% from baseline), weakness, chronic diarrhea, and fever. Wasting is thought to be caused by a combination of factors including: (1) the body's on-going immunologic response to HIV; (2) the number and severity of opportunistic infections in any one individual; (3) inadequate nutrition secondary to poor oral intake or malabsorption of nutrients due to diarrheal disorders; and (4) any androgen deficiency present. Successful treatment depends on anti-retroviral therapy, treatment of secondary infections and tumors, adequate nutrition, and measures to correct underlying androgen deficiency (Reiter, 1996).

Emotional Disorders

The psychological reaction to impairments caused by HIV depends chiefly on the severity and rate of progression of the particular impairment, the underlying personality of the affected individual, including self-image and coping style, any neuropsychiatric changes caused by HIV itself, and the reaction of those around the patient to the condition. The extent of the patient's social support network and quality of psychological care available are crucial factors. Emotional disturbances are common, the most common of which are depression and anxiety (Basu, Chwastiak, & Bruce, 2005).

Emotional problems increase when a previously stable person infected with HIV develops an AIDS-defining disease. Loss of health, earning power, enjoyable activities, and sex life, coupled with having to experience premature old age and disability produce profound depression and suicidal ideation. The primary psychological effects of HIV/AIDS intensify a person's physical impairments. Disturbances of sleep, appetite, and weight are only a few of the physical effects that can be a direct result of the emotional manifestations associated with HIV disease. Undiagnosed and untreated mental illnesses already present in an individual are compounded by the knowledge of having to face a life with HIV/AIDS (Basu et al., 2005).

Social Factors

Social factors can exert significant effects on health and rehabilitation. A person's ethnic and cultural background, marital status, family support system, educational level, financial capability, and vocational background have an effect on the provision of rehabilitation services. Understanding the social aspects that influence the daily life of a person with HIV/AIDS is important since the disease is transmitted mostly through sexual contact and shared needle behaviors, both of which are fundamentally social phenomena (Friedman, Kippax, Phaswana-Mafuya, Rossi, & Newman, 2006).

A great challenge facing rehabilitation for a person with HIV infection or disease is that of overcoming the social limitations associated with HIV/AIDS. The HIV epidemic has elicited very strong responses from society as HIV transmission involves forms of behavior that are either illegal or socially taboo. The groups at greatest risk for becoming infected with HIV and developing AIDS, men who have sex with men and intravenous drug users, have traditionally been the subject of legal sanctions and social stigma. Further, HIV/AIDS affects a disproportionate number of African-Americans and Latinos, racial and ethnic groups already the subject of various social limitations and prejudices (Darbes, Crepaz, Lyles, Kennedy, & Rutherford, 2008; An et al., 2012).

Vocational Limitations

Vocational rehabilitation services for persons with HIV/AIDS makes an individualized approach to rehabilitation crucial. Although no single method of evaluation can be applied universally, three questions should be stressed. Is the individual able to return to his or her previous job or occupation? Are the skills or abilities of the person transferable to a new job? In conjunction with the medical and emotional factors, what type of rehabilitation training needs to be conducted to facilitate reemployment? (Matheson, 1984).

Young adults are most commonly affected by HIV/AIDS, ranging from 20 to 40 years of age. Although they may later seek disability benefits, people living with HIV/AIDS can remain in the workforce, although accommodations may be needed. Prior to the advent of effective antiretroviral therapies, many persons could not continue working at their prior levels of activity. They had to quit their jobs because of functional impairments; some resigned or were fired after the employer learned about their condition. Now, more individuals with HIV/AIDS are maintained on effective antiretroviral medications and can continue to work but may need vocational assessment and rehabilitation.

During vocational evaluation, physical, emotional, and social factors associated with HIV/AIDS need to be kept in mind. Individuals have different levels of medical stability given the different side effects from antiretroviral medications they are taking. Unlike impairments that reach a level of permanence before the process of vocational rehabilitation begins, impairments associated with HIV/AIDS are progressively and inherently unstable. A challenging factor in the vocational environment may be the lack of physical endurance to work a full day. A rehabilitation counselor can assess physical tolerance for work by ascertaining daily energy patterns and energy requirements expended in the home. Assistance in home management activities may save energy that can be used for work.

Individuals can develop various cognitive impairments secondary to those which affect the central nervous system. Moderate to severe degrees of AIDS dementia complex manifested by memory deficits, lack of coordination, and poor concentration ability create difficulties in the work environment. Cognitive impairments may exist in any person infected with HIV and neuropsychological testing should be part of rehabilitation evaluation.

The presence of skin lesions on the face or other exposed surfaces of the body from Kaposi's sarcoma are physical sources of embarrassment for patients which may impede rehabilitation. Changes in facial appearance due to fat redistribution secondary to antiretroviral medications can lead to reluctance to participate in the work environment. The application of cosmetics to cover skin lesions may help a person overcome reluctance to enter the workforce.

Lastly, two social factors are particularly disabling for someone attempting to re-enter the workforce after being diagnosed with HIV. The most important factor relates to the incorrect belief that individuals infected with HIV pose a communicable disease risk in the workplace. The only possible risk of HIV transmission in the workplace is if an accident occurs resulting in blood from the individual infected with HIV coming into direct contact with the non-intact skin of a co-worker who is uninfected. Another social factor is the prejudicial treatment individuals with HIV infection face based on others' judgments or misconceptions about their sexual behavior or drug use. This prejudice may severely limit vocational rehabilitation.

Rehabilitation Potential

Rehabilitation potential for persons affected by HIV depends in large part on the level of their underlying immunodeficiency, the presence of any physical limitations arising from specific disorders, and complications from multi-drug treatments. Individuals with greater degrees of immunodeficiency, as measured by increases in their HIV viral load, or in reductions in their level of CD4+ T-lymphocytes, will have less residual capacity for rehabilitation. Severity of physical impairments frequently worsens with increased immunodeficiency. Many persons with HIV disease and severe immunodeficiency, however, manifest significant capabilities for rehabilitation. The development of effective antiretroviral therapies in the mid-1990s has greatly enhanced rehabilitation potential.

Since HIV/AIDS primarily affects previously healthy young adults, these individuals maintain fairly high rehabilitation potential. A minority are in the category of limited rehabilitation potential, usually those who remain untreated or who have had the condition for many years. The vast majority of persons have sufficient physical, mental, emotional, and educational capabilities to respond favorably to vocational rehabilitation. Rehabilitation counselors should note, that by 2012, half of the U.S. population living with HIV/AIDS will be older than 50 years of age (Mills, Barnighausen, & Negin, 2012).

An additional positive factor contributing to rehabilitation potential is the absence of severely disabling neuromuscular impairments such as spinal cord damage, loss of appendages, and reduction in arm or leg mobility. Most ambulatory individuals with HIV/AIDS have adequate residual neuromuscular capacity to engage in sedentary or higher exertional levels of work, and those with energy-restricting disorders usually maintain sufficient capacity to engage in sedentary to light work levels.

The rehabilitation counselor needs to conduct a comprehensive assessment of a person's strengths, capacities, and skills. As medical science improves the quality and length of life for those with HIV/AIDS, rehabilitation professionals will be called upon more frequently to help restore the individual's ability to live and work successfully, and to the fullest extent.

Case Study

Mr. James Dexter is 29 years of age and works in an oil refinery. Mr. Dexter did not finish high school, completing most of the 12th grade. His job title of equipment mechanic (petroleum production), *Dictionary of Occupational Titles (D.O.T.)* # 629.381-014 (United States Department of Labor, 1991), puts him in charge of the installation, maintenance, and repair of oil well drilling machinery and equipment. He uses hand tools and power tools, and reads diagrams and schematics to repair equipment such as pumps, transmissions, and diesel engines. All oil refinery mechanics run tests to insure that the equipment is fully functional. One to two years are required for proficiency in this field, which requires occasional lifting of 50 pounds and repetitive lifting and carrying of 25 pounds. Mr. Dexter worked as an oil-field equipment mechanic for six years.

Before this job, Mr. Dexter worked in the construction field as a Construction Worker II (construction), D.O.T# 869.687-026, a position which did not involve any skills but required lifting up to 120 pounds occasionally and 50 to 75 pounds repetitively. The job responsibilities included loading and unloading of building materials, tools, and supplies. Also involved were digging, spreading, and leveling dirt and gravel using a pick and shovel. Mr. Dexter held this job for four years.

In 2010, Mr. Dexter developed a painful tingling sensation on the left side of his chest, followed the next day by water blisters in the same area. He was diagnosed with shingles (herpes zoster). His physician advised him that herpes zoster was a sign of an impaired immune system. He thought no more about it; after four weeks, the shingles disappeared.

In late 2010, James began to develop feelings of fatigue at work, especially when climbing the cracking towers at the oil refinery. Gradually, his fatigue worsened and his work performance began to decline. James never felt rested. His boss told him to "shape up" or he would be fired. In January 2011, his fatigue became severe and he lost 11 pounds. When he developed shortness of breath, a dry cough, and a fever, Mr. Dexter saw a physician, who diagnosed him with pneumonia. He was admitted to the hospital.

A thorough medical and social history revealed that, except for a broken leg in 2003, Mr. Dexter had been in good health all his life. James has been married for several years and has three young children but he and his wife have had marital difficulties. During a period of about two years, when he and his wife were separated, Mr. Dexter had sexual contacts with other women.

Mr. Dexter's pneumonia turned out to be caused by *Pneumocystis carinii*. His doctors became suspicious that he was infected with HIV and ordered an HIV antibody test which was positive. He was found to be severely immunodeficient with a CD4+ T-lymphocyte count of 127 (CDC CD4+ T-Lymphocyte Category 3) and an HIV viral load of 250,000 copies (normal is *undetectable*). His wife tested negative for the HIV antibody.

During hospitalization, James experienced intermittent diarrhea with no diagnosed cause. He lost about 30 pounds and developed CMV retinitis in the left eye which left him with a 50% visual loss in that eye, even after treatment with medication; he was hospitalized for a total of six weeks. Upon hospital discharge, James was sent home on three antiretroviral medications. After a tumultuous three weeks, his wife moved out with the children and filed for divorce. James considered suicide. His physician recommended emotional counseling, but Mr. Dexter turned it down.

After six months of convalescence, James began to feel better. His CD4+ T-lymphocyte count rose from 127 to 487, and his HIV viral load became undetectable. James decided to return to work. He has been experiencing pain in the muscles of his upper legs, which his physician thinks may be a myopathy due to his medications. Mr. Dexter believes he can work an eight-hour shift. The physician has restricted him light work activity.

Mr. Dexter wants to return to his previous job because he feels confident and physically fit enough to do the work. Concerned about his ability to support himself and his family, he desires to return to work as soon as possible. Recently, the oil company terminated his employment.

Questions

1. What is the nature of James Dexter's HIV-related disease and what are the possible physical limitations associated with his medical condition that may influence his rehabilitation potential?
2. What emotional limitations does Mr. Dexter have that need to be addressed during the process of rehabilitation?
3. Discuss the social limitations of James' medical condition.
4. What is this client's rehabilitation potential? Discuss the possibility of him returning to his previous job.

5. Provide a vocational profile including age category, educational level, exertional level of previous work, occupationally significant characteristics, and work skills. Note if any of Mr. Dexter's skills are transferable and, if so, to what jobs.
6. Identify types of rehabilitation training that will facilitate his reemployment.

References

An, Q., Hernandez A, Prejean J, German E. J., Thompson H., & Hall H. I. (2012). Geographical differences in HIV infection among Hispanics or Latinos—46 states and Puerto Rico. *Morbidity and Mortality Weekly Report, 61*(40), 805–810.

Baden L. R., & Dolin, R. (2012). The road to an effective HIV vaccine. *New England Journal of Medicine, 366*(14), 1343–1344.

Basu, S., Chwastiak, L. A., & Bruce, R. D. (2005). Clinical management of depression and anxiety in HIV-infected adults. *AIDS, 19*, 2057–2067.

Centers for Disease Control and Prevention. (1981). Surveillance case definition for the acquired immunodeficiency syndrome. *Morbidity and Mortality Weekly Report, 30*, 305.

Centers for Disease Control and Prevention. (1987). Revision of the CDC surveillance case definition for acquired immunodeficiency syndrome. *Morbidity and Mortality Weekly Report, 36*, 1S–15S.

Centers for Disease Control and Prevention. (1992). 1993 revised classification system for HIV infection and expanded surveillance case definition for AIDS among adolescents and adults. *Morbidity and Mortality Weekly Report, 41*(RR-17), 1–19.

Centers for Disease Control and Prevention. (2006a). Twenty-five years of HIV/AIDS—United States, 1981-2006. *Morbidity and Mortality Weekly Report, 55*(21), 585–589.

Centers for Disease Control and Prevention. (2006b). Revised recommendations for HIV testing of adults, adolescents, and pregnant women in health-care settings. *Morbidity and Mortality Weekly Report, 55* (NoRR-14).

Cohen, M. S., Shaw, G. M., McMichael A. J., & Haynes B. F. (2011a). Acute HIV-1 infection. *New England Journal of Medicine, 364*, 1943–1954.

Cohen, M. S., Chen, X. Q., McCauley, M., Gamble, T., Hosseinipour, M. C., Kumarasamy, N., . . . Celentano, D. (2011b). Prevention of HIV-1 infection with early antiretroviral therapy. *New England Journal of Medicine, 365*(6), 493–505.

Daily, J. P. (1997). Postexposure prophylaxis for HIV. *AIDS Clinical Care, 9*(8), 59–66.

Darbes L., Crepaz, N., Lyles C., Kennedy G., & Rutherford, G. (2008). The efficacy of behavioral interventions in reducing HIV risk behaviors and incidence in sexually transmitted diseases in heterosexual African Americans. *AIDS, 22*, 1177–1194.

Dube, M. P., & Sattler, F. R. (1998). Metabolic complications of antiretroviral therapies. *AIDS Clinical Care, 10*(6), 41–44.

Dybul, M., Fauci, A. S., Bartlett, J. G., Kaplan, J. E., Pau, A. K., & Panel on Clinical Practices for Treatment of HIV. (2002). *Annals of Internal Medicine, 137*, 381–433.

Friedland, G. H. (1990). Early treatment for HIV: The time has come. *New England Journal of Medicine, 322*, 1000–1002.

Friedman, S. R., Kippax, S. C., Phaswana-Mafuya, N., Rossi, D., & Newman, C. E. (2006). Emerging future issues in HIV/AIDS social research. *AIDS, 20*, 959–965.

Gottlieb, M. S., Schroff, R., Schanker, H. M., Weisman, J. O., Fan, P. T., Wolf, R. A., & Saxon, A. (1981). Pneumocystis carinii pneumonia and mucosal candidiasis in previously healthy homosexual men: Evidence of a new acquired cellular immunodeficiency. *New England Journal of Medicine, 305*, 1425–1431.

Grubb, J. R., Moorman A. C., Baker, R. K., Masur, H., & the HOPS Investigators. (2006). The changing spectrum of pulmonary disease in patients with HIV infection on anti-retroviral therapy. *AIDS, 20,* 1095–1107.

Hammer S. M. (2011). Antiretroviral treatment as prevention. *New England Journal of Medicine, 365*(6), 561–562.

Hammer S. M. (2013). Baby steps on the road to HIV eradication. *New England Journal of Medicine, 369*(19), 1855–1856.

Havlir, D. V. (2008). HIV integrase inhibitors—Out of the pipeline and into the clinic. *New England Journal of Medicine, 359,* 416–418.

Health Resources and Services Administration (HRSA). (2012). *HRSA care action.* Retrieved from http://hab.hrsa.gov/newspublications/careactionnewsletter/hab_test_and_treat_january_careaction_pdf.pdf

Hutter, G., Nowak D., Mossner M., Ganepola, S., Müßig, A., Allers, K., ...Thiel E. (2009). Long-term control of HIV by CCR5 Delta32/Delta32 stem-cell transplantation. *New England Journal of Medicine, 360,* 692–698.

Johnston, M. I., & Fauci, A. S. (2008). An HIV vaccine – Challenges and prospects. *New England Journal of Medicine, 359,* 888–890.

Joint United Nations Programme on HIV/AIDS (UNAIDS). (2012). *UNAIDS World AIDS Day Report 2012.* Retrieved from http://www.unaids.org/en/resources/campaigns/20121120_globalreport2012/

Koziel, M. J., & Peters, M. G. (2007). Viral hepatitis in HIV infection. *New England Journal of Medicine, 356,* 1445–1454.

Larder, B. A., Darby, G., & Richman, D. D. (1989). HIV with reduced sensitivity to zidovudine (AZT) isolated during prolonged therapy. *Science, 243,* 1731–1734.

Lenhard, J. M., Furfine, E. S., Jain, R. G., Ittoop, O., Orband-Miller L. A., Blanchard S. G., ... Weiel, J. E. (2000). HIV protease inhibitors block angiogenesis and increase lipolysis in vitro. *Antiviral Research, 47*(2), 121–129.

Marcus, R., & Centers for Disease Control (CDC) Cooperative Needlestick Surveillance Group (1988). Surveillance of healthcare workers exposed to blood from patients infected with the human immunodeficiency virus. *New England Journal of Medicine, 319,* 1118–1122.

Marsden, M. D., & Zack, J. A. (2009). Eradication of HIV: Current challenges and new directions. *Journal of Antimicrobial Chemotherapy, 63,* 7–10.

Matheson, L. (1984). *Work capacity evaluation: Interdisciplinary approach to industrial rehabilitation.* Anaheim, CA: Employment and Rehabilitation Institute of California.

Mills E. J., Barnighausen T., & Negin J. (2012). HIV and aging—Preparing for the challenges ahead. *New England Journal of Medicine, 366*(14), 1270–1273.

Nguyen A. T., Feasley C. L., Jackson K.W., Nitz T. J., Salzwedd K., Air G. M., & Sakalian M. (2011). The prototype HIV-1 maturation inhibitor, bevirimat, binds to the CA-SP1 cleavage site in immature Gag particles. *Retrovirology 8*(11), 101–114.

Palella, F. J., Delaney, K. M., Moorman, A. C., & the HIV Outpatient Study Investigators. (1998). Declining morbidity and mortality among patients with advanced human immunodeficiency virus infection. *New England Journal of Medicine, 338,* 853–860.

Piot, P., & Quinn, T. C. (2013). Response to the AIDS pandemic—A global health model. *New England Journal of Medicine, 368,* 2210–2218.

Poveda, E., Briz, V., Quinones-Mateu, M., & Soriano, V. (2006). HIV tropism: Diagnostic tools and implications for disease progression and treatment with entry inhibitors. *AIDS, 20,* 1359–1367.

Reiter, G. S. (1996). The HIV wasting syndrome. *AIDS Clinical Care, 8*(11), 89–96.

Richman, D. D., Morton, S. C., Wrin, T., Hellman, N., Berry, S., Shapiro, M. F., & Bozzette, S. A. (2004). The prevalence of antiretroviral drug resistance in the United States. *AIDS, 18,* 1393–1401.

Rodriguez, W. (1998). Musculoskeletal manifestations of HIV disease. *AIDS Clinical Care, 10*(7), 49–52.

Rosenberg, E. (1997). Primary HIV infection and the acute retroviral syndrome. *AIDS Clinical Care, 9*(3), 19–25.

Social Security Administration (SSA). *Social Security for people living with AIDS.* SSA Publication No. 05-10019, February 2005. ICN 454510. Retrieved from http://www.socialsecurity.gov/pubs/10019.html

Stebbing J., Gazzard, B., & Douek D. C. (2004). Where does HIV live? *New England Journal of Medicine, 350,* 1872-1880.

Stix, G. (June, 2006), A new assault on HIV. *Scientific American,* 77–79.

Thomas, C. F., & Limper, A. H. (2004). Pneumocystis pneumonia. *New England Journal of Medicine, 350,* 2487–2498.

United States Department of Labor. (1991). *Dictionary of Occupational Titles* (4th ed., revised). Washington, D.C.: Author.

Walensky, R. P., Paltiel, A. D., Losina, E., Mercincavage, L. M., Schackman, B. R., Sax, P. E., . . . Freedberg, K. A. (2006). The survival benefits of AIDS treatment in the United States. *Journal of Infectious Diseases, 194,* 11–19.

Walmsley, S. L., Antela A., Clumeck, N., Duiculescu D., Eberhard, A., Gutierrez F., . . . Nichols, G. for the SINGLE Investigators (2013). Dolutegravir plus Abacavir—Lamivudine for the treatment of HIV-1 Infection. *New England Journal of Medicine, 369,* 1807–1818.

Weber, R., & the Data Collection on Adverse Events of Anti-HIV Drugs Study Group. (2006). Liver-related deaths in persons infected with the human immunodeficiency virus. *Archives of Internal Medicine, 166,* 1632–1641.

Wong, J. K., Ignacio, C. C., Torriani, F., Havlir, D., Fitch, N. J. S., & Richman, D. D. (1997a). In vivo compartmentalization of HIV: Evidence from the examination of pol sequences from autopsy tissues. *Journal of Virology, 71,* 2059–2071.

Wong, J. K., Hezareh, M., Gunthard, H. F., Havlir, D., Ignacio, C. A., Spina, C. A., & Richman, D. D. (1997b). Recovery of replication-competent HIV despite prolonged suppression of plasma viremia. *Science, 278,* 1291–1295.

On-Line References. The Internet hosts thousands of Web pages devoted to HIV infection and AIDS. Typically, these pages are more current than other sources of AIDS-related information. The United Nations' HIV/AIDS web site at http://www.unaids.org/en/ provides a current global perspective on HIV/AIDS. The U. S. Centers for Disease Control and Prevention offer the latest statistics about HIV/AIDS in the U. S. at http://www.cdc.gov/hiv/topics/surveillance/basic.htm. Current information about AIDS clinical drug trials is available at http://aidsinfo.nih.gov/. The state of current vaccine research is located at http://www.iavi.org/Pages/default.aspx

About the Author

John J. Howard, M.D., M.P.H., J.D., is Professorial Lecturer in Environmental and Occupational Health, School of Public Health and Health Services, The George Washington University, Washington, D.C. Dr. Howard is board-certified in internal medicine and occupational medicine. He is admitted to the practice of medicine and law in California and the District of Columbia.

Chapter 8

HEARING LOSS, DEAFNESS, AND RELATED VESTIBULAR DISORDERS

Shawn P. Saladin, Ph.D., C.R.C.
Sandra Hansmann, Ph.D.

Introduction

The ability to hear is a critical sensory function, yet hearing loss is the most common sensory disability. Although it can be challenging to accurately quantify the number of individuals who have hearing loss and other auditory disorders, one trend is clear—hearing loss among adults and children is increasing exponentially (National Research Council, 2005). By the year 2015, the number of people with hearing loss in the United States will reach nearly 13 million. The inability to hear has far reaching social and health related consequences and negatively impacts speech, language, academic, social, and vocational development (Luft, 2013).

This chapter reviews selected medical, psychosocial, and vocational aspects of major disorders of the auditory and vestibular systems that impact hearing and communication, specifically focusing on Deafness, hearing loss, and disorders associated with hearing loss. A brief overview of the anatomy of the ear is provided, followed by a discussion of basic hearing evaluation and classification techniques. Next, the chapter describes common disorders of the auditory system, followed by a description of several related conditions of the vestibular system. Treatment, management, and aural rehabilitation options are reviewed. The chapter explores functional limitations and related psychosocial and vocation implications of hearing loss and the rehabilitation potential of individuals who are Deaf or hard of hearing.

Anatomy of the Ear

To understand hearing disorders, it is helpful to have a basic understanding of anatomy of the human ear and the process through which sound waves are perceived as sound by the brain. The human ear includes two distinct but interrelated systems that provide important sensory functions— the auditory system (pertaining to the detection of sound) and the vestibular system (pertaining to balance, proprioception, and the detection of movement and acceleration).

The auditory system of the ear consists of three principle sections including the outer ear, middle ear, and inner ear (as shown in Figure 1). Sounds may consequently be conducted through the air into the outer, middle, and inner ear structures, or through the bones around the ear. Dysfunction in any one of the primary areas of the ear can result in difficulty hearing or the inability to hear.

The outer ear consists of the *pinna*, the externally visible part of the ear which is also called the *auricle*, and the ear canal up to the *tympanic membrane*, also known as the *eardrum*. Sound energy is collected by the pinna and then directed into the outer ear canal and onward to the tympanic membrane. The elastic cartilage of the pinna has an intricate funnel-like shape that facilitates the effective collection and transmission of sound energy into and through the ear canal (Koga, 2004). *Audition*, or hearing, begins when sound waves of various frequencies are created by vibrations in the environment. These vibrations travel through the atmosphere and reach the pinna.

FIGURE 1
The Auditory System

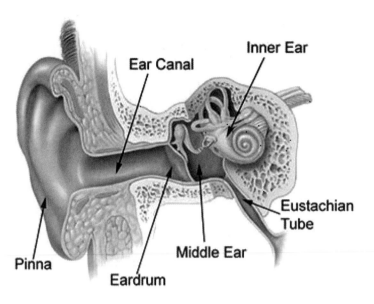

Source: Kaiser Permanente. (2012). *The basics of how we hear.* Retrieved from http://kphearingservices.com/hearinghealth/understandinghearingloss.html

The middle ear functions to transfer and amplify vibratory energy deeper into the inner ear, where it can be perceived as sound. It is an air-containing space that includes the inside of the tympanic membrane and the *ossicular chain*, made up of three very small bones known collectively as *ossicles* and individually as the *malleus, incus,* and *stapes*. The ossicles are often referred to as the hammer, anvil, and stirrup. The tympanic membrane seals the middle ear. In hearing, sound waves vibrate the tympanic membrane which then presses against and vibrates the ossicles. The incus lies between the malleus (attached to the middle ear) and the stapes, articulating the two. The middle ear also connects to the back of the nose and throat through the *eustachian tube*, which functions to maintain equal pressure between the middle ear and the external environment.

The inner ear is a complex fluid-filled structure that converts vibratory sound energy into nerve impulses perceivable by the brain. The inner ear contains a membranous structure, the *labyrinth*, which is surrounded by bone and is filled with perilymphatic fluid. The inner ear is involved in both auditory and vestibular functions, and its major structures include the *vestibule* and *semicircular canals*, and the *cochlea*. The stapes footplate in the middle ear is attached to the base of the *cochlea*, a crucial structure of the inner ear. The cochlea is a small, spiral structure that includes the *organ of Corti* to convert sound from mechanical vibrations into electrical signals through a process known as *transduction*. Transduction is performed by specialized sensory cells inside the organ of Corti— the inner and outer *hair cells* which include *stereocilia,* cellular projections that look like fine hairs. The movement of the stapes vibrates the stereocilia above and is connected to the auditory nerve root. In audition, the inner ear is of little use without an intact and functional *cranial nerve VIII* or *auditory nerve* to pass signals to the brain stem and brain. The brain plays a key role in the identification, localization, and understanding of sound (Martin & Clark, 2011). The vestibule contains the *utricle* and *saccule*, which help facilitate balance.

Hearing Assessment

Several considerations are relevant to assessment and categorization of hearing loss, including degree of severity, configuration, onset, and progression (Tye-Murray, 2008). Accordingly, the assessment of hearing ability may encompass a variety of subjective, objective, and alternative methodologies. Severity is quantified through tests of hearing ability, which have become increasingly accurate and standardized through use of commercial audiometers, devices for measuring pure tone air and bone conduction of sound. While a number of methods are available, pure tone audiometry, speech audiometry, and tympanometry are commonly encountered measures in rehabilitation and related settings.

Pure Tone Audiometry

Pure-tone audiometry is an established standardized method for evaluating hearing loss (American National Standards Institute, 2003). Audiometers are used to assess hearing and measure in *decibels* and *hertz*. Decibels (dB) measure the intensity or loudness of a sound, while the tone or pitch of a sound is expressed as hertz (Hz). Using pure-tone audiometry, an *audiologist* uses an *audiometer* to generate and measure the softest pure tone sound a person can hear to establish an *auditory sensitivity threshold* (National Research Council, 2005). The American National Standards Institute (1996, 2003) defined threshold as "the lowest input level at which responses occur in at least 50% of a series of ascending trials" (American National Standards Institute, 1996, p. 10).

During a test, the individual responds to high and low pure tones delivered over a wide range of frequencies. The audiologist repeats each sound at increasing lower volume until no sound can be heard. This type of testing, termed *air conduction testing*, relies on the transfer of sound waves to the inner ear through air. *Bone conduction audiometry* is an alternative procedure that uses a sound vibrator fitted to the bone behind each ear. Bone conduction testing covers a wide range of high and low sound frequencies repeated at decreasing volume (National Research Council, 2005).

Speech Audiometry and Tympanometry

Speech audiometry is conceptually similar to pure tone audiometry. It is used to determine the softest speech sounds a person can hear in each ear at approximately 50% accuracy, known as the speech awareness threshold (SAT) or speech reception threshold (SRT). Audiometric testing results are documented on an *audiogram* to provide a visual representation of severity of hearing loss in each ear. An important aspect of both audiograms and tympanograms is the information they provide about the configuration of an individual's hearing loss. *Tympanometry* is a measure of the stiffness of the eardrum and is used to evaluate middle ear function. This test is helpful in detecting fluid in the middle ear, negative middle ear pressure, tympanic membrane perforations, and disruption of the ossicles.

Configuration of Hearing Loss

Hearing *configuration* refers to the specific location, consistency, and quality of an individual's hearing difficulties. Determining the configuration of a person's hearing loss provides a more holistic view of hearing ability. Initially, a person may be described as having hearing loss in either one ear, termed a *unilateral hearing loss*, or as having a *bilateral hearing loss*, when both ears are affected. If the degree or severity of hearing loss is the same in both ears, the person has a *symmetrical* loss; if the degree differs in each ear, the loss is *asymmetrical* (Nicolosi, Harryman, & Kresheck, 2004). Configuration also includes the amount of hearing loss present at low, mid, and high frequencies (Tye-Murray, 2008). For example, a person who has difficulty hearing low frequencies, but no difficulties at higher frequency levels has a low-frequency hearing loss.

Definitions of Hearing Loss and Deafness

As with many health conditions, hearing loss severity may range from a very mild loss to profound Deafness. Before the field of audiology was developed, differences along the hearing loss continuum were imprecisely defined. Even today, precise definitions of Deafness and hearing loss vary. Not all definitions of hearing loss rely exclusively on numeric data, using instead functional self-reports or observations of hearing ability. As a result, there are both medical and cultural definitions related to hearing loss.

Medical Definitions

Most medical definitions of hearing loss rely on the average of audiometric test results at three specific frequencies, most often at 500, 1000, and 2000 Hz. Known as the pure tone average (PTA), this number is a basic indicator of how much hearing a person has in each ear independently without any type of amplification device (Hull, 2001). In general, six levels of hearing loss are calculated. Normal hearing ability is typified by sensitivity thresholds of 0 dB to 25 dB. ***Mild*** hearing loss is usually diagnosed when PTA results demonstrate a 26 dB to 40 dB threshold, while ***mild-to-moderate*** hearing loss is diagnosed in individuals who have a sensitivity threshold of 41 dB to 55 dB. An individual with a 56 dB to 70 dB threshold has a ***moderate*** hearing loss; with threshold ranges from 71 to 90 dB, a person has a ***severe*** hearing loss. Persons with a 90 decibel threshold or greater have a ***profound*** hearing loss. Diagnostic weight is given to the results of the better ear. People with hearing in the mild to moderate categories are considered ***hard of hearing*** while those with hearing loss assessed in the severe and profound categories are considered ***Deaf*** (Tye-Murray, 2008).

Cultural Definitions

Audiometric and functional definitions focus on severity and functional impact of hearing loss. Cultural definitions of Deafness, however, are grounded in personal choices about self-identification and language use. Thus, an individual may be identified as culturally Deaf, although he or she may only have a mild or moderate hearing loss from an audiological standpoint. The converse may also be true; a person may have an audiologically profound hearing loss but not identify with Deaf culture (Padden & Humphries, 2006). The term ***Deaf*** is capitalized when referring to people with hearing loss who identify themselves as part of the Deaf cultural group (Lane, Hoffmeister, & Bahan, 1996).

The cultural definition of Deafness represents a life and world view that is manifested by beliefs, values, and traditions unique to Deaf people and expressed through the use of American Sign Language (ASL). Within Deaf culture, the term ***hearing impaired*** is rejected because it reflects an illness-oriented medical paradigm that pathologizes Deaf people and negates the cultural component of Deafness. Deaf culture makes no distinction between person-first language and more Deaf-centric phrases such as ***Deaf person***, finding either option acceptable (Lane et al., 1996). This chapter uses the terminology and grammar preferred by the Deaf cultural community.

Onset and Progression of Hearing Loss

Onset and progression are important dimensions of hearing loss classification. Onset encompasses both the rapidity of hearing loss, and the life stage at which onset occurs. Progression refers to the course of the hearing loss. If a person's hearing loss occurs quickly and unexpectedly, it is considered a ***sudden*** hearing loss. If hearing status worsens slowly over time, an individual is said to have a ***progressive*** loss. A person may also have a ***fluctuating*** hearing loss, one that alternates in severity. When no such variability exists, the hearing loss is considered ***stable*** (Martin & Clark, 2011).

Hearing loss occurs at any life stage. When a person is Deaf or hard of hearing from birth or in the first days of life, the person has a ***congenital*** hearing loss. This may include ***pre-lingual*** hearing loss which refers to hearing loss occurring prior to development of speech. Pre-lingual hearing loss occurs before the age of two or three years (Kral & O'Donoghue, 2010). If hearing problems develop later in childhood or adulthood, an individual has an ***acquired*** hearing loss that is ***post-lingual***, because it has occurred after development of speech. Post-lingual hearing losses may be additionally classified as ***prevocational***, occurring when an individual is school aged (Tye-Murray, 2008). ***Late deafened*** is a term used to describe people whose hearing loss occurs well into adulthood.

Types of Hearing Loss

Deafness and hearing loss occur due to a wide variety of genetic, obstructive, neural, age-related, and environmental factors, several of which are discussed later in this chapter. Regardless of exact etiology, hearing loss is described as ***sensorineural***, ***conductive***, or ***mixed***. Hearing loss stemming from conditions of the inner ear or auditory nerve is sensorineural. Most often, sensorineural hearing loss is due to damage to the pathway for sound impulses from the hair cells of the inner ear to the auditory nerve and the brain (Katz & White, 2001). Damage may occur as a result of noise exposure, viruses, head trauma, and other causes.

Conductive hearing loss most often originates in the outer and middle portions of the ear. Most conductive hearing problems result from some form of interference that results in the inability of sound waves to conduct from the pinna into the ear to vibrate the tympanic membrane and inner ear structures (Kiessling et al., 2003). Examples of conditions that may result in a conductive hearing loss include blockage by wax, a punctured eardrum, an ear infection, and congenital or acquired irregularities in the outer and middle ear. A mixed hearing loss simply results from a combination of both conductive and sensorineural losses.

Specific Etiologies

The population of people with hearing loss and other auditory disorders is very diverse. Two accepted etiological categories of hearing loss are *acquired* and *genetic*. Acquired hearing loss is sometimes labeled *non-genetic hearing loss* and may be sensorineural, conductive, or mixed. Acquired hearing loss is related to a number of causes such as chronic infections, acoustical injury, occupation hearing loss, and aging. Other causes may include head injuries, inner ear disorders, and exposure to toxins (Martin & Clark, 2011). Genetic hearing loss is caused by differences or changes in genes; it may be inherited or occur as the result of an isolated gene mutation, and may be conductive, sensorineural, or mixed (Nance, 2003). This chapter section reviews several of the most common causes of acquired hearing loss, followed by an overview of key genetically linked causes of hearing loss.

Chronic Ear Infection

Infections of the middle ear and middle ear structures are called *otitis media (OM)*. Causes of the condition include bacterial infection, injury to the eardrum, and presence of fluid in the ear. Symptoms include a sensation of pressure in the ear, dizziness, and discharge. Ear pain may be present and range from mild to severe. Chronically occurring OM is defined as a perforation of the tympanic membrane that is permanent and occurs with or without permanent changes to the middle ear.

Injury

Injuries to either the external or internal structures of the ear can result in significant hearing-related problems. The external ear may be damaged in accidents. If the pinna is no longer able to adequately gather sound energy, hearing ability can be significantly impacted. Internally, the tympanic membrane may be punctured by penetrating objects such as cotton swabs, pencils, or other small sharp objects. Sudden pressure changes, including pressure changes associated with explosions can rupture the eardrum, such as in swimming and diving accidents. When the tympanic membrane is punctured, dislocation of the ossicular chain may occur, and the stapes footplate may fracture. Sudden hearing loss usually accompanies perforation of the eardrum, along with dizziness and ringing sensations in the ear. Most perforations close completely without medical intervention (National Research Council, 2005).

Noise-induced hearing loss (noise exposure seriously injuring the inner ear) (NIHL), is a common yet preventable health concern (Koga, 2004). Occupational, recreational, and accidental causes of noise-related hearing loss may include sound exposure through either continuous or impulse noise exposure. Continuous exposure occurs when an individual is frequently in environments that include noisy on-going sounds such as industrial machinery or loud music. It is often associated with employment settings in adults and with recreational settings in adolescents. Impulse exposure occurs when a person is exposed to sharp loud bursts of sound, such as gunshots or explosive blasts (Tambs, Hoffman, Borchgrevink, Holmen, & Engdahl, 2006). While NIHL has been closely linked to the volume, duration, and type of noise exposure, it is often due to a more complex interaction of factors, including age, psychological well-being, and lifestyle.

Otosclerosis

Otosclerosis is a common cause of hearing loss and can develop in late adolescence and early adulthood; it may develop rapidly during pregnancy. Primarily, otosclerosis results in a conductive hearing loss, but sensorineural loss may occur. As previously discussed, normal hearing results when sound enters the ear, vibrates the eardrum, and in turn, the malleus, incus, and stapes. Movement of the stapes vibrates fluids within the ear to stimulate the auditory nerve for hearing. This process can be impeded by *otosclerosis*, involving hardening or fixation of the stapes.

Presbycusis

Presbycusis refers to age-related hearing loss. It is actually a multidimensional disorder that spans not only hearing loss but also decreased auditory sensitivity. Presbycusis may cause social, psychological, and communication problems (Hull, 2001).

As humans age, both the external and internal structures of the ear undergo changes. During the aging process, the external ear, or pinna, may become less firm and elastic, while skin may thin and wrinkle, and hair growth inside the ear may increase. These changes act simultaneously to impact the effectiveness of the ear as a sound collection mechanism. Middle ear structures, including the tympanic membrane and ossicular chain, become more rigid with age, thus decreasing vibratory response, while the hair cells and cochlea of the inner ear may also deteriorate (Hull, 2001).

Ototoxicity

Ototoxicity refers to the negative effects some medications, solvents, and other substances have on the nerves and organs of the ear. Literally meaning ear poisoning, ototoxicity can result in deafness. A number of industrial chemicals are classified as ototoxic, including mercury, styrene, and carbon disulfide. Most individuals do not come into contact with these substances unless they work in occupations where they are in direct contact with industrial chemicals. More typically, people are exposed through medications (National Research Council, 2005). A number of non-prescription medications have ototoxic effects, but those derived from salicylic acid are most common. Aspirin is a popular salicylate; an estimated 50 billion tons are consumed annually worldwide (Prepageran & Rutka, 2004). In most instances, the ototoxic effects of salicylates are the result of long-term, high dose use. Usually, these effects are temporary, while in rare circumstances permanent hearing loss and other complications result, including balance dysfunction.

Prescription medications used in treatment for cancer, severe infection, and following organ transplantation can have ototoxic properties, especially with prolonged use or at high dosages. Chemotherapeutic and immunosuppressant medications can damage the hair cells of the inner ear, resulting in sudden deafness or permanent high frequency hearing loss and tinnitus (Gratton & Smyth, 2004). Some classes of antibiotics, especially when administered intravenously, may result in profound, irreversible sensorineural hearing loss

Vestibular Disorders

The vestibular system of the inner ear is responsible for orientation of sound location and balance. The system works in conjunction with visual images and head movement to send information to the brain regarding the physical orientation of the individual. Disturbances to this system, even when minor, may result in a variety of nonspecific sensations. **Tinnitus** is a condition characterized by the perception of sounds that originate in the head or ears rather than the environment itself (Sindhusake et al., 2003). More severe disruptions of the vestibular system may result in **vertigo** — the sensation of movement, usually rotational, when no actual movement is occurring. **Ménière's disease** is a complex disorder that combines symptoms of tinnitus, vertigo, and progressive hearing loss (Baloh & Jen, 2012).

Tinnitus

Tinnitus is one of the most prevalent disorders of the vestibular system. It is estimated that 36 to 50 million people in the United States have experienced some form of this disorder. Tinnitus is caused by damage to the nerve endings in the inner ear and may be symptomatic of other problems of the ear, including elevated blood pressure, diabetes, thyroid problems, injuries, and infections (Sindhusake et al., 2003). Symptoms of tinnitus include ringing, buzzing, or whining sounds originating in the head or ears. The sounds may be intermittent or continuous; intensity may vary from a dull rumble to a high whine or buzz. Most people do not report being overly disturbed or distressed by these symptoms, and may only be able to perceive the sounds in very quiet environments. Rarely, people experience severe symptoms that interfere with all aspects of life.

Vertigo

Vertigo is both a vestibular dysfunction and a symptom of other similar dysfunctions, including labyrinthitis or inner ear inflammation, tumors, brain hemorrhages or stroke, migraines, and multiple sclerosis. Imagined sensations of vertigo may be categorized as either subjective or objective. Abnormal eye movements and vision changes, hearing loss, nausea, tinnitus, imbalance, and gait disturbances are typical of the disorder. Symptoms may last just minutes, or may linger for hours, be either intermittent or continuous, and range from mild to severe (Ruka, 2004). Treatment of vertigo involves management of the underlying cause, whenever possible (Baloh & Jen, 2012).

Ménière's Disease

Ménière's disease is a disorder related to volume and pressure changes in the inner ear fluids. The early course of the condition can be mild and episodic, but over time progresses to a more severe unilateral hearing loss with worsening vertigo and tinnitus. Generally, a diagnosis is made following two or more clear episodes of spontaneous vertigo lasting a minimum of 20 minutes, with at least one episode of a sensation of fullness in the affected ear (Pullen, 2006).

Treatment Strategies

Once the underlying causes of auditory or vestibular disturbances are addressed, treatment and management of residuals may be considered. Treatment and management strategies for hearing loss, Deafness, and related vestibular disorders are dependent on the type, severity, and etiology of the condition (Eng & Learner, 2011; Luft, 2013). In this section, key treatment and management devices and strategies for hearing loss and vestibular disorders are reviewed.

Treatment and management of hearing loss is vital. The most common hearing management method involves use of assistive listening devices. Assistive listening devices are beneficial in the social and emotional areas, and include ***hearing aids*** and ***cochlear implants***.

Hearing Aids

Hearing aids are the most common listening device used to treat and manage hearing disorders. Simply stated, a hearing aid is a self-contained system used to amplify sound. They use a microphone to detect sounds, an amplifier to increase the level of sounds, and several filters to modify sound to the needs of the user and reduce background noise. Hearing aids are generally prescribed for people whose hearing thresholds are 25 dB or greater in the better ear, and are usually not sought until the person experiences noticeable difficulties in daily living (National Research Council, 2005). These difficulties become more pronounced at approximately a 40 dB threshold, or the point at which background noise markedly impacts hearing ability.

Air conduction or bone conduction hearing aids are available in a wide variety of styles and shapes, may use air or bone conduction to transmit sound, and are either analog or digital (Martin & Clark, 2011). Air conduction hearing aids use a receiver to amplify sound and direct it into the ear canal using vibratory sound waves moving through air. Bone conduction hearing aids are suitable for individuals who have conductive loss related to the middle ear, but have inner ear functioning.

Analog hearing aids generate signals that are analogous, or similar, to the sound energy they receive and then amplify those signals for use (Martin & Clark, 2011). Modern hearing aids operate by receiving and modifying sound signals (***signal processing***). Analog aids amplify all environmental sounds similarly and are thus appropriate for a variety of types of hearing loss. Programmable analog hearing aids use a microchip to store different settings; the person changes the level of amplification needed in different listening environments.

Digital hearing aids use technology that converts sounds waves into binary code to represent the frequency, intensity, and patterns of the signal, a function termed *digitized sound processing.* The processing determines if the signal is useful sound or unwanted noise with extreme speed, providing an undistorted signal and improved filtering of background sounds. Many digital hearing aids are not completely digital, but rather combine aspects of analog and digital technology (Martin & Clark, 2011). Current trends, however, are focused increasingly on completely digital devices.

The primarily goal of use of a hearing aid is to achieve the best auditory functioning possible. Binaural hearing aids often improve speech clarity and volume, enhance perception of directional sound, and lessen the perception of background noise. Unilateral or *monaural* hearing aids are selected when hearing loss exists in only one ear.

Many health-related and psychosocial factors impact the selection of hearing aids, including the appearance, comfort, and financial considerations. Hearing aid models are tailored to different functional and aesthetic needs, and range from behind-the-ear devices to aids that fit completely inside the ear canal. Analog devices are the least costly type of hearing aid, a crucial advantage for many consumers. Digital and hybrid models are preferred by many consumers due to better performance in managing background noise, despite their significantly higher cost (Wood & Lutman, 2004).

Cochlear Implants

In the past, hearing aids have been the only available option for sound amplification for people who are Deaf or hard of hearing. Today however, rehabilitation options have dramatically changed with the advent of cochlear implant technology. "*Cochlear implants*, a recent breakthrough, are surgically implanted devices available for children and adults who present with severe to profound hearing losses" (Eng & Learner, 2011, p. 219). They are prosthetic devices implanted in the inner ear that bypass the external, middle, and inner ear hair cells, and uses electrical impulses to stimulate the auditory nerve directly through electrical impulses. Essentially, a cochlear implant performs the function of hair cells by stimulating the auditory nerves.

Cochlear implant systems have both external and internal components and require at least four basic parts: an external microphone, signal processor, transmitter, and electrodes. The system receives sound through an external microphone, converts sound to magnetic impulses, and sends them to an audio processor connected to a transmitter beneath the skin. The transmitter converts the magnetic impulses to electrical impulses and sends them through the skin to a series of electrodes that have been implanted within the cochlea. The electrical signals stimulate the auditory nerves and are perceived as sound.

Surgical implantation criteria include personal traits, including cultural and educational background, age, and preferred method of communication. These factors can play a more influential role in surgery than any physical factors. The age at which an individual undergoes cochlear implantation, the length and severity of deafness prior to implantation, and whether the person possesses useful speech reading skills are critical factors that influence cochlear implant outcomes. In general, individuals who are younger with shorter-term hearing loss and speech reading abilities have more successful outcomes than people with more adverse profiles, individuals who are prelingually deaf, and those who have exclusively used manual communication.

Aural Rehabilitation

Hearing aids and cochlear implants provide auditory feedback that may foster spoken language development in some consumers who are Deaf or hard of hearing due to improvement in speech perception (Pantelemidou, Herman, & Thomas, 2003). Aural rehabilitation plays a significant role in the treatment and management of Deafness and hearing loss. For adults, aural rehabilitation focuses predominantly on the impact of hearing loss on communication and the procedures used to improve communication effectiveness (Hull, 2001).

Several methods of aural rehabilitation are centered on use of residual hearing and visual cueing with reinforcement for the development of auditory awareness and speech. ***Auditory methods*** use residual hearing abilities, with or without assistive devices, with special attention to the development of listening skills. Techniques that focus on fostering awareness of the physical motion of speech and related sensations are considered ***kinesthetic methods***. Increasingly, sophisticated computer-assisted systems are being used in kinesthesis (Pantelemidou et al., 2003). ***Oral methods*** combine assistive listening devices, speech reading, and kinesthesis to develop speaking abilities. ***Speech reading*** (inaccurately termed lip reading) allows an individual to comprehend speech by observing lip and facial movements along with body gestures to determine what is being spoken and in what context.

Aural rehabilitation includes other types of services, including training in ***manual communication***. Manual methods of aural rehabilitation exist in contrast to oral strategies, embracing rather than discouraging the use of non-verbal communication. Manual communication training prepares the individual to communicate through non-verbal techniques such as finger spelling and signed languages including American Sign Language (ASL) and Signed English. ***Total communication*** is a highly inclusive rehabilitation option that involves selecting the most effective and appropriate strategies from all methods to maximize both expressive and receptive communication.

Functional Limitations

Functional limitations related to deafness and hearing loss are largely dependent on pre-lingual versus postlingual occurrence, severity of hearing loss, presence or absence of other complicating factors such as a vestibular disorder or a secondary disability, and other situational factors. It is clear, however, that audition and communication difficulties are the primary functional limitation across all categories and configurations of hearing loss.

If an individual has a mild hearing loss, he or she will likely experience a slight difficulty in understanding speech when background noise is present. A person who has a mild-to-moderate loss will have some problems understanding conversation in group settings, and may need face-to-face communication to comprehend at least half of a conversation. A moderate hearing loss results in significant difficulty in group settings and in face-to-face verbal conversations. People who have severe hearing losses are not likely to recognize voices or environmental noises, while individuals who have profound hearing losses may only detect sounds through vibrations and are likely to use manual or visual methods of communication. Significant hearing limitations may result in marked difficulties in reading, writing, and comprehending English (Gallaudet Research Institute, 2003).

People who have prelingual severe or profound hearing losses have considerable functional limitations in expressive and receptive language (Kral & O'Donoghue, 2010). For individuals with sensorineural hearing losses, comprehension in noisy environments is more difficult than for people with conductive hearing loss. Conductive hearing losses do not usually result in functional deficits that are as significant as those associated with sensorineural hearing loss. People who also have severe tinnitus or vertigo may experience additional frustration, anxiety, and a notable disturbance of attention and ability to listen.

Psychosocial Implications

Deaf or hard of hearing individuals often face significant isolation and social alienation due to functional limitations in audition and communication. Speech comprehension problems can result in a marked inability to participate in reciprocal conversations and social interactions (Gallaudet Research Institute, 2003). The major psychosocial implications experienced by people who are Deaf or hard of hearing are social and familial isolation.

Feelings of isolation due to communication barriers within the family and society are prevalent. The impact of communication barriers for people who are Deaf and hard of hearing may begin at a very early age, especially if hearing loss occurred pre-lingually. The vast majority of parents and siblings of Deaf and hard of hearing children are hearing, resulting in incomplete communication within the family. Nearly a third of

Deaf and hard of hearing children have difficulties with social interaction and behavior (Gallaudet Research Institute, 2003), probably as a result of communication barriers in the home.

Many people with hearing loss report negative experiences with the hearing world. Such experiences result in emotional and behavioral problems. Research indicates that nearly half of Deaf and hard of hearing people experience mental health conditions attributed to difficulties in communication.

Vocational Implications

The broad vocational implications of functional limitations experienced by people who are Deaf or hard of hearing include unemployment and underemployment. Historically, jobs that require higher levels of reading, frequent interaction with coworkers, customers or clients, and use of the telephone have not traditionally been open to people who are Deaf or hard of hearing. They tend to have trade jobs related to transportation, farming, and machine operation and are less likely to be in more lucrative professional areas. In some instances, Deaf individuals have faced significant bias from employers, and been shut out of the workforce completely. The cumulative effect of chronic unemployment and underemployment is markedly negative at the end of one's working years; the median net worth of people with hearing losses as they enter retirement is considerably less than reported for people without hearing loss (Brodwin, Parker, & DeLaGarza, 2010; Lucas, Schiller, & Benson, 2004). Limited abilities in detecting environmental sounds, difficulties in communicating with others, and occupational hearing requirements have resulted in limitations in job placement and have notable vocational implications.

Environmental Sounds

The ability to detect sounds such as warning bells, alarms, and door chimes, to locate the source of sounds, and to make distinctions among various sounds are critical in some work settings. Abilities to localize sounds and discriminate between sounds is especially crucial if an individual is working with or near machinery, so functional limitations in detecting environmental stimuli may result in work setting safety concerns (National Research Council, 2005). For example, the inability to hear or localize warning buzzers, alarms, or bells is a vocational limitation which could, if unnoticed, result in injury to the person or others in the work environment (Arlinger, 2003). Problems with balance, dizziness, and tinnitus impact a person's ability to function effectively in hazardous environments. General vocational precautions include avoidance of ladders, scaffolds, heights, dangerous machinery, and driving.

Occupational Hearing Requirements

Problems hearing can significantly impede employment in professions with specific job entry requirements. In some instances, individuals may be completely excluded from certain professions such as military service and law enforcement. While hearing may be important in many work settings, even severe or profound hearing loss does not prevent employment. Most young adults who are Deaf or significantly hard of hearing are employed at some level (Brodwin et al., 2010).

Accommodations

Accommodations are those modifications, adjustments, auxiliary aids, and services used in home, work, and recreational settings to reduce barriers and diminish functional limitations. In the absence of accommodations, people who are Deaf or hard of hearing may be unintentionally excluded from almost all communicative interactions with the hearing world. A variety of available options for accommodations and assistive devices are available for use in activities of daily living and in work settings (Brodwin et al., 2010). Assistive communication technology, modifications of the environment, and use of communication strategies are particularly beneficial options for reasonable accommodation.

Assistive Technology

Bryant and Bryant (2011) have defined assistive technology (AT) as "the applications of science, engineering, and other disciplines that results in processes, methods, or inventions that support people with disabilities" (p. 2). Currently, a wide variety of AT is available. Technologies used by hearing people are useful to people with hearing loss, such as web-based chat, electronic mail, and text messaging. Additional communication technologies have been developed for people who are Deaf or hard of hearing including text-based telephone relay systems and video relay systems.

Telecommunication Devices for the Deaf

As early as 1874, telephone access for Deaf and hard of hearing users has been an issue. Unfortunately, early communication technologies were rarely efficient, increasing communication barriers for people who were Deaf or hard of hearing. To increase and facilitate communication between the Deaf and hearing populations, the teletypewriter (TTY), also called the telecommunications device for the Deaf (TDD), was developed, allowing people to type and receive messages over telephone lines. These systems continue to operate as a link between three parties. In such a system, the person with a hearing loss or speech impairment uses the teletypewriter to type out messages, while the hearing person uses a telephone, and a relay operator conveys the messages to each through the appropriate voice or text format (Grossman, 2001).

Video Relay Services (VRS)

VRS is an alternative to TTY/TDD relay service communication. It is a visual communication system requiring at least three basic components: a video monitor such as a television or computer screen, a video camera, and a high-speed broadband line. Like the TTY/TDD system, VRS uses a third-party relay operator, but in the VRS system, the operator is also a sign language interpreter. People who communicate with sign language see and are seen by the interpreter through cameras linked to monitors. Using videophones, VRS is also used among people who use manual languages without a relay operator (Grossman, 2001). Studies have shown that across all areas, participants demonstrated preference for the VRS over text-based services, despite the slightly higher cost of equipment. Participants noted that quality of the service was faster and more professional using the VRS system, and reported greater positive impact on their quality of life.

Assistive Listening Devices (ALDS)

The National Institute on Deafness and other Communication Disorders (NIDCD) is a comprehensive resource for current information on this ever changing technology. ALDS are any devices that will help a person hear or communicate in an enhanced manner. There are digital and wireless varieties. Hearing loops consist of a wire which circles a room, a microphone, and a receiver. There are similar systems in which the individual wears a loop.

There are also FM systems. The difference between the hearing loop and the FM system is the way the sound is transmitted. The FM system transmits sound directly to a receiver. In many cases, this is a portable system where a microphone is given to a presenter or set up in the middle of a table and the person receiving is using his or her telecoil or hearing aid boot-type receiver to hear the sound.

A more complicated system is the infrared system. This system transmits sound into light which is sent to a receiver worn by an individual; the light is decoded and converted back to a magnetic signal which is picked up by the person's telecoil. The infrared system does not transmit through walls which makes it useful in situations where confidentiality is necessary. Sound is transmitted to the listener clearly and free of distracting noise in the environment (NIDCD, 2011).

Environmental Modifications

Across home, work, and leisure settings, individuals who are Deaf or hard of hearing may encounter situations in which a response to sounds in the environment is compulsory. Modifications to the environment that promote awareness of such environmental sounds and provide safety measures are valuable for Deaf and hard of hearing. Telephones, doorbells, and fire alarms may be linked to visual alerting devices, such as flashing lights. Tactile alerting devices, such as vibrating pagers are also useful.

Noisy environments are often difficult. In many settings, individuals who are Deaf or hard of hearing benefit from noise reduction to promote use of residual hearing in communication. Quiet surroundings have less hearing interference due to background noise, and individuals may manage extraneous noises effectively through sound absorbing carpeting, upholstery, or panels. Well-lit surroundings are beneficial, as are surroundings free of objects or other barriers to visual sight lines, allowing for clearly visible manual communication or speech-reading (Geyer & Schroedel, 1999).

Communication Strategies

For successful communication with persons who have hearing loss, it is necessary to establish and maintain attention and eye contact. It is acceptable to wave your hand or gently tap individuals who are Deaf or hard of hearing to gain their attention. One should articulate clearly, although over-articulation distorts the shape of the speaker's mouth and hinders speech reading. Speaking quickly or too slowly may hinder speech reading and distort conversational cues. It is important not look down or face away from a person who is Deaf or hard of hearing during communication; speakers should avoid obstructing the mouth while talking.

Some persons use sign language exclusively, while others may use spoken language or a combination of both. Those who communicate manually often have difficulty participating in situations where few or no other people use sign language, and a qualified sign language interpreter may be required to facilitate communication. Sign language training for family members and friends will significantly reduce isolation and improve home and community inclusion; sign language classes for employers and co-workers may serve as an accommodation (Geyer & Schroedel, 1999). When using interpreter services, it is appropriate for the hearing speaker to address the Deaf or hard of hearing person directly, and not look instead at the interpreter.

Job Restructuring

Job restructuring is an effective reasonable accommodation that relates to communication strategies, and typically involves redistribution or exchange of job duties or job assignments, redeveloping of job processes, and eliminating any non-essential job functions. For example, in work where speech communication is not essential, individuals may communicate through alternative means such as text messaging, electronic mail, or written memos (Geyer & Schroedel, 1999). Using support personnel to accomplish non-essential job functions, such as incidental telephone use, is an element of job restructuring (National Research Council, 2005). Changing the way meetings are conducted or providing transcripts of meetings are examples of changes to process. The selection of jobs and work environments not requiring an ability to hear is another possible job structuring strategy.

Issues in Job Accommodations

The Americans with Disabilities Act of 1990 (ADA) mandates collaboration among employees and employers in determining and providing reasonable job accommodations. A growing body of research suggests that people who are Deaf or hard of hearing face a number of challenges in obtaining accommodations. Employers exhibit greater willingness in providing job accommodations to workers in more advanced positions, such as managers than to workers in lower status positions. Differences in hearing status may also account for variations among workplace accommodations provided or authorized by employers. In general, persons who are Deaf are more likely to request and receive accommodations than those who are hard of hearing (Geyer & Schroedel, 1999). Size of the company or organization influences provision of accommodation, with larger employers providing accommodations more readily than smaller companies.

Summary

Understanding the unique needs of a person with hearing loss is a complex and sometimes challenging rehabilitation task. To serve the needs of people with hearing loss, rehabilitation professionals must possess an understanding of critical dimensions of hearing, listening, and communication, and the impact these factors have on service provision. Although terms such as hearing, listening, and communicating are often used interchangeably, these concepts are actually unique. **Hearing** is best described as a passive function that involves the perception of environmental sound. Hearing includes having an awareness of sound, ability to locate sounds, as well as the capacity to discern the quality of sound as well as make distinctions related to pitch and volume. ***Listening*** is an active and purposeful process undertaken with the intention of experiencing sound. ***Communication*** is another process, one that requires bi-directional or multi-directional exchanges of information which includes hearing, listening, and comprehension (Kiessling et al., 2003).

The primary functional limitation of hearing loss is communication. Assistive listening devices, communication technologies, environmental modifications, and reasonable accommodation are available and may effectively address these limitations. Such options should be explored as part of comprehensive rehabilitation planning and service provision. Many people who are Deaf or hard of hearing have useful residual hearing abilities, and successfully use devices such as hearing aids or cochlear implants; some individuals are skilled in speech reading, while others are fluent in sign language. Each person has unique strengths on which to build. Despite the many challenges encountered by people who are Deaf or hard of hearing and by professionals who serve them, the opportunities for rehabilitation are abundant.

Case Study

Alan Parchman is a 42 year-old married male with three children, ages 12, 15, and 16. He has been working at a chemical plant as a kettle operator and tender since graduating from high school. Mr. Parchman's job has required frequent exposure to both noise and ototoxic chemicals.

Three years ago, Mr. Parchman began to notice a decrease in hearing ability and developed intermittent severe tinnitus. Due to concerns about losing his position or being placed on unpaid medical leave, he did not report these symptoms to his employer. About six months ago, Mr. Parchman's symptoms worsened significantly, and at his wife's urging, he sought evaluation by his general practitioner.

His physician noted that Mr. Parchman had difficulty understanding speech in the office environment. She referred him to an audiologist for further evaluation. The audiological results demonstrated a pure tone average (PTA in the right ear of 60 dB, and a PTA in the left ear of 55 dB). Mr. Parchman further demonstrated 82% word understanding in the right ear, and 78% word understanding in the left ear. The tympanogram was within normal limits. Mr. Parchment was diagnosed with sensorineural hearing loss due to noise and ototoxic chemical exposure and was scheduled for a hearing aid fitting.

Questions

1. What level of hearing loss does this consumer have? Identify other characteristics of the hearing loss.
2. What transferable skills does this individual have; identify occupations using these skills?
3. If the consumer decided to remain in his current job, how would you as the rehabilitation counselor approach this decision? Provide supporting arguments.
4. What is this person's vocational profile?
5. Identify the consumer's likely functional limitations and recommend accommodations.
6. What are the implications of this type of hearing loss in regard to possible future functional limitations?

References

American National Standards Institute. (1996). *Specification for audiometers* (ANSI S3.6-1996). New York, NY: Author.

American National Standards Institute. (2003). *Maximum permissible ambient noise levels for audiometric test rooms* (ANSI S3.1-1999). New York, NY: Author.

Americans with Disabilities Act of 1990, P.L. 101-336, U.S.C. § 12101 *et seq.*

Arlinger, S. (2003). Negative consequences of uncorrected hearing loss – A review. *International Journal of Audiology, 42*(2), 2S17–2S20.

Baloh, R. W., & Jen, J. (2012). Hearing and equilibrium. In L. Goldman & A. I. Schafer (Eds.). *Goldman's Cecil textbook of medicine* (24th ed., pp. 2461–2469). Philadelphia, PA: Elsevier Saunders.

Brodwin, M. G., Parker, R. M., & DeLaGarza, D. (2010). Disability and reasonable accommodation. In E. M. Szymanski & R. M. Parker (Eds.), *Work and disability: Contexts, issues, and strategies for enhancing employment outcomes for people with disabilities* (3rd ed., pp. 281–323). Austin, TX: Pro-ed.

Bryant, D. P., & Bryant, B. R. (2011). *Assistive technology for people with disabilities* (2nd ed.) New York, NY: Pearson.

Eng, N., & Learner, P. K. (2011). Speech, language, and swallowing disorders. In S. R. Flanagan, H. H. Zaretsky, & A. Moroz (Eds.), *Medical aspects of disability: A handbook for the rehabilitation professional* (4th ed., pp. 195–222). New York, NY: Springer.

Gallaudet Research Institute. (2003). *Regional and national summary report of data from the 2002-2003 annual survey of deaf and hard of hearing children and youth*. Washington, DC: Author.

Geyer, P. D., & Schroedel, J. G. (1999). Conditions influencing the availability of accommodations for workers who are deaf or hard-of-hearing. *Journal of Rehabilitation, 65*, 42–50.

Gratton, M. A., & Smyth, B. J. (2004). Ototoxicity of platinum compounds. In P. S. Roland & J. A. Rutka (Eds.), *Ototoxicity* (pp. 60–75). London, England: BC Becker.

Grossman, R. B. (2001). Dynamic facial expressions in American Sign Language: Behavioral, neuroimaging, and facial-coding analyses for deaf and hearing subjects. *Dissertation Abstracts International, 62*(01), (UMI No. AAT 3001497).

Hull, R. H. (2001). What is aural rehabilitation? In R. H. Hull (Ed.), *Aural rehabilitation: Serving children and adults* (4th ed., pp. 3–17). New York, NY: Singular.

Kaiser Permanente. (2012). *The basics of how we hear*. Retrieved from http://kphearingservices.com/hearinghealth/understandinghearingloss.html

Katz, J., & White, T. P. (2001). Introduction to the handicap of hearing impairment. In R. H. Hull (Ed.), *Aural rehabilitation: Serving children and adults* (4th ed., pp. 21–39). New York, NY: Singular.

Kiessling, J., Pichora-Fuller, M. K., Gatehouse, S., Stephens, D., Arlinger, S., Chisolm, T., . . . von Wedel, H. (2003). Candidature for and delivery of audiological services: Special needs of older people. *International Journal of Audiology, 42*(2S), 92–101.

Koga, K. (2004). The hearing mechanism: A guide for laymen. In J. Suzuki, T. Kobayashi, & K. Koga (Eds.), *Hearing impairment, an invisible disability: How you can live with a hearing impairment* (pp. 8–13). Hicom, Japan: Springer.

Kral, A., & O'Donoghue, G. M. (2010). Profound deafness in childhood. *New England Journal of Medicine, 363*(15), 1438–1450.

Lane, H., Hoffmeister, R., & Bahan, B. (1996). *A journey into the Deaf world*. San Diego, CA: Dawn Sign.

Lucas, J. W., Schiller, J. S., & Benson, V. (2004). *Summary health statistics for U. S. adults: National health interview survey, 2001: Vital & health statistics, 10*(218). (DHHS Publication No. PHS 2004-1546). Hyattsville, MD: U. S. Department of Health and Human Services.

Luft, P. (2013). Independent living services for Deaf and hard of hearing students: Results of a national survey of school programs. *Journal of Applied Rehabilitation Counseling, 44*, 18–27.

Martin, F. N., & Clark, J. G. (2011). *Introduction to audiology* (11th ed.). New York, NY: Pearson.

Nance, W. E. (2003). The genetics of deafness. *Mental Retardation and Developmental Disabilities Research Reviews, 9*, 109–119.

National Institute on Deafness and other Communication Disorders (NIDCD). (2011). *NIDCD fact sheet: Assistive devices for people with hearing, voice, speech, or language disorders*. Retrieved from http://www.nidcd.nih.gov/staticresources/health/hearing/NIDCD-Assistive-Devices-FS.pdf

National Research Council. (2005). *Hearing loss: Determining eligibility for Social Security benefits*. Washington, DC: National Academies.

Nicolosi, L., Harryman, E., & Kresheck, J. (2004). *Terminology of communication disorders: Speech language hearing* (5th ed.). Baltimore, MD: Lippincott Williams and Wilkins.

Padden, C., & Humphries, T. (2006). *Inside Deaf culture*. Cambridge, MA: Harvard University.

Pantelemidou, V., Herman, R., & Thomas, J. (2003). Efficacy of speech intervention using electropalatography with a cochlear implant user. *Clinical Linguistics & Phonetics, 17*(4-5), 383–392.

Prepageran, N., & Rutka, J. A. (2004). Salicylates, nonsteroidal anti-inflammatory drugs, quinie, and heavy metals. In P. S. Roland & J. A. Rutka (Eds.), *Ototoxicity* (pp. 28–41). London, England: BC Becker.

Pullen, R. L., Jr. (2006). Spin control: Caring for a patient with inner ear disease. *Nursing, 36*(5), 48–51.

Ruka, J. A. (2004). Physiology of the vestibular system. In P. S. Roland & J. A. Rutka (Eds.), *Ototoxicity* (pp. 20–27). London, England: BC Becker.

Sindhusake, D., Mitchell, P., Newall, P., Golding, M., Rochtchina, E., & Rubin, G. (2003). Prevalence and characteristics of tinnitus in older adults: The Blue Mountains Hearing Study. *International Journal of Audiology, 42*(5), 289–294.

Tambs, K., Hoffman, H. J., Borchgrevink, H. M., Holmen, J., & Engdahl, B. (2006). Hearing loss induced by occupational and impulse noise: Results on threshold shifts by frequencies, age, and gender from the Nord-Trondelag Hearing Loss Study. *International Journal of Audiology, 45*(5), 309–317.

Tye-Murray, N. (2008). *Foundations of aural rehabilitation: Children, adults, and their family members* (3rd ed.). Clifton Park, NY: Cengage Learning.

Wood, S. A., & Lutman, M. E. (2004). Relative benefits of linear analogue and advanced digital hearing aids. *International Journal of Audiology, 43*(3), 144–155.

About the Authors

Shawn P. Saladin, Ph.D., C.R.C., is an Associate Dean, College of Health Sciences and Human Services at the University of Texas, Pan American. He is a Certified Rehabilitation Counselor and Certified Public Manager. As a person who is Deaf and communicates through both oral and signed modalities, he is skilled in American Sign Language (ASL), total communication, and Signed English. His research interests include assistive technology, Deaf-hearing relationships, and employment of people who are Deaf or hard of hearing.

Sandra Hansmann, Ph.D., is assistant professor, Department of Rehabilitation at the University of Texas, Pan American. She serves as the hard of hearing specialist for the Services to Individuals who are Deaf or Hard of Hearing undergraduate concentration program. Dr. Hansmann has conversational skills in ASL and Signed English, and is co-principal investigator of the Center of Academic Excellence and its Director of Research and Sustainability. Her research agenda is focused on health sciences-human services higher education and distance education.

Chapter 9

VISUAL DISABILITIES

Bill Takeshita, O.D., F.A.A.O., F.C.O.V.D.
Robin Langman, M.S., C.R.C.
Rebekah Brod, M.A., M.F.T.

Introduction

Vision is a complex and fascinating process of the human body. Although vision can be described as being analogous to a camera, it involves much more. The eyes are a matrix of millions of cells that convert light information into electrical signals. Two-thirds of the brain is involved in the complex process of vision (Kanski & Bowling, 2011). The visual centers of the brain communicate with the motor, auditory, language, speech, and executive processing areas of the brain to impact reading, facial recognition, spatial awareness, and problem solving.

In a matter of milliseconds, vision allows us to gather information about the surrounding environment at distances well beyond the reach of the arms and fingers. The central visual system allows us to identify details and enables us to read, identify faces, and perform fine motor tasks. The peripheral visual system provides the brain with continuous information to assist with independent mobility in familiar and unfamiliar areas. Integration of both central and peripheral visual information allows adults with normal vision to perform tasks efficiently and independently (Kanski & Bowling, 2011).

Blindness and loss of vision are frightening and emotionally stressful events. Vision impairment causes functional difficulties with reading, driving, walking, and working independently and may also cause emotional, psychological, social, and financial difficulties (Corn & Erin, 2010). In the United States, over 70% of adults between the ages of 20 and 65 who are visually impaired are unemployed (Congdon et al., 2004; Mitchell, 2004). The absence of employment can exacerbate emotional, psychological, and financial difficulties of patients with vision impairment and contribute to the development of other problems. To provide training and promote maximum productivity and independence at home and in the workplace, rehabilitation counselors play a pivotal role in developing treatment plans that may involve ophthalmologists, optometrists, psychologists, orientation and mobility specialists, and teachers for the visually impaired. In this chapter, the many different aspects of vision are described, along with diseases and disorders that impact the functional abilities of individuals.

Vision Impairment and Disability

The rehabilitation counselor must have a thorough understanding of the degree of vision impairment and functional vision of a client before developing a vocational plan. This can be challenging because the counselor must rely on medical reports, chart notes, and information provided by the client. Unfortunately, medical reports and chart records may describe the diagnosis without reflecting the client's visual strengths and limitations.

In the United States, eye care professionals, the Social Security Administration, and government agencies have adopted the definitions set forth by the World Health Organization (1994) to provide a uniform definition of vision impairment and set standards to determine qualifications for government services and benefits.

Definitions of Visual Impairment

- *Functionally blind* describes individuals who are not able to perceive light.
- *Legal blindness* is visual ability with a best-corrected acuity of 20/200 or worse in the better eye, or the widest diameter of peripheral vision measuring 20 degrees or less in the better eye.
- *Visually impaired* or *partially sighted* describes individuals with a best-corrected visual acuity of 20/70 to 20/180 in the better eye, or a peripheral field of vision between 21 degrees and 140 degrees.
- *Fully sighted* describes people with a best-corrected visual acuity of 20/40 or better in the best eye.

Although the definitions of functionally blind, legal blindness, and visually impaired or partially sighted are often used in medical reports, they do not completely describe a client's functional vision. These definitions only consider visual acuity and peripheral vision. Clarity of sight, depth perception, eye-hand-foot coordination, color vision, day and night vision, and visual processing skills are some of the visual sub-skills that affect visual functions (Corn & Erin, 2010). Deficits in a specific skill can have significant ramifications regarding the client's ability to perform one task but may not affect another. It is crucial to define vision impairment as it relates to specific occupations or job tasks (Brodwin, Parker, & DeLaGarza, 2010).

Prevalence of Visual Loss

According to the American Community Survey (Erickson, Lee, & von Schrader, 2013), the number of non-institutionalized males and females, ages four through age 20 in the United States who were reported to have a visual disability in 2011 was the following:

- Total = 656,300
- Girls = 308,600
- Boys = 347,700

The number of non-institutionalized males and females of all ages in the United States reported to have a visual disability in 2011 was as follows:

- Total = 6,636,800
- Women = 3,665,200
- Men = 2,971,600
- Age 18-64 = 3,372,400
- Age 65 and older = 2,743,600

Eye Care Professionals

A counselor works with eye care professionals to obtain information regarding the client's functional vision. In the United States, optometrists and ophthalmologists are licensed to diagnose and treat diseases and disorders of the visual system. Optometrists are considered to be the primary eye care professional in health systems. If the patient requires surgery or additional medical treatment, the optometrist refers the patient to an ophthalmologist (Kanski & Bowling, 2011).

The Eye Examination

The general eye examination involves a case history, measurement of the distance and near clarity of sight, screening of neurological function, inspection of the health of the eyes, and refraction to determine the need for corrective lenses (Corn & Erin, 2010). This section describes information obtained with the eye examination and specific tests performed to quantify various visual skills and functional implications.

Case History

The case history is one of the most informative components of the eye examination. A medical history and results from prior eye examinations provide clues to explain the patient's symptoms and complaints. Questions regarding vision problems of family members help the examiner gain insight into the possible patterns of genetic eye conditions and prognosis.

Visual Acuity Testing

A Snellen eye chart is the most common test used to measure clarity of sight. It is typically placed 20 feet from the patient, who is then directed to identify letters of varying sizes with each eye. Each letter on the Snellen chart, called an optotype, has a specific size. The physician records the distance from the chart to the patient. A patient who identifies the 20-size letter from 20 feet has 20/20 visual acuity, whereas a person who can only read the 200-size letter from 20 feet has 20/200 acuity. If the individual is not able to read the 200-size letter from 20 feet with either eye with the best corrected vision, he or she is considered to be legally blind. The patient with 20/200 acuity has difficulty identifying faces, and reading street signs and chalkboards (Kanski & Bowling, 2011).

Visual Field Testing

Visual field testing measures the width or area of vision a person can see. Glaucoma, retinitis pigmentosa, and cerebral vascular accidents can cause loss of peripheral vision and affect a person's mobility, night vision, balance, and spatial orientation. Macular degeneration and diabetic retinopathy affect central field of vision and may cause blurred sight, blind spots in the central vision, reduced contrast vision, and diminished color vision. Visual field defects in the central vision affect one's ability to read, identify faces, drive, and carry out other activities needed at school and work (Sheth et al., 2012).

Visual field defects are not always noticed by the patient. If the location of a visual field defect is different in both eyes, one eye can compensate for the other. The visual field defect may be mild and may not cause an absolute blind spot but rather appear faded.

The most sophisticated method of testing peripheral vision is through the use of computerized perimetry. In this test, the patient is positioned in front of a large dome in which lights of varying sizes and intensities flash in different parts of the central and peripheral fields. Low vision specialists use this information to map out regions of the eye that have the highest sensitivity and use lenses and prisms to deflect images onto functional fields of vision.

Refraction

Refraction is a test that determines the optimal prescription to sharpen a person's sight. Myopia (nearsightedness) is a condition where light rays focus in front of the macula, causing blurred distance sight. Hyperopia (farsightedness) is when the light rays focus behind the macula, causing blurred near vision. Astigmatism is another refractive error where the shape of the eye is distorted, causing distorted vision. Eye doctors prescribe glasses with prescription lenses that focus the light rays on the central retina (macula) to produce clarity of sight. Contact lenses and refractive surgery also correct myopia, hyperopia, and astigmatism.

Color Vision Testing

Color vision is generally tested with pseudoisochromatic plates, which display numbers of different colors on backgrounds of varying colors. Color vision deficiencies are more common among males than females and affect a person's ability to differentiate between similar colors. For instance, they may confuse red and burgundy. Someone with a color vision deficiency, for example, may have trouble distinguishing red from burgundy. Individuals with complete color blindness, on the other hand, are unable to identify any colors and their vision can be thought of as similar to watching a black and white television. People with complete color blindness also often have blurred sight and sensitivity to bright light.

Eye Teaming and Binocular Vision Testing

Binocular vision involves the ability to coordinate the eyes. Eye coordination testing is administered to patients who complain of double vision, frequent loss of place when reading, and eye strain. Each eye has six extra-ocular muscles that control the movement of the eyes along with one internal muscle, which changes the shape of the internal crystalline lens to focus on near and distant objects. Abnormal coordination of these muscles results in a crossed or turned eye (strabismus), double vision (diplopia), poor depth perception, blurred sight, headaches, and eye strain. Trauma, tumors, amyotrophic lateral sclerosis (ALS), Parkinson's disease, diabetes, multiple sclerosis, and myasthenia gravis can affect eye movement and hinder a person's ability to perform daily activities (Falvo, 2014).

Parts of the Eye

Orbit

The orbit, often called the eye socket, houses and protects the eyeball from direct trauma. It consists of several bones that are susceptible to fracture during trauma. Six ocular muscles of the eye have tendons that are attached to the orbit. This provides the foundation which allows for eye movement. Brain tumors, thyroid disease, and trauma to the orbit itself can restrict the movement of the eyes, and cause diplopia (double vision), affecting the positioning of the eyes.

Eyelids

The eyelids lubricate and protect the cornea and the anterior portion of the eye. Whenever an individual blinks, various glands produce tears to lubricate the eyes. Trauma, tumors, and neurological disorders can affect the function of the eyelids. Incomplete closure of the eyelids causes dry eyes, blurred vision, sensitivity to light and glare, and eye pain.

Cornea, Sclera, and Conjunctiva

The cornea is the transparent structure in the front of the eye. The vision of patients with a corneal scar is similar to looking through frosted glass; patients with corneal scars have blurred sight and extreme sensitivity to light. A patient with corneal disease may benefit from laser treatment, as well as corneal transplantation surgery. Some patients with myopia and astigmatism benefit from refractive surgery, a procedure that alters the shape of the cornea to eliminate the need for glasses (Kanski & Bowling, 2011).

Iris, Pupil, and Anterior Chamber

The iris is the colored muscular tissue of the eye. A round opening called the pupil in the center of the eye regulates the amount of light entering the eyes. The pupils dilate in dim illumination and constrict in bright illumination. Trauma to the iris, aniridia, and iritis (inflammation of the iris) cause sensitivity to light (photophobia) and moderate to severe eye pain. Chronic inflammation of the iris (iritis) produces severe sensitivity to light, blurred vision, and disabling eye pain (Kanski & Bowling, 2011).

Crystalline Lens

Behind the iris is a transparent focusable lens called the crystalline lens. The crystalline lens changes its shape when the ciliary muscle contracts and relaxes, enabling the eye to focus at different distances. With aging, the lens loses the ability to change shape and patients may then require glasses for reading. Cataracts involve the clouding of the transparent lens leading to blurred sight.

Vitreous

The vitreous, located behind the lens and iris, is filled with a gel-like substance called vitreous humor. Light must pass through the pupil, crystalline lens, and vitreous humor before it can focus on the retina. Scar tissue and blood can interfere with the manner that light focuses on the retina, causing blurred sight, reduced peripheral vision, poor color vision, and distorted vision (Kanski & Bowling, 2011).

Retina

The retina is the light-sensing tissue that consists of millions of rod and cone cells that absorb light and send electrical signals through the optic nerve to the brain. Cone cells are located in the centermost region of the retina. The macula is the area of the retina that consists entirely of cone cells and is responsible for clarity of sight, color vision, spatial contrast sensitivity, and ability to adapt to different lighting conditions. Macular degeneration, diabetic retinopathy, and Stargardt's disease negatively affects the macula and one's

FIGURE 1
Eye

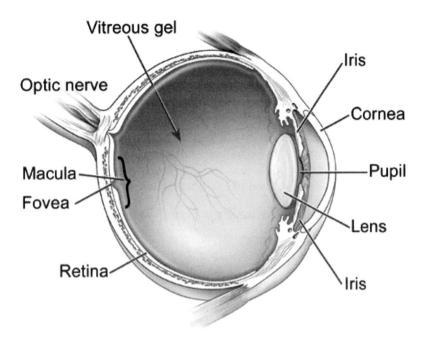

Source: National Eye Institute. (2014). Diagram of the eye. Retrieved on May 18, 2014 from http://www.nei.nih.gov/health/eyediagram/eyeimages3.asp

ability to read. These conditions can cause blurred central vision. Rod cells are located on the periphery of the retina and provide peripheral vision, perception of movement, night vision, and low spatial contrast sensitivity, used for mobility. Retinitis pigmentosa, Leber's congenital amaurosis, and retinopathy of prematurity affect peripheral vision and cause problems with walking and seeing at night (Gerstenblith et al., 2012).

Optic Nerve

The optic nerve is a bundle of nerve fibers that send information from the rod and cone cells to the visual cortex of the brain. Abnormalities of the optic nerve are diagnostic of eye diseases such as glaucoma, optic nerve hypoplasia, optic nerve atrophy, as well as systemic illnesses, such as multiple sclerosis, brain tumors, and increased intra-cranial pressure. Eye injuries and trauma to the head also cause optic nerve damage. Optic nerve disorders lead to varying degrees of blurred sight, color blindness, peripheral and central visual field defects, and total blindness (Sheth et al., 2012).

Low Vision Rehabilitation

Low vision rehabilitation has been shown to be extremely beneficial for adults with sub-normal vision (Crandell, Jr. & Robinson, 2007). Low vision specialists are doctors who design, customize, and prescribe visual aids and provide training to help patients with low vision perform their desired goals independently. Individuals are generally referred to low vision specialists by ophthalmologists when medical and surgical treatments no longer correct vision.

The low vision examination identifies visual strengths and limitations and offers possible solutions. Specialized glasses, filters, prisms, and technology are used to help a person read, write, use a computer, cross the street independently, and perform other activities.

Customized Low Vision Aids

Low vision specialists develop glasses and visual aids to maximize the individual's visual strengths and compensate for their weaknesses (Corn & Erin, 2010). Telescopes and high-powered lenses magnify images to allow a person to see small print, while prisms are used to reduce eyestrain, headaches, and double vision caused by binocular vision disorders. Filters and colored lenses reduce glare, maximize the perception of colors, increase contrast, and simulate lighting conditions that provide the best acuity. Additionally, prisms and eccentric viewing training can be incorporated to deflect the image onto the most usable areas of the retina, maximizing overall visual function.

Bioptic Spectacles

Bioptic spectacles are glasses that contain a small telescope to improve visual acuity, helping individuals see traffic signals and street signs, and to read a computer screen. Bioptic glasses are one of the most useful low vision aids enabling people to read small print and perform specialized work tasks, such as reading the labels of items on store shelves and the numbers on a cash register.

High-Powered Reading and Writing Glasses

Glasses with specialized lenses magnify reading materials up to six times (Crandell, Jr. & Robinson, 2007). They may be customized to reduce glare, increase contrast, and are available in bifocal forms to allow a person to focus on both far and near vision.

Visual Field Expanding Glasses

Prisms, reverse telescopes, and amorphic lenses can be incorporated into the design of glasses to help individuals with reduced peripheral vision due to glaucoma, retinitis pigmentosa, and traumatic head injury or stroke. Reverse telescopic glasses shrink the peripheral vision into the usable field of vision to help individuals see better. Orientation and mobility training is highly recommended for patients with reduced peripheral vision.

Telescopes

Hand held telescopes are helpful when a person has blurred distance sight. Monocular telescopes can focus on both distant and near objects. To assist with independent mobility, adults with low vision use telescopes to read bus numbers, street signs, and traffic signals. They are also helpful for students and employees who have to read text from the board or see PowerPoint presentations.

Magnifiers

Magnifiers are available with their own light source and are very useful in helping people read mail and text on grocery items or other small objects. Magnifiers are fairly affordable and come in magnification powers up to 12 times.

Electronic Video Magnifiers

Electronic video magnifiers are particularly helpful for people with low vision. They are available in desktop and portable forms to allow individuals to have access to books, newspapers, documents, photographs, and medications. Video magnifiers offer more magnification, a brighter image, and a wider field of view than optical hand magnifiers. In addition, video magnifiers are capable of changing the colors of the text and background to reduce glare and magnify up to 85 times. Some video magnifiers help to focus on distant objects such as overhead projections, whiteboard displays, and PowerPoint presentations. A number of video magnifiers can also read text aloud.

Common Causes of Vision Impairment

Diabetic Retinopathy

Diabetic retinopathy is the leading cause of blindness among adults between the ages of 20 to 74; there are 5.5 million Americans who have this condition (Erickson et al., 2013). Diabetic retinopathy is a progressive disease in which the retina is damaged due to prolonged lack of oxygen. The onset of vision problems among those with diabetes is usually during adulthood (Unger, 2007).

The prevalence of diabetic retinopathy is directly related to the duration of the disease. For those with Type I (insulin dependent diabetes mellitus), more than 90% demonstrate evidence of diabetic retinopathy within 15 years. Sixty to 80% of individuals with Type II (non-insulin dependent diabetes) show signs of diabetic retinopathy after the same time period (American Diabetes Association, 2013).

Diabetic retinopathy slowly causes damage to the cells of the retina and initially causes the loss of peripheral vision and night vision. In the later stages of the disease, it affects the macula, causing blurred sight, sensitivity to glare, and fluctuating vision. Individuals with diabetes can help stabilize their vision with proper control of blood sugar. Low vision aids are helpful for those who have diabetic retinopathy-related visual impairment.

Optic Atrophy

Optic atrophy is a rare condition in which some or all of the optic nerve fibers have been damaged, resulting in mild to severe loss of vision. This can be present at birth or develop from various conditions. Optic atrophy is caused by lack of oxygen (anoxia, hypoxia), trauma, inflammation, vitamin deficiency, drug toxicity, demyelinating diseases such as multiple sclerosis, and increased intra-cranial pressure (Sheth et al., 2012). Persons may have blurred sight, red-green color blindness, reduced contrast sensitivity, limited depth perception, poor eye-hand-foot coordination, and large blind spots in the visual field. Visual loss related to optic atrophy causes difficulties with reading, walking, driving, and performing a wide variety of tasks. The optic nerve cannot be transplanted because of the millions of nerves within the optic tract. Low vision aids and assistive technology are very helpful for those with this condition.

Glaucoma

Glaucoma affects 2.3 million people in the United States (Erickson et al., 2013). In glaucoma, the intra-ocular pressure is too high, causing damage to optic nerve fibers. In a normal eye, aqueous humor is continually produced and drained through a structure called the trabecular meshwork, located in the anterior chamber angle. In open angle glaucoma, the trabecular meshwork does not drain aqueous fluid normally, resulting in an increase in intra-ocular pressure. Elevation of pressure is slow and is generally not noticeable in vision until significant loss has occurred. Small blind spots in the mid-peripheral field of vision initially develop and later progress to cause severe peripheral vision loss, reduced night vision, tunnel vision, and blindness. Advanced glaucoma creates difficulties with walking, reading, writing, and performing activities under dim illumination.

Glaucoma is common among adults of specific sub-groups. It is more prevalent among adults over age 40, African-Americans, Hispanics, and those with a family history of glaucoma (Allingham, Damji, Freedman, Moroi, & Rhee, 2010).

Glaucoma is a chronic disease. As a result, daily medication is required to sustain a healthy level of intra-ocular pressure. Compliance with therapy is frequently a problem because symptoms often are not immediate when medications are discontinued (Allingham et al., 2010). An individual with glaucoma needs a consultation with a low vision specialist to prescribe visual aids, including visual field expanders, high powered reading glasses, night vision aids, computer and assistive technology, and specific lighting for the workplace and home.

Retinitis Pigmentosa

Retinitis pigmentosa (RP) is a variety of degenerative eye conditions that affect the cells of the retina causing night blindness, reduced peripheral vision, sensitivity to glare, and blurred sight (Hartong, Berson, & Dryja, 2006). Symptoms generally develop between the first and second decade of life. In severe forms of retinitis pigmentosa, individuals lose nearly all their peripheral vision and are left with a small central island of vision. They are considered legally blind due to the absence of peripheral vision. Some people maintain 20/20 visual acuity, while others have blurred sight and a blue-yellow color vision deficiency.

Patients with RP tend to have many functional problems. Night blindness is the most common occurrence. Adults with night blindness may have trouble finding their chairs in dimly lit restaurants or movie theatres, and may avoid going out at night. As peripheral vision deteriorates, driving and walking become increasingly difficult. Low vision aids are helpful for individuals with RP. Visual field expanding glasses help people compensate for the reduced peripheral vision, while night vision glasses enhance mobility at night. Low vision spectacles improve visual acuity for distance and reading, while specialized filters enhance contrast vision and allow patients to adapt more readily to different lighting conditions. Desk lamps, track lighting, and full spectrum fluorescent light fixtures enhance illumination level. Orientation and mobility training is essential for independent mobility (Hartong et al., 2006).

Macular Degeneration and Stargardt's Disease

Macular degeneration, a disease of the central retina, is a leading cause of vision impairment in this country. Two million Americans are affected by this condition (Erickson et al., 2013). The macula (central retina) is a small region of the retina responsible for detailed clarity of sight, color, depth perception, and adaptation to light and glare. There are two main forms of macular degeneration. Dry (atrophic) macular degeneration is the most common and occurs when the cells of the macula atrophy due to age. When it occurs in teenagers and young adults, it is called Stargardt's disease. The second form is called wet (disciform) macular degeneration. In this form, abnormal blood vessels develop under the retina forming a sub-retinal neovascular membrane that result in sub-retinal hemorrhages. Leakage of blood under the macula can result in a sudden loss of central vision (Sheth et al., 2012). Symptoms of macular degeneration include blurred distant and near sight, sensitivity to glare and bright light, poor contrast vision, reduced stereoscopic depth perception, and color vision problems. People with this disability experience difficulty driving, reading, and performing tasks requiring fine dexterity.

Research studies are investigating the use of gene therapy and stem cells to treat dry macular degeneration and Stargardt's disease. Anti-oxidant vitamins and protection from the harmful rays of the sun have been reported to be beneficial for people with both types of macular degeneration. Low vision aids and video magnifiers are particularly helpful. Laser photocoagulation, photo dynamic therapy, and intra-ocular injections of anti-angiogenic medications help patients with wet macular degeneration (Sheth et al., 2012).

Head Injury, Neurological Vision Impairment, and Traumatic Eye Injuries

Head injury, blunt trauma, sports, and employment-related injuries are common causes of vision loss among adults. There are approximately 2.5 million eye injuries in the United States annually; 50,000 of these injuries result in permanent lose of partial or total vision (Erickson et al., 2013). Penetrating injuries to the cornea and globe of the eye can result in total blindness due to retinal detachment, glaucoma, optic nerve damage, and ocular inflammation. In other cases, symptoms include blurred sight, distorted vision, severe sensitivity to glare, blind spots in the central and peripheral fields of vision, eye movement problems, and double vision. These eye problems interfere with reading, depth perception, eye-hand-foot coordination, balance, and mobility.

Traumatic brain injuries (TBI) cause significant vision problems, including double vision, poor depth perception, severe sensitivity to light, and profound visual processing difficulties (Panek, 2002). Patients have difficulty perceiving size, shape, depth, and have problems performing basic tasks, such as placing a cap on a water bottle. Some people with TBI have visual neglect, where they ignore all objects on one side of their midline, including their own body; they may not comb half their hair, as well as leave food untouched on one side of the plate.

Cerebrovascular accidents (stroke) cause symptoms similar to traumatic head injury. When the stroke or injury affects the right side of the brain, there may be no peripheral vision on the left side with either eye and weakness on the left side of the body. Neurological involvement to the right occipital and parietal lobes of the brain often significantly impact visual perception; as a result, the individual has poor depth perception, difficulty recognizing faces, and impaired visual-spatial perception skills. Conversely, strokes and injuries to the left occipital and parietal lobes of the brain cause a loss of peripheral vision on the right side of each eye, reduced motor function on the right side of the body, and affect language, reading, speech, word recognition, and ability to remember sequences of information (Sheth et al., 2012).

Cataracts

Cataracts affect nearly 22 million Americans (Erickson et al., 2013). A cataract occurs when the internal lens of the eye becomes clouded or opaque. Cataracts may be present at birth or develop at any age as a result of trauma, diabetes, steroid use, and aging (Kanski & Bowling, 2011). They cause a wide variety of vision problems ranging from blurred sight, reduced color vision, glare sensitivity, reduced peripheral vision, double vision, and sometimes total blindness. Dense cataracts that significantly impair vision may be surgically removed and an artificial lens implanted in the eye to restore focusing power. When cataracts develop after the age of seven and there is no other eye pathology, individuals typically regain normal vision after surgery.

However, adults who are born with congenital cataracts may continue to have sub-normal vision even after cataract extraction surgery. Limitations include blurred vision, nystagmus (uncontrollable shaking of the eyes), strabismus (mis-aligned eyes), and severe sensitivity to glare. Visual acuity can range from 20/40 to 20/200. Low vision aids and assistive technology help enhance remaining vision.

Congenital Causes of Vision Impairment

Albinism

Albinism is a congenital, inherited condition that affects the pigmentation and color of the eyes and may also affect the skin and hair (Sheth et al., 2012). Individuals with albinism have a very high degree of functional vision because they have generally learned to adapt to their vision impairments. These persons usually have visual acuity ranging from 20/70 to 20/200, and have normal peripheral and color vision. People with albinism tend to have better vision at night and respond well to tinted contact lenses, specialized filters, and low vision aids to improve both their distance and near clarity of sight. Computer and assistive technology, orientation and mobility training, and independent living skills training are helpful for those with albinism who have severe sensitivity to light (Brodwin, Siu, & Cardoso, 2012).

Retinopathy of Prematurity

Retinopathy of Prematurity (ROP) is a congenital condition that develops as a response to premature birth. It primarily affects the retina of newborn children born before 32 weeks of gestation and those weighing less than two pounds. Children with ROP may develop abnormal blood vessels in the retina which form scar tissue and can pull or detach the retina, causing blindness. The scar tissue in the eye often alters the shape of the eye causing it to be elongated, resulting in high myopia. ROP is related to exposure of a newborn to concentrated oxygen.

Functional Limitations

Emotional Adjustment

While discovering new ways to accomplish tasks which formerly required sight, some clients experience a conflicting desire to deny that any change in method or lifestyle need occur. There are feelings of loss, sadness, and anger after learning of permanent visual impairment. Adjusting to vision loss is an emotional process and clients must find ways to express their feelings and adapt to this radical change

(Kinash, 2006). Losing one's sight involves creating a new identity. Life can return to normal once the client begins to use other senses and find alternative ways of doing activities (Guide Dogs for the Blind, 1999).

Family and friends may find it difficult to accept a loved one's vision loss. They may become overprotective, thus limiting an individual's ability to function independently. The period of greatest emotional stress usually occurs at the onset of visual loss. While sudden loss of vision is extremely traumatic, it may be easier to cope with than the uncertain, slow visual loss seen in many chronic ocular diseases.

Age plays an important part in the way the person reacts emotionally to loss of sight. Younger people are more resilient from the severe emotional sequelae generated by loss of sight. Middle-aged individuals are at greater risk of having severe psychological difficulties, perhaps because of other stresses associated with changes occurring during mid-life. Another variable is the overall degree of visual loss; the more profound the visual loss, the slower and more challenging the adjustment (Crandell, Jr. & Robinson, 2007).

The stages of grieving outlined by Dr. Elizabeth Kubler-Ross apply to vision loss as with most disabling conditions. Denial, anger, bargaining, depression, and acceptance are the major steps of reaction to visual loss. Not everyone goes through all the stages or in this order (Kubler-Ross & Kessler, 2005).

Carroll (1961) outlined secondary losses that occur with loss of sight, including diminished physical integrity, decreased visual contact with the environment, loss of a means of communication, and reduced mobility. With some loss of physical integrity, the individual may no longer feel like a *whole* person, resulting in feelings of isolation and withdrawal from one's social network. The sighted person easily recognizes characteristics of distant objects including size, shape, position, speed, and direction; persons with visual impairment have lost part or all of this recognition ability (Crandell, Jr. & Robinson, 2007). This limitation evokes fear and anxiety. Body language, facial expressions, and shadows suggesting the time of day are instances of what is absent when a person no longer has vision.

Visual disability refers to one's inability to perform tasks visually. Both physical and psychological factors are important when defining functional status of individuals with visual impairment. A person with total visual loss but with newly acquired competencies may still achieve physical, emotional, and financial independence, as well as social integration (Kinash, 2006).

Physical Adjustment

Loss of sight is a major disruptive factor in daily living. Inability to perform essential tasks such as reading, driving, and recognizing faces poses barriers to successful employment, along with fatigue, depression, and anxiety. Visual loss negatively impacts most activities, and places stress on the individual's daily life.

Use of one's other senses frequently compensates for loss of visual acuity. Orientation and mobility specialists train clients to navigate with the assistance of white canes or guide dogs. Orientation and mobility play a vital role in an individual's perception of personal freedom and independence. Factors that contribute to the degree of orientation and mobility include residual vision, age at onset of visual loss, posture and balance, intelligence, body image, space orientation, auditory tactile abilities, and personality (Panek, 2002). Substantial loss of peripheral field of vision is more debilitating than loss of central vision.

A white cane is the primary mobility aid used by persons who are blind or visually impaired. It is recommended that training begin following diagnosis; yet, clients with some progressive eye disorders may decide to wait until vision loss impacts mobility. Those in need of aid must first acknowledge loss of vision to be comfortable using a white cane, a clear identifier of a person with vision impairment both to the individual and to others. Clients are taught to walk safely down the street by rhythmically touching the tip of the cane side-to-side in front of them to obtain advanced knowledge of what is ahead.

While many people prefer to use a red-tipped white cane for ambulation, some feel more comfortable relying on a guide dog (Guide Dogs for the Blind, 1999). Traveling with a guide dog differs from using a cane in that the dog navigates around obstacles, stops for stairs and other changes in elevation, and avoids overhead obstructions. The guide dog and owner work together as a team.

Vocational Adjustment

Vocational skills are a major component of successful independent functioning. The capability to perform job tasks well and provide for one's self and family greatly enhances self-esteem, reduces financial concerns, and diminishes family conflict. In addition to remaining visual capabilities, those with visual impairment can function independently by using physical dexterity, non-visual job skills, natural talents, and refinement of the senses (Panek, 2002).

Advances in assistive technology play a major part in enabling persons with vision impairment to perform essential job tasks. The rehabilitation counselor plays a significant role in assessing assistive technology needs and potential accommodations that enable clients to succeed in the workforce (Brodwin et al., 2012). Counselors can help dispel employer misconceptions about the capabilities of people with visual impairment.

Rehabilitation Potential

The general goal of rehabilitation is optimal physical functioning, economic independence, and social integration. Potential for rehabilitation depends on the physiology of the impairment (amount, type, and progression), conditions of the immediate environment, attitude and motivation, and use of residual vision. Since it is the auditory system that is the mainstay of mobility for clients with severe visual impairment, it is necessary for the counselor to determine the status of the person's auditory system. Duration and severity of disability, degree of personal adjustment, and positive or negative attributes of the family and the environment influence vocational rehabilitation of people with visual impairment (Carroll, 1961).

Rehabilitation efforts focus on providing the best possible use of residual vision (*vision enhancement*), and assisting with development of non-visual skills that can substitute for lost visual function (*vision substitution*). Vision enhancement involves use of magnifiers, telescopic aids, colored filters, and computer and video-generated magnification screens. These devices generally present an enlarged image that is more readily seen. Braille, an example of vision substitution, is a tactile system. Braille typewriters make it easier for people to take class notes, write, and read. Software is available that converts computerized text into Braille which can then be embossed on a Braille printer.

Computers and assistive technology can help enhance residual vision. Advances in technology allow patients with vision impairment to read, write, and perform job tasks and daily living activities independently (Brodwin et al., 2012). Thorough assessment of the client's need for assistive technology is beneficial. A vocational evaluator can assess the actual worksite to determine which aids promote optimum performance of essential job functions.

An effective technology for clients with low vision is video magnifiers, also known as closed-circuit televisions (CCTVs). This equipment provides significant magnification and offers a brighter, sharper, and wider field of view than magnifiers and glasses. Other models can be interfaced with a computer and allow the user to share the same screen to see text both on the computer and on paper (Kinash, 2006). There are now video magnifiers that can also scan the reading material and read the text out loud for the person.

Hand-held video magnifiers are useful for people with low vision to read print when they do not have access to a desktop magnifier. These video magnifiers produce a bright and sharp image on LCD screens. Distance and near focusing video magnifiers allow the user to see distant objects and reading material in a magnified view at work, school, and home (Crandell, Jr. & Robinson, 2007). This equipment is portable and useful for clients who are attending conferences, lectures, and presentations.

Many clients with low vision who are re-entering the workplace need assistance in seeing the print on a computer screen. Specialized glasses maximize sight at the distance of a computer screen, while a larger computer monitor facilitates seeing. Users can magnify the text on the computer screen or they can use the speech output to listen to what is on the screen. There are also software programs that are designed specifically to magnify the computer screen, read text aloud, and scan documents with the computer.

Working age adults who require additional help to see a computer screen may benefit from special computer software for the visually impaired (Brodwin et al., 2010; Falvo, 2014). Software magnification programs magnify all images on the computer screen and can also change the color of the background and text to help people with poor contrast vision and those with severe sensitivity to glare.

Screen reading programs help people who are functionally blind, as well as those who experience eye strain after reading for short periods of time. These programs can read text aloud from the screen thus allowing clients to access information from the Internet, type documents, and perform other software applications. Scanning software programs are available that allow users to scan books, letters, and other documents. The text is displayed in a magnified view on the computer screen and read aloud. Other technological advances include software programs that convert printed text into Braille, voice recognition software, telephone voice-controlled Internet access, and talking personal data assistants (PDAs) (Crandell, Jr. & Robinson, 2007).

Smart-phones enable people with low vision to be more independent. These telephones incorporate global positioning systems that help people travel independently and find places of interest easily. There are applications for cell phones that can identify currency, colors, bar codes, and even geographical landmarks. With accessible cell phones, individuals who are blind can access text messages, e-mail, and the Internet.

Conclusion

Approximately 55% of adults with visual impairment (defined as having difficulty seeing words or letters even with optical correction) are gainfully employed. This figure drops to 48% for persons who cannot see words or letters (Brodwin et al, 2010). Through careful interviewing and assessment, counselors can enhance the rehabilitation potential of many of these clients. Vocational rehabilitation counselors can enable their clients to choose realistic, practical, and attainable goals through the provision of rehabilitation services in a holistic manner. A variety of resources are available within the community. These include Braille foundations, low vision centers, service organizations (e.g., Lions' Clubs), centers for the partially sighted, college programs and services, and public school programs with specialists who have knowledge of community services available for persons with visual impairments.

Case Study

Ms. Alexa Bitari is a 51-year old Caucasian female diagnosed with (dry) macular degeneration. She has never been married and lives alone. Ms. Bitari's best corrected vision is reported as 20/40 (right eye) and 20/300 (left eye). Her central vision is compromised in both eyes due to macular degeneration. The client reports that her vision loss interferes with personal grooming and managing her finances, causing difficulties performing essential functions of her job. To be able to read, Alexa needs bright light and large print with 3.5 magnification. She reports no hospitalizations or medications, and a lack of major emotional problems or substance abuse issues.

Ms. Bitari graduated from high school and earned a bachelor's degree in the field of communications. Subsequently, she obtained clerical skills training at a local business college and took classes related to advancement in the entertainment field. For the past 25 years, Alexa has worked for a large entertainment firm as an administrative secretary. This position was in the corporate graphics design department and was recently eliminated due to downsizing. Ms. Bitari is currently working within the clerical pool and will have to interview for a new position to remain with the employer. Attitudes prevail throughout the entertainment industry that very few jobs can be performed by someone who is visually impaired. Alexa recognizes that the entertainment industry is populated by mostly young workers; she is concerned that she will be viewed as "washed up," especially if she discloses that she is coping with vision loss due to macular degeneration.

Despite her long tenure with the employer and excellent clerical skills, Ms. Bitari believes she will not be retained by the company in a permanent position because of her disability. She enjoys working in the entertainment industry, especially the challenging, fast-paced, and at times, glamorous working environment. Because she has trouble using the computer and reading file labels, Ms. Bitari fears that her request for accommodation will be denied. Alexa is worried that she will begin making errors on the job if her eye condition worsens.

In her most recent position as an administrative secretary, Ms. Bitari was responsible for typing purchase orders and correspondence, answering telephones and making appointments, coordinating meetings, and performing other staff responsibilities. An administrative secretary lifts and carries a maximum of ten pounds, with frequent lifting of less than five pounds. Most of the work is conducted while sitting. It takes approximately one year to acquire the skills needed for this position. Ms. Bitari has consulted with a rehabilitation counselor regarding the requirements and potential reasonable accommodations that will be needed for retaining a position with her current employer.

Questions

1. Discuss possible limitations, both physical and psychosocial, for individuals with low vision or blindness.
2. Describe Mr. Bitari's job as an administrative secretary in terms of physical exertion and skill levels. Provide a vocational profile.
3. As Ms. Bitari's rehabilitation counselor, describe the steps you would take to identify appropriate rehabilitation technology services.
4. Given the size of Alexa's employer, discuss how you would propose she be accommodated through assistive technology.
5. If Ms. Bitari is unable to continue working for her present employer, as her counselor, what alternatives will you recommend? Include short-term and long-term goals.

References

Allingham, R. R., Damji, K. F., Freedman, S., Moroi, S. E., & Rhee, D. J. (Eds.). (2010). *Shields textbook of glaucoma* (6th ed.). Philadelphia, PA: Lippincott Williams & Wilkins.

American Diabetes Association. (2013). Clinical practice recommendations 2013: Standards of medical care in diabetes. *Diabetes Care* (Supplement 1), S5.

Brodwin, M., Parker, R. M., & DeLaGarza, D. (2010). Disability and reasonable accommodation. In E. M. Szymanski & R. M. Parker (Eds.), *Work and disability: Contexts, issues, and strategies for enhancing outcomes for people with disabilities* (3rd ed., pp. 281–323). Austin, TX: Pro-ed.

Brodwin, M. G., Siu, F. W., & Cardoso, E. (2012). Users of assistive technology: The human component. In I. Marini & M. Stebnicki (Ed.), *The psychological and social impact of illness and disability* (6th ed., pp. 331–339). New York, NY: Springer.

Carroll, T. J. (1961). *Blindness: What is it, what it does, and how to live with it.* Boston, MA: Little, Brown.

Congdon, N., O'Colmain, B., Klaver, C. C., Klein, R., Munoz, B., Kempen, J., . . . Mitchell, P. (2004). Causes and prevalence of visual impairment among adults in the United States. *Ophthalmology, 122*, 477–485.

Corn, A. L., & Erin, J. N. (Eds.). (2010). *Foundations of low vision: Clinical and functional perspectives* (2nd ed.). New York, NY: AFB Press.

Crandell, Jr., J. M., & Robinson, L. W. (2007). *Living with low vision and blindness: Guidelines that help professionals and individuals understand vision impairment.* Springfield, IL: Charles C Thomas.

Erickson, W., Lee, C., & von Schrader, S. (2013). *Disability statistics from the 2011 American Community Survey*. Ithaca, NY: Cornell University Employment and Disability Institute.

Falvo, D. (2014). *Medical and psychosocial aspects of chronic illness and disability* (5th ed.). Burlington, MA: Jones and Bartlett Learning.

Gerstenblith, A.T., Rabinowiltz, M. P., Barahimi, B. I., Fecarotta, C. M., Friedberg, M. A., & Rapuano, C. J. (2012). *The Wills Eye Manual: Office and emergency room diagnosis and treatment of eye disease* (6th ed.). Philadelphia, PA: Lippincott Williams & Wilkins.

Guide Dogs for the Blind. (1999). *At a glance: An educational resource guide*. San Rafael, CA: Author.

Hartong, D. T., Berson, E. L., & Dryja, T. P. (2006). Retinitis pigmentosa. *Lancet, 368*, 1795–1809.

Kanski, J. & Bowling, B. (2011). *Clinical ophthalmology: A systematic approach* (7th ed.). London, England: Butterworth-Heinemann.

Kinash, S. (2006). *Seeing beyond blindness*. Greenwich, CT: IAP-Information Age.

Kubler-Ross, E., & Kessler, D. (2005). *On grief and grieving: Finding the meaning of grief through the five stages of loss*. New York, NY: Scribner.

Mitchell P. (2004). Causes and prevalence of visual impairment among adults in the United States. *Ophthalmology, 122*, 477–485.

Panek, W. C. (2002). Visual disabilities. In M. G. Brodwin, F. A. Tellez, & S. K. Brodwin (Eds). *Medical, psychosocial, and vocational aspects of disability* (2nd ed., pp. 157–169). Athens, GA: Elliott & Fitzpatrick.

Sheth, V. S., Marcet, M. M., Chiranand, P., Bhatt, H. K., Lamkin, J. C., & Jager, R. D. (Eds.). (2012). *The Massachusetts eye and ear infirmary illustrated manual of ophthalmology* (4th ed.). Philadelphia, PA: Lippincott Williams & Wilkins.

Unger, J. (Ed.). (2007). *Diabetes management*. Philadelphia, PA: Saunders.

World Health Organization. (1994). *International classification of impairments, disabilities, and handicaps: A manual of classification relating to the consequences of disease*. Geneva, Switzerland: Author.

About The Authors

Bill Takeshita, O.D., F.A.A.O., F.C.V.D., is a low vision optometrist who received his doctorate from the Southern California College of Optometry. He is a fellow of the American Academy of Optometry and the College of Optometrists in Vision Development. Dr. Takeshita lectures throughout the country on low vision and vision development. Currently, he is Chief of Optometric Services at the Center for the Partially Sighted in Los Angeles, California and Director of Low Vision Services at the Braille Institute of America, Los Angeles.

Robin Langman, M.S., C.R.C., received her Master of Science degree in rehabilitation counseling from California State University, Los Angeles. She is a Certified Rehabilitation Counselor and completed a Certificate in Assistive Technology through California State University, Northridge. Ms. Langman is employed by the State of California, Department of Rehabilitation as a vocational rehabilitation counselor.

Rebekah Ketover Brod, M.A., M.F.T., is a licensed marriage and family therapist with a private practice in Santa Monica, California. Ms. Brod received her Master's Degree in Counseling from Antioch University in Santa Monica, California. Additionally, Rebekah is a professional chef.

Acknowledgements

Special thanks for assistance to Garry Brod and Marissa Langman.

Chapter 10

CHRONIC PAIN MANAGEMENT

Ashley T. Du, M.S.
John Lindberg, M.D.
Brendon W. Bluestein, Ph.D.

Introduction

Pain is one of the most common reasons for physician visits, use of medication, and cause of work disability (Institute of Medicine, 2011). Pain management represents one of the most difficult healthcare issues facing the medical profession and general population. Chronic pain is described as persistent pain which lasts more than three to six months and sometimes for years (American Chronic Pain Association [ACPA], 2013). In 2011, approximately 100 million adults in the United States were affected by chronic pain; about 50 million Americans today are either partially or totally disabled by it. The annual national economic cost associated with chronic pain is $560-630 billion (ACPA, 2013; Institute of Medicine, 2011). Chronic pain has been ranked as the third greatest healthcare problem in this country, following heart disease and cancer. Annual costs related to pain management are higher than those for heart disease, cancer, and diabetes combined (Pizzo & Clark, 2012).

Though advances have been made in pain management, chronic pain is still an overlooked problem in the United States (Pizzo & Clark, 2012). The rate of disability due to low back pain has increased by 14-fold. This chapter summarizes the theoretical and practical aspects of treating chronic pain. Emphasis is placed on the multifactorial nature of pain and the need to treat each patient as an individual within a biopsychosocial environment.

The following topics are discussed in this chapter: definition of pain, medical evaluation of chronic pain disorders, psychosocial assessment, medical management of chronic pain, patient involvement in treatment, and vocational aspects and rehabilitation. The chapter concludes with a case study of an individual with chronic pain.

Definition of Pain

Pain is a universal experience that is unique and subjective to each individual. A widely accepted definition given by the International Association for the Study of Pain (IASP) (1986) is the following: "Pain is an unpleasant sensory and emotional experience associated with actual or potential tissue damage, or described in terms of such damage. Pain is always subjective" (p. S217). Pain is classified by nociceptive, neuropathic, and sometimes undetermined causes. Nociceptive pain is due to ongoing tissue injury; neuropathic pain results from damage to the brain, spinal cord, or peripheral nerves (ACPA, 2013). Common origins of chronic pain are motor vehicle accidents, sports injuries, migraines, diabetes, arthritis, and shingles (Davis, 2010). Less understood pain disorders include phantom-limb pain, central pain (e.g., post-stroke pain), atypical facial neuralgias (pain not corresponding to a specific nerve disorder), fibromyalgia (non-specific aching pain, tenderness, and stiffness around joints and soft tissue), and enthesopathies (pain at the site of a tendon or muscle attachment). The IASP definition of pain includes those experienced in mental disorders that have no known noxious somatic source of the pain. Examples are pain as a symptom of mood disorders (depression and unresolved grief reactions), conversion disorders (e.g., hysterical neurosis), and delusional states.

Due to the subjectivity of pain and lack of objective diagnoses and treatments, healthcare providers and insurance companies encounter difficulties serving individuals with chronic pain. A subjective experience, the sensation of pain is an interaction between pain signals from the nervous system and a host of psychosocial factors such as past pain experiences and emotional responses (Pizzo & Clark, 2012).

Other than diagnosis, distinguishing between acute and chronic pain may be the most important factor influencing a treating clinician's options. Most researchers define acute pain as pain that lasts for less than six months (short-term pain), and chronic pain as pain that goes on for longer than six months (long-standing pain) (Banks & Mackrodt, 2005; Smith, 2007). The terms, *acute* and *chronic*, refer to the period of time the pain has lasted, not the severity of the problem or intensity of the pain (ACPA, 2013).

Impacting all aspects of life, chronic pain is complex, debilitating, and influenced by a variety of psychosocial factors. Rehabilitation often includes a team of healthcare providers and a carefully developed and implemented plan. Focus of care differs for patients experiencing acute versus chronic pain. Acute pain is typically managed with rest, immobilization of the particular joint(s), medication to reduce inflammation or provide analgesia, physical therapy, massage, pain control medications, surgery, exercise, and other health strategies. Interventions for acute pain are oriented towards resolution or return to baseline health and functioning.

While acute pain treatment strives for a cure, chronic pain treatment focuses on a longer-term solution aimed at managing pain by teaching the patient techniques on how to actively manage symptoms. Interventions such as injections, adjunctive medications, implanted devices, cognitive and behavioral techniques, relaxation strategies, and exercise are common methods used. The healthcare provider reorients the individual to achieve quality of life despite pain, while pursuing long-term strategies for pain reduction. Unfortunately, chronic pain often becomes a central issue in the person's life. Individuals with chronic pain frequently have observable alterations in their behaviors, including anxiety, depression, anger, and excessive use of medications and medical services.

Medical Evaluation of Chronic Pain Disorders

Assessment/Evaluation

Assessment of chronic pain requires a comprehensive and multidisciplinary approach (Smith, 2007). Given the prevalence of chronic pain, a major challenge that faces the United States health care system is the limited education medical students receive about chronic pain. Illustrated in a survey of 117 medical schools, deficiencies in pain management training pervade across all medical specialties; professionals are inadequately trained in the field to counsel patients with pain (Pizzo & Clark, 2012). According to these researchers, pain management needs to be taught to all medical professionals. The medical history of an illness may be pertinent to the cause of the pain. Specifying the location, frequency, intensity, and radiation of pain forms the foundation of most medical assessments. Just as important are how the pain began, what aggravates it, and what helps alleviate it. These are crucial questions prior to making a definitive diagnosis. The treating physician should investigate coexisting diseases or symptoms that appear unrelated but, on further evaluation, may point to previously undiscovered pathology (Clark & Treisman, 2004).

Examples of Common Chronic Pain Disorders

Complex Regional Pain Syndrome

This syndrome has had many names including causalgia, shoulder-hand syndrome, and most often, reflexive sympathetic dystrophy. Sensitivity to touch, tissue swelling, burning pain, excessive sweating, and changes in bone and skin are common symptoms of the syndrome (Reflex Sympathetic Dystrophy Syndrome Association, 2013). Trauma to an extremity usually precedes the onset of symptoms. Treatment outcome improves with early recognition, along with aggressive treatment of the sympathetic nervous system abnormality.

Fibromyalgia Syndrome

This disorder is marked by a presentation of chronic, diffuse muscular pain. Diagnosis is confirmed by finding of specific, localized tender points. Insomnia, headaches, and irritable bowel syndrome are common associated problems. Fibromyalgia is resistant to treatment and is a chronic condition in which minimal improvement is typical. People who have this condition need to remain as active as possible, while avoiding activities that exacerbate symptoms.

Arthropathies

Arthritic conditions such as osteoarthritis and rheumatic arthritis are common chronic pain conditions. Other arthropathies include systemic lupus erthymatosus and ankylosing spondylitis. Multiple joint involvements are typical, although only one joint may be involved with a chronic, progressive course. Diagnostic tests are beneficial for categorizing the arthritis and enhancing treatment options. With social support and encouragement, as well as effective coping strategies, adjustment issues such as anxiety and depression tend to decrease and outlook improves.

Phantom Limb Pain

Phantom limb sensation typically follows an amputation. The individual feels sensations that the amputated limb is still present. An adjustment period after an amputation is normal and phantom limb typically diminishes over time (Falvo, 2014). Some people, however, experience *phantom limb pain*, described as moderate to severe chronic pain in the amputated area which can reach a point where it becomes disabling. Medical treatment includes nerve blocks, surgical removal of neuromas, and chronic pain management (Clark & Treisman, 2004).

Neuropathies

These disorders often lead to chronic pain. Polyneuropathies, such as diabetic peripheral neuropathy, cause severe distal lower extremity pain that is resistant to treatment. A single traumatic nerve injury can be disabling if high intensity chronic pain becomes resistant to treatment. Carpal tunnel syndrome and cubital tunnel syndrome are neuropathies that are common and the result of cumulative traumas.

Lumbar Spine Disorders

According to the Centers for Disease Control and Prevention (CDC) and the National Center for Health Statistics, lower back pain is the most reported cause of chronic pain (Institute of Medicine, 2011). Some conditions have a primary symptom of chronic low back pain. Spinal stenosis, failed back syndrome, and chronic musculoligamentous strain are examples. General diagnoses such as *chronic low back pain* or *lumbago* are confusing to patients and healthcare providers alike. Vague diagnoses promote inaccurate treatment approaches for a broad range of these disorders. Successful formulation of a treatment plan and education of the patient with chronic low back pain necessitates a specific diagnosis (Polatin, Kinney, Gatchel, Lillo, & Mayer, 1993).

Headaches

Migraines and other severe headaches are common presenting pain complaints with a multitude of causes (Institute of Medicine, 2011). The headache is frequently a primary concern; yet, it may be a secondary symptom of a cervical spine disorder. Treatment of neck disorders frequently resolves headaches. Treatments include medications, biofeedback, stress reduction, and dietary changes (National Institute of Neurological Disorders and Stroke, 2013).

Psychosocial Assessment

In preparation for treatment of acute and chronic pain, the clinician assesses the complete physical and psychological status of the individual (Davis, 2010; Smith, 2007). The intake should focus on the individual's current and historical reports of pain. A three-part evaluation process begins with classification of the pain experience, followed by patient feedback, and development of treatment goals.

Adequate understanding of the pain complaints includes an assessment of the duration (acute vs. chronic), location, cause, frequency, and intensity of pain. The McGill Pain Questionnaire (Melzack, 1975) is still the most widely used instrument addressing these factors. However, the resulting data will lack coherence without a detailed psychosocial history that places the pain complaints in the appropriate context. The following should be addressed during chronic pain evaluations (Institute of Medicine, 2011; Melzack, 1975):

1. Orientation and neurocognitive status
2. Depression and the potential for suicide
3. Anxiety and post-traumatic stress disorder
4. Substance abuse
5. Pain behaviors (assess systemic reinforcers and punishers)
6. Status of litigation
7. Beliefs about pain
8. Consequences of pain reduction
9. Expectations of treatment

Regardless of the specific syndrome, chronic pain is recognized as a *biopsychosocial* disorder. Biopsychosocial assessment is used to identify the individual's attitudes, emotions about pain, environmental circumstances, and knowledge and beliefs about treatments (Institute of Medicine, 2011). According to Block, Kremer, and Kremer (2005), "there is now fairly strong literature demonstrating that, at least for some medical interventions, psychosocial variables are more potent indicators of treatment outcome than medical variables" (p. 219). As patients continue to experience chronic pain, they develop a constellation of beliefs. These attitudes become the psychological modulators of pain. Cognition and perceptions interact with affective, behavioral, and environmental factors in the interpretation of pain. As

FIGURE 1
The Cycle of Pain and Influence

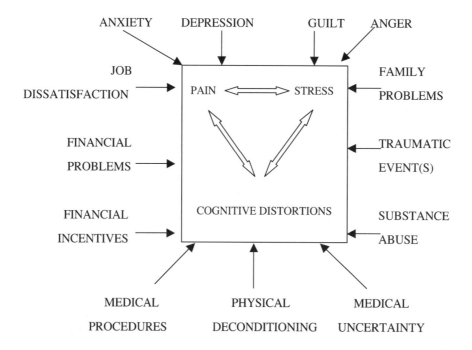

Source: Gatchel, R. J., & Turk, D. C. (1996). *Psychological approaches to pain management: A practitioner's guide.* New York, NY: Guilford.

depicted in Figure 1, pain, stress, and their cognitive interpretations create affective, social, occupational, and physical disruption.

Medical Management of Chronic Pain

Treatment of chronic pain can be a complicated process because many attempts often have to be made to find a treatment that is effective. Furthermore, many people with chronic pain do not know where to go for help, and when they do, they become discouraged and frustrated at the trial and error process of finding effective treatment or because of a practitioner's perceived insensitivity (Pizzo & Clark, 2012). Throughout this section, emphasis is placed on the need for a multidisciplinary team approach that blends a variety of treatments for each patient.

Treatment Modalities

Physical Therapy

Therapists utilize a variety of physical therapy modalities as adjuncts to overall treatment plans. Application of heat and cold, electrical stimulation, and ultrasound relax underlying tissues; this assists injured tissues to become more amenable to other treatments. Physical therapy is considered the first approach during the acute phase of pain. If pain persists despite several weeks of physical therapy, other modalities are prescribed for the person to administer at home. Individuals experiencing chronic pain commonly use heat or cold to alleviate symptoms of pain. Transcutaneous electrical nerve stimulation (TENS) is helpful for short-term pain relief (Davis, 2010). By carrying a small battery-operated unit attached to a belt, this portable device can provide effective pain relief at the job site and at home.

Manual Techniques

Massage, manipulation, manual adjustments, and physical therapy may relieve common ailments that cause both acute and chronic pain. These techniques may be applied to increase function, control pain, or help speed recovery (Institute of Medicine, 2011). Research shows that spinal manipulation can be more effective than bed rest, topical gels, traction, or no treatment (ACPA, 2013). Myofascial pain syndrome benefits from specific massage techniques which can be curative. During the acute phase of pain, these techniques attempt to correct the underlying problem.

Medications

For many clinicians, medication is the primary treatment of choice for chronic pain. Medications are used to treat the underlying condition and alleviate pain. Principles of pain management include strategic use of medications, conservative dosages, and frequent review of the necessity for continuing medications (Smith, 2007). The following is a review of the major medication categories used for chronic pain management.

Anti-Inflammatory Medication

Reducing inflammation is a goal of many chronic pain treatments. When an injury occurs, inflammatory cells respond, causing pain. Medications to treat inflammation heal tissues while concurrently alleviating pain. Nonsteroidal anti-inflammatory medications (NSAIDs) comprise the majority of pain relieving medications. They serve two roles: as a pain reliever and an anti-inflammatory agent (Davis, 2010).

Narcotic Analgesic Medications

Narcotics are one of the most prescribed medications for chronic pain (Davis, 2010). Narcotic analgesics are divided into two categories: opiates (alkaloids found in opium-like morphine) and opioids (fully synthetic and semi-synthetic derivatives of opiates like oxycodone and hydrocodone). They are used for acute pain, post-surgical pain, and pain related to malignancy. Controversy exists concerning the use of long-term narcotic analgesics due to addiction concerns. However, studies show that when used appropriately, often along with a combination of other medications, narcotic analgesic medications can be a beneficial component of pain management (Falvo, 2014; Gharibo & Khan, 2011).

Non-Narcotic Analgesic Medications

To prevent drug dependence on narcotic medications, non-narcotic analgesic medications are used for chronic pain management. The most commonly used non-narcotic analgesic is acetaminophen, which is sold without a prescription (more commonly known as Tylenol) (ACPA, 2013). The daily maximum dose of acetaminophen is 4000 mg; taking more than the maximum suggested dose or long-term use increases the risk of liver damage.

Muscle Relaxants

These medications are used during acute pain when muscle contractions are the predominant symptom. Muscle relaxants are sedating and are a concern when driving or when performing other high-risk activities. Careful caution should be taken when this category of drugs is used along with opioids (ACPA, 2013). Side effects make long term use difficult, especially when a person experiences cognitive deficits. Muscle relaxants are frequently avoided for chronic pain management.

Antidepressant Medications

Neurotransmitters, such as serotonin and norepinephrine, play a key role in depression and are also used for chronic pain (ACPA, 2013). Antidepressants neurochemically alleviate depression, directly relieve pain, and improve sleep by adjusting brain chemical levels (Clark & Treisman, 2004; Davis, 2010). This class of medication is helpful for fibromyalgia, headache, and pain due to nerve damage, but is less helpful for musculoskeltal injuries.

Injections

A multitude of injected medications exist for short-term pain relief. Injections are considered invasive and are not recommended until less invasive treatments are exhausted. Repetitive injections over an extensive time are contraindicated due to possible side effects (ACPA, 2013). Chronic pain programs use injections strategically as an adjunct within a comprehensive program.

Implanted Devices

Morphine pumps and intraspinal drug infusion therapy are used for chronic spine pain that has been resistant to other treatment modalities (Banks & Mackrodt, 2005). An implanted catheter releases small amounts of morphine or other medications into the spine, allowing pain relief with small timed doses (ACPA, 2013). Spinal cord stimulators are used for chronic pain, including pain in the extremities, secondary to radiculopathy. Spinal cord stimulators are only considered when all other methods have been unsuccessful (Davis, 2010).

Exercise

There is strong evidence that exercise is beneficial for individuals with chronic pain and should be a part of any pain management program. Building and maintaining strength, flexibility, and endurance, while increasing function and range of motion helps alleviate discomfort and pain (ACPA, 2013). The chronic pain cycle commonly deconditions a person, secondary to the sedentary lifestyle of bed rest and medications for the treatment of minor exacerbations. Exercise is a method used to prevent this unnecessary slide into a deconditioned state of health (Smith, 2007). The act of exercise, however, is often difficult for the individual with chronic pain and health care professionals need knowledge about designing an appropriate exercise program. Tai chi, yoga, and aquatics are possible exercise modalities that may be included in a comprehensive rehabilitation program for people with chronic pain (ACPA, 2013).

Biopsychosocial Treatment Management

As noted previously, treatment choice is dependent upon diagnosis, biopsychosocial background, and treatment goals. Pain interventions should be multidisciplinary and begin as soon as possible from the time of injury (Gharibo & Khan, 2011). The most effective chronic pain management programs provide medical intervention, physical therapy, occupational therapy, psychological treatment, and vocational therapy

(McCarberg & Passik, 2005). Biopsychosocial treatment of chronic pain syndromes relies on cognitive-behavioral techniques and self-regulation.

Operant Conditioning

Current psychological interventions in pain management are based on the conceptual understanding of operant pain (Fordyce et al., 1973). As *respondent pain* leads to altered accommodative behavior, expression of pain is shaped by behavioral reinforcement. Operant intervention occurs on two levels. Behavior is extinguished by withholding reinforcement, including switching to fixed medication intervals and eliminating social attention for pain. Concurrently, *well behaviors* are reinforced and attention is given for behaviors that are incompatible with pain. As with other psychological methods of pain management, self-regulation strategies (e.g., relaxation and biofeedback) are based upon operant conditioning theory.

Cognitive-Behavioral Techniques

Cognitive-behavioral techniques are based on the assumption that a person's thoughts and beliefs influence pain. For instance, a person's negative feelings about pain can increase sensitivity to pain and decrease activities that may alleviate pain (ACPA, 2013). Patients with chronic pain often fear that steps toward progress will lead to reinjury, worsening pain, failure, and loss of financial support. Thoughts, behaviors, emotions, and physiology affect one another. Four goals of cognitive-behavioral techniques follow (Smith, 2007; Turk, Meichenbaum, & Genest, 1983):

1. **Act rather than react.** Assist patients to perceive problems as manageable by developing problem-solving skills instead of being consumed by emotional reactions.
2. **Monitor.** Increase self-monitoring of thoughts, emotions, and behaviors in response to changes in physiology or the environment.
3. **Just do it.** Change behaviors regardless of feelings or belief in the response.
4. **Develop flexibility.** Maintain and develop effective coping strategies and continually adapt them.

Cognitive restructuring and self-regulation techniques are part of a comprehensive treatment plan for individuals who have chronic pain. Strategies of cognitive behavioral techniques enhance coping skills and confidence, as well as self-efficacy for managing pain (Institute of Medicine, 2011).

Self-Regulation Strategies

Current developments of self-regulation strategies are diverse and multimodal, and include regulating physiological states and autonomic responses to the environment. Active strategies for regulation include relaxation, biofeedback, hypnosis, and guided imagery.

Relaxation. Relaxation exercises include techniques such as diaphragmatic breathing, progressive muscle relaxation, guided imagery, and cue-controlled relaxation (ACPA, 2013). These techniques, along with biofeedback or hypnotic induction, often form the foundation of treatment. Progressive muscle relaxation increases awareness of the level of tension or relaxation.

Biofeedback. Biofeedback focuses on training the mind to control body functions to help reduce anxiety and stress reactions by controlling muscle tension, breathing, and heart rate (Davis, 2010). Equipment is used to measure muscle tension, hand temperature, and skin conductance to help teach patients about their bodies responses and how to relax (ACPA, 2013).

Hypnosis. When considering hypnosis, it is important to assess the person's attitudes and expectations concerning the nature and practice of this therapy. Direct induction procedures include (a) eliciting the patient's full cooperation, (b) focusing attention on the clinician's voice, (c) turning attention inward, and (d) suggesting dissociation. Once dissociation has been established, therapeutic suggestions are made to alleviate pain symptoms (Barber, 1996).

Guided imagery. Guided imagery incorporates relaxation techniques with clinician-directed or self-directed suggestions (Araoz, 1985). It is an internally mediated sensory (typically visual) experience of focused attention (Burte & Acer, 1997). Association of pain and relaxation to positive images promotes control over an abstract concept, along with dissociation from the experience of pain.

Patient Involvement in Treatment

One of the most challenging aspects of pain management is patient compliance and involvement in treatment. Faced with the perceived simplicity of psychological techniques, the patient is often skeptical about the efficacy of treatment (Falvo, 2014; Gordon & Dahl, 2004). With the burgeoning emphasis on medically-based pain management, patients may ascribe the following to psychological techniques. They may believe that therapists are discounting medical procedures, suggesting that the pain is not real, but rather "all in their head." Given this, even the individual who participates in treatment has difficulty succeeding with psychological techniques. Success indirectly confirms this belief, while failure provides assurance to the patient that the pain is real.

While enhancing the person's motivation for treatment is difficult, there is a great imperative for patient involvement in medication, physical rehabilitation, and psychological treatment. Responsibility for treatment is shifted from the professional to the patient; the patient is given the lead in treatment and management of his or her pain. The professional takes the role of *coach*, encouraging responsibility while assisting the person to develop a sense of efficacy through use of empowering presentation styles, reframing, role playing, metaphors, paradoxes, and challenging irrational ideation (Turk et al., 1983). If the professional's desire for improvement is greater than that of the patient, the treatment is likely to fail. Individuals need to be encouraged to develop realistic and practical goals to meet their specific needs and interests (Pizzo & Clark, 2012).

Vocational Aspects and Rehabilitation

Systemic factors influencing rehabilitation are as complex as they are powerful. Priorities of insurance companies are often in conflict with those of patients. Financial concerns of the insurer may be in opposition to the provision of effective vocational rehabilitation services. A main priority of the insurance industry is to save finances and maximize profit by limiting services provided. Limiting care in the short term reduces costs to the employer, removes non-eligible employees from the system, keeps financial settlements lower, and limits the responsibility of the company, impeding successful outcomes.

Early intervention in vocational rehabilitation increases motivation of injured workers. Employer interest and involvement, as well as an understanding of chronic pain, helps facilitate return to work. Reasonable accommodations for workers with chronic pain are variable and depend upon individualized assessment (Brodwin, Parker, & DeLaGarza, 2010). Key factors to success include a motivated worker, an involved employer, and a successful pain management treatment program. Williams et al. (1998) found that job satisfaction is a strong predictor of pain management success and eventual return to work. Employees who report high levels of dissatisfaction were two and a half times more likely to incur job-related back injuries than employees who reported work satisfaction. Individuals who blame their employers for the accident had poorer treatment outcomes (Gharibo & Khan, 2011). The rehabilitation counselor can best improve employment opportunities for those who have chronic pain by implementing a comprehensive evaluation of a person's capabilities and limitations, analysis of the types of worksite accommodations needed, and assessment of potential assistive devices.

Early intervention enhances the motivation of an employee to remain on the job if currently working or to return to work if on disability. Through participation in a chronic pain management program, identifying the causes of pain, understanding the side effects of medication, and assessing pain factors at work, the client can more effectively work with a counselor toward successful rehabilitation. Side effects of medication may require modification of certain work duties and in some cases, a change in medication regimen may alleviate problematic side effects that affect work functions. Employers who comprehend the dynamics of chronic pain are more willing to consider reasonable accommodation and job modification. Accommodations and job modifications are as variable as chronic pain itself (Brodwin et al., 2010).

Conclusion

The factors and wide-ranging effects of chronic pain give healthcare practitioners no simple solutions. Rather, a comprehensive rehabilitation team needs to take into account all aspects of the individual and how pain uniquely affects him or her. Multi-disciplinary treatment programs with a *biopsychosocial* emphasis are approaches that have the greatest chance for success.

Understanding the psychosocial aspects of chronic pain is often more important than the diagnosis or degree of pathology when predicting success. Though at times professionals would like to view pain as a purely mechanical problem that needs to be *fixed*, the more successful approach involves widening one's scope to include the multifactorial nature of pain. Through proactive rehabilitation, the counselor can assist the employee to remain on the job, minimize consequences of impairment, and effectively work with the employer to understand the importance of accommodation in diminishing disability and increasing job productivity.

Case Study

Mr. Thomas Malone is 29 years of age, married, and has a child three years of age. His wife is a physical therapist, employed full time by a medical clinic. After completing high school, Thomas attended a trade school for one year to become a respiratory therapist. During trade school, he was employed part-time as an orderly in a local community hospital. At times when the hospital was short staffed, he worked in the pharmacy as a pharmacy clerk, and also in the substance abuse clinic as a counselor aide.

The work of a respiratory therapist requires lifting up to 50 pounds occasionally and repetitive lifting and carrying of 10-20 pounds. The work takes one to two years to learn proficiently. The job of orderly requires lifting up to 100 pounds and can be learned in three to six months. A pharmacy clerk lifts and carries small items up to a maximum of 20 pounds. The position takes one to three months to learn. Counselor aide is sedentary work involving brief on-the-job training.

Upon completion of the respiratory therapy training program, Mr. Malone secured employment as a respiratory therapist for the same community hospital where he had been employed. After working for two years, Thomas injured his back while helping lift a patient. For the next nine months, he received comprehensive multidisciplinary treatment first for acute, and then for chronic low back pain.

Presently, Mr. Malone's chronic pain has diminished from moderately severe to moderate pain. His treating physician restricts him to a maximum of light work activities.

Questions

1. Provide a vocational profile for Mr. Malone, including age category, educational level, and work history. Include the skill and exertional levels for each job.
2. Discuss the differences between acute and chronic pain.
3. Describe a comprehensive, multidisciplinary treatment program for chronic pain.
4. Explore the psychosocial factors involved in chronic pain and its relevance to this case.
5. How would you approach vocational rehabilitation for this client?
6. Assess the various treatment modalities used for chronic pain.
7. Develop several vocational rehabilitation plans for Tom Malone.

References

American Chronic Pain Association (ACPA). (2013). *ACPA resource guide to chronic pain medicine and treatment*. Retrieved from http://www.theacpa.org/uploads/ACPA_Resource_Guide_2013_Final_011313.pdf

Araoz, D. L. (1985). *The new hypnosis*. New York, NY: Brunner/Mazel.

Banks, C., & Mackrodt, K. (Eds.). (2005). *Chronic pain management. Part 1*. Philadelphia, PA: Whurr.

Barber, J. (1996). *Hypnosis and suggestion in the treatment of pain: A clinical guide.* New York, NY: W. W. Norton.

Block, A. R., Kremer, E. F., & Kremer, A. M. (2005). Chronic pain syndromes. In H. H. Zaretsky, E. F. Richter, & M. G. Eisenberg (Eds.), *Medical aspects of disability: A handbook for the rehabilitation professional* (3rd ed., pp. 213–239). New York, NY: Springer.

Brodwin, M. G., Parker, R. M., & DeLaGarza, D. (2010). Disability and reasonable accommodation. In E. M. Szymanski & R. M. Parker (Eds.), *Work and disability: Contexts, issues, and strategies for enhancing employment for people with disabilities* (3rd ed., pp. 281–323). Austin, TX: Pro-ed.

Burte, J. M., & Acer, K. M. (1997, May). *Guided Imagery.* Paper presented at the meeting of the American Academy of Pain Management, Las Vegas, NV.

Clark, M. R., & Treisman, G. J. (2004). *Pain and depression: An interdisciplinary patient-centered approach.* New York, NY: Basel.

Davis, J. L. (2010). *Chronic pain relief: New treatments.* Retrieved from http://www.webmd.com/pain-management/features/chronic-pain-relief-new-treatments

Falvo, D. (2014). *Medical and psychosocial aspects of chronic illness and disability* (5th ed.). Burlington, MA: Jones and Bartlett.

Fordyce, W. E., Fowler, R. S., Lehmann, J. F., Delateur, B. J., Sand, P. L., & Trieschmann, R. B. (1973). Operant conditioning in the treatment of chronic pain. *Archives of Physical Medicine and Rehabilitation, 54,* 399–408.

Gharibo, C. G., & Khan, M. F. (2011). Chronic pain syndromes. In S. R. Flanagan, H. H. Zaretsky, & A. Moroz (Eds.). *Medical aspects of disability: A handbook for the rehabilitation professional* (4th ed., pp. 147–158). New York, NY: Springer.

Gordon, D., & Dahl, J. (2004). Quality improvement challenges in pain management. *Pain, 107,* 1–4.

Institute of Medicine. (2011). *Relieving pain in America: A bluebook for transforming prevention, care, education, and research.* Washington, DC: National Academies.

International Association for the Study of Pain. (1986). Classification of chronic pain: Descriptions of chronic pain syndromes and definitions of pain terms. *Pain, 13,* S1–S225.

McCarberg, B., & Passik, S. D. (Eds.). (2005). *Expert guide to pain management.* Philadelphia, PA: American College of Physicians.

Melzack, R. (1975). The McGill Pain Questionnaire: Major properties and scoring methods. *Pain, 1,* 277–299.

National Institute of Neurological Disorders and Stroke. (2013). *Headache: Hope through research.* Bethesda, MD: Author.

Pizzo, P. A., & Clark, N. M. (2012). Alleviating suffering 101— Pain relief in the United States. *New England Journal of Medicine, 366,* 3.

Polatin, P. B., Kinney, R. K., Gatchel, R. J., Lillo, E., & Mayer, T. G. (1993). Psychiatric illness and chronic low back pain. *Spine, 18,* 66–77.

Reflex Sympathetic Dystrophy Association. (2013). *About CRPS.* Retrieved from http://www.rsds.org/2/what_is_rsd_crps/

Smith, H. S. (2007). *Pain management. Part 1.* Philadelphia, PA: Saunders.

Turk, D. C., Meichenbaum, D., & Genest, J. (1983). *Pain and behavioral medicine: A cognitive behavioral perspective.* New York, NY: Guilford.

Williams, R. A., Pruitt, S. D., Doctor, J. N., Epping-Jordan, J. E., Wahlgren, D. R., Grant, I., . . . Atkinson, J. B. (1998). The contribution of job satisfaction to the transition from acute to chronic low back pain. *Archives of Physical Medicine and Rehabilitation, 79*(4), 366–374.

About the Authors

Ashley T. Du, M.S., received her Master of Science degree in counseling, with options in rehabilitation and school counseling leadership. Her interests are in the areas of chronic pain management and in providing the most effective counseling and rehabilitation services for students. Ms. Du specializes in transitional counseling with an emphasis in college and career.

John Lindberg, M.D., specializes in treatment and management of chronic pain patients. He is a board certified physiatrist by the American Board of Physical Medicine and Rehabilitation. Dr. Lindberg is Medical Director of the Chronic Pain Management Program at Casa Colina Center for Rehabilitative Medicine in Pomona, California. Additionally, Dr. Lindberg is Medical Director of Rehabilitation Medicine at Citrus Valley Medical Center in Covina, California.

Brendon W. Bluestein, Ph.D., is a clinical psychologist with a specialty in behavioral analysis and chronic pain management. He practices in Fort Meade, Maryland. Dr. Bluestein was the Coordinator of the Chronic Pain Program at Casa Colina Center for Rehabilitative Medicine. While a Captain in the United States Army, he served as a psychologist at Walter Reed Hospital and worked in pain management with paratroopers and pilots in Alabama and Georgia.

Chapter 11

INTEGRATIVE MEDICINE

Hua Gu, Ph.D., L.Ac.
Sandra K. Brodwin, M.S., C.R.C.

Introduction

Alternative and complementary medicines, together with East Asian and other forms of traditional medicine, have attracted the attention of people worldwide. In 2002, the National Library of Medicine classified alternative medicine under the term complementary therapies: therapeutic practices which are not currently considered an integral part of conventional medical practice. These interventions are not often taught in American medical schools and are not available in American hospitals. It is accepted that a number of diseases remain incurable by Western medicine. With all its successes, Western medicine has its limitations, such as alleviating symptoms, the side effects of medications, high costs of treatment, inaccessibility of facilities and treatment, and so forth. Alternative medicine is part of a solution to some of these inadequacies (Bishop & Lewith, 2013).

The Federal government's lead research agenda for the study of Complementary and Alternative Medicine (CAM) is the National Center for Complementary and Alternative Medicine (NCCAM). When Western medicine began to address the growing trend toward CAM treatment, the National Institute of Health (NIH) formed a policy panel that defined CAM as "a broad domain of healing resources that encompasses all health systems, modalities, and practices, and their accompanying theories and beliefs, other than those intrinsic to the politically dominant health system of a particular society or culture in a given historical period." Most CAM practices are guided by four common principles: prevention, natural healing, active learning, and holistic approaches. Doctors who are embracing CAM therapies, combining them with mainstream medical therapies, often use the term *integrative medicine* to refer to their practices (Mayo Clinic, 2010). In its 2011-2015 strategic plan, NCCAM Director Josephine P. Briggs stated, "Symptoms matter, and few would dispute the fact that modern medicine does not always succeed in alleviating them. Few would also dispute the need for better approaches for encouraging healthy lifestyle choices. These are places in which I believe CAM-inclusive approaches offer promise."

What we now define as *alternative or integrative medicine* was first discussed by Chinese philosophers over 3,000 years ago (Pham, Yoo, Tran, & Ta, 2013). Foundational differences between Western and Eastern medical models has made it difficult for medical providers in the United States to embrace the idea of health as a state of balance between the physical, mental, social, and super-natural environment. Western medicine tends to approach disease by assuming it is due to an external force, such as a virus or bacteria, or a slow degeneration of the functional ability of the body. Disease, in the eyes of Western medicine, is either physical or mental. The Eastern approach, on the other hand, assumes that each part of the body is intimately connected. Each organ is viewed as having a mental as well as a physical function (Carteret, 2011).

The goal of CAM treatment practices is to promote health and prevent or manage conditions. Between 1990 and 2007, more adults turned to CAM to treat conditions including back pain, neck pain, joint pain, stiffness, anxiety, and depression (the latter two are commonly associated with chronic pain) via acupuncture, deep breathing exercises, massage therapy, meditation, naturopathy, and yoga.

NCCAM classifies CAM therapies into these categories: Whole Medical Systems, Mind-body Medicine, Biologically-based Practices, Manipulative and Body-based Practices, and Energy Therapy. **Whole Medical Systems** is based on the idea that a system is not just a single practice or remedy but many practices that center on a philosophy, such as the power of nature or the presence of energy in one's body. Homeopathy uses minute doses of a substance that causes symptoms to stimulate the body's self-healing response. Naturopathy focuses on noninvasive treatments to help the body do its own healing and uses a variety of practices, such as massage, acupuncture, herbal remedies, exercise, and lifestyle counseling. **Mind-body** techniques target strengthening the paths of communication between the mental and physical states of being, enabling them to function in harmony. Examples of mind-body connection techniques include meditation, prayer, and relaxation and art therapies (Ernst, Pittler, & Wider, 2006; Mayo Clinic, 2010).

Biologically-based practices include dietary supplements and herbal remedies using ingredients found in nature. Examples of herbs are ginseng, ginkgo, and Echinacea. Other dietary supplements include selenium, glucosamine sulfate, and SAMe. Herbs and supplements can be taken as teas, oils, syrups, powders, and tablets or capsules. The methods of **Manipulative and Body-based** practices use human touch to move or manipulate a specific part of the body. They include chiropractic and osteopathic manipulation and massage. **Energy Therapy** is based on balancing the body's flowing energy force. When this energy flow is blocked or unbalanced, the individual can become sick. This energy is referred to as chi, prana, or life force. Energy Therapies include qi gong, therapeutic touch, reiki, and magnet therapy (Moroz & Schulman, 2011).

It is not possible in one chapter to capture all the pertinent information on the total spectrum of Complementary and Alternative (Integrative) Medicine. Therefore, the authors have chosen the most commonly used of these therapies in the United States: **Whole Medical Systems** (i.e., Traditional Chinese Medicine-Acupuncture and Homeopathy), **Manipulative and Body-based** (i.e., Chiropractic Medicine), and **Biologically-based** (i.e., Biofeedback/Neurofeedback).

Whole Medical Systems

Traditional Chinese Medicine – Acupuncture

Traditional Chinese Medicine (TCM) is one of the most ancient forms of medicine and embodies achievements accumulated over millennia (Tan et al., 2007). Practice of this ancient form of medicine began in earnest in the United States in the early 1970s after President Richard Nixon visited China in 1972. TCM is based on a personalized and holistic approach to health and disease. Herbal remedies and acupuncture are the treatments most commonly used by TCM practitioners. Other TCM practices include moxibustion, cupping, massage, mind-body therapy, and dietary therapy. In this chapter, the focus is on the practice of acupuncture.

Overview and History

The *Yellow Emperor's Internal Classic*, the oldest known work of Chinese medical theory, was compiled around the first century BCE (Before the Common Era) on the basis of shorter texts from different medical lineages. Written in the form of dialogues between the legendary Yellow Emperor and his ministers, it offers explanations on the relation between humans, their environment, and the cosmos; on the contents of the body; on human vitality and pathology; on the symptoms of illness; and on how to make diagnostic and therapeutic decisions in light of all these factors. Unlike earlier texts, such as *Recipes for Fifty-Two Ailments*, excavated in the 1970s from a tomb that had been sealed in 168 BCE, the Yellow Emperor's internal classic rejected the influence of spirits and the use of magic. It was also one of the first books in which the cosmological doctrines of Yingyang and the Five Phases were brought to a mature synthesis (Gu, 1989).

Traces of therapeutic activities in China date from the Shang Dynasty (14th – 11th centuries BCE). Though the Shang did not have a concept of *medicine* as distinct from other fields, their oracular inscriptions on bones and tortoise shells refer to illnesses that affected the Shang royal family. These included eye disorders, toothaches, bloated abdomen, and so forth, which Shang elites usually attributed to curses sent by their ancestors.

In 600 BCE, TCM doctors began practicing bone-setting along with palpation, observation, and measurement. Hua Tou of the Eastern Han Dynasty, performed orthopedic surgery and used herbs for anesthesia. Between 341 and 265 BCE, TCM practitioners used wood splints to stabilize fractures and avoid surgery. Splints enabled doctors to treat and rehabilitate their patients simultaneously. From 206 to 112 BCE, functional exercises and rehabilitation were widely used in the therapy of trauma and bone/joint diseases. Physicians asked patients to do exercises similar to other animals, such as the monkey, bear, bird, and rhino called the *five animal exercises*. These exercises are used today after surgery to assist in the healing process (Wax & White, 2000).

TCM practices a complete system between treatment and rehabilitation based on the theory of Qi and blood, Yin and Yang, internal organs, and the five elements and meridians within the body. The concept of Qi was first introduced in TCM in the 5th Century BCE. Body movement is key to maintaining Qi circulation. If the body is injured and not able to move, the Qi will stagnate and cause problems. In 475 to 221 BCE, the first TCM book was written describing Qi as consisting of blood, brain, spinal cord, joints, and muscles (Beijing College of Traditional Chinese Medicine, 2011).

When Qi or blood circulation is interrupted, injury or disease occurs. To protect the body with proper Qi and blood movement, TCM emphasizes prevention with acupuncture, herbs, and exercises. Generally speaking, the word Qi connotes both substance and function, two different but closely related concepts that cannot be entirely separated. Each function must be based on a certain substance and vice versa (Beijing College of Traditional Chinese Medicine, 2011).

Patterns of Use

As noted by Gu (1989), the theory of *yin-yang* is that every object or phenomenon in the universe consists of two opposite aspects: yin and yang, which are at once in conflict and act interdependently. This relationship is the universal law of the material world, the principle and source of existence, and the root cause for the flourishing and perishing of living things. These relationships between yin and yang are extensively used in TCM to explain the physiology and pathology of the human body, and serve as a guide for diagnosis and treatment in clinical work.

The theory of the five elements indicates that wood, fire, earth, metal, and water are basic materials constituting the material world. There exists among them an interdependence and inter-restraint that determines their state of constant motion and change. The theory of the five elements explains the symbiotic and counter active relationship of yin-yang. Using the theory of the five elements and yin-yang, TCM is classified into different categories: natural phenomena, tissues and organs of the human body, and human emotions (Gu, 1989, 2010).

The internal organs connect in the body through channels and collaterals with the various tissues and organs of the superficial portion of the body to create organic integrity (Teppone & Avakyan, 2007). In the network of channels and collaterals, the channels pertain to the respective organs; the collaterals are their minor branches which are distributed throughout the body. Along each channel are points for applying acupuncture. The efficacy of acupuncture in prevention and treatment of disease is due to regulating and strengthening the defensive function and helping restore relative balance within the human body, as well as that between the body and its environment. Points are the specific sites through which the Qi of the organs and channels is transported to the body surface. When the body is affected by a disease, the treatment will center on puncturing the corresponding points on the body surface.

Seven emotional factors are classified in TCM: joy, anger, melancholy, meditation, grief, fear, and fright (Ots, 1990). These factors are reflections of the human mental state as induced by various stimulations in the environment. They are physiological phenomena that do not cause disease under normal conditions. However, if the emotions are very intense and persistent or the individual is hypersensitive to the stimulations, they may result in drastic and long-standing changes in emotion, which can lead to chronic physical problems or disease. Traumatic injuries, for example, can cause stagnant blood or phlegm and induce pain or deformity (Xinnong & Deng, 2010).

The four diagnostic methods in TCM include: inquiring about the patient's condition; inspection, or examining the expression, color, and appearance of the tongue; auscultation or listening; and palpation (feeling the patient's pulse) (Gu, 1989). The palpation of pulse means not only the speed, but also the quality (thready, wiry, or slippery) (Zhiya, 2002).

Identifying a syndrome entails further analysis and synthesis of the clinical data obtained using the four diagnostic methods. The differentiation of diseases can be derived from eight principles: exterior and interior, cold and heat, deficiency and excess, and yin and yang (Langevin et al., 2004). Disorders of channels may affect the corresponding organs, and disorders of the organs are reflected at the corresponding channels. Channels connect with organs and exteriorly with the body surface where points are distributed.

Herbal medicine is a part of TCM; there are roughly 13,000 medicinals used in China and over 100,000 medicinal recipes recorded in the ancient literature. Plant elements and extracts are by far the most common elements used. In the classic *Handbook of Traditional Drugs* from 1941, 517 drugs were listed. Out of these, only 45 were derived from animal parts, and 30 were based on minerals. For many plants used as medicinals, detailed instructions have been handed down not only regarding the locations and areas where they grow best, but also regarding the best timing of planting and harvesting them.

There are many differences between Chinese medicine and conventional medicine (Gu, 1989). Conventional medicine tries to locate where the problem specifically originates, such as organ level (heart, liver, kidney), cell level, or even molecular level. Rather, Chinese medicine focuses on the whole body and tries to balance the body with acupuncture and herbs. Sometimes TCM concentrates on the result and may not seek to understand what happened inside the body. Acupuncture helps induce the body's own healing power to regain balance (Beijing College of Traditional Chinese Medicine, 2011).

Professionals working in the area of acupuncture attend formal training. The intensity and length of training varies, including certificate or diploma programs and degree programs – bachelor's, master's, and doctorate degrees.

Homeopathy

Homeopathy ("home-ee-AH-pah-thy") is derived from the Greek words *homios* (similar) and *pathos* (suffering) and focuses on stimulating the body's natural healing properties to cure or alleviate illness or disease. A practitioner of homeopathy treats a patient by introducing a substance into the body that induces symptoms identical to those caused by the disease to stimulate healing energy. Homeopathy is based on Hippocrates' Law of Similars, otherwise known as the philosophy that *like cures like* (Yuan & Bieber, 2003). Homeopathic remedies are dilutions of natural substances from plants, minerals, and animals. Once the patient's initial symptoms are resolved, the practitioner treats underlying symptoms.

Overview and History

In the late 1700s, Samuel Hahnemann, a physician, chemist, and linguist in Germany, developed homeopathy as an approach to treating illness (Haller, 2005). This was at a time when the most common medical treatments included bloodletting, purging, and blistering, using harsh substances such as sulfur and mercury. At the time, few effective medications existed to treat patients, and knowledge about the effects of existing treatments was limited.

Hahnemann was interested in developing a less-threatening approach to medicine. It is alleged that Hahnemann stumbled upon his first major discovery while translating an herbal text about the use of cinchona bark to cure malaria. Curious, an otherwise healthy Hahnemann ingested some cinchona bark. He developed symptoms very similar to those experienced by sufferers of malaria. This led Hahnemann to consider that a substance may create symptoms that it can also relieve. He began experimenting with other single, pure substances on himself and, in more dilute forms, on healthy volunteers. He kept meticulous records of his experiments and participants' responses, and he combined these observations with information from clinical practice, the known uses of herbs and other medicinal substances, and toxicology, eventually treating the sick and developing a homeopathic clinical practice (Yuan & Bieber, 2003).

Hahnemann added two additional elements to homeopathy: *potentization* and the idea that treatment should be selected based upon a total picture of an individual and his or her symptoms, not solely upon symptoms of a disease. Potentization holds that diluting a substance with vigorous shaking at each step of dilution makes the remedy more, not less, effective by extracting the vital essence of the substance. If dilution continues to a point where the substance's molecules are gone, homeopathy holds that the *memory* of them - that is, the effects they exerted on the surrounding water molecules - may still be therapeutic. Homeopaths evaluate not only a person's physical symptoms but emotions, mental states, lifestyle, nutrition, and other aspects. In homeopathy, different people with the same symptoms may receive different homeopathic remedies (Yuan & Bieber, 2003).

Boston-born physician Hans Burch Gram introduced homeopathy into the United States in 1825. European immigrants trained in homeopathy made the treatment increasingly available in America. In 1835, the first homeopathic medical college was established in Allentown, Pennsylvania. By the turn of the 20th Century, 8% of all American medical practitioners were homeopaths; there were 20 homeopathic medical colleges and more than 100 homeopathic hospitals in this country (Andrasik & Lords, 2009).

In the 1960s, the popularity of homeopathy increased in North America. In 1999, over six million Americans reported using homeopathy. In 1994, the World Health Organization reported that homeopathy had been integrated into the national health care systems of numerous countries including Germany, the United Kingdom, India, Pakistan, Sri Lanka, and Mexico (Jonas, Kaptchuk, & Linde, 2003).

Patterns of Use

Many who seek homeopathic care use it to alleviate chronic medical conditions; most treat themselves with homeopathic products and do not consult professional care. Those who do seek professional help experience a lengthy first visit during which the provider takes an in-depth assessment which guides the selection of one or more homeopathic remedies. During follow-up visits, patients report how they are responding to the remedy or remedies to help the practitioner make decisions about further treatment (Kessler et al., 2001).

A homeopathic remedy is prepared by diluting a substance through a series of steps. Providers refer to the *Homeopathic Pharmacopoeia of the United States* to match symptom profiles of patients with the appropriate remedy. Homeopathy asserts that this process can maintain the healing properties of a substance regardless of how many times it has been diluted. Many homeopathic remedies are so highly diluted that none of the original natural substance remains. The U. S. Food and Drug Administration recognizes homeopathic dilutions as official drugs and regulates the manufacturing, labeling, and dispensing of homeopathic medications.

Research has been conducted to address this dilemma. Researchers have found that homeopathic remedies give off electromagnetic signals; each homeopathic substance has a specific dominant frequency (del Giudici & Preparata, 1990). It is theorized that homeopathic remedies convey the electromagnetic message to the body that matches the frequency of the illness, stimulating the healing properties of the body: one subtle energy (remedy) affects another subtle energy (human energy field). As in other CAMs, this subtle energy field in the body is called the *vital force*.

In the United States, homeopathic training is offered through diploma and certificate programs, short courses, and correspondence courses. It is also a component of medical education in naturopathy, a medical system that originated in Europe which aims to support the ability of the body to heal itself through the use of dietary and lifestyle changes together with CAM therapies such as herbs, massage, and joint manipulation. Most homeopathy in North America is conducted along with another health care practice for which the practitioner is licensed, such as conventional medicine, naturopathy, chiropractic, dentistry, or acupuncture.

Manipulative and Body-Based

Chiropractic

As with acupuncture practitioners, the goal of chiropractic is to support the natural ability of the body to heal itself. The Greek word *chiropractor* means done by hand. Chiropractic is a health care approach that focuses on the relationship between the body structure, primarily the musculoskeletal system and its functioning. Although practitioners may use a variety of treatment approaches, they mainly perform manipulation (an ancient healing art) with the goal of correcting alignment. Chiropractors are the second largest group of primary care providers in this country (World Federation of Chiropractic, 2012).

Overview and History

The word *chiropractor* combines the Greek words *cheir* (hand) and *praxis* (action) to describe a treatment done by hand. Hands-on therapy, especially adjustment of the spine, is central in chiropractic care. No one culture has been identified as the originator of chiropractic. It has been found in the ancient cultures of China, Japan, Polynesia, India, Egypt, Tibet, and in the Aztec, Inca, Maya, Sioux, and Winnebago cultures of the Americas. Through the 17th Century, there are medical records throughout the cultures of Europe detailing the use of traction applied to parts of the body while pressure was applied on a specific area of the spine. Hippocrates, considered to be the father of medicine, was a practitioner of manipulation. Practitioners of bone setting during the Middle Ages and the Renaissance performed manipulation (Bergman & Peterson, 2011).

Therapeutic manipulation practice was founded in the late 19th century. While Andrew Still watched his wife and their three children die, he became convinced that the body needed to heal itself, but had to be structurally sound to accomplish the healing. He decided that healing would take place when the *life force* could be accessed. The life force could be released when the spine was manipulated to relieve mechanical pressure on blood vessels and nerves. If the nerves were impinged in any way, blood flow was reduced resulting in pain, necrosis, and impingement of the healing life force (Still, 2009).

While some procedures associated with chiropractic care can be traced back to ancient times, the modern profession of chiropractic was founded by Dr. Daniel Palmer in 1895 in Davenport, Iowa. Palmer, a self-taught healer, believed the body has a natural healing ability. Misalignments of the spine interfere with the flow of energy needed to support health. Palmer theorized that the key to health is to normalize the function of the nervous system, especially the spinal cord. As with acupuncture providers, chiropractors perform diagnosis by visual inspection and palpation in addition to x-ray and other diagnostic methods. Chiropractic is the leading complementary and alternative medicine model. Acupuncturists, nutritionists, homeopaths, and naturopaths combined do not equal the number of chiropractors in the United States (Singer, 2013).

Patterns of Use

People seek chiropractic care primarily for pain conditions such as back and neck pain, headache, musculoskeletal conditions, menstrual pain, and asthma. According to the 2007 National Health Interview Survey, which includes a comprehensive survey of the use of complementary health practices by Anericans, about 8% of adults (more than 18 million) and nearly 3% of children (more than two million) had received chiropractic care within the past year.

A 1999 national survey on use of CAM found that 20% of adults in the United States had received chiropractic care at some point during their lives. Those surveyed reported using chiropractic treatment for the following reasons: combining chiropractic services with conventional medical treatments would help (53%); conventional medicine would not help (40%); chiropractic would be interesting to try (32%); a conventional medical professional suggested it (20%); and conventional medical treatments were too expensive (10%) (Ni, Simile, & Hardy, 2002).

Chiropractic is based on these key concepts: (a) the body has a powerful self-healing ability; (b) the body's structure (primarily the spine) and its function are closely related; and (c) this relationship affects health. Therapy aims to normalize this relationship between structure and function and assist the body as it heals. Chiropractic has two main groups: *straights*, now the minority, emphasize vitalism, innate intelligence, and spinal adjustments, and consider subluxations, complexes of functional, structural, and/or pathological articular changes that compromise neural integrity and may influence organ system function and general health. *Mixers* are more open to mainstream and alternative medical techniques such as exercise, massage, nutritional supplements, and acupuncture (Tetrault, 2004). This treatment modality is the most frequently used of the CAMs. However, many providers of chiropractic treatment do not associate it with CAM, but with Western conventional medicine (Davis, Mackenzie, Coulter, Whedon, & Weeks, 2012). This treatment modality is the most frequently used of all types of CAM.

The theory of chiropractic is that misaligned spinal vertebrae interfere with nerve function, resulting in altered physiologic conditions which contribute to pain and disease. A common diagnosis to support this theory is subluxation, an impinged nerve as a result of misalignment in the spine, causing pain (Gatterman, 2005). Chiropractic belief is that this misalignment also prevents body defenses from performing appropriately. By adjusting the spinal joints, subluxation is resolved, restoring normal nerve function and optimal health. Chiropractic has expanded to include improving joint mobility and alleviating restricted movement as a result of spinal fixation (Mirtz, Morgan, Wyatt, & Greene, 2009).

During the initial visit, chiropractors take a health history and perform a physical examination, with a special emphasis on the spine. Other examinations or tests, such as x-rays, may be performed. If chiropractic treatment is considered appropriate, the practitioner develops a treatment plan. During follow-up visits, practitioners may perform one or more of the many different types of adjustments used in chiropractic care. Centered mainly in the spine, a chiropractic adjustment (sometimes referred to as a manipulation) involves using the hands or a device to apply a controlled, sudden force to a joint, moving it beyond its passive range of motion. The goal is to increase range and quality of motion in the area being treated, and to aid in restoring health. Other hands-on therapies also are used (Ernst et al., 2006).

Adjustment procedures, including adjustments, manipulations, and mobilization, are the defining technique of chiropractic treatment. Terms associated with chiropractic include: adjustment, manipulation, and mobilization. These terms relate to joint movement, which can be divided into active end range (how far the patient can, with muscular effort, move a joint in a particular direction), passive end range (at the end of the active end range, a clinician can safely move the joint further), anatomic end range, and paraphysiologic joint space which exceeds the passive end range but not the anatomic end range (Andrasik & Lords, 2009). *Manipulation* is passive movement of the joint past the passive end range but not the anatomic end range. *Mobilization* is the clinician-assisted passive movement within the anatomic end range resulting in an increased overall range-of-joint motion. Over 150 chiropractic techniques are currently being used (Cox, 2011).

The effects of manipulation are classified as either mechanical or neurological. Mechanical manipulations are defined in terms of the subluxation – spinal joint strain or sprain with local and referred pain and muscle spasm. Neurological manipulations include both direct and indirect effects on the function of the peripheral nervous system and the central nervous system because of spinal dysfunction.

Chiropractors may combine the application of spinal adjustments with several other treatments, such as application of alternating temperatures, electrical stimulation, and rehabilitative exercise. Chiropractors may also prescribe lifestyle changes including adjustments to the patient's diet.

To practice within the United States, a chiropractor must earn a Doctor of Chiropractic (D.C.) degree from a college accredited by the Council on Chiropractic Education (CCE, 2013). CCE is the agency certified by the U. S. Department of Education to accredit chiropractic colleges. Admission to a chiropractic college requires a minimum of 90 semester hour credits (approximately three years) of undergraduate study, primarily in the sciences. Chiropractic training is a four-year academic program that includes both classroom work and direct experience caring for patients. Coursework typically includes instruction in the biomedical sciences, as well as in public health and research methods. Some chiropractors pursue an additional two to three-year residency for training in specialized fields.

Biologically-Based Practices

Biofeedback/Neurofeedback

Biofeedback/neurofeedback is a treatment technique in which patients are trained to improve their health by using signals from their own bodies (Collura, 2012). While physical therapists may use biofeedback, for example, to help stroke survivors regain movement in paralyzed muscles, psychologists may use it to help clients reduce tension and anxiety. Specialists in different fields sometimes use biofeedback to help patients cope with pain. Using biofeedback machines, clinicians detect a patient's internal bodily functions, which they then use to gauge and direct the progress of treatment. A biofeedback therapist acts as a coach, helping the patient set goals and limits on what to expect and how to improve performance.

Overview and History

In the early part of the 20th century in Germany, J. H. Schultz developed a technique called autogenic training in which verbal instructions are used to guide a person to a different, more relaxed and controlled physiological state. Years later, an American, Edmund Jacobson, developed the technique of progressive relaxation training, a series of muscle activities designed to teach people how to control tension and relaxation through awareness of reducing muscle tension and stress. During the 1960s and 1970s, gradual awareness of Eastern yogic traditions involving voluntary physiologic adjustments began to emerge in the Western world attracting the attention of a few key researchers. Gurus taught these researchers that by using relaxation and control, they could change a number of variables previously thought to be autonomously regulated, including blood pressure, heart rate, and body temperature. These functions are managed by the autonomic nervous system (ANS), so named precisely because it was thought that such functions could not be voluntarily altered (Collura, 2012).

The ANS has two divisions—the *sympathetic* and the *parasympathetic*. The sympathetic nervous system regulates the flight/fight response. The parasympathetic nervous system calms and relaxes and manages body functions. The two work in tandem in a reciprocal relationship. Canon and Selye, two researchers who focused on the body's response to stress, brought an increase in the general awareness of the role of stress in physical diseases and mental disorders (Robertson, Biaggioni, Burnstock, Low, & Paton, 2011).

Yogic practices, such as *hatha yoga*, became established in the United States as techniques for physical relaxation and enhancement of conscious control over physiology. Additionally, meditation techniques stimulated the elaboration of the relaxation and attention training techniques influencing and controlling the body with the conscious mind to promote relaxation and manage pain and stress. A number of these techniques, combined with biofeedback/neurofeedback, enhance learning physiological self-regulation (mind-body control).

Patterns of Use

The word *biofeedback* was coined in the late 1960s to describe laboratory procedures then being used to train experimental research subjects to alter brain activity, blood pressure, heart rate, and other bodily functions that normally are not controlled voluntarily. Research has demonstrated that biofeedback/neurofeedback help in the treatment of many diseases and painful conditions. It has shown that people have more control over so-called involuntary bodily function than researchers once thought possible. It has also been shown that nature limits the extent of such control. Scientists are now trying to determine just how much voluntary control a person can exert (Rajeswaran, 2012).

At the highest level of organization, each life form may possess an innate biologic field (biofield), a complex, dynamic field of energy involved in maintaining an organism's integrity regulating its physiologic and biochemical responses and allowing it to develop, heal, and regenerate (Rubik, 2002). Both life force and biofield proponents agree that a form of life-giving energy flows through the body, and illness arises as a result of blockages, excesses, or irregularities in this flow.

Samples of commonly used measures of the biofield include electrocardiogram (ECG) and electroencephalogram (EEG) to assess the function of the heart and brain. Corresponding magnetic field measurements of the heart and brain have been discovered: magnetocardiogram (MCG) and magnetoencephalogram (MEG). The MEG allows for localizing the activity of a region of the brain the size of a pea. Lie detectors and biofeedback use galvanic skin response (GSR) to measure the electrical conductance between electrodes on the skin. Thermography, an accepted diagnostic procedure in conventional Western medicine, measures the emission of infrared radiation from the body (Rajeswaran, 2012).

Biofeedback generally involves using measures derived from peripheral physiology rather than EEG results, measures such as skin temperature, muscle tension, skin conductance, heart rate, and breathing. All these are subject to management of the CNS and refer back to the brain. Each specialty area in biofeedback has its unique strengths (Larsen, 2012).

Biofeedback patients are taught a form of relaxation exercise which allows them to identify the circumstances that trigger their symptoms. While some may be taught how to avoid or cope with stressful events, most are encouraged to change their habits. The majority of patients who choose to use biofeedback are trained in special techniques aimed at giving them self-control. Biofeedback is a tool that reminds physicians that behavior, thoughts, and feelings profoundly influence physical health.

A biofeedback therapist is required when the problems that are experienced become greater than a person can handle. Biofeedback can be seen as a journey toward increased self-awareness. Despite a strong self-help component, it is prudent that biofeedback be conducted under the care of a trained mental health professional, and only after medical evaluation has determined that a more serious condition will not be neglected by the training. Initially, the biofeedback/neurofeedback therapist will do a history of past health and current symptoms. The biofeedback practitioner guides the trainee by designing an individualized program for improved health, encouraging regular practice, monitoring results, and supporting the training process in various ways, including advice regarding complementary interventions (Yucha & Montegomery, 2008).

Specialists who provide biofield services range from psychiatrists and psychologists to dentists, internists, nurses, and physical therapists. Most rely on many other techniques in addition to biofield practices. The most widely used biofield treatment is biofeedback.

References

Andrasik, F., & Lords, A. O. (2009). Biofeedback. In L. Freeman (Ed.), *Mosby's complementary and alternative medicine: A research-based approach* (3rd ed., pp. 189-214). St Louis, MO: Mosby Elsevier.

Beijing College of Traditional Chinese Medicine. (2011). *Essentials of Chinese acupuncture* (3rd ed.). Beijing, China: Foreign Languages.

Bergman, T., & Peterson, D. (2011). *Chiropractic technique: Principles and procedures* (3rd ed.). St. Louis, MO: Elsevier.

Bishop, F. L., & Lewith, G. T. (2013). Patients' preconceptions of acupuncture: A qualitative study exploring the decisions patients make when seeking acupuncture. *BMC Complementary and Alternative Medicine, 13*(1), 13–102.

Carteret, M. (2011). Traditional Asian health beliefs and healing practice. *Dimensions of Culture: Cross-Cultural Communications for Healthcare Professionals*. Retrieved July 26, 2013 from http://www.dimensionsofculture.com

Collura, T. F. (2013). *Technical foundations of neurofeedback*. New York, NY: Taylor & Francis.

Council on Chiropractic Education Accreditation Standards: Principles, processes, and requirements for accreditation (CCE). (2013). Scottsdale, AZ: Council on Chiropractic Medicine.

Cox, J. M. (2011). *Low back pain: Mechanism, diagnosis, and treatment* (7th ed.). Philadelphia, PA: Lippincott Williams & Wilkins.

Davis, M. A., Mackenzie, T. A., Coulter, I. D., Whedon, J. M., & Weeks, W. B. (2012). The United States chiropractic workforce: An alternative or complement to primary care? *Chiropractic & Manual Therapies 20*(1), 20–35.

del Giudici, E., & Preparata, G. (1990). Superradiance: A new approach to coherent dynamical behaviors of condenses matter, frontier perspectives. *Medical Hypotheses, 44*(6), 527–535.

Ernst, E., Pittler, M. H., & Wider, B. (Eds.). (2006). *The desktop guide to complementary and alternative medicine: An evidence-based approach* (2nd ed.). St. Louis, MO: Mosby Elsevier.

Gatterman, M. I. (Ed.). (2005). *Foundations of chiropractic: Subluxation* (2nd ed.) St. Louis, MO: Mosby Elsevier.

Gu, H. (1989). *Clinical traditional Chinese medicine: Orthopedic Volume*. Guangxi, China: Chinese Medical Science.

Gu, H. (2010). Acupuncture treatment for piriformis syndrome following lumbar diskectomy. *Journal of Medical Acupuncture, 22*(3), 203–206.

Haller, J. S. (2005). *The history of American homeopathy: The academic years*. London, England: Haworth.

Jonas, W. B., Kaptchuk, T. J., & Linde, K. (2003). A critical overview of homeopathy. *Annals of Internal Medicine, 138*(5), 393–399.

Kessler, R. C., Davis, R. B., Foster, D. F., Van Rompay, M. I., Walters, E. E., Wilkey, S. A.,...Eisenberg, D. M. (2001). Long term trends in the use of complementary and alternative medical therapies in the United States. *Annals of Internal Medicine, 135*(4), 262–268.

Langevin, H. M., Badger, G. J., Povolny, B. K., Davis, R. T., Johnston, A. C., Sherman, K. J., . . . Kaptchuk, T. J. (2004). Y*in* scores and y*ang* scores: A new method for quantitative diagnostic evaluation in traditional Chinese medicine research. *Journal of Alternative and Complementary Medicine, 10*(2), 389–395.

Larsen, S. (2012). *The neurofeedback solution: How to treat autism, ADHD, anxiety, brain injury, stroke, PTSD, and more*. Rochester, VT: Healing Arts.

Mayo Clinic. (2010). *Mayo Clinic book of alternative medicine: Integrating the best of natural therapies with conventional medicine* (2nd ed.). New York, NY: Oxmoor.

Mirtz, T. A., Morgan, L., Wyatt, L. H., & Greene, L. (2009). An epidemiological examination of the subluxation construct using Hill's criteria of causation. *Chiropractic & Osteopathy, 17*(13), 1–7.

Moroz, A., & Schulman, R. A. (2011). Complementary and alternative medicine. In S. R. Flanagan, H. H. Zaretsky, & A. Moroz (Eds.), *Medical aspects of disability: A handbook for the rehabilitation professional* (4th ed., pp. 595–609). New York, NY: Springer.

Ni, H., Simile, C., & Hardy, A. M. (2002). Utilization of complementary and alternative medicine by United States adults: Results from the 1999 National Health Interview Survey. *Medical Care, 40*(4), 353–358.

Ots, T. (1990). The angry liver, the anxious heart, and the melancholy spleen: The phenomenology of perceptions in Chinese culture. *Culture, Medicine, and Psychiatry, 14*(1), 21–58.

Pham, D. D., Yoo, J. H, Tran, B. Q., & Ta, T. T. (2013). Complementary and alternative medicine use among physicians in Oriental medicine hospitals in Vietnam: A hospital-based survey. *Evidence-Based Complementary and Alternative Medicine,* 392191.

Rajeswaran, J. (2012). *Neuropsychological rehabilitation: Principles and applications*. New York, NY: Elsevier.

Robertson, D., Biaggioni, I. Burnstock, G., Low, P. A., & Paton, J. F. R. (2011). *Primer on the autonomic nervous system* (3rd ed.). Salt Lake City, UT: Academic.

Rubik, B. (2002). The biofield hypothesis: Its biophysical basis and role in medicine. *Journal of Alternative and Complementary Medicine, 8*(6), 703–717.

Singer, D. C. (2013). *Equal rights for all chiropractors*. Arlington, VA: American Chiropractic Association.

Still, A. T. (2009). *Philosophy of osteopathy* (Classic Reprint). Charleston, SC: BiblioBazaar.

Tan, G., Craine, M. H., Bair, M. J., Garcia, M. K., Giordano, J., Jensen, M. P.,...Tsao, J. C. (2007). Efficacy of selected complementary and alternative medicine interventions for chronic pain. *Journal of Rehabilitation Research and Development, 44*(2), 195–222.

Teppone, M., & Avakyan, R. (2007). Modern view on the theory of channels, collaterals, and organs. *Medical Acupuncture, 19*(1), 43–48.

Tetrault, M. (2004). *Global professional strategy for chiropractic*. Tustin, CA: Chiropractic Diplomatic Corps.

Wax, W. A., & White, K. R. (2000). A short history of a long tradition. *American Journal of Nursing, 100*(9), 40–45.

World Federation of Chiropractic (2012). *The current status of the chiropractic profession: Report to the World Health Organization*. Toronto, Canada: Author.

Xinnong, C., & Deng, A. (2010). *Chinese acupuncture and moxibustion* (3rd ed.). Beijing, China: Foreign Languages.

Yuan, C. S., & Bieber, E. J. (Eds.). (2003). *Textbook of complementary and alternative medicine*. London, England: Taylor and Francis.

Yucha, C., & Montgomery, D. (2008.) *Evidence-based practice in biofeedback and neurofeedback.* Wheat Ridge, CO: Association for Applied Psychophysiology and Biofeedback.

Zhiya, Z. (2002). *Advanced textbook on traditional Chinese medicine and pharmacology* (Vol. 1). Middle Island, NY: New World.

About the Authors

Dr. Hua Gu, Ph.D., L.Ac., is an integrative medical practitioner with a practice in Woodland Hills, California. He received his Master's and Doctoral Degrees in Integrative Medicine from China Academy of Traditional Chinese Medicine, Beijing, China. After receiving his medical degree, Dr. Gu practiced as a surgeon in integrated Chinese and conventional medicine. Dr. Gu published three books and over a dozen papers in medical journals, including the *New England Journal of Medicine.* He is the founder of the American Acupunture Academy, Los Angeles, which specializes in education, integrating biomedicine and traditional Chinese medicine. Dr. Gu served as the Chief Research Scientist with West Coast Spine Institute, where he operated research programs of spine disc herniation, stenosis, and biomechanics; created databases for research; evaluated patients with orthopedic neurological disorders; and reviewed, abstracted, and summarized personal injury and workers' compensation cases.

Sandra K. Brodwin, M.Ed., M.S., C.R.C., is a part-time lecturer in the Rehabilitation Counselor Education Program at California State University, Los Angeles, and a grant writer in the areas of disability, rehabilitation, and domestic violence. As a vocational rehabilitation counselor, she has provided reasonable accommodation, job restructuring, employer consultation, and a full range of rehabilitation services for employees on short-term and long-term disability due to chronic illness and injuries. Ms. Brodwin has published book chapters and journal articles on the subjects of medical aspects of disabling conditions, counseling, disability, job analysis, and rehabilitation.

Chapter 12

TRAUMATIC BRAIN INJURY

Stacey Hunter Schwartz, Ph.D.
Michelle Ranae Wild, M.A.

Introduction

Traumatic brain injury (TBI) involves sudden physical damage to the brain. Males ages 14 to 24 years are at the highest risk of TBI, followed by infants and the elderly. Males are twice as likely as females to sustain TBI because of differences in risk exposure and lifestyle. Each year, an estimated 1.7 million people sustain TBI (Faul, Xu, Wald, & Coronado, 2010). About 275,000 Americans are hospitalized and 52,000 die as a result of TBI each year (Centers for Disease Control and Prevention [CDC], 2013a). Approximately 1.1 million Americans are treated for brain injuries and released from emergency rooms; of these, 99,000 individuals sustain moderate to severe brain injuries resulting in lifelong disabling conditions. About 75% of TBIs are concussions or other forms of mild injury (CDC, 2013a). After one traumatic brain injury, the risk for a second injury is three times greater; after a second TBI, the risk for a third injury is eight times greater (Kraus & McArthur, 1999). CDC (2013b) estimated that at least 5.3 million Americans currently have long-term or lifelong need for help to perform activities of daily living as a result of TBI.

A traumatic brain injury produces an injury to one's core sense of self. Persons with TBI undergo such dramatic cognitive and personality changes that they seem, both to themselves and those closest to them, to be different people than they were pre-injury. Many persons with TBI regard their post-injury experiences as their second lives. At the same time, some have called TBI an *invisible disability* because the physical appearances of many persons with TBI do not change as a result of their head injury. While persons with other disabilities may feel frustrated because they are treated as different, individuals with TBI often feel frustrated because others treat them as if they were the same as before the injury. This disjunction between appearance and functionality complicates adjustment.

Rehabilitation is particularly challenging for other reasons as well. Counselors usually rely on their clients for information regarding their skills, abilities, and limitations. Like other individuals with new disabilities, people with TBI experience a state of psychological denial about the extent and ramifications of their deficits; additionally, they may have a neurologically induced failure to recognize the deficiencies. They may have become cognitively incapable of knowing their limitations. Others with TBI do not remember what they were like before their injuries, or have an idealized memory of their pre-injury capabilities. Consequently, some people with TBI insist on unrealistic goals for rehabilitation.

Other people with TBI are able to set realistic goals, but implementing those goals presents challenges. Deficits in attention or auditory processing interfere with successful educational and vocational planning (Rios, Periàñez, & Munoz-Céspedes, 2004). Counseling may be unproductive because the client is unable to distinguish relevant from irrelevant information. Other clients show great insight and understanding while in counseling sessions, but forget the content of the sessions soon after each session ends. For these reasons and others, rehabilitation presents unique challenges to rehabilitation counselors.

Etiology

Brain injuries result from a variety of causes, including vehicle collisions, falls, stabbings, gunshots, infections, tumors, and strokes. Although a survivor of an automobile accident and a survivor of an aneurysm may experience similar symptoms, benefit from the same cognitive strategies, and face the same vocational outcomes, the two may qualify for different assistance programs. The labels used by those who study or work with persons with TBI relate to the causes of injury; outcomes tend to be similar across causal groups, based on the severity of injury and location within the brain (Reilly & Bullock, 2005).

Causes of brain injury can be divided into two categories. Traumatic injuries are those caused by something outside the body, such as by the impact of an automobile accident or penetration of a bullet. Atraumatic injuries are those that occur because of internal causes, such as a cerebrovascular accident (stroke) or infection. Consequences of brain injury detailed in this chapter apply to survivors of traumatic as well as atraumatic brain injury.

The Brain Injury Association, formerly the National Head Injury Foundation, defines traumatic brain injury as "an insult to the brain, not of degenerative or congenital nature, but caused by an external physical force that may produce a diminished or altered state of consciousness, resulting in an impairment of cognitive abilities or physical functioning." Vehicle accidents are the leading cause of TBI, accounting for 50% of all injuries. Falls are the second leading cause, accounting for more than 20%. Alcohol is a significant risk factor, with more than 50% of persons intoxicated at the time of traumatic brain injury (Kraus & McArthur, 1999; Kreutzer, Witol, & Marwitz, 1996).

Closed Head Injury

In a closed head injury, the skull is not penetrated. Damage usually occurs when the brain experiences rapid acceleration and deceleration because of a blow to the head, such as in a motor vehicle accident or a fall. The brain hits against the skull in an initial impact called the *coup*. Next, the brain stem turns and twists on its axis causing localized or widespread damage to the brain. The brain then rebounds and hits the opposite side of the skull (the *contre coup*). Consequently, in a closed head injury, damage often occurs to diffuse areas of the brain. Swelling and bleeding, problems that frequently occur with open head injuries, also cause injury to various areas of the brain.

Loss of consciousness may result, but in other instances, the survivor remains conscious and there are no outer signs of brain injury. The medical team concentrates on and provides treatment for more obvious wounds. Later on, the person with TBI and those who attempt to offer help may have a difficult time identifying and documenting that an injury occurred.

Severity of injury is a good predictor of eventual outcome, but many people who sustain what are considered mild injuries nonetheless suffer life-altering deficits. Consequences of mild TBIs are particularly pronounced among persons whose careers involve high-level cognitive demands. The American College of Rehabilitation (ACR) has developed a definition of such injuries. Although the definition adopts the somewhat understated term *mild* traumatic brain injury, it clearly communicates the idea that these non-coma type injuries are serious with permanent consequences. According to the ACR definition of mild traumatic brain injury, a permanent brain injury can occur under any of the following four conditions: any period of loss of consciousness, a loss of memory for events immediately before or after the accident (amnesia), an alteration in mental state at the time of the accident (e.g., feeling dazed, disoriented, or confused), or focal neurological deficit(s) (Mild Traumatic Brain Injury Committee, 1993).

Blast Injuries

Traumatic brain injuries caused by explosions (blast injuries) have become known as the signature injury of the wars in Afghanistan and Iraq. According to brainlinemilitary.org (2012), over 244,000 service members sustained TBIs between 2000 and the first quarter of 2012. Blast-related TBIs are typically caused by the impact of improvised explosive devices (IEDs). The impact of a blast can produce unique multi-system injuries that may be life-threatening.

Blast injuries are caused by one of two categories of explosions or a combination of the two. High-order explosives (HE) cause a supersonic over-pressurization shock wave, which can impact multiple body systems such as the brain, lungs, ears, and gastrointestinal tract. The shock wave may significantly impact individuals near the explosion site. Low-order explosives (LE) cause a subsonic explosion without the over-pressurization shock wave. It is possible for service members to be exposed to both in a single explosive episode. Improvised Explosive Devices have become well known during these wars and may fall within the HE or LE categories, or both.

According to the CDC (2012), the four basic mechanisms of blast injury are labeled primary, secondary, tertiary, and quaternary. The primary mechanism is associated with the high over-pressurization of the blast wave as it impacts body structures and causes multi-system injuries as described above, including injuries to the brain, such as concussion, hemorrhage, and diffuse axonal injury. The secondary mechanism is associated with flying debris and shrapnel from the explosion, resulting in a variety of possible penetrating wounds. Effects of individuals being thrown by the wind generated by the blast are part of the tertiary mechanism which causes a variety of brain injuries. Injuries not caused by the first three mechanisms are considered quaternary.

Brain injuries caused by HE blasts are often characterized as mild traumatic brain injuries and cause common symptoms such as headache, fatigue, poor concentration, depression, anxiety, and insomnia. However, it is important to note that the nature of blast injury and its potential for significant multi-system injuries differentiate this type of injury from non-blast-related injuries. Brain injuries include both closed and open brain injuries.

Open Head Injury

In an open head injury, verification of TBI is not difficult. The person's brain matter has been penetrated, such as by stabbing or gunshot. Skull fractures, visible brain matter, and obvious bleeding indicate the trauma. Often, the patient goes into a coma or a physician pharmacologically induces a coma immediately following the trauma. This type of head injury is more likely to damage a specific area of the brain. Additional risks exist as well; some patients develop infections or need to have their lost skull material replaced with artificial plates (Zink & McQuillan, 2005).

Atraumatic Brain Injury

A category of brain injury which receives less attention in the literature, but which some experts say is growing, is atraumatic causes of brain injury. Atraumatic injuries are those that occur due to internal causes. Examples include arterial-venous malformations (blood vessels with weaknesses present at birth) and infections in the brain, both of which can result in cerebrovascular accident. In recent years, more people are benefiting from new surgical procedures which help increase survival of people with vascular injuries. Similarly, persons who have brain tumors survive more often today because of advances in oncology. Meningitis (inflammation of the brain and spinal cord) and cardiac arrest leading to anoxia (where the brain has been completely deprived of oxygen for a period of time) or hypoxia (where the brain has been partially deprived of oxygen) also cause serious diffuse brain damage (Thurman, Alverson, Dunn, Guerrero, & Sniezek, 1999).

Functional Limitations

Because the brain is such a critical organ that performs a wide variety of necessary functions, injury to the brain causes a host of deficits. No one survivor is likely to exhibit all the functional limitations described below. As causal agents, severity of injury and location of injury vary as do resulting cognitive deficits. Even the number of locations of injury and severity at those locations are not necessarily determinative of functional outcome. Impairment of life processes related to deficits also depends on the client's personal lifestyle and career demands (Im, Hibbard, Grunwald, Swift, & Salimi, 2011; Rios et al., 2004). The description of deficits (below) is helpful in understanding the potential consequences of TBI; each client must be assessed for the particular injuries and resulting deficits. Table 1 summarizes the types of sequelae and deficits that commonly follow TBI.

TABLE 1
Various Categories of Deficits

Physical	Balance difficulties, fatigue, pain, hemiparesis, uneven gait, ataxia, apraxia, decreased motor speed, seizure disorders, sensory deficits
Cognitive	Impairments in attention/concentration, memory, visual or auditory perceptual processing, verbal reasoning, critical thinking/logic, language, awareness
Psychosocial	Personality changes, emotional lability, flat affect, depression, substance abuse, frustration intolerance, impulsivity/disinhibition, lack of initiative

Physical

Traumatic events like automotive accidents and falls may result in physical impairments (such as immobility caused by bone fractures), which are unrelated to the brain. There also may be physical consequences resulting directly from the brain injury, as described below.

Balance

Many people have difficulty with balance and coordination immediately following injury. In some, dizziness and unsteadiness are permanent conditions. Special retraining programs exist for these problems.

Fatigue

For several reasons, extreme mental and physical fatigue are common after TBI, as are sleep disorders. Ouellet, Beaulieu-Bonneau, and Morin (2006) found that over half of patients with mild to severe brain injuries reported symptoms of insomnia. Tasks which were formerly easy become far more mentally challenging and, consequently, physically exhausting. For example, four hours of concentrated activity may necessitate several hours of rest.

Pain

Individuals with TBI frequently report persistent headaches. Those with concussions often have neck and back pain and require ergonomically correct workstations to reduce pain complaints. There may be increased sensitivity to pain.

Hemiparesis

Each side of the body is controlled by the opposite side of the brain. Therefore, injury to the motor strip of one hemisphere affects movements on the opposite side of the body. For example, the left side of the body may be paralyzed because the right hemisphere has been injured. Although a leg or arm may not itself be injured, the brain may not be able to control that leg or arm properly, resulting in dysfunctions of movement (Kraus & McArthur, 1999).

Other Disorders of Movement

Many persons have permanent impairment of movement caused by an inability of the brain to control the extremities. The individual experiences impaired gait, ataxia (jerky movements), apraxia (uncontrolled movements), muscle spasticity, tremors, and impaired fine motor control.

Decreased Motor Speed

Many people feel as though they are moving in slow motion. Their brain signals travel at a slower pace and tasks take longer. These individuals appear to have a few seconds delay between when they decide to move and when they carry out the planned action.

Seizure Activity (traumatic epilepsy)

Following TBI, recurrent seizures are possible (17% of all cases) (Reilly & Bullock, 2005). Most of those who experience seizures have their first seizure within 24 hours of injury. Usually, seizures are controllable with anti-convulsive medication. For the rare individual, however, continuing seizures may provide the greatest obstacle to rehabilitation.

Cognitive

Repeated mild TBIs occurring over an extended period (i.e., months and even years) can result in cumulative neurological and cognitive deficits while repeated mild TBIs occurring within a short period (i.e., hours, days, or weeks) can be catastrophic or fatal. People with TBI are likely to need assistance to perform activities of daily living. TBI can cause epilepsy, and increases the risk for conditions such as Alzheimer's disease, Parkinson's disease, and other disorders affecting the brain (National Institute of Neurological Disorders & Stroke, 2002). Cognitive deficits are divided into some common classification areas, although the distinction is somewhat artificial. In real-world experiences, it is difficult to find a task that draws exclusively upon a single, distinct skill. Almost every activity involves two or more of the cognitive skills described below.

Attention/Concentration and Arousal

Some persons with TBI find it difficult to focus and maintain attention on a task (Rios et al., 2004). Persons may have difficulty becoming sufficiently aroused (i.e., alert) to focus on a specific activity, and they may have a shortened attention span.

Some are unable to shift mental tasks (alternating attention) or follow multi-step directions. As an illustration, assume that Sam has TBI but is able, with effort, to focus on a particular work task. If the telephone rings, interrupting his attention for even a minute or two, Sam might be unable to return to the prior task on which he had been working. Many tasks involve divided attention, such as driving which requires that a person is able to concentrate on steering while also obeying speed limits, monitoring other drivers, and perhaps navigating a new route, all while listening to the radio and having a conversation. Driving is often impossible after TBI.

Memory

Television shows and movies about persons with TBI usually depict memory loss as the chief cognitive deficit of TBI. These media depictions are misleading both in the narrow focus on memory loss and the dramatization of the type of memory loss that occurs. While memory loss is common, the type of loss depicted in the media (where the person awakens from a coma and needs to be informed about events that have occurred) is uncommon. Retrospective amnesia (long term memory loss), the inability to remember all that happened before the injury, seldom occurs.

Far more common is anterograde amnesia (short-term memory loss). For example, many persons cannot remember new information, such as what they had for breakfast that same morning. Individuals may have prospective amnesia (inability to remember future plans). Some persons cannot keep track of their appointments, and even struggle to use memory aids, such as day and week planning tools (e.g., Day Timer). Such tools, while helpful for persons with TBI, assume the user will remember to write down appointments, remember where to write the appointments, and remember to look at the planning guide with regular frequency. Intensive training may be necessary to establish what will become vital organizational habits. Fortunately, new technologies, discussed below, have emerged which make memory compensation easier and more consistent (Gillespie, Best, & O'Neill, 2012).

Perception/Visual Processing

Some persons have problems with spatial orientation. They get lost in a parking lot, going home or to work, or even in their own home environment. These individuals can lose the ability to deal with smaller-scale spatial relations, as well. For example, they may find themselves unable to figure out which container is an appropriate size for storing leftovers or may have difficulty wrapping gifts. They struggle with visual field cuts, in which a large portion of their visual field is missing.

Sensory Deficits

Other sensory deficits include visual processing difficulties (e.g., neglect of one side of the visual field), sensitivity to light, loss of hearing, and loss of the senses of smell or taste.

Verbal Reasoning

Many persons have problems understanding conversations. They cannot identify the main idea of written or spoken communication, distinguish relevant from irrelevant details, detect similarities and differences, or understand analogies. They struggle to organize ideas, important papers, and their lives. Many have difficulty paying bills, even if sufficient funds are available, because of organizational or comprehension difficulties.

Critical Thinking/Logic

One individual with TBI might declare an inability to return to work despite having received a medical clearance. On the contrary, another person may attempt to return to work without recognizing the presence of severe cognitive deficits. Judgment and the ability to process information accurately with consistency and speed can be impaired, as well as an inability to make decisions (Rios et al., 2004).

Language

Persons with TBI often have communicative disturbances (aphasia). Individuals may have difficulty expressing thoughts (i.e., expressive aphasia), such as having word-finding problems. For example, one might say, "that thing you write with" to communicate the word "pen." Other speech problems stem from physical impairments, including speech that is unclear when the person has decreased control of the muscles in the lips, tongue, and jaw, or because he or she has developed poor breathing patterns. Dysarthria, where motor function interferes with correct formation of sounds, produces slurred speech that is extremely difficult to understand. In addition, some persons have problems understanding others (i.e., receptive aphasia).

Unawareness

Anosognosia is a failure to recognize one's own impairment. It can be difficult to distinguish anosognosia from psychological denial, a normal defense mechanism. Giacino and Cicerone (1998) found evidence that three factors underlie lack of awareness of deficits following TBI: (a) diminished awareness of deficits secondary to impaired cognition, especially memory and reasoning deficits; (b) psychological reaction and denial of deficits; and (c) a relatively *pure* inability to recognize areas of impaired functioning as a direct consequence of brain injury.

Psychosocial

Various psychological, behavioral, and emotional changes are common following TBI, especially major depression and anxiety disorders. Major depression and substance abuse disorders are more likely to remit than anxiety disorder (Im et al., 2011). These conditions and others of a psychosocial nature are discussed below.

Personality Changes

TBI frequently exacerbates negative pre-injury personality traits. For example, someone who had a short temper now has angry, emotional outbursts. One adult daughter said of her father after his TBI, "He's Dad, just more Dad." A man who was formerly self-confident is now annoyingly arrogant and critical of others. Conversely, family members often report that the shy have become outgoing, and vice versa. A common complaint of family members is that the survivor has become intensely egocentric.

Emotional Lability

Heightened emotional responses or reactions are common. Some feel unable to control mood swings from moment to moment. They laugh or cry for no apparent reason and at inappropriate times.

Flat Affect

Some survivors show a complete lack of emotions. For example, they report a sense of puzzlement that they neither feel elation at happy times, nor anxiety in stressful times.

Depression

Major depression is present in about 40% of individuals who have been hospitalized for TBI (Jorge & Starkstein, 2005). TBI may be accompanied by loss of defining personality traits, career, status, income, relationships, or feelings of competency. Persons with TBI have a high divorce rate, lose many of their friends, and suffer family estrangements. They discover that, after the initial burst of rapid gains from rehabilitation, progress levels off. Some deficits are temporary, while others are permanent. Consequences of TBI have emotional costs not only for the person who is injured, but also for families.

Substance Abuse

Hibbard, Uysal, Kepler, Bogdany, and Silver (1998) investigated TBI survivors eight years post-injury and found that a significant percent had substance abuse disorders prior to injury. Kreutzer et al. (1996) compared drinking rates after TBI with large-sample studies on non-TBI populations and found that young persons with TBI had pre-injury drinking patterns similar to those in the general population. There was evidence of a decline in alcohol use at initial follow-up, but pre-injury and secondary follow-up show similar alcohol use patterns. Post-injury illicit drug use rates remained relatively low, falling below 10% at both follow-up intervals. The findings suggested that men with moderate to heavy pre-injury alcohol use and those taking prescribed medications are at greatest risk for long-term alcohol use.

Decreased Frustration Tolerance

After TBI, people may become frustrated more easily than they did before their injuries. For example, they may realize that particular tasks on which they are working seem elementary. They could competently perform the activities before injury, yet post-injury may be unable to perform them with ease or at all.

Impulsivity/Disinhibition

People have many thoughts each day that they do not express, or urges on which they do not act. The frontal lobes within the brain keep individuals from acting on these ideas. Without this check system, people with TBI may ask inappropriate personal questions of co-workers, make sexual advances, touch others inappropriately, act in an aggressive manner, or make prejudicial remarks.

Lack of Initiative

Some individuals with brain injury lack initiative, as is common with frontal lobe injuries. Such persons may be content to watch television all day. They respond with apathy.

Treatment

An individual with signs or symptoms of moderate or severe TBI needs immediate medical attention. Priorities of treatment are to maintain passages to the airway, breathing, and circulation. Medical professionals attempt to stabilize the person and focus on preventing further injury; concerns include ensuring the brain has sufficient blood supply, maintaining blood flow, and monitoring blood pressure.

Imaging Tests

Neuroradiological tests using computer-assisted scans can help assess the areas and extent of damage to the brain. The most common imaging test is called computed axial tomography (CT or CAT) scan. It uses a computer to combine X-rays of thin *slices* of the brain into one unified three-dimensional image. Magnetic resonance imaging (MRI) tests rely on a magnet and radio waves to produce computerized images of the brain. Unfortunately, many mild brain injuries involve such subtle damage that tests may not detect the injury (Belanger, Vanderploeg, Curtiss, & Warder, 2007),

New forms of imaging continue to develop. Single-photon emission computed tomography (SPECT) scans are used to form cross-sectional images of the brain using images from a camera which detects the presence of radioactive particles that have been injected into the blood. Positron emission tomography (PET) scans similarly use radioactive particles, but PET scans produce data regarding metabolic activity, not anatomic data. Diffusion tensor imaging (DTI) holds promise as a technique which may detect more subtle damage. DTI is a type of MRI that measures fluid movement in the brain, and can show where normal fluid flow is not occurring (Nakayama et al., 2006).

Depending on type and severity of injury, rehabilitation typically includes physical therapy, speech therapy, occupational therapy, and cognitive therapy. These therapies are described below.

Physical Therapy (PT)

After a coma, many patients need to learn to walk again. It may take weeks, months, or years for a patient to progress from using a wheelchair to a walker, to a cane, and finally to ambulate unassisted. Some persons never progress past wheelchair use. Nevertheless, because the physical impairments are most visible, survivors frequently put the bulk of their energy into PT, sometimes to the detriment of other therapies.

Speech Therapy

Beginning with relearning how to swallow (while in the hospital), TBI patients frequently receive a wide spectrum of therapy from speech and language pathologists. Depending on location of injury, a speech therapist helps the patient learn to speak again and may assist with developing word-finding skills or forming sounds. Many speech therapists teach cognitive remediation skills.

Occupational Therapy (OT)

Occupational therapists help with such skills as learning to button a shirt with one hand to compensate for hemiplegia, or increasing independence by structuring an environment using memory cues. OT addresses learning to drive post-injury by teaching compensatory strategies for coping with physical and visual deficits.

Cognitive Therapy/Retraining/Remediation

Cognitive retraining principally occurs in five settings: hospitals (especially immediately after injury), neuropsychologists' offices, speech therapy clinics, therapeutic milieu settings such as the New York University Rusk Institute, and in educational settings such as the Coastline Community College Acquired Brain Injury Program in Orange County, California.

The cognitive retrainer begins by assessing cognitive functioning and prescribing cognitive remediation. Such treatment includes tasks designed to help individuals utilize their cognitive strengths to compensate for limitations. This involves teaching new strategies for common tasks. The cognitive retrainer seeks to stimulate progress for those activities with which the person is having difficulties. By stimulating these activities, the cognitive retrainer attempts to build new neural pathways to replace damaged areas, although it is currently believed that after childhood, no new brain cells develop. The dendrites or fibers on each neuron, however, can grow and be functional. From this, neuropsychologists have developed the theory of neural plasticity, which posits that a new neural pathway can be developed to take over a brain function that has been lost because of damage to the area (Reilly & Bullock, 2005).

Assistive Technology for Cognition

Assistive Technology for Cognition (ATC) refers to any technology that assists cognitive function during task performance (Gillespie et al., 2012). ATC devices vary from low-tech (e.g., watch alarms) to high-tech (e.g., smart phones). High-tech ATC devices range from specialized augmentative and alternative communication devices that can cost several thousand dollars to commonly used smart devices (e.g., iPod Touch, iPhone, tablets) that may cost several hundred dollars. Gillespie et al. (2012) found that ATC devices can effectively support many common cognitive functions associated with brain injury, including those related to memory, attention, organization, planning, and time management. Sohlberg and Turkstra (2011) stated, "The increasing use of technology to help individuals compensate for cognitive impairments is one of the most notable advances in neuropsychological rehabilitation in recent years." The common use of such devices among the general population serves to destigmatize their use as a compensation tool for people with brain injuries.

The popularity of smart devices, the vast number of applications (apps) available, and their relatively low cost (as compared to specialized ATC devices) all work together to increase their viability as ATC devices. Smart devices being used as ATC devices at this time include the iPod Touch, smartphones (Apple, Android, and Windows), tablets, Kindle Fire, and Nook. Amazingly, Nielsen Wire (2012) reported that 55% of U.S. mobile phone owners have a smartphone. In addition, over 22 million tablets have been sold in the U.S. in the first half of 2012. Smart devices are becoming commonplace.

Although smart devices vary in size, storage capacity, number of available add-on apps, and price, they all provide a number of similar features and come with several native apps that can be used to assist with cognitive issues resulting from brain injury. These include a calendar, contacts (address book), camera, maps, task lists, e-mail, browser, and notes. These apps play a role in assisting with a variety of daily activities such as scheduling appointments, storing contact information (including pictures of the contact), and creating to-do lists. All smart devices have add-on apps available from their respective *app stores*. The Apple App Store and the Android Google Play Store have the largest collection of free and for-pay apps, quickly nearing a million. Add-on apps are available in many categories that can help with brain-injury related issues.

Memory compensation is one of the primary advantages of using ATC after brain injury. Gillete and DePompei (2008) noted that people with brain injury who use traditional paper notebooks do not perform as well as those who use hand-held computers programmed to prompt the performance of various common tasks. Additionally, they found that personal data assistant (PDA) use not only improved survivors' functioning, but also improved their sociability, self-esteem, and independence (Gentry, Wallace, Kvarfordt, & Lynch, 2008; Gilete & DePompei, 2008). The systematic training of brain injury survivors, caregivers, and rehabilitation professionals is essential to successful implementation of smart device technology. Although there are any number of books and manuals related to using the various smart devices, there are limited resources currently available for training individuals with brain injury to use smart devices as cognitive prosthetics. ID 4 the Web (http://id4theweb.com) provides training resources specifically structured as learning tools for those with brain injury. The training resources emphasize the Making Cognitive Connections® approach which teaches the fundamental technical skills necessary to operate a smart device while drawing attention to the cognitive skills. The Making Cognitive Connections® approach integrated into the various training resources allows users to focus on the cognitive skills required to use the device and how those same cognitive skills apply to their everyday lives.

Rehabilitation Features

Rehabilitation Outcomes

Cognitive retraining is a relatively new field, having first gained prominence in the 1980s. Chestnut et al. (1999) conducted a systematic review of over 3,000 studies to evaluate evidence for the effectiveness of rehabilitation methods throughout the phases of recovery. They found significant practice variations occur across clinics and professionals. While some studies have demonstrated highly individualized treatment and assessment, others have shown that standardization of treatment is possible and results in positive outcomes.

It is difficult to know when an individual has reached maximum recovery and improvement (O'Keeffe, Dockree, Moloney, Carton, & Robertson, 2007). Many physicians believe that the outer limits of functional improvement are between six months and one to two years following TBI. Yet, cognitive retraining has produced successes as long as 20 years post-injury.

Factors Affecting Outcome

A variety of factors affect outcome. Severity of injury is the strongest predictor of recovery. Professionals working with TBI survivors measure severity of injury using several methods. First, TBI experts use length of coma to predict outcomes. Studies indicated that the longer the coma, the more likely the outcome will be worse. Second, duration of post-traumatic amnesia is used to predict outcomes. The longer it takes to start remembering daily events, the more negative the outcome. Unfortunately, some people never regain ability to remember daily events (Zink & McQuillan, 2005).

Age correlates negatively with outcomes. The older a person is at time of injury, the worse the outcome. Research has established a relationship between age and increased psychosocial limitations, especially in persons over the age of 60. Consequences of TBI worsen with age.

Researchers (Faul et al., 2010; Jorge & Starkstein, 2005) have determined that higher pre-injury educational level correlates with better outcomes. Most persons with TBI have difficulty learning new information, but a good portion of pre-injury knowledge and skills can be left intact. Persons who were well educated before injury frequently need to learn new ways to organize and access their previous knowledge and cognitive skills.

A final predictor of good outcome is pre-injury work history. Those who have poor work histories before their injuries are likely to have even greater problems post-injury.

Vocational Rehabilitation and Placement

There is wide variance in outcomes after TBI. Some people with TBI recover fully and return to their former routines. Others are able to learn compensatory strategies and perform modified versions of their former routines; still others retrain for new occupations. Some will require structured work settings or find volunteer positions. Unfortunately, some return home to nonproductive lives.

It seems clear for some persons with severe brain injuries that a reasonable rehabilitation long-term goal is supported employment or volunteer work designed to increase life activities (Brodwin, Parker, & DeLaGarza, 2010). Other persons with TBI are able to return to some form of work. Briel (1996) and Sherer et al. (1998) addressed supported employment programs. Briel described an approach for promoting the effective use of compensatory strategies at the job site through supported employment programs. Self-awareness is essential for succeeding at work. Characteristics of supported employment that can promote successful return to work include: community placement and integration, competitive hiring and wages, zero exclusion policy, holistic assessment, emphasis on choice and job matching, intervention after placement, co-worker and employer education, long-term follow along, job completion guarantee (through job coaching), and intensive ongoing analysis of program outcomes.

Because the disability is not visible and often misunderstood, the employer and the TBI survivor must cooperate to work out appropriate accommodations. For example, the employee may require written instructions from the employer or may need to be assigned only one or a few tasks at a time. The employer must have knowledge of the employee's strengths and limitations (Brodwin et al., 2010). For example, a mechanic may still be able to diagnose what is wrong with an automotive engine by listening to it and observing its functioning, even though the person is no longer able to reassemble the engine. An attorney might be able to assist with legal strategizing, but be unable to remember what steps have been taken or which forms have been filed with the court. Persons who process information slowly take longer to perform assigned tasks. Some employers can work around this deficit, but not if impulsivity makes accuracy poor. Therefore, persons with TBI need to be trained to work more slowly when accuracy is essential.

Individuals whose TBI has caused them to lose their inhibitions often struggle to successfully return to work (Brodwin et al., 2010; O'Keeffe et al., 2007). Most jobs require working with others. Impulsive sexual remarks, racial slurs, and low frustration tolerance are not the characteristics of those who succeed in most employment contexts. Job coaching may help in these situations.

Conclusion

Each year, TBI changes the lives of over a million people. Those at highest risk are young males. In TBI, injury is classified as closed head injury and open head injury. A variety of deficits such as physical impairments, pain, fatigue, mobility disorders, seizures, cognitive dysfunctions, speech impairments, and changes in personality are found. These can be devastating and challenging to the injured persons, family members, physicians, and helping professionals. Individuals may experience not only trauma to the brain but alterations in body image, changes in personality, age-related and role-related problems, and financial difficulties. Immediate attention to their physical and psychosocial needs, in addition to maintaining the focus on early rehabilitation and prevention of recurring injury or complications, are imperative to the recoveries of people with TBI.

Case Study

Mr. Randall Owens is 47 years of age, African-American, with an Associate of Science Degree in the Building and Construction Trades from a trade college. While on a construction site, he fell 25 feet from the roof of a house, landing on his right side. He was unable to speak for approximately five minutes and was moving in and out of a comatose state. Paramedics transported Mr. Owens to a local trauma center where a CT scan revealed cerebral contusions, intracranial air in the subarachnoid space of the frontal lobe, punctate hemorrhages in the frontal lobe, a right orbital fracture, a fracture at the base of the skull, right frontal skull fracture, right temporal skull fracture, and temporal bone fracture.

Discharged home after eight days of hospitalization, Mr. Owens received outpatient physical therapy and speech therapy. Eight months later, he initiated outpatient full-time day treatment at a comprehensive post-acute rehabilitation center where an evaluation indicated the following problems: minimally decreased visual processing speed, reduced binocular vision, diminished convergence skills, impaired depth perception, decreased strength in both upper extremities, word finding errors, decreased verbal fluency, diminished auditory and visual recall, and decreased abstract reasoning. Through participation in a full-time day-treatment program for two weeks, Randall was able to transition to a part-time program at a rehabilitation center. Two weeks later, he was discharged.

Six months later (1½ years after injury), Randall was struggling to operate his own construction company, started years before the injury. The physical demand of working 12-hour days was difficult; there were problems remembering details of jobs, sequencing the steps of the jobs, and communicating effectively with clients, vendors, and his two employees. He reported, "I want to get my life back. I want the motivation and the desires I used to have to work and enjoy life. I feel like I have lost control of my life."

Mr. Owens recognized that he might need to work for someone else instead of operating his own business. He enrolled in a community college-based cognitive retraining program, which taught him compensatory strategies to use for memory, sequencing, and communication deficits. With help, he learned to identify and accept his limitations, emphasize his strengths, and set realistic expectations. While enrolled in the program, he became employed at a large home-improvement store. Randall found he could utilize his past experience as a contractor by working in the window and door department helping customers and writing orders. Able to concentrate on a rather isolated portion of the building process, he was less overwhelmed, receiving a promotion to department assistant manager. He was successful and satisfied with his position.

Questions

1. Identify possible functional limitations of traumatic brain injury, including physical, cognitive, and psychosocial.
2. Define emotional lability and its potential impact on job performance.
3. Some individuals with brain injury have problems with impulsivity and make inappropriate remarks (including sexual remarks and racial slurs). Discuss implications of this for vocational rehabilitation.
4. Evaluate cognitive retraining from the standpoint of this case.
5. Describe other possible vocational rehabilitation plans for this client.
6. Discuss supported employment for clients with severe head trauma and whether this is applicable to this case. You may want to refer to the chapter on intellectual disabilities in this book for information on supported employment.

References

Belanger, H. G., Vanderploeg, R. D., Curtiss, G., & Warder, D. L. (2007). Recent neuroimaging techniques in mild traumatic brain injury. *Journal of Neuropsychiatry and Clinical Neuroscience, 19*(1), 5–20.

Brainline Military. (2012). *About traumatic brain injury*. Retrieved November 17, 2012, from http://www.brainlinemilitary.org/categories/abouttbi.php

Briel, L. W. (1996). Promoting the effective use of compensatory strategies on the job for individuals with traumatic brain injury. *Journal of Vocational Rehabilitation, 7*(3), 151–158.

Brodwin, M. G., Parker, R. M., & DeLaGarza, D. (2010). Disability and reasonable accommodation. In E. M. Szymanski & R. M. Parker (Eds.). *Work and disability: Contexts, issues, and strategies for enhancing outcomes for people with disabilities* (3rd ed., pp. 281–323). Austin, TX: Pro-ed.

Centers for Disease Control and Prevention (CDC). (2012). *Explosions and blast injuries: A primer for clinicians*. Retrieved November 17, 2012, from http://www.bt.cdc.gov/masscasualties/explosions.asp

Centers for Disease Control and Prevention (CDC). (2013a). *Get the stats on traumatic brain injury in the United States*. Retrieved July 7, 2013, from http://www.cdc.gov/traumaticbraininjury/pdf/Bluebook_factsheet-a.pdf

Centers for Disease Control and Prevention (CDC). (2013b). *What are the potential effects of TBI?* Retrieved July 7, 2013, http://www.cdc.gov/traumaticbraininjury/outcomes.html

Chestnut, R. M., Carney, N., Maynard, H., Mann, N. C., Patterson, P., & Helfand, M. (1999). Summary report: Evidence for the effectiveness of rehabilitation for persons with traumatic brain injury. *Journal of Head Trauma Rehabilitation, 14*(2), 176–188.

Faul, M., Xu, L., Wald, M. M., & Coronado, V. G. (2010). *Traumatic brain injury in the United States: Emergency department visits, hospitalizations, and deaths*. Atlanta, GA: Centers for Disease Control and Prevention, National Center for Injury Prevention and Control.

Gentry, T. W. J., Kvarsordt, C., & Bodisch, L. (2008). Personal digital assistants as cognitive aids for individuals with severe traumatic brain injury: A community-based trial. *Brain Injury, 22*(1), 19–24.

Giacino, J. T., & Cicerone, K. D. (1998). Varieties of deficit unawareness after brain injury. *Journal of Head Trauma Rehabilitation, 13*(5), 1–15.

Gilette, Y., & DePompei, R. (2008). Do PDAs enhance the organization and memory skills of students with cognitive disabilities? *Psychology in the Schools, 45*(7), 665–677.

Gillespie, A., Best, C., & O'Neill, B. (2012). Cognitive function and assistive technology for cognition: A systematic review. *Journal of the International Neuropsychological Society, 18*, 1–19.

Hibbard, M. R., Uysal, S., Kepler, K., Bogdany, J., & Silver, J. (1998). Axis I psychopathology in individuals with traumatic brain injury. *Journal of Head Trauma Rehabilitation, 13*(4), 24–39.

Im, B., Hibbard, M., Grunwald, I., Swift, P., & Salimi, N. (2011). Traumatic brain injury. In S. R. Flamagan, H. H. Zaretsky, & A. Moroz (Eds.), *Medical aspects of disability: A handbook for the rehabilitation professional* (4th ed., pp. 65–87). New York, NY: Springer.

Jorge R. E., & Starkstein, S. E. (2005). Pathophysiologic aspects of major depression following traumatic brain injury. *Journal of Head Trauma Rehabilitation, 20*(6), 475–487.

Kraus, J. F., & McArthur, D. L. (1999). Incidence and prevalence of and costs associated with traumatic brain injury. In M. Rosenthal, J. S. Kreutzer, E. R. Griffith, & L. B. Pentland (Eds.), *Rehabilitation of the adult and child with traumatic brain injury* (3rd ed., pp. 3–18), Philadelphia, PA: F. A. Davis.

Kreutzer, J. S., Witol, A. D., & Marwitz, J. H. (1996). Alcohol and drug use among young persons with traumatic brain injury. *Journal of Learning Disabilities, 29*(6), 643–651.

Mild Traumatic Brain Injury Committee of the Head Injury Interdisciplinary Special Interest Group of the American Congress of Rehabilitation Medicine. (1993). Definition of mild traumatic brain injury. *Journal of Head Trauma Rehabilitation, 8*(3), 86–87.

Nakayama, N., Okumura, A., Shinoda, J., Yasokawa, Y.T., Miwa, K., Yosihmura, S. I., & Iwama, T. (2006). Evidence for white matter disruption in traumatic brain injury without macroscopic lesions. *Journal of Neurology, Neurosurgery, and Psychiatry, 77*(7), 850–855.

National Institute of Neurological Disorders & Stroke. (2002). *Traumatic brain injury: Hope through research*. Bethesda, MD: National Institutes of Health.

Neilsen Wire. (2012, July 12). *Two-thirds of new mobile buyers now opting for smartphones*. Message posted to http://blog.nielsen.com/nielsenwire/online_mobile/two-thirds-of-new-mobile-buyers-now-opting-for-smartphones/

O'Keeffe, F., Dockree, P., Moloney, P., Carton, S. & Robertson, I. H. (2007). Awareness of deficits in traumatic brain injury: A multidimensional approach to assessing metacognitive knowledge and online awareness. *Journal of the International Neuropsychological Society, 13*(1), 38–49.

Ouellet, M. C., Beaulieu-Bonneau, S., & Morin, C. M. (2006). Insomnia in patients with traumatic brain injury: Frequency, characteristics, and risk factors. *Journal of Head Trauma Rehabilitation, 21*(3), 199–212.

Reilly, P. L., & Bullock, R. (Eds.). (2005). *Head injury: Pathophysiology and management* (2nd ed.). London, England: Arnold.

Rios, M., Periàñez, J. A., & Munoz-Céspedes, J. M. (2004). Attentional control and slowness of information processing after severe traumatic brain injury. *Brain Injury, 18*(3), 257–272.

Sherer, M., Bergloff, P., Levin, E., High, W. M., Oden, K. E., & Nick, T. G. (1998). Impaired awareness and employment outcome after traumatic brain injury. *Journal of Head Trauma Rehabilitation, 13*(5), 2–61.

Sohlberg, M. M., & Turkstra, L. S. (2011). *Optimizing cognitive rehabilitation: Effective instructional methods*. New York, NY: Guilford.

Thurman, D., Alverson, C., Dunn, K., Guerrero, J., & Sniezek, J. (1999). Traumatic brain injury in the United States: A public health perspective. *Journal of Head Trauma Rehabilitation, 14*(6), 602–615.

Zink, E. K., & McQuillan, K. (2005). Managing traumatic brain injury. *Nursing, 35*(9), 36–43.

About the Authors

Stacey Hunter Schwartz, Ph.D., is Executive Director of Independence, Inc. in Lawrence, Kansas, a non-profit center for independent living providing advocacy, peer support, training, and other services. Dr. Schwartz was Dean of Instruction for Special Programs at Coastline Community College in Costa Mesa, California. She served as instructor, counselor, and director of the Acquired Brain Injury Program, which provides cognitive retraining. This led to the development of the Coastline Community College web-based Cognitive Retraining Specialist vocational training program and the Comprehensive Cognitive-Retraining Curriculum for Adults and Adolescents with Acquired Brain Injury.

Michelle R. Wild, M.A., is a professor at Coastline Community College and has taught in Coastline's Acquired Brain Injury Program for over 25 years. She received the David R. Pierce Faculty Technology award, sponsored by Microsoft Corporation and the American Association of Community Colleges. Ms. Wild has authored workbooks on the use of Apple-based, Android-based, and Windows-based smart devices as cognitive prosthetics. Her materials are in use in schools, rehabilitation facilities, and VA hospitals around the country, and are also available for active duty military personnel.

Chapter 13

STROKE

Andrew D. Barreto, M.D.
Frances W. Siu, Ph.D., C.R.C.

Introduction

Yearly, about 130,000 Americans die from stroke. One in every 19 deaths in this country is due to stroke (Centers for Disease Control and Prevention [CDC], 2013). It is the 4th leading cause of death. Stroke is also a leading cause of incapacitation and long-term disability. Unfortunately, one-third of all people who have stroke are under age 65 (Go et al., 2013).

Stroke (also known as cerebral vascular accident [CVA]) is a medical emergency characterized by the rapid loss of brain function due either to interruption of its blood supply (ischemic stroke) or bleeding into the brain from rupture of a blood vessel (hemorrhagic stroke). Ischemic strokes account for approximately 80% and hemorrhagic strokes 20%. Both types result in reduction of oxygen and nutrition to the brain which leads to the symptoms of stroke and resultant brain damage (Barreto et al., 2012). Many of these are recurrent strokes in patients whom have already had a prior CVA. A stroke can result in temporary or permanent neurological dysfunction (Go et al., 2013). Stroke occurs in people of all ages, but predominantly among those over 60 years of age.

Approximately half of all cerebral vascular events are transient ischemic attacks (TIA), a condition of temporary neurological deficit usually lasting 20-40 minutes without permanent brain damage and full recovery of all functions (American Stroke Association [ASA], 2013). Importantly, TIA symptoms mimic those of stroke and should be treated as emergencies. Symptoms which persist longer than 24 hours or result in permanent brain damage are always defined as stroke. This brain damage can be imaged using either computed tomography (CT) or magnetic resonance imaging (MRI) scans. Since 1995, the Federal Drug Administration (FDA) approved medication which has improved treatment for ischemic stroke and reduced resulting disability (CDC, 2012; 2013). At the turn of the millennium, novel treatments and cutting-edge technology continue to be discovered and tested in clinical trials. Specialized emergency care and stroke centers have proven to be effective in further improving care (Anderson et al., 2013). This chapter provides an overview of stroke as a disability. It begins with etiology, followed by anatomy of the brain, categories of stroke, diagnosis, complications and limitations, and concludes with treatment, prevention, and rehabilitation potential of stroke survivors.

Etiology and Statistics

Risk Factors and Costs

The two major categories of stroke risk factors are labeled modifiable and non-modifiable. Modifiable risk factors are under control of the patient, while non-modifiable are beyond one's control. Modifiable risk factors for stroke include the following: hypertension, cigarette smoking, heart disease, Type II diabetes mellitus, excessive alcohol intake, high LDL cholesterol, drug abuse (especially cocaine and amphetamines), and carotid artery atherosclerosis (cholesterol build-up causing blockage of an artery). The most important modifiable risk factor which contributes to the highest rate of stroke is hypertension, as many clinical studies have proven that blood pressure reduction results in lower rates of stroke (ASA, 2013; CDC, 2013). Non-modifiable stroke risk factors include age, a history of prior stroke or transient ischemic attack, male gender, race, certain genetic disorders of blood clotting, and a family medical history of stroke or cardiovascular disease. About half of Americans have one of the three following risk factors for stroke: high blood pressure, high LDL cholesterol, and smoking (Grysiewicz, Thomas, & Pandey, 2008). Patients who have a history of TIAs are nine times more likely to have subsequent strokes than those without (ASA, 2013). Each year, there are 795,000 strokes in the United States; of these, 185,000 are recurrent and 610,000 are first strokes. African-Americans have higher rates of stroke, partly because higher rates of diabetes and high blood pressure are found within this population. This is especially true of African-Americans who live in the *stroke-belt*, an area in the southeastern United States where stroke incidence leads the nation (Go et al., 2013). In this country, stroke costs an estimated $38.6 billion a year. This figure includes health care services, medications, and missed work days (CDC, 2013). These costs will, of necessity, continue to rise.

Signs and Symptoms

Stroke is defined by the *sudden* onset of neurological deficits. Although some patients may have warning signs (TIAs) that appear before an actual stroke, many strokes occur without warning. Some of these symptoms include sudden (a) numbness or weakness in the face, arm, or leg, which usually occurs on one side of the body, (b) severe headache with unknown cause, (c) vision impairment in one or both eyes, (d) confusion, such as having trouble understanding or speaking, and (e) trouble walking and problem with motor coordination. As discussed above, when these symptoms dissipate rapidly, the patient may have had a TIA (CDC, 2012, 2013). The diagnosis is stroke if the symptoms persist for at least 24 hours from onset or when neuroimaging demonstrates brain damage.

Anatomy of the Brain

Stroke occurs within the brain, the control center for the majority of body functions. The cerebral cortex, the largest part of the brain, is responsible for language abilities and personality. The brainstem and cerebellum control automatic functions such as heartbeat, breathing, and coordination. A wide range of symptoms and deficits results from damage to various areas of the brain. Blood is transported to the brain from the heart via arteries, and is returned to the heart through veins. Stroke is primarily caused by interruptions in either the arterial circulation of the brain or, less commonly, abnormalities in the venous circulation. The four major arteries that supply the brain include two carotid arteries in the front of the neck and two vertebral arteries in the back of the neck supplying the posterior lobes of the brain and brain stem. Each artery supplies a specific area of the brain. When an artery is occluded, lack of oxygen (ischemia) leads to abnormalities of brain function and, if persistent, results in death of brain cells supplied by the involved artery. The brain can tolerate only four minutes of anoxia (a lack of oxygen) before brain cells begin to die. It has been estimated that for every minute the brain lacks oxygen, 1.9 million brain cells (neurons) are lost (Saver, 2006). Inside the skull, the internal carotid artery splits into the middle cerebral arteries and anterior cerebral arteries. These arteries supply the parietal lobe and portions of the frontal lobe and anterior portion of the temporal lobe. If the dominant hemisphere middle cerebral arteries are blocked (usually the left brain), language and speech are affected. Blood from the anterior cerebral artery supplies the anterior frontal lobe. Small perforating arteries provide the blood supply to areas deep within the brain (e.g., the thalamus and basal ganglia). In the back of the brain, two vertebral arteries combine to form a basilar artery, which supplies blood to the brainstem and cerebellum. The terminal branches of the vertebrobasilar system supply the visual cortex. These small arteries are susceptible to rupture from long-standing hypertension. Collateral circulation generally does not occur in the blood supply of the central nervous system, even though it is present in most areas of the body. When collateral circulation does develop, arterial interconnections occur between major arterial systems – that is, when one artery is blocked, the area needing oxygen obtains blood from another major artery.

Categories of Stroke

The two main categories of stroke are (a) ischemic stroke due to blood vessel blockage, and (b) intracranial hemorrhage stroke caused by blood vessel rupture. Etiology, diagnosis, and treatment differ for these two types of stroke. The following section reviews the different types of stroke in both categories.

Ischemic Stroke

Ischemic stroke is the most common type of stroke, accounting for approximately 75-80% of all events (Zivin, 2012b). It results from blockage of an artery due to a blood clot. The origination of the blood clot can be multifactorial, but the two major categories are cerebral embolus and cerebral thrombus (Hemmen et al., 2010).

Cerebral Embolus

When a plaque or particle travels from the heart or a larger artery and lodges in a smaller artery, obstruction of blood flow causes an embolic stroke. If the obstruction persists for over a few minutes, brain cells (neurons) begin to die. The death of brain cells and tissue lead to functional limitations. However, if the arterial obstruction lasts for a brief period and permits full recovery, the condition is described as a TIA. Sources of emboli are typically the heart, ascending aorta or aortic arch, and carotid arteries. Cerebral emboli are usually caused by atherosclerotic vascular disease (hardening of the arteries) in which a small portion of atherosclerotic plaque breaks off and travels to the blood vessels within the brain. Embolic stroke may also be caused by a blood clot originating in the heart (Grysiewicz et al., 2008). In people over 60 years of age, atherosclerotic vascular disease and cardiac disease are the most common causes of ischemic stroke. Cerebral embolus is less common in younger people, but might be associated with blood clotting disorders known as coagulopathy.

Cerebral Thrombus

Another form of stroke, caused by a blood clot, develops from atherosclerotic plaque in the wall of a vessel (Zivin, 2012b). Years of uncontrolled hypertension, tobacco abuse, and high cholesterol may cause lineatherosclerosis or *hardening of the arteries*. Build-up of cholesterol plaque can result in a fracture causing a local clumping of platelets occluding a vessel. The resultant mix of platelets and fibrin, a thrombus, does not travel; rather, it causes an arterial obstruction at the site of origin. Depending on the length and severity of the obstruction, resulting disability can vary from partial to full recovery (Hemmen et al., 2010).

Intracranial Hemorrhage Stroke

Intracranial hemorrhage, occurring in approximately 15-20% of strokes, is caused by a ruptured blood vessel (Zivin, 2012a). The focus of this section includes three main forms of intracerebral hemorrhage (ICH): (a) hypertensive hemorrhage due to uncontrolled high blood pressure, (b) subarachnoid hemorrhage due to aneurysm rupture (a congenital weakness and ballooning of the vessel wall), and (c) rupture of a vascular malformation (usually a congenital lesion).

Cerebral Hypertensive Hemorrhage

Long-standing uncontrolled hypertension can lead to damage in the arteries of the brain (as well as other organs, such as the kidneys and eyes). The resulting damage, called lipohyalinosis, affects the small blood vessels in the brain. Lipohyalinosis is a progressive process that weakens the wall of an artery, in turn increasing the risk of rupture. The most common sites of cerebral hypertensive hemorrhage occur in deep structures supplied by the small, penetrating arteries affected by lipohyalinosis. These structures include the basal ganglia and pons. In addition, the cerebellum (the portion of the brain responsible for coordination) is subject to hemorrhage. Morbidity and mortality for hypertensive hemorrhage is extremely high; one-third of these individuals die within a month. Potential treatments for these strokes have focused on limiting the size and rate of bleeding, surgical removal of the hemorrhage, as well as rapidly lowering the blood pressure upon emergency room admission (Anderson et al., 2013). To date, these interventions have failed to improve outcomes from this type of stroke. However, one trial of rapid blood pressure lowering demonstrated promising results after lowering the systolic blood pressure to <140mm Hg and a second similar trial is on-going (Anderson et al., 2013; Qureshi & Palesch, 2011). Since emergency treatment options for hypertensive hemorrhage are generally lacking, the focus remains on preventative strategies, specifically control of hypertension.

Aneurysmal Subarachnoid Hemorrhage

An aneurysm is an out-pouching of a blood vessel due to thinning of the arterial wall. It is usually located at the branching points of cerebral blood vessels. Approximately 85% of cerebral aneurysms develop in the middle cerebral artery, as well as the anterior and posterior communicating arteries. Roughly 20% of those who experience aneurysm have additional aneurysms in the future (ASA, 2013). Aneurysm formation is more likely to occur in individuals with long-standing high blood pressure. Weakened arterial walls can rupture, resulting in subarachnoid hemorrhage (SAH). Patients with aneurismal-SAH are typically younger than their ischemic stroke cohort (typically 40-60 year olds) (Grysiewicz et al., 2008). Risk factors for aneurysmal rupture include: size of the aneurysm (larger aneurysms are higher risk), excessive alcohol intake, tobacco abuse, and other congenital abnormalities, such as fibromuscular dysplasia and polycystic kidney disease. Patients who undergo aneurysmal ruptures usually present with severe headache and focal neurological deficits. Aneurysmal SAH is a catastrophic condition affecting 30,000 people in the United States yearly. Sixty percent of these individuals either die or suffer permanent disability; fifty percent of the survivors with favorable outcomes experience considerable neuropsychological dysfunction (Falvo, 2014). Cerebral vasospasm (i.e., narrowing of proximal arterial segments) complicates 20-50% of cases, and is the major cause of disability and death associated with aneurysmal SAH. The spasm of the vessel itself, which complicates SAH, can also lead to ischemic stroke.

Cerebral Vascular Malformation

Cerebral vascular malformation, also known as arterial venous malformation (AVM), is characterized by congenital abnormalities of blood vessels in the brain. AVM, tangled networks of blood vessels, consist of arteries that directly empty into veins without the normal intervening capillaries that support brain tissue. These lesions, usually present at birth, tend to become apparent later in life when they leak or bleed. It is only half of all vascular malformations, however, which eventually become apparent in this manner. AVM rupture typically occurs abruptly without symptoms and results in neurological deficits (Reddy et al., 2009).

Diagnosis

Physicians diagnose stroke by finding acute neurological symptoms, abnormalities seen during a clinical neurological examination, aided by imaging techniques. Upon arrival at the hospital, all patients who have had a stroke receive a CT scan or MRI of the brain, which evaluates for intracranial hemorrhage, establishes ischemic stroke from hemorrhagic, and eliminates other possible causes of the neurological symptoms (e.g., brain tumors). Specialized centers for the treatment of stroke can rapidly evaluate the cerebral arteries using either ultrasound or arteriography (injection of intravenous contrast dye to visualize the anatomy of the cerebral circulation). These studies assist the clinician with diagnosis, cause, and treatment. Additional studies obtained during hospitalization include a cardiac evaluation, including electrocardiogram and echocardiogram. Once it is determined that the patient is having a stroke, appropriate management is undertaken (Barreto et al., 2012; Falvo, 2014).

Complications and Limitations

Cerebrovascular diseases, such as stroke, follow a spectrum of severity. Frequently, small strokes occur resulting in mild or non-noticeable residual deficits. Contrastingly, a stroke classified as severe is a devastating occurrence. One-third of individuals with severe strokes die within two weeks. Mortality rates increase with advancing age and the presence of other comorbid diseases such as hypertension, heart disease, and diabetes. Approximately one-third of CVAs result in significant neurological deficit, while one-third of individuals have minor or no deficits. A stroke can affect any part of the brain and symptoms vary depending on size and location of the damage. When brain tissue is damaged, far reaching deficits occur including paralysis, cognitive decline, language difficulty, behavioral and mood changes, and psychological effects, such as depression. Those surviving a severe stroke are at much higher risk for other medical complications, including pneumonia and blood clots in the legs. Medical complications can result in death. Other long-term complications of stroke include development of contractures, seizure disorders, bowel and bladder problems, and spasticity of muscles.

Neurological Deficits

In general, when the stroke occurs on one side of the brain, the opposite side of the body is affected. Brainstem strokes caused by abnormalities of the posterior circulation (i.e., vertebral or basilar arteries) can be associated with crossed neurological findings. These patients display abnormalities both ipsilateral (affecting the same side) to the side of the stroke involving the face, and contralateral (affecting the opposite side) to the side of the stroke involving the body. After a stroke, typical neurological deficits range from paralysis, to hemiparesis, to minimal or unnoticeable deficits (Eisenberg & Rashbaum, 2011). An overview of physiological effects and physical limitations related to post-stroke neurological deficits follows. Typical clinical residual findings of middle cerebral artery (MCA) stroke include abnormalities of the motor and sensory cortex leading to spastic hemiparesis and sensory loss, respectively. If the stroke occurs in the right MCA territory, the patient may suffer from anosognosia (also known as neglect), a state in which the individual does not recognize the affected side of the body as belonging to himself or herself. In such cases, the person is unable to perceive objects on either the right or left side of the central field of vision and is unaware of the deficit. When the stroke occurs in the right side of the brain, visual-spatial deficits result. Individuals with visual-spatial problems may incorrectly interpret visual information and have difficulty orienting to the surrounding environment. A stroke on the left side of the brain may result in paralysis to the right side of the face, arm, and leg. Lesions of the left MCA affect the language centers, causing speech or comprehension impairment. When the speech center is affected, the condition is known as aphasia. Patients with aphasia have difficulty sounding words, understanding words, or both; these different forms of aphasia are termed expressive, receptive, and global aphasia. Anosognosia and aphasia seriously impair vocational rehabilitation. Dysphagia, a swallowing disorder, occurs in up to 65% of stroke survivors. If not identified and managed, this condition can lead to poor nutrition, pneumonia, and increased disability. Posterior circulation strokes involving the vertebral and basilar arteries can be fatal. Basilar artery occlusion is known for its extreme mortality rates, as high as 80% (ASA, 2013). These patients initially present with declining mental status, coordination difficulties (ataxia), double vision (diplopia), severe dysarthria (slurred speech), dysphagia (difficulty swallowing), and trouble controlling saliva. Patients with posterior circulation strokes often require mechanical (artificial) ventilation with a breathing tube. Depending on the extent of the stroke, patients can have severe global weakness or even quadriplegia (weakness in all extremities).

Paralysis

The complete loss of function of one or more muscle groups due to damage to the brain is referred to as paralysis. Depending on the area and size of damage, post-stroke survivors may experience weakness, as well as loss of muscle function and sensation.

Paresis

Paresis refers to weakness of muscle strength. Paresis can be localized, and often follows a pattern. For example, localized paresis of one side of the face may result due to damage of the brain tissues that leads to inflammation of the facial nerve affecting that side of the face.

Hemiplegia

This is a common consequence of stroke. It involves paralysis on one side of the body. A person is said to have right hemiplegia if the right side of the body is paralyzed. As mentioned earlier in this chapter, the lesion causing paralysis is typically located in the opposite hemisphere of the brain. When the stroke occurs on the left side of the brain, paralysis limits functions of limbs on the right side of the body. This condition usually has more impact on the upper extremity than the lower extremity. The extent of paralysis is dependent on the site and size of the lesion. These individuals can have deficits in ability to solve problems. Visual-spatial deficits occur when the stroke takes place in the right brain. An individual with visual-spatial problems may incorrectly interpret visual information and have difficulty with environmental orientation. A stroke on the left side of the brain may result in paralysis to the right upper and lower extremities (Duncan et al., 2011).

Aphasia

When the dominant hemisphere of the brain (in the majority of people, this is the left side) is damaged, a language disturbance can result (CDC, 2012; 2013). This language problem is called aphasia and it can take several forms. First, the ability to understand might be affected by the stroke (receptive aphasia). Patients will appear confused since they will not understand the words or commands being spoken to them. Other patients might be able to understand, but not be able to get words out (expressive aphasia). Expressively aphasic (Broca's aphasia) patients typically appear frustrated since they know what they want to say, but are not able to form sentences. In some cases, both reception and expression are affected and these patients are mute and unable to comprehend (global aphasia).

Cognitive Deficits

Strokes cause a wide variety of cognitive deficits. It is common to find survivors of stroke having difficulties in memory retention, especially of newly acquired information. Results of such accidents include slowed retention and disorganized processing of information. Intellectual deficits, behavioral changes, and problem-solving difficulties, can result. Intellectual deficits are minimized and others circumvented with relearning and through job accommodations. For example, patients with memory difficulty can use a notepad to record information. Specific intellectual tasks crucial to an individual vocation can be reassigned to other employees, if unable to be accomplished by the person. If job modification cannot accommodate the extent of intellectual impairment, use of transferable skills or retraining needs assessment. The most common psychological problem found among stroke survivors is depression. This may be related to the degree of functional disability and can impact a person's ability for rehabilitation (Thomas & Lincoln, 2006). Common symptoms of depression include (a) persistent sadness and anxiety, (b) feelings of hopelessness, (c) loss of interest, (d) fatigue and lack of energy, (e) insomnia or hypersomnia, (f) loss or increase of appetite and weight changes, and (g) difficulties in concentrating, remembering, and decision-making (ASA, 2013). Treating depression can improve the stroke survivor's mood and physical recovery. Treating depression may enhance cognitive and intellectual recovery. In addition, social support from family, friends, stroke support groups, and rehabilitation professionals remains a crucial part of recovery for stroke survivors dealing with depression. Emotional lability (partial loss of emotional control) may be experienced and expressed clinically as various emotional states, such as crying, sudden laughter, depression, and anger. Such emotions change rapidly and for no apparent reason; the individual may additionally express emotions considered inappropriate for particular situations. Persons with stroke may also show irritability, frustration, insecurity, hesitancy, anger, hostility, depression, flat affect, and generalized indifference. In addition to affecting the patient, stroke impacts family members and caregivers. The results of a stroke are physically, financially, and practically demanding, as well as emotionally distressing for all involved. Feelings of sadness, grief, exhaustion, fear, and anger are common reactions to increased dependence and vulnerability following a stroke. The disruption in family relationships that can result from a stroke, in addition to resulting heightened conflicts and loss of supportive ties, can be decreased with help from available support groups (Palmer & Glass, 2003).

Treatment

Emerging treatments for ischemic stroke and hemorrhagic stroke vary. Regardless of the type of stroke, timing is an important aspect of treatment. Emergency medical care must be provided at the onset of stroke symptoms. The sooner treatment is delivered, the less severe the resulting disability limitations. Brain damage and other negative results can be significantly reduced through prompt emergency care (Reddy et al., 2009).

Medications

With ischemic stroke, pharmacologic thrombolytic therapy can be administered (within three hours) which aims to dissolve the clot causing the obstruction and unblock the artery. Tissue plasminogen activator (tPA) is the most commonly administered thrombolytic. Delivered intravenously, tPA has been shown in a large clinical trial to improve functional outcomes by dissolving blood clots and restoring blood flow (National Institute of Neurological Disorders and Stroke rt-PA Stroke Study Group, 1995). Benefit was maintained at 12 months after stroke (Kwiatkowski et al., 1999). As expected, there was a risk of bleeding when stroke patients received tPA, but this risk was outweighed by its benefit. Patients who received tPA were 30% more likely to achieve minimal or no neurological symptoms when compared to those who received the placebo.

If a narrowed carotid artery in the neck proves to be the cause of either a TIA or an ischemic stroke, a patient can undergo surgery called carotid endarterectomy (CEA). This procedure removes plaque from the carotid artery, reopens the blocked artery, and improves blood flow. CEA reduces subsequent risk of ischemic stroke. An alternative to traditional CEA surgery, carotid artery stenting, has been proven effective (Brott et al., 2010).

Treatments for hemorrhagic stroke are minimal. Researchers have failed to show that drugs which can reduce bleeding lead to improved outcomes (Mayer et al., 2008; Zivin, 2012a). Surgical decompression or blood removal also has failed to prevent disability or death. However, for subarachnoid hemorrhage, a neurosurgeon can perform aneurismal clipping around the base of the aneurysm to occlude the aneurysm and prevent future rupture and reduce risk of subsequent stroke.

Physical and Occupational Therapy

For patients who have post-stroke hemiplegia or hemiparesis, physical therapy provides strengthening exercises for both the upper and lower extremities. Occupational therapy provides range-of-motion activities and splints which assist in preventing contractures and spasticity. Programs can be oriented toward recovery of occupational modalities and may utilize orthotic devices, such as leg braces, which help the person ambulate. Once the counselor and client have decided on a return to work objective, special orthotic devices can help the person perform specific job functions (Brodwin, Parker, & DeLaGarza, 2010).

Medical Advances

The brain was once thought to be a static, non-repairable organ. Although neurons do not regenerate, recent brain-imaging techniques have given researchers and physicians new understanding of the ability of the brain to adapt and regain function after stroke. Brain-plasticity, one such adaptation, is the ability of one area of the brain to take over the function of a damaged region. Brain cells surrounding the damaged area assume the functions of the damaged cells. Recent rehabilitation advances include (a) constraint-induced therapy, restricting the use of the unaffected limb while intensively training the affected limb; (b) focused-use therapy that includes thousands of passive movement repetitions to help the injured brain relearn how to use the impaired limb; (c) electrical stimulation that uses low voltage electricity to stimulate muscles weakened or paralyzed by stroke; and (d) biofeedback which involves putting a sensor over a target muscle (Eisenberg & Rashbaum, 2011; Falvo, 2014). In biofeedback, when the target muscle moves, the electrical activity generated is sensed by the device, providing immediate feedback to the individual. Although the science is currently in the preliminary phase, research on stem cell implants has been initiated. It is hypothesized that delivery of stem cells to a stroke patient could stimulate other cells to grow in the brain and form new connections to help restore motor function (Chu et al., 2008).

Prevention

Preventing a first-time stroke (primary prevention) and recurrent stroke (secondary prevention) are the goals of neurologists specializing in stroke. Targets that provide protection include: blood pressure reduction, antiplatelet medications (e.g., aspirin), cholesterol reduction, diabetes control, smoking cessation, and blood thinners for heart arrhythmias. Because compliance with medication and resulting side effects is challenging for some individuals, vocational rehabilitation counselors are key in providing support and assistance (Brodwin et al., 2010; Gilbride & Stensrud, 2012). Familiarity with medications and their side effects, especially when considering return to work, is crucial to successful rehabilitation.

Blood Pressure Control

Blood pressure reduction remains the most critical means of avoiding stroke. Long-term damage to the arteries that results from unmanaged hypertension increases the risks of stroke. Numerous clinical studies have shown a reduction in stroke when blood pressure was reduced with antihypertensive medications (Officers and Coordinators for the ALLHAT Collaborative Research Group, 2002; Dahlöf, Devereux, & Kjeldsen, 2002; PROGRESS Collaborative Group, 2001). Aspirin and the combination of aspirin plus extended-release dipyridamole help prevent recurrent stroke. Management of high cholesterol decreases the risk of stroke and heart disease.

Diet and Exercise

The maintenance of a healthy diet low in saturated fats and high in complex grains, fruit, and vegetables reduces the risk of stroke. Many metabolic changes occur during dietary restriction including (a) lower blood pressure; (b) reduced arterial stiffness, cholesterol points, and triglyceride level; (c) slower age-related decline in functional and cognitive capacities; (d) enhanced resistance to stress; and (e) improved ability to adapt to stress at the cellular level (ASA, 2013; CDC, 2012). Along with a healthy diet, exercise is an important part of a healthy lifestyle. Recommendations include at least an hour of moderately intense daily exercise, which may be distributed throughout the day. Exercise is crucial for the individual's health and promotes proper functioning of blood vessels, improves delivery of oxygen to muscle tissues, and increases the good-to-bad cholesterol ratio.

Smoking and Drug Use

Tobacco and illicit drugs should be avoided since they are addictive and have deleterious effects on blood vessels. Damage to the arteries can lead to accelerated atherosclerosis. Along with the medical community, the American Heart and Stroke Associations have bolstered their oppositions to smoking and illicit drugs, as both are associated with the development of cerebrovascular disease.

Rehabilitation Potential

Rehabilitation is a crucial part of recovery, improving the outlook for survivors of stroke. Approximately half of stroke survivors experience some permanent disability; the success of rehabilitation depends on several key factors. Such factors include (a) timing of treatment, (b) extent and size of brain injury, (c) intensity and frequency of therapy, (d) availability of companionship and emotional support, and (e) the stroke survivor's personal outlook and attitude (ASA, 2013; CDC, 2012; 2013). Maximum return of function after a stroke can require a six-month recovery period; counselors must take this into account before determining an individual's rehabilitation potential. Early intervention helps maintain and encourage the person's return to work, keeping in mind that maximum return of function does not occur immediately. The goal of stroke rehabilitation is to help the survivor maximize independence. The level of independence reached after rehabilitation is different for each individual, depending on the size and extent of stroke and previous functioning. Physical, speech, and occupational therapy aid in recovery. Individuals can improve independence in many areas such as mobility, communication, swallowing, cognitive and behavior modifications, and self-care. Below, are a few characteristics of rehabilitation unique to stroke survivors.

Passive Exercise

Manually-assisted movement serves two primary purposes. First, the repetitive movements help prevent spasticity and contractures which are limiting and painful for stroke patients. Development of contractures can lead to skin breakdown and infections. The inability to flex and extend muscles due to contractures inhibits caregivers from providing effective bowel and bladder care. Second, passive movement of the affected limbs may aid the brain in reorganization and recovery of function. This conventional forced-use therapy is performed in thousands of repetitions with the help of a physical therapist or caregiver (Eisenberg & Rashbaum, 2011; Falvo, 2014).

Assistive Devices and Technology

Canes, walkers, and motorized carts increase mobility after stroke. Hoists used at home and some worksites assist lifting and care of the person. Mechanical devices aid pushing and pulling work activities. A variety of work-related equipment is adaptable for one-hand operations. Various types of orthotic devices improve hand function. Use of a computer minimizes writing. Desk and file cabinets may be arranged to diminish limitations. Often, simple accommodations provide for access by wheelchair users. Various accommodations can be recommended, depending on the particular work site and functional needs of the individual (Brodwin et al., 2010; Gilbride & Stensrud, 2012).

Technology has improved the range and availability of adaptive devices for post-stroke survivors. For individuals with limited strength or hand dexterity, low-tech devices are available such as doorknob-turners which slip over a doorknob to allow the door to be opened with lever action. Fine motor skill impairments cause changes in the individual's daily routine. Assistive devices, such as those that allow buttons to hook, make the resumption of independence easier. High-tech technology includes computers with specialized programs that speak for people with severe aphasia or enhance vision. Such programs allow survivors to express their needs and wants with greater ease. Computerized robotic gait trainers allow patients to be mobile at early stages (Brodwin et al., 2010). Funding for such technology can be assisted by programs like Medicaid, Medicare, Social Security Disability Insurance (SSDI and SSI), state rehabilitation work incentive programs, and private insurance (ASA, 2013).

Increased Dependency on Caregivers

As a result of physical and cognitive deficits, stroke survivors may need assistance from caregivers. These individuals are likely to be immediate family members. Because stroke is characterized by its sudden onset, change of roles and family dynamics occurs quickly and without preparation, causing emotional distress. Stroke survivors with high levels of emotional support demonstrate enhanced levels of recovery. Lack of perceived support is associated with the presence and severity of depression. Survivors and family members can experience positive effects after stroke, such as increased compassion and empathy for others, self-confidence, attention to relationships, spiritual growth, reassessment of personal values, and enhanced sense of meaning of life (Palmer & Glass, 2003).

Psychosocial Factors

Studies of post-stroke outcomes focus on recovery of physical function and reduction of medical complications. Some studies cite psychosocial factors, such as motivation, as a key to successful vocational rehabilitation (Brodwin et al., 2010; Gilbride & Stensrud, 2012; Szymanski, Enright, & Hershenson, 2012). Socioeconomic issues also effect return to gainful employment. Workers with higher education levels and professional, managerial, and technical jobs successfully return to work at a significantly higher rate than those with lower levels of education and unskilled manual job experience. Vocational programs that offer a multidisciplinary approach to stroke rehabilitation have had great success in rehabilitation and successful employment. A key to success is careful coordination of comprehensive services by a multidisciplinary team made up of rehabilitation counselors, physicians, therapists, psychologists, and social workers.

Conclusion

As the most common cause of long-term disability, stroke impacts all aspects of a person's life, as well as the lives of family and friends. Disability adjustments range from attending to medical and financial needs to physical and psychological adaptations to addressing loss of interpersonal relationships and employment. Recovery from stroke is a challenging journey that can last the rest of the patient's life. Rehabilitation counselors, working together with a multidisciplinary team of healthcare providers, can improve the quality of life of the individual and aid his or her family in coping with the complications of stroke.

Case Study

La Shaun Jackson is a 59-year old African American widow with an adopted 15-year old boy who has a record of substance abuse and juvenile delinquency. She has worked as a claims processor for the Internal Revenue Service (IRS) in Fresno, California for over five years. Prior to returning to school to earn her Associate of Arts degree in accounting, she held a secretarial position for 15 years at a small import-export firm. Several long term clerical and retail store sales positions were listed on her resume before and immediately after she moved from Illinois to California.

Ms. Jackson has had hypertension and chronic headaches for 13 years and has been struggling with an overweight problem throughout her life. Since her husband died five years ago, her weight has continued to increase, along with her blood pressure. A year ago, she experienced a mild hemorrhagic CVA. No surgery was contemplated. Her hypertension was controlled by medication. As a result of the hemorrhage, La Shaun has hemiplegia on the dominant side (right side) of her body and face; she has moderately slurred speech, and she was unable to recognize or identify sensory stimuli, resulting in neglect of one side of her body. The trauma caused physical limitations and concurrent emotional problems.

A multidisciplinary rehabilitative program began almost immediately after La Shaun's medical condition stabilized. Rehabilitative therapy was started in the acute-care hospital within the first month following the stroke. After eight months of intensive care and physical therapy, Ms. Jackson regained 80% of her cognitive and physical functioning. Her physician released her to work in an environment with minimal stress. The position must be sedentary with some time allowed for physical therapy at a nearby clinic.

Questions

1. Provide a vocational profile for Ms. La Shaun Jackson. Identify additional information you need to help this client.
2. How does La Shaun's age affect your provision of rehabilitation services? Explain your response both for her and other older working individuals. Discuss age discrimination and other stereotypical factors relevant to this and other cases.
3. Outline the rehabilitation services you intend to provide, including when to begin and the time frame for each step in the process.
4. How would you counsel Ms. Jackson if she has mixed feelings about returning to work?
5. Would you counsel her differently if she was 20 years younger?

References

American Stroke Association (ASA). (2013). *Stroke statistics, guidelines, and prevention*. Retrieved from http://www.strokeassociation.org

Anderson, C. S., Heeley, E., Huang, Y., Wang, J., Stapf, C., Delcourt, C., . . . Chalmers, J. (2013). Rapid blood-pressure lowering in patients with acute intracerebral hemorrhage. *New England Journal of Medicine, 368*(25), 2355–2365.

Barreto, A. D., Alexandrov, A. V., Lyden, P., Lee, J., Martin-Schild, S., Shen, L., . . . Grotta, J. C. (2012). The Argatroban and tissue-type plasminogen activator stroke study: Final results of a pilot safety study. *Stroke, 43*(3), 770–775.

Brodwin, M. G., Parker, R. M., & DeLaGarza, D. (2010). Disability and reasonable accommodation. In E. M. Szymanski & R. M. Parker (Eds.), *Work and disability: Contexts, issues, and strategies for enhancing employment opportunities for people with disabilities* (3rd ed., pp. 281–323). Austin, TX: Pro-ed.

Brott, T. G., Hobson, R. W. II, Howard, G., Roubin, G. S., Clark, W. M., Brooks, W., . . . Meschia, J. F. (2010). Stenting versus endarterectomy for treatment of carotid-artery stenosis. *New England Journal of Medicine, 363*(1), 11–23.

Centers for Disease Control and Prevention (CDC). (2012). Prevalence of stroke – United States, 2006-2010. *Morbidity and Mortality Weekly Report*. Atlanta, GA: Author.

CDC. (2013). *Stroke facts*. Retrieved from http://www.cdc.gov/stroke/facts.htm

Chu, K., Jung, K. H., Kim, S. J., Lee, S. T., Kim, J., Park, H. K., . . . Roh, J. K. (2008). Transplantation of human neural stem cells protect against ischemia in a preventive mode via hypoxia-inducible factor-1á stabilization in the host brain. *Brain Research, 1207*, 182–192.

Dahlöf, B., Devereux, R. B., & Kjeldsen, S. E. (2002). Cardiovascular morbidity and mortality in the Losartan Intervention for Endpoint Reduction in Hypertension Study (LIFE): A randomized trial against atenolol. *Lancet, 359*, 995–1003.

Duncan, P. W., Sullivan, K. T., Behrman, A. L., Azen, S. P., Wu, S. S., Nadeau, S. E., . . . Hayden, S. K. (2011). Body-weight-supported treadmill rehabilitation after stroke. *New England Journal of Medicine, 364*(21), 2026–2036.

Eisenberg, M., & Rashbaum, I. (2011). Stroke. In S. R. Flanagan, H. H. Zaretsky, & A. Moroz (Eds.), *Medical aspects of disability: A handbook for the rehabilitation professional* (4th ed., pp. 549–567). New York, NY: Springer.

Falvo, D. R. (2014). *Medical and psychosocial aspects of chronic illness and disability* (5th ed.). Burlington, MA: Jones & Bartlett.

Gilbride, D., & Stensrud, R. (2012). People with disabilities in the workplace. In R. M. Parker & J. B. Patterson (Eds.). *Rehabilitation counseling: Basics and beyond* (5th ed., pp. 259–284). Austin, TX: Pro-ed.

Go, A. S., Mozaffarian, D., Roger, V. L., Benjamin, E. J., Berry, J. D., Borden, W. B., . . . Turner, M. B. (2013) Heart disease and stroke statistics – 2013 update: A report from the American Heart Association. *Circulation, 127*, e6–e245.

Grysiewicz, R. A., Thomas, K., & Pandey, D. K. (2008). Epidemiology of ischemic and hemorrhage stroke: Incidence prevalence, and risk factors. *Neurologic Clinics, 26*, 871–895.

Hemmen, T. M., Raman, R., Guluma, K. Z., Meyer, B. C., Gomes, J. A., Cruz-Flores, S., . . . Lyden, P. D. (2010). Intravenous thrombolysis plus hypothermia for acute treatment of ischemic stroke (ICTuS-L): Final results. *Stroke, 41*(10), 2265–2270.

Kwiatkowski, T. G., Libman, R. B., Frankel, M., Tilley, B. C., Morgenstern, L. B., Lu, M., . . . Brott, T., for the National Institute of Neurological Disorders and Stroke Recombinant Tissue Plasminogen Activator Stroke Study Group. (1999). Effects of tissue plasminogen activator for acute ischemic stroke at one year. *New England Journal of Medicine, 340*, 1781–1787.

Mayer, S. A., Brun, N. C., Begtrup, K., Broderick, J., Davis, S. M., Diringer, M. N., . . . Steiner T. (2008). FAST Trial Investigators. Efficacy and safety of recombinant activated Factor VII for acute intracerebral hemorrhage. *New England Journal of Medicine, 358*, 2127–2137.

National Institute of Neurological Disorders and Stroke rt-PA Stroke Study Group. (1995). Tissue plasminogen activator for acute ischemic stroke. *New England Journal of Medicine, 333*, 1581–1587.

Officers and Coordinators for the ALLHAT Collaborative Research Group. (2002). Antihypertensive and Lipid-Lowering Treatment to Prevent Heart Attack Trial (ALLHAT). Major outcomes in high-risk hypertensive patients randomized to angiotensinconverting enzyme inhibitor or calcium channel blocker vs. diuretic. *Journal of the American Medical Association, 288*, 2981–2997.

Palmer, S., & Glass, T. A. (2003). Family function and stroke recovery: A review. *Rehabilitation Psychology, 48*(4), 255–265.

PROGRESS Collaborative Group. (2001). Randomized trial of a perindopril-based blood-pressure-lowering regimen among 6105 individuals with previous stroke or transient ischemic attack. *Lancet, 358*, 1033–1041.

Qureshi, A. I., & Palesch Y. Y. (2011). Antihypertensive treatment of acute cerebral hemorrhage (ATACH) II: Design, methods, and rationale. *Neurocritical Care, 15*, 559-576.

Reddy, C., Chae, J., Lew, H., Lombard, L., Edgley, S., & Moroz, A. (2009). Stroke management in the acute care setting. *Physical Medicine and Rehabilitation: The Journal of Injury, Function, and Rehabilitation, 1*, s4–s12.

Saver, J. L. (2006). Time is brain – Quantified. *Stroke, 37*(1), 236–263.

Szymanski, E. A., Enright, M. S., & Hershenson, D. B. (2012). An ecological approach to the vocational behavior and career development of people with disabilities. In R. M. Parker & J.B. Patterson (Eds.), *Rehabilitation counseling: Basics and beyond* (5th ed., pp. 199–258). Austin, Tx: Pro-ed.

Thomas, S. A., & Lincoln, N. B. (2006). Factors relating to depression after stroke. *British Journal of Clinical Psychology, 45*(1), 49–61.

Zivin, J. A. (2012a). Hemorrhagic cerebrovascular disease. In L. Goldman & A. I. Schafer (Eds.), *Goldman's Cecil medicine* (24th ed., pp. 2320–2326). Philadelphia, PA: Elsevier Saunders.

Zivin, J. A. (2012b). Ischemic cerebrovascular disease. In L. Goldman & A. I. Schafer (Eds.), *Goldman's Cecil medicine* (24th ed., pp. 2310–2319). Philadelphia, PA: Elsevier Saunders.

About the Authors

Andrew D. Barreto, M.D., is a cerebrovascular neurologist who specializes in stroke at the University of Texas-Health Science Center in Houston. Dr. Barreto is an Assistant Professor at the University of Texas-Houston Medical School and is involved with all aspects of management of stroke, including emergency treatment, hospital care, and clinic follow-up. Research interests of Dr. Barreto include the use of ultrasound technology and novel adjunctive medical treatments aimed at enhancing stroke treatment.

Frances W. Siu, Ph.D., C.R.C., is an Assistant Professor and Undergraduate Coordinator of the Rehabilitation Services Program at California State University, Los Angeles (CSULA). She received her Ph.D. in Special Education and Counseling, option in Rehabilitation Counselor Education, from the University of Texas at Austin, her M.S. in rehabilitation counseling and B.S. in psychology, both from CSULA. Research interests of Dr. Siu include medical aspects of disability, multicultural issues, and violence against people with disabilities. She has published over 20 articles and book chapters, and given over 50 professional presentations on violence against people with disabilities, rehabilitation education, and rehabilitation services.

Chapter 14

EPILEPSY

Robert T. Fraser, Ph.D., C.R.C.
John W. Miller, M.D., Ph.D.
Erica K. Johnson, Ph.D., C.R.C.

Introduction

Several well-known individuals in history including Socrates, Leonardo de Vinci, Charles Dickens, Thomas Edison, and Julius Caesar had active seizure conditions. The word *epilepsy* derives from the Greek word meaning *to be seized* and is an umbrella term that refers to a wide variety of seizure conditions. A seizure involves a transient disruption of the normal activity of the brain through neuronal instability or firing in an abnormally rapid manner. This excessive electrical discharge results in a seizure. A seizure may be confined to one area of the brain (focal seizure) or take place throughout the entire brain (generalized seizure). Epilepsy is defined as: (a) two unprovoked seizures more than 24 hours apart, (b) one unprovoked seizure under circumstances where there is a greater than 75% probability of future seizures, or (c) at least two seizures in a reflex epilepsy setting (Fisher et al., 2005).

The extent to which seizure disorders affect brain functioning depends on the location, spread, and duration of seizures. Consequently, some seizures only impair brain functioning slightly, while other seizures result in a complete disruption of normal brain activities. Risk factors are diverse but include hypertension, substance abuse, depressive illness, and being in a lower socioeconomic group (Deray, Resnick, & Alvarez, 2004). Direct causes of epilepsy include genetic disorders, malformations of the brain, traumatic brain injury, anoxia (insufficient oxygen), brain tumors, infectious diseases, parasitic infections, stroke and other vascular diseases, and substance abuse. Only 1-2% of people in the general population have a risk of developing epilepsy, but the risk increases to 6% by age 25 if a parent has epilepsy (Devinsky, 2008). A seizure is a discrete event and is a symptom of brain dysfunction (Wiebe, 2012).

This chapter discusses classification of seizures, diagnosis and treatment, functional and psychosocial aspects, vocational limitations, potential for rehabilitation, and job development. The chapter concludes with a case study analysis of an individual who has a partial complex seizure disorder.

Classification

Seizures are classified by review of clinical symptoms, electroencephalogram (EEG), and video EEG monitoring. Seizures were classified by the International League Against Epilepsy (ILAE) Commission on Classification and Terminology and are summarized in Table 1.

The two most important seizure types are as follows:
1. **Generalized seizures** that begin in both cerebral hemispheres.
2. **Partial (focal) seizures** that begin in one location of one cerebral hemisphere.
    a) **Simple partial seizures** (1981) or focal seizures without impairment of consciousness (2010).
    b) **Complex partial seizures** (1981) or focal seizures with impairment of consciousness (2010).
    c) **Partial seizures secondarily generalized** (1981) or focal seizures evolving into a bilateral convulsive seizure (2010).

TABLE 1
Classification and Terminology for Seizures, 1981 and 2010

Nomenclature of the International Classification of Epileptic Seizures (1981)	Revised Nomenclature (2010)
I. Partial Seizures (seizures that begin locally)	**I. Focal Seizures**

A. Simple Partial (without impaired consciousness)
  1. With motor symptoms
  2. With somatosensory or special sensory symptoms
  3. With autonomic symptoms
  4. With psychic symptoms
	A. Focal without impairment of consciousness or awareness
	  1. With observable motor components
	  2. Involving subjective sensory phenomena only
	  3. With observable motor or autonomic components
	  4. Involving subjective psychic phenomena only

B. Complex Partial (with impaired consciousness)
  1. With impaired consciousness only
  2. With automatisms
	B. Focal with Impairment of Consciousness or Awareness

C. Partial
  1 Secondarily generalized
	C. Focal
	  1. Evolving to a bilateral, convulsive seizure (involving tonic, clonic, or tonic and clonic components)

II. Generalized Seizures
A. Absence
	II. Generalized Seizures
	A. Absence
	  1. Typical
	  2. Atypical
	  3. With special features

B. Generalized Tonic-Clonic
C. Myoclonic
	B. Tonic-Clonic
	C. Myoclonic
	  1. Myoclonic
	  2. Myolonic atonic
	  3. Myoclonic tonic

D. Akinetic E. Atonic F. Tonic G. Clonic	D. Atonic E. Atonic F. Tonic G. Clonic
III. Unclassified Seizures	**III. Unknown Seizures**

Source: Berg, A. T., Berkovic, S. F., Brodie, M. J., Buchhalter, J., Cross, J. H., van Emde Boas, W., . . . Scheffer, I. E. (2010). Revised terminology and concepts for organization of seizures and epilepsies: Report of the ILAE Commission on Classification and Terminology, 2005-2009. *Epilepsia, 51,* 676-685.

Generalized Epilepsy

These conditions involve both cerebral hemispheres, as well as deeper areas of the brain (i.e., thalamus and brain stem structures). They are sub-categorized into three major types: (a) tonic-clonic or convulsive seizures, (b) absence seizures, and (c) myoclonic seizures.

Convulsive (generalized tonic-clonic) Seizures

This form of generalized seizure, sometimes called *grand mal seizure,* is the stereotypic seizure with which most people are familiar. It may begin with a tonic phase, during which the body becomes rigid for a few seconds. A clonic phase follows during which there are rhythmic symmetric movements of the arms and other body regions. The entire seizure generally lasts about one to three minutes (Fraser, Miller, & Johnson, 2011b). Although most convulsions last just a few minutes, an individual may have a continuous prolonged seizure, or repeated seizures without regaining consciousness. This is called *status epilepticus* and requires emergency medical intervention when the seizure exceeds five minutes. First aid for tonic-clonic seizures involves turning a person's body on its side to prevent choking and protecting the head from hitting hard surfaces. People cannot *swallow their tongue* during seizures. Depending on the severity of the seizure, it may leave some individuals disoriented and fatigued afterwards. Some individuals may return to work immediately, while others may require a full day of rest before returning.

Absence Seizures

These seizures, sometimes called *petit mal seizures*, last only a few seconds and involve a brief disruption of consciousness. The individual may appear like they are staring, have small rhythmic movements of the eyelids, and autonomic symptoms (e.g., pupil dilation). This type of epilepsy may begin in childhood (Childhood Absence Epilepsy) or at puberty (Juvenile Absence Epilepsy), and often remits in adulthood. This category involves less than 5% of all epilepsy cases (Pellock, Bourgeois, & Dodson, 2008; Wiebe, 2012). Absence seizures are often not identified for years, and may not be diagnosed unless convulsions occur. Absences interfere with learning and make it dangerous to drive a motor vehicle, so early treatment is essential. From a functional perspective, absence seizures may be minimally vocationally limiting. Exceptions occur when an individual is experiencing many seizures of this type throughout the day or has a physically high risk occupation, where even brief losses of consciousness affect job performance.

Myoclonic Seizures

Myoclonic seizures consist of sudden contractions of the limbs or trunk that may lead to convulsions. This is most commonly encountered in a genetic form of epilepsy, called Juvenile Myoclonic Epilepsy (Wiebe, 2012). This syndrome occurs in more than 10% of patients in adult epilepsy clinics, and is most often seen shortly after awakening and triggered by sleep deprivation.

Partial (Focal) Seizures

These seizures are divided into three categories: (a) simple partial seizures with unimpaired consciousness; (b) complex partial seizures with impaired consciousness; and (c) partial seizures evolving into secondarily generalized seizures. Approximately 60% of people with epilepsy have seizures which are classified as partial seizures (Fraser et al., 2011b; Leppik, 2006).

Simple Partial Seizures

These seizures may involve motor, sensory, autonomic, or a combination of symptoms without impaired consciousness or responsiveness. They are linked specifically to the affected area of the brain. Many simple partial seizures last less than 30 seconds; because consciousness is not impaired, this is often not a significant problem in regard to simple job performance.

Complex Partial Seizures

Impairment of consciousness accompanies complex partial seizures; these seizures are more commonly associated with temporal or frontal lobe functioning (Wiebe, 2012). This type of seizure may have an associated aura or warning prior to a convulsion that can involve an odor, aphasia, dizziness, nausea, headache, unusual stomach sensation, or a déjà vu experience. Common events include the individual having repetitive motor movements, fumbling with one's hands or clothing, lip-smacking, or aimless wandering. Complex partial seizures without motor components also occur, and consist of impaired consciousness with motionless staring. These seizures are impairing due to unpredictable loss of consciousness.

From a functional perspective, complex partial seizures are impairing due to unpredictable loss of consciousness and the associated unusual behavior. It is fortunate when an individual has a brief aura or warning before a seizure, allowing the person to take safety precautions or alert others of an impending seizure.

Partial (focal) Seizures Evolving into Secondarily Generalized Seizures

Some individuals have focal seizures, which sometimes spread into generalized seizures. Convulsive seizures may have an even greater risk of injury than complex partial seizures. Sometimes smaller partial seizures may go unrecognized and untreated.

Psychogenic Nonepileptic Episodes

These events mimic seizures but are the result of panic attacks, conversion disorders, dissociative events, or other diverse psychological causes. The most definitive way to diagnose nonepileptic seizures is long-term video/EEG monitoring. Approximately 20-30% of patients evaluated at epilepsy centers have nonepileptic seizures (Devinsky, 2008).

Diagnosis and Treatment

Diagnosis

When individuals initially experience seizures, they generally consult a primary care physician first. If the person does not achieve seizure control within three months, the individual is then referred to a general neurologist. If seizure control cannot be achieved after 12 months by the general neurologist, a referral is made to an epilepsy specialist.

Neurological consultation includes a physical examination and patient history, metabolic studies, EEG testing, and other evaluations. When a patient starts having seizures, neuroimaging, usually with magnetic resonance imaging (MRI) of the head, is used to look for lesions that might be the cause of seizures (Wiebe, 2012). The EEG may reveal epileptiform abnormalities which confirm a seizure diagnosis and helps determine if the seizures are focal or generalized.

As recommended by the National Association of Epilepsy Centers (2010), when the general neurologist does not achieve seizure control within 12 months, referral to an epilepsy center should be made. These centers are staffed with neurologists who specialize in epilepsy treatment and are located within a health center that has specialized teams devoted to the medical and psychosocial needs of persons with epilepsy.

Treatment Principles and Medications

It is desirable that individuals use one medication (monotherapy), if possible, to control symptoms. When effective, one drug is easier to manage, and has less potential toxicity. Brodie and Kwon (2002) found that 47% of patients with new onset epilepsy responded to the first antiepileptic medication, 13% to the second, but only 1% to a third monotherapy choice. By adding a second medication, only 3% achieved control of seizures. A dosage should be established that maintains seizure control without unacceptable adverse effects. Table 2 overviews pharmacological data on the major antiepileptic drugs.

Toxic levels of medication (excessive drug concentrations) can result in double vision, lethargy, cognitive impairment, coordination difficulties, and other medical symptoms. Drug side effects may require medical intervention. Non-compliance with medication is a major issue, and in some communities, up to 90% of patients can be found with medication levels below therapeutic ranges (Leppik, 2006).

Another treatment approach which is used if medications are not effective is a vagal nerve stimulator. The vagal nerve stimulator is implanted in the chest and stimulates the vagal nerve at a steady cycle and at seizure onset. Approximately 30-35% of those using the stimulator achieve greater than 50% seizure reduction, another third have some benefit with seizure frequency reduced 20-50%, but only 1% achieve complete control (Devinsky, 2008).

Surgery

Surgery is considered only when thorough trials of appropriate antiepileptic medications fail to control seizures. When seizures impair independent living, school performance, work capacities, or social activities in a substantial way, the physician may recommend a surgical consultation. For surgery to occur, a series of diagnostic tests that include neuropsychological and continuous video EEG monitoring are conducted so

TABLE 2
Seizure Types and Indicated Antiepileptic Drugs

Seizure Type	Effective Antiepileptic Drugs (Listed alphabetically)	
Simple partial or complex partial	**Primary Drugs**	**Secondary Drugs**
	Carbamazepine (Tegretol, Carbatrol)	Clonazepam (Klonopin)
	Lacosamide (Vimpat)	Ezogabine (Potiga)
	Lamotrigine (Lamictal)	Felbamate (Felbatol)
	Levetiracetam (Keppra)	Gabapentin (Neurontin)
	Oxcarbazepine (Trileptal)	Methsuximide (Celontin)
	Phenytoin (Dilantin)	Phenobarbital (Luminal)
	Pregabalin (Lyrica)	Primidone (Mysoline)
	Topirimate (Topamax)	Tiagabine (Gabitxil)
	Zonisamide (Zonegran)	Valproic acid (Depakene)
Secondarily generalized tonic-clonic	**Primary Drugs**	**Secondary Drugs**
	Carbamazepine	Ezogabine
	Lacosamide	Felbamate
	Lamotrigine	Gabapentin
	Levetiracetam	Phenobarbital
	Oxcarbazepine	Primidone (Mysoline)
	Phenytoin	
	Pregabalin	
	Topiramate	
	Valproic acid	
	Zonisamide	
Generalized tonic-clonic (generalized from onset)	**Primary Drugs**	**Secondary Drugs**
	Lamotrigine	Clonazepam
	Levetiracetam	Felbamate
	Topiramate	
	Valproic acid	
	Zonisamide	
Generalized absence	**Primary Drugs**	**Secondary Drugs**
	Ethosuximide (Zarontin)	Acetazolamide (Diamox)
	Lamotrigine	Clonazepam
	Levetiracetam	Felbamate
	Topirimate	Methsuximide
	Valproic acid	
	Zonisamide	
Generalized myoclonic	**Primary Drugs**	**Secondary Drugs**
	Clonazepam	Acetazolamide
	Lamotrigine	Felbamate
	Levetiracetam	Methsuximide
	Topiramate	
	Valproic acid	

that the medical staff and patient have an understanding of the site of origin of the seizures, and the risks of removing that area. Some individuals and families choose to accept risks of minor memory or language deficits for possible seizure-free or ameliorated status.

The outcome in temporal lobe surgery for those with hippocampal sclerosis is 60-70% seizure free, 20-25% with greater than 85% seizure reduction, and 10-15% with no worthwhile improvement (Devinsky, 2008).

Medical Prognosis for Patients with Epilepsy

Long term follow-up of childhood epilepsy (Sillanpää & Schmidt, 2006) noted that 67% eventually achieved seizure control. An important prognostic indicator for the eventual control of seizures is the duration of uncontrolled seizures. Other factors include cognitive and neurological impairment, known cause (remote symptomatic epilepsy), seizure type, and age of onset.

Functional and Psychosocial Aspects

Functional Issues

Unless seizures are due to stroke or other acquired brain impairment, individuals with epilepsy generally have no physical limitations and are fully independent in eating, walking, personal hygiene, and dressing. At times, adverse effects of antiepileptic medication may impair the individual's physical and intellectual functioning. Even low-grade toxicity can produce awkwardness of gait, coordination problems, and eye-focusing difficulties. Other adverse effects include problems in physical functioning and cognitive issues such as memory and attention span. These effects may improve with alteration in drug regimen. While independent living is a possibility for most people with the condition, driving is prohibited for people with uncontrolled epilepsy (Fraser et al., 2011b; Wiebe, 2012).

Psychosocial Issues

Individuals with epilepsy may have one or more of the specific emotional problems that occur from having a seizure disorder. There are three prominent features of adjustment that persons with epilepsy encounter:

1. Epileptic seizures are episodic, where the person is functioning normally one minute and not the next. The time, place, and circumstances are often unknown; the individual has to live with a great degree of ambiguity, fear, and anxiety.
2. The epileptic seizure itself is often an alien, unusual, and frightening spectacle to observers. Bystanders may not know how to safely respond to a person during a seizure.
3. Not only does the individual usually lose control during the seizure, but he or she also does not have control of the initiation of the seizure. All societies desire and respect predictability and regularity. This is particularly true in the United States, a society that stresses self-control and responsibility.

Psychological adjustment in epilepsy involves multi-etiological considerations (Hermann et al., 2006). Neurological concerns include seizure severity/frequency, duration of epilepsy, and neuropsychological impairment. Psychosocial considerations involve parenting style, available social support, vocational/educational functioning, and perceived stigma. Adolescents with epilepsy are particularly at risk of poor mental health and associated suicidality (Nilsson, Ahlbom, Farahmand, Asberg, & Tomson, 2002; Rodenburg, Wagner, Austin, Kerr, & Dunn, 2011).

Anxiety and depression are common in adult epilepsy and significantly affect quality of life. Research conducted by de Souza and Salgado (2006) indicated that depression was diagnosed in 41% of women with epilepsy and 22% of men with this disability. Research at the University of Washington Epilepsy Center (Fraser, Trejo, Clemmons, & Freelove, 1987) indicated that across neurological, demographic, cognitive, and psychosocial variables, levels of anxiety and depression were most significantly related to early dropouts from an epilepsy vocational rehabilitation program. Financial status and lack of adjustment to seizures were also significantly related.

The Centers for Disease Control and Prevention (CDC-P) promotes a public health agenda related to epilepsy with an emphasis on self-management and self-determination in clinical and community care. Self-management programs are patient education programs that involve patients as active participants in treatment. Daily management of the illness is the responsibility of the patient, as opposed to medical providers. Wellness management skills become a focus of intervention (Fraser et al., 2011a; Lorig, Ritter, Laurent, & Plant, 2006).

DiIorio et al. (2009a, 2009b) developed an internet-based intervention, WebEase, based on the transtheoretical model of behavior change, social cognitive theory, and motivational interviewing (Miller & Rolnick, 2013). Three patient behavioral areas are addressed: medication, stress, and sleep management. Significant results were seen in epilepsy self-management, sleep quality, self-efficacy, and social support.

Self-management interventions appear to hold promise in their ability to improve patients' social and emotional functioning, health adherence, and quality of life. Involving the client in the identification of self-management needs to be emphasized (Johnson et al., 2012).

Vocational Limitations and Rehabilitation Potential

Seizure Status

A review of functional seizure-related considerations is necessary when determining employment potential. For those who do not achieve seizure control, employability is most affected by seizure type, related symptoms, duration, frequency, and pattern of occurrence. For example, a person can have generalized tonic-clonic seizures on a weekly basis, but have them nocturnally (at night) in a way that does not affect employment.

Neuropsychological and Psychosocial Assessment

Seizures are not always the primary issue of epilepsy. Concerns about brain functioning and psychosocial adjustment are prevalent among those referred for specialized epilepsy medical and vocational assessment. Dodrill (1978) established a comprehensive battery of 16 neuropsychological measures directly related to brain impairment and epilepsy. Additionally, psychosocial adjustment difficulties are identified through use of the Washington Psychosocial Seizure Inventory as an initial screening device (Dodrill, Batzel, Queisser, & Temkin, 1980).

Batzel, Dodrill, and Fraser (1980) established that this test battery differentiated well between the unemployed (64% of test scores outside normal limits), the underemployed (53% of the battery outside normal limits), and the employed (only 22%). Research by Hermann et al. (2006), Oyegbile et al. (2004), and Rausch, Le, and Langfitt (1997) indicated that common cognitive concerns for individuals with epilepsy include attentional issues, speed of mental processing/cognitive flexibility, memory and learning, and executive functioning. Individuals with known brain injury, other neurological insult, or recurrent severe seizures over a number of years need periodic neuropsychological testing. Testing should be customized when possible to specific job goal demands (e.g., aspects of memory, problem solving, speed of information processing, motor functioning language).

Work History and Prior Training

The rehabilitation counselor carefully reviews employment history and determines reasons for any job changes or termination. At times, the individual had adequate abilities but lost employment due to discrimination because of seizure occurrences at work. Conversely, some clients identify seizures as the reason for job termination when difficulties at work were more related to lack of abilities or interpersonal functioning. Information from family members, prior employers, and other third parties is helpful in clarifying job performance issues. For some clients with epilepsy and associated brain impairment, on-the-job training and supported employment are more effective avenues to placement than formal academic or technical training. On-the-job training can be effective for people who have had negative experiences in the school environment.

Considerations for the Rehabilitation Counselor

The rehabilitation counselor carefully reviews employment history and determines needed job accommodations or changes. It is important not only to address the client's strengths and limitations, but also suitable employment options that will provide a safe work environment. Each client must be evaluated individually, with job skills and experience carefully assessed. Assets and limitations of clients vary widely. It is not so much the type of seizure that influences the person's functioning level as the frequency of seizures. Frequently occurring absence seizures can pose more problems than well-controlled tonic-clonic epilepsy. The counselor should consider these crucial questions concerning seizure status (Bishop, 2004; Fraser et al., 2011a, 2011b):

- What type of seizures and specific symptoms does the client have? What is the seizure activity during and after the seizure? If there is a loss of consciousness, how much time is involved?
- How well controlled are the seizures? If the client has active seizures, when do they occur?
- Does the client have a warning or aura before a seizure? How consistent are the warnings and how much time do they provide the client?
- Are there certain precipitants (e.g., flickering lights, stress, fatigue, substance use) to seizure events?
- Is the client on the right type or level of medication for the seizure type? Is there consistent medication compliance? Does the client complain of side effects from medication? How specialized was the medical evaluation? Did a general practitioner, neurologist, or epileptologist (neurologist specializing in epilepsy) perform the evaluation?
- When was the last medical evaluation?
- What is involved in the recovery period following a seizure? What is a reasonable time in which a client can return to work?
- Does the client have any other physical, mental, or sensory disabilities? If so, have they been evaluated in the area of disability (e.g., cognitive concerns requiring neuropsychological evaluation)?

These issues can be more impairing than the seizures.

The above information is helpful in establishing daily functional capacities. Motor performance can be slowed, primarily in cases involving repeated severe seizure activity over time, but also as a result of side effects or toxicity from medication and other acquired brain impairment.

When beginning vocational rehabilitation services, the counselor should carefully evaluate the client's financial needs. Those on federal subsidy such as Supplementary Security Income (SSI) or Social Security Disability Income (SSDI), may need to seek part-time work instead of full time work to avoid jeopardizing their benefits. They may need to use either the Plan for Achieving Self-Support (PASS) or Impairment-Related Work Expenses (IRWE) work incentive programs to establish capacity for self-support.

For people with epilepsy, ability to drive is often affected. In most states, a specific seizure-free period must occur. If driving is not possible, access to public transportation is crucial.

Job Development and Placement
Service Methodology

Interpretation of assessment data and individual counseling is helpful. The philosophy of the National Epilepsy Foundation vocational programs is that of shared responsibility between employment services staff and clients. The philosophical emphasis is on personal empowerment and independence.

Most clients benefit from job-seeking skills training provided within a job club format. The job club setting provides emotional support and encouragement in addition to teaching basic skills and ongoing organization of job search activities. Reinforcing information from individual counseling sessions within the group setting helps assure that clients retain information (Miller & Rollnick, 2013).

Disclosure and Accommodation

The issue of whether to disclose epilepsy to a potential employer is a topic for discussion within the job club setting. Although an individual may have a seizure condition that does not affect job performance, the majority of clients with epilepsy prefer to disclose their condition to perspective employers. Job seekers with seizure conditions have a responsibility to consider various work-related factors. These include type of seizure, frequency of occurrence, and risks associated with specific job duties. A related issue is whether the person experiences an aura or warning before a seizure occurs. For some with no significant safety issues in the workplace, disclosure is less of a concern (Bishop, 2004).

People with frequent seizures occurring during the workday need to discuss their epilepsy with prospective employers. Some individuals have decided not to disclose their seizure condition on the job application but discuss it during the interview process. This enables them to describe their skills and aptitudes in relation to the job before mentioning their seizure status. Other individuals decide to disclose epilepsy immediately upon receipt of a job offer or after being hired. There is no one strategy that is appropriate for all (Fraser et al., 2011b). The ADA Amendments Act of 2008 states that employers cannot discriminate because of a person's disability. If the seizure disorder does not affect job performance, the job seeker can choose not to disclose.

Applicants should be capable of discussing their seizure conditions clearly, positively, and succinctly, in terms that are understood by the layperson, keeping the information brief and job-related. For example, people who have absence seizures may describe periods lasting a few seconds in which they may look distracted. Following the seizure, they are able to resume work quickly. A job seeker with a seizure condition needs to practice disclosure to present information comfortably and clearly to prospective employers (Saunders, Leahy, McGlynn, & Estrada-Hernandez, 2006). A successful placement program includes active job development and a job bank from interested companies with integration of employers on an advisory board.

Interacting with Employers

Information can be presented to the employer to affect positive hiring (Fraser et al., 2011a; Miller & Rollnick, 2013). The following considerations can guide the vocational counselor and prospective job candidate.

Work and Job Performance

With today's safety standards, it is rare that machinery will require special modifications for people with epilepsy. Plastic guards on hazardous machinery or rubber matting on a concrete floor are examples of inexpensive jobsite modifications. In other cases, assigning driving tasks to a different worker produces simple job restructuring. Both jobsite modifications and job restructuring are examples of reasonable accommodations. Most studies suggest attendance and performance records for those with epilepsy are equal to or better than the general working population (McLellan, 1987).

Accident Rates

Risch (1968) demonstrated the actual time lost due to seizures was approximately one hour for every 1,000 hours worked for individuals with active seizure conditions. According to research completed by Sands (1961), when comparing workers' compensation cases over a 13-year period in New York, accidents caused by sneezing or coughing on the job were twice as frequent as those related to seizure occurrences.

Insurance Rates

Hiring a person with epilepsy does not increase industrial insurance rates. These rates are linked to hazards of specific occupational classifications. Health insurance providers generally link rates to age and gender in larger companies, while among smaller companies the providers usually pool claim experiences and no one employer is penalized. Epi-Hab, an earlier sheltered work system for those with seizure disorders, reported receiving significant insurance premium reductions due to outstanding safety records

(Risch, 1968). People with epilepsy generally refrain from drinking alcohol or using illegal drugs since these aggravate their conditions. Thus, they are often safer on the job than typical employees.

Predictors of Successful Placement

Factors that influence successful vocational rehabilitation can be considered across different categories: demographic, neuropsychological, and psychosocial. The National Epilepsy Foundation has found that individuals with less than one seizure per month, 12 years of education, no additional disabilities, and the capacity to drive, are more successful. Other factors associated with employment outcome include the recency and substantiveness of employment (months employed pre-program) before program entry, previous salary earned, and compliance with an anticonvulsant medicine regimen.

Existing Programs

The Rehabilitation Services Administration (RSA) has always advocated for and supported vocational rehabilitation on a national level for clients with epilepsy. Some state-funded vocational rehabilitation programs will assign clients with epilepsy to specialized counselors with particular expertise. Rehabilitation counselors seeking additional information can contact the National Epilepsy Foundation as to local resources (www.epilepsyfoundation.org), or for legal advocacy assistance relating to employment.

Intervention spans a wide range in epilepsy vocational rehabilitation. Some clients with clear goals, adequate training and experience, and well controlled seizures may need simple advisement, while others require vocational and neuropsychological evaluation, situational assessment, job placement, and even jobsite support.

Case Study

Roger is a 28-year-old Latino male with partial complex seizures. He is the only child in a traditional rural Mexican-American family. His family tends to be over-protective of Roger because of his seizures. Since his late teens, Roger's general practitioner has been treating him with Phenobarbital; yet, adequate seizure control has never been achieved. He seeks vocational rehabilitation services while still recovering from third degree burns (deep partial-thickness burns) he sustained while working as a sous chef in a neighborhood restaurant. This is the second burn he has experienced while at work. Roger explains that his seizure condition is disconcerting, but he has *more or less* become accustomed to it. Seizures occur once every two to three months.

This individual is a high school graduate with one semester of college. Results of aptitude testing suggest he has superior intelligence. He has an interest in engineering and completed several years of architectural drafting coursework while in high school. Due to lack of funding, Roger states he was unable to continue his college education.

Presently, Roger is unsure what to do. He is financially compromised and must leave the rental home he shares with roommates to move back with his family. There are no vocational plans and Roger describes minimal social involvement within his community. An avid user of his home computer and the internet, Roger believes he has developed expertise in this area.

Questions

1. What do we need to know about Roger's seizure type?
2. What are the issues related to his current medication and medical care? What should the referral sequence be to optimize his care?
3. Is Roger a possible candidate for epilepsy surgery? Explain.
4. Should this client attempt to return to his job at the restaurant? Support your response.
5. What are the potential vocational rehabilitation counseling issues related to Roger's situation?
6. Identify community resources that may be helpful to this individual's psychosocial well-being.
7. Describe cultural considerations relevant to this case and implications of the family's overprotective approach to this individual's epilepsy.

References

Batzel, L. W., Dodrill, C. B., & Fraser, R. T. (1980). Further validation of the WPSI Vocational Scale: Comparisons with other correlates of employment in epilepsy. *Epilepsia, 21*, 35–42.

Berg, A. T., Berkovic, S. F., Brodie, M. J., Buchhalter, J., Cross, J. H., van Emde Boas, W., . . . Scheffer, I. E. (2010). Revised terminology and concepts for organization of seizures and epilepsies: Report of the ILAE Commission on Classification and Terminology, 2005-2009. *Epilepsia, 51*, 676–685.

Bishop, M. (2004). Determinants of employment status among a community-based sample of people with epilepsy: Implications for rehabilitation interventions. *Rehabilitation Counseling Bulletin, 47*(2), 112–122.

Brodie, M. J., & Kwan, P. (2002). Staged approach to epilepsy management. *Neurology, 58*(Suppl. 5), 52–58.

de Souza, E. A. P., & Salgado, P. C. B. (2006). A psychosocial view of anxiety and depression in epilepsy. *Epilepsy & Behavior, 8*, 232–238.

Deray, M., Resnick, T., & Alvarez, L. (2004). *Complete pocket reference for the treatment of epilepsy*. Miami, FL: CPR Educational Services.

Devinsky, O. (2008). *Epilepsy: Patient and family guide* (3rd ed.). Philadelphia, PA: F. A. Davis.

DiIorio, C., Escoffery, C., McCarty, F., Yeager, K. A., Henry, T. R., & Koganti, A. (2009a). Evaluation of WebEase: An epilepsy self-management Web site. *Health Education Research, 24*, 185–197.

DiIorio, C., Escoffery, C., Yeager, K. A., McCarty, F., Henry, T. R., & Koganti, A. (2009b). WebEase: Development of a web-based epilepsy self-management intervention. *Preventing Chronic Disease: Public Health Research, Practice, and Policy, 6*, 1–7.

Dodrill, C. B. (1978). A neuropsychological battery for epilepsy. *Epilepsy, 19*, 611–623.

Dodrill, C. B., Batzel, L. W., Queisser, H. R., & Temkin, N. R. (1980). An objective method for the assessment of psychological and social problems among epileptics. *Epilepsia, 21*, 123–135.

Fisher, R. S., Boas, W. V. E., Blume, W., Elger, C., Genton, P., Lee, P., & Engel, J. (2005). Epileptic seizures and epilepsy: Definitions proposed by the International League Against Epilepsy (ILAE) and the International Bureau for Epilepsy (IBE). *Epilepsia, 46*, 470–472.

Fraser, R. T., Johnson, E. K., Miller, J. W., Temkin, N., Barber, J., & Caylor, L. (2011a). Managing epilepsy well: Self-management needs assessment. *Epilepsy & Behavior, 20*, 291–98.

Fraser, R. T., Miller, J. W., & Johnson, E. K. (2011b). Epilepsy. In S. R. Flanagan, H. H. Zaretsky, & A. Moroz (Eds.), *Medical aspects of disability: A handbook for the rehabilitation professional* (4th ed., pp. 177–194). New York, NY: Springer.

Fraser, R. T., Trejo, W., Clemmons, D. C., & Freelove, C. (1987, November). *Psychosocial adjustment of early dropouts compared to competitive placements*. Paper presented at the annual meeting of the American Epilepsy Society, San Francisco, CA.

Hermann, B. P., Seidenberg, M., Dow, C., Jones, J., Rutecki, P., & Bhattacharya, E. (2006). Cognitive prognosis in chronic temporal lobe epilepsy. *Annals of Neurology, 60*, 80–87.

Johnson, E. K., Fraser, R. T., Miller, J. W., Temkin, N., Barber, J., & Caylor, L. (2012). A comparison of self-management needs: Provider and patient perspectives. *Epilepsy and Behavior, 25*, 150–155.

Leppik, I. E. (2006). *Contemporary diagnosis and management of the patient with epilepsy* (6th ed.). Newtown, PA: Handbooks in Health Care.

Lorig, K. R., Ritter, P. L., Laurent, D. D., & Plant, K. (2006). Internet-based chronic disease self-management: A randomized trial. *Medical Care, 44*, 964–971.

McLellan, D. L. (1987). Epilepsy and employment. *Journal of Social and Occupational Medicine, 3*, 94–99.

Miller, L., & Rollnick, S. (2013). *Motivational interviewing: Helping people change* (3rd ed.). New York, NY: Guilford.

National Association of Epilepsy Centers. (2010). *Guidelines for essential services, personnel, and facilities in epilepsy centers*. Minneapolis, MN: Author.

Nilsson, L., Ahlbom, A., Farahmand, B.Y., Asberg, M., & Tomson, T. (2002). Risk factors for suicide in epilepsy: A case control study. *Epilepsia, 43,* 644–651.

Oyegbile, T. O., Dow, C., Jones, J., Bell, B., Rutecki, P., & Sheth, R. (2004). The nature and course of neuropsychological morbidity in chronic temporal lobe epilepsy. *Neurology, 62,* 1736–1742.

Pellock, J. M., Bourgeois, B. F. D., & Dodson, W. E. (Eds.). (2008). *Pediatric epilepsy: Diagnosis and therapy* (3rd ed.). New York, NY: Demos Medical.

Rausch, R., Le, M. T., & Langfitt, J. L. (1997). Neuropsychological evaluation: Adults. In J. Engel & T. A. Pedley (Eds.), *Epilepsy.* Philadelphia, PA: Lippincott-Raven.

Risch, F. (1968). We lost every game . . . but. *Rehabilitation Record, 9,* 16–18.

Rodenburg, R., Wagner, J. L., Austin, J. K., Kerr, M., & Dunn, D. W. (2011). Psychosocial issues for children with epilepsy. *Epilepsy & Behavior, 22,* 47–54.

Sands, H. (1961). Report of a study undertaken for the Committee on Neurological Disorders in Industry. *Epilepsy News, 7*(abstract), 1.

Saunders, J. L., Leahy, M. J., McGlynn, C., & Estrada-Hernandez, N. (2006). Predictors of employment outcomes for persons with disabilities: An integrative review of potential evidence-based factors. *Journal of Applied Rehabilitation Counseling, 37*(2), 3–20.

Schaul, N. (1987). Epilepsy surgery. *New York Journal of Epilepsy, 5,* 14–15.

Sillanpää, M., & Schmidt, D. (2006). Natural history of treated childhood-onset epilepsy: Prospective, long-term population-based study. *Brain, 129*(3), 617–624.

Wiebe, S. (2012). The epilepsies. In L. Goldman & A. I. Schafer (Eds.), *Goldman's Cecil medicine* (24th ed., pp. 2283–2294). New York, NY: Elsevier Saunders.

About the Authors

Robert T. Fraser, Ph.D., C.R.C., is Professor within the University of Washington, Department of Neurology, a joint appointment with Neurological Surgery and Rehabilitation Medicine in Seattle, Washington. Dr. Fraser began the Vocational Services Unit of the University of Washington Regional Epilepsy Center in 1976, which has expanded to provide vocational services for the Department of Neurology.

John W. Miller, M.D., Ph.D., is Professor of Neurology and Neurological Surgery at the University of Washington. He has been Director of the University of Washington Regional Epilepsy Center at Harborview Medical Center in Seattle, Washington since 1999. Previously, he was Director of the Washington University Comprehensive Epilepsy Center in St. Louis, Missouri.

Erica K. Johnson, Ph.D., C.R.C, is Senior Instructor and Clinical Director at Western Washington University, Department of Human Services and Rehabilitation Counseling, and Research Consultant at the University of Washington Health Promotion Research Center since 2008. Dr. Johnson has been a practitioner and researcher in the areas of vocational rehabilitation counseling, rehabilitation and neuropsychology, and neurological disabilities since 1993.

Chapter 15

NEUROLOGICAL DIAGNOSES

David B. Peterson, Ph.D., C.R.C.
Thomas VanVleet, Ph.D.

Introduction

Neurology is a specialty of medicine concerned with the study and treatment of the nervous system and related disorders. The practice of neurology requires specialized knowledge of anatomy and physiology of the nervous system, and familiarity with many diseases encountered in general medicine. Neurologists may partner with other professionals, such as neuropsychologists, who are experts in evaluating brain-behavior relationships. Through a wide array of assessment techniques, neuropsychologists interpret the brain's myriad processes of thought, memory, judgment, decision-making or *goal-directed behavior,* and motor function (Lezak, Howieson, Bigler, & Tranel, 2012). This chapter provides a general orientation and overview of a very complex topic. The complexities of the neurological system challenge the expertise of the most experienced health professionals. Thus, consultation with neurologists, neuropsychologists, or other related health professionals is recommended. While there are many aspects of brain functioning that are not well understood, considerable advances have occurred in recent years, and there is a growing confidence among neuroscientists that "a real understanding is beginning to emerge" (Beaumont, 2008, p. 3).

This chapter familiarizes rehabilitation counselors with basic aspects of the neurological examination and frequently diagnosed neurological illnesses and conditions. It is not intended to be an all-inclusive discussion of neurology. Standard textbooks are referenced for in-depth inquiry (Beaumont, 2008; Brust, 2011; Greenberg, Aminoff, & Simon, 2014; Hauser & Josephson, 2013; Lezak et al., 2012; Ropper, Samuels, & Klein, 2014).

Neurological Examination

Individuals with complaints suggesting disease of a neurological origin (e.g., headaches, motor weakness, pain, sensory disturbance, vertigo, and difficulties in cognition and speech) seek help from their treating physicians. After a preliminary evaluation, the family practitioner may refer the patient to a neurologist for further evaluation. The neurologist attempts to determine the source of the abnormality within the nervous system and assesses possible etiology. Causes or origins of the problem may include trauma, tumor, immunological response, stroke, inherited dysfunction, or any of a great number of other disease processes. Based on the evaluation, history of the illness, and specialized testing, the neurologist establishes a specific diagnosis (Biller, Gruener, & Brazis, 2011; Papadakis, McPhee, & Rabow, 2014).

The neurologist begins the examination by obtaining a thorough medical history. A neurological evaluation is made that includes a systematic examination of mental status, cranial nerves, gait and station, cerebellum, and motor and sensory function. Based upon the data, the neurologist may order laboratory tests, imaging procedures, or neuropsychological testing.

Mental Status

The mental status examination evaluates the patient's orientation (e.g., time, place), short-term memory, reasoning, comprehension and communication, and problem solving ability. It reveals gross abnormalities of mental functioning, including difficulties in speech. When dysfunction exists, return to typical functioning is dependent on the cause or course of the dysfunction and may improve, worsen, or remain unchanged over time. During acute, subacute, and post acute recovery, neuropsychological testing is used to further monitor treatment progress; once the condition is stable, additional testing is used to estimate the individual's extant functional capacity (Lezak et al., 2012).

Cranial Nerves

Examination of cranial nerves involves evaluation of the nerves that attend the areas of the face, including sense of smell, vision, eye movement, face movement, and sensation. Of particular importance are visual disturbances and disturbances in the motoric aspects of speech (dysarthria).

A frequently encountered neurological finding from an examination of the eyes is *homonymous hemianopia*. In this condition, a portion of the visual field becomes blind (i.e., nasal half of the field of vision of one eye and the temporal half of the other or right-sided or left-sided blindness of the corresponding sides in both eyes). In either situation, there is blindness in one half of each eye with vision unaffected in the other half of each eye (Brust, 2011). This condition may result from damage to the cranial nerve or primary occipital cortex.

With abnormalities of the facial nerve, there are disturbances of facial movements that may cause difficulties in articulation (e.g., poor pronunciation or slurred speech) and produce a functional limitation in speech (*dysarthria*).

Gait and Station

Disorders of gait and station include disturbances of walking, such as *ataxia* or gross incoordination of muscle movements, spasticity, or *steppage gait* (i.e., high-stepping gait so that the toe clears the ground). Gait disturbance causes limitations in the ability to walk, particularly for long distances. If a significant gait disturbance is present, vocational rehabilitation needs to be directed toward work involving limited ambulation (e.g., sedentary work).

Cerebellar Function

The cerebellum controls movement and coordination. Damage to the cerebellum may manifest as jerky movements, intention tremors (tremors only during deliberate movement), and loss of balance and proprioception (position sense), especially with the eyes closed (Beaumont, 2008). Damage to the posterior cerebellum may also result in impairment of executive functions such as planning, set-shifting, verbal fluency, abstract reasoning, and working memory; difficulties with spatial cognition including visual-spatial organization and memory; personality change with blunting of affect or disinhibited and inappropriate behavior; and language deficits including agrammatism and dysprosodia (Schmahmann & Sherman, 1998)

Motor and Sensory Function

During the motor and sensory function evaluation, the neurologist systematically tests reflexes and muscle tone in each group of muscles. For example, the neurologist often uses a nylon monofilament or a vibrating instrument to examine sensory response. *Proprioception*, or the ability to tell where a finger or toe is in relation to the rest of the body, is also queried.

The motor system consists of upper motor neurons (nerve connections from the central nervous system to the spinal cord) and lower motor neurons (nerve connections from the spinal cord to muscle fibers in the periphery). Upper motor neuron dysfunction occurs in illnesses involving the cortex and brain stem. This often produces abnormalities involving at least one limb or one-half of the body. There is a characteristic loss of strength, increase in reflexes (hyperflexia), and spasticity associated with these disorders (Greenberg et al., 2014). Lower motor neuron diseases involve the nerve roots, peripheral nerves, or both. They cause a smaller area of deficit that affects a specific group of muscles, resulting in abnormal muscle functioning. Characteristically, there is muscle weakness, lack of muscular tone (hypotonicity), and loss of reflexes (areflexia). The sensory system has central and peripheral nervous system components. In disease within the peripheral nervous system, a small area of the skin may show decreased sensation corresponding with abnormality of the specific nerve or nerve root that supplies that given skin area (Brust, 2011).

Electrophysiology

Electroencephalogram (EEG)

Neurologists or other physicians may request an electrophysiological test called the electroencephalogram (EEG). An EEG involves the use of electrodes placed on the scalp to provide amplification and summation of regional brain activity. This information is used to explore suspected pathological processes, particularly seizure disorders.

Electromyography (EMG)

Another physiological test employed in neurology is **electromyography** (EMG), which involves the insertion of small needles into various muscles to amplify the electrical activity inherent in those muscles. EMG examination reveals abnormalities suggestive of muscle or nerve disease. This procedure aids in diagnosis and location of potential disturbances of a particular nerve, nerve root (radiculopathy), or muscle (myopathy). A **nerve conduction study** is a test that delivers small electric shocks via electrodes placed on the skin. Electrical stimulation is then followed as it travels along the nerve. Motor and sensory nerve fibers are tested and is most useful for identifying mononeuropathy (e.g., carpal tunnel syndrome) and peripheral neuropathy.

Neuroimaging Techniques

Advances in neuroimaging technology have allowed physicians to construct detailed visualizations of brain structures and vasculature, blood flow and related metabolic activity, and basic neurochemical composition. Neuropsychological assessments are used in combination with these technologies to help identify impairment and residual functioning.

Computerized Tomography (CT)

Cross-sectional images of the brain and spinal cord are captured via neuroimaging techniques such as computerized tomography (CT) or computerized axial tomography (CAT) scans. These scans employ x-rays directed from different angles through the brain to the x-ray film on the other side. Many images are combined by computational methods to provide a gross overview of brain areas. Relatively inexpensive and widely available, it has limited ability to image abnormalities, and has lower resolution relative to other methods (e.g., magnetic resonance imaging, MRI), but tends to be a first-line of inquiry before more advanced and expensive imaging techniques (Longo et al., 2011).

Magnetic Resonance Imaging (MRI)

An MRI creates a more precise image of the brain (i.e., higher resolution) by using a powerful magnetic field in which radio waves are used to align the nuclear magnetization of hydrogen atoms. This process allows for greater contrast between soft tissues of the body than CT scans. MRI provides a high resolution, three-dimensional image of the brain. Recent advances in MRI technology enable mapping of the connections between brain areas (white matter) and is referred to as diffusion tensor imaging (DTI).

Functional MRI (fMRI)

Functional MRI (fMRI) goes a step beyond showing clear structures of the brain to illustrating brain function. fMRI detects neuronal activity through the *haemodynamic response*, which is associated with the concentration of oxygen in the blood. fMRI is used to determine which brain areas are most active during a particular cognitive operation; images taken seconds apart can suggest dynamic brain function in association with different cognitive processes. Brain images taken during various stages of a cognitive process are later compared to suggest areas of the brain associated with specific tasks or functions. Recent advances in fMRI have led to the examination of *patterns of connectivity* between related brain areas or *brain networks*, and can be acquired while the patient is resting in the MRI scanner (i.e., *resting state functional connectivity*) (Grefkes & Fink, 2011).

Positron Emission Tomography (PET)

Positron emission tomography scans can also image brain function, but at a much slower pace than the fMRI. This technique uses a positron-emitting radionuclide (tracer) to detect regions of greater activity. Further, PET scans may be employed to determine the relative distribution of neurotransmitters (chemical messengers) in the brain. A related technique that allows the construction of three-dimensional images from two-dimensional images based on gamma ray technology is the single-photon emission computed tomography (SPECT).

Abnormalities of the Brain

Clinical data suggest specific behaviors associated with areas of the brain and understanding of these relationships is evolving with advances in neuroscience (Beaumont, 2008; Lezak et al., 2012). Historically, there has been an inherent difficulty in building a sound scientific basis in this area of inquiry. Lesions could not ethically be introduced into the human brain; researchers have to make the best use of the clinical data available to them in the normal course of healthcare. Recent advances in functional neuroimaging have allowed neuroscientists to test hypotheses in the healthy brain regarding the role of discreet function areas and their associated networks across cognitive domains. Neuroscientists have also begun to use a *virtual lesion* technique known as Transcranial Magnetic Stimulation (TMS), whereby an innocuous magnetic field is applied to the scalp temporarily disrupting function of the underlying brain area. Historically, clinical cases and data from advanced neuroscientific methods have provided converging evidence to elucidate the function of many brain areas (Hallett, 2000). However, most cognitive operations are not performed by any single area of the brain. While elementary operations forming the basis of cognition may be localized to discreet brain areas, many such local operations are involved in any given cognitive task. Thus, a set of distributed brain areas must be evaluated in the performance of even simple cognitive tasks (Brust, 2011).

Subcortical Structures

Much of what is known about deep subcortical brain function was learned from animal research models. Clinical studies of humans with damage to deep subcortical structures are difficult, as major functional impairments of consciousness and/or basic drives are typically present. Damage to the brain stem, mesencephalon, and the diencephalon can be catastrophic. A notable exception is research examining the role of the thalamus and basal ganglia; together with frontal and parietal cortex, these areas form a number of interconnected cortical-subcortical circuits involved in such diverse cognitive operations as response selection, learning, attention, and routine motor operations (Alexander, DeLong, & Strick, 1986).

Frontal Lobes

Functioning associated with the frontal lobes includes a broad variety of behaviors with a central function related to the management of goal-directed behavior (i.e., executive functions). The frontal lobes have also been associated with the ability to think abstractly; the ability to form and change mental sets; consider different aspects of a situation; take apart and put together (synthesize) the elements of an object or idea; and plan, monitor, and correct on-going goal-directed behaviors. These functions are essential to independent living and work; damage to the frontal lobes can impair these abilities with dramatic consequences. Severe frontal lobe damage can cause dull emotional affect and lack of initiative and spontaneity. Other frontal lobe-related abnormalities include poor self-monitoring (e.g., inattention to personal hygiene) and socially inappropriate and impulsive behavior. These symptoms have been associated with a frontal lobe syndrome that is quite debilitating and may require substantial and long-term care (Beaumont, 2008; Longo et al., 2011).

Four frontal lobe sections are associated with different functional limitations to injury, beginning from the top of the head and moving down toward the eye orbits. These are the motor and pre-motor cortex, prefrontal cortex, Broca's area, and orbital cortex. Damage to the motor cortex may result in loss of voluntary control over specific parts of the body and possibly fine-motor control (e.g., movements of the hands, fingers, face). Lesions in the pre-motor cortex result in difficulty with coordinating gross body reflexes and movements, verbal and design fluency, and spelling. Lesions in the prefrontal cortex may affect planning and programming of sequences of behavior, problem-solving, perceptual judgment, memory, and attention. The relationship among these regions parallels the primary, secondary, and tertiary cortex relationships described earlier (Beaumont, 2008).

Located in the left frontal lobe, Broca's area, when damaged, can result in impairment of expressive communication (see also receptive speech as it relates to the temporal lobe discussion below). Finally, the orbital cortex region of the frontal lobes relates to aspects of personality and social behavior. Motor vehicle accidents causing bilateral damage to the orbital cortex can result in dramatic personality changes, problems with anger management, and inappropriate social behavior.

Parietal Lobes

Abnormalities of the parietal lobes result in a wide range of symptoms, from misperception of sensory events, loss of or deficits related to attention, and problems with navigation or mapping of the body in relationship to the environment. Lesions in the parietal lobes can result in contralateral (side opposite a lesion) or ipsilateral (same-side) loss or alteration of sensation for parts of the body. The loss or change may be total or may only involve a single feature of sensation, such as touch, pressure, temperature, or pain. In addition to sensations perceived by the skin, damage to the parietal lobes may affect ability to perceive information about body position and movement. Parietal lesions may cause apraxia (loss of intentional movement) (Beaumont, 2008; Ropper et al., 2014).

Disease of the left parietal lobe produce problems with language functions, including reading (dyslexia) and writing (alexia). It can cause difficulty with recognizing objects both visually and through the sense of touch (visual or tactile agnosia). Diseases of the right parietal lobe cause difficulty with mathematical calculations (acalculia), as spatial representation is helpful in solving more complex math problems.

Spatial neglect is a parietal lobe condition associated with failure to pay attention to a particular area of space, typically the half of space opposite the parietal lesion. Most often persistent symptoms of neglect occur following damage to the right parietal lobe. Patients who have spatial neglect may present with scratching and bruising on the side of the body opposite the lesion due to bumping into things on that side. They may shave only one side of the face or forget to completely dress one side of the body.

Temporal Lobes

Damage to the temporal lobes impact all aspects of auditory perception; traumatic brain injuries that lead to skull fracture and associated damage in the temporal region cause hearing loss or deafness. The temporal lobes impact some aspects of visual perception (given its connections with the occipital lobes). Reception and comprehension of language is associated with Wernike's area, in the left hemisphere, at the junction of the temporal, parietal, and occipital lobes. Damage to Wernike's area produces receptive or Wernicke's aphasia, compromising the ability to receive and comprehend written and spoken language. Lesions in the right temporal lobe cause difficulty with musical ability. The temporal lobes also influence affective, emotional, and personal experience, having close physical connections with the limbic system described earlier. Damage to these structures produce personality changes, psychosis, and changes in sexual behavior (Beaumont, 2008).

The temporal lobes, along with some subcortical structures are involved in encoding and retrieving long-term memory. Typically, lesions in the left temporal lobe impact verbal memory, while lesions in the right temporal lobe impact spatial memory. Korsakoff's disease and Wernike-Korsakoff syndrome are bilateral diseases of the temporal lobes that create difficulty with retaining new information, or cause anterograde amnesia. Korsakoff's disease is caused by thiamine deficiency often brought about by chronic alcoholism or infection. Wernike-Korsakoff syndrome is caused by a diffuse disease of the brain called Wernike's encephalopathy (Beaumont, 2008).

Occipital Lobes

Abnormalities of the occipital lobes affect elementary aspects of visual sensation and perception. Homonymous hemianopsia, visual distortions, and blindness result from lesions in either occipital lobe. Disease of both lobes cause cortical blindness where the pupils remain reactive, but the individual cannot see or react to visual stimuli, called Anton's syndrome, which may include a lack of awareness of the deficit. Smaller areas of damage cause gaps in vision (scotomas). Sometimes, the entire visual field is affected except for the very center or macular region of vision (Beaumont, 2008; Lezak et al., 2012).

Disorders of the Central Nervous System

Disorders of the central nervous system (CNS) are diverse and complex. Disorders reviewed elsewhere is this text include traumatic brain injury, spinal cord injury, multiple sclerosis, intellectual disability, cerebral palsy, and epilepsy. A few remaining disorders of the central nervous system are reviewed here, including dementias, aphasias, Parkinson's disease, Huntington's disease, and motor neuron disease.

Dementias

Dementias involve the decline of general cognitive ability, particularly memory and executive function typically in older adulthood. They can be degenerative or nondegenerative.

Nondegenerative Dementias

Nondegenerative dementias have a number of causes, including infection, chronic drug or alcohol abuse, cerebrovascular accidents (strokes), and autoimmune disease (e.g., lupus). Various types of infection affect the CNS. Patterns of infection include a focal inflammation site (cerebritis) or abscess, most frequently bacterial in origin. Bacterial and viral inflammations of the meninges (membranes enveloping the brain and spinal cord) cause meningitis. Meningoencephalitis, usually viral in origin, affects the brain and meninges. Most CNS infections result in residual deficits, such as personality change, sleep disturbance, decreased cognition, and seizures. When complications occur, damage to cranial nerves and brain tissue result in permanent deficits.

Hardening of the arteries (arteriosclerosis) and hypertension (high blood pressure) are disorders which predispose an individual to arterial vessel abnormalities that may result in a rupture causing a cerebrovascular accident (CVA). Functional impairment depends upon the location and size of the area affected. Depending on the type of vascular compromise, strokes can produce either focal or diffuse brain damage. Based on severity, CVAs result in loss or diminished use of one side of the body due to paralysis (hemiplegia). Speech disturbance often occurs with damage to the dominant hemisphere of the brain (see Aphasias). Even in mild cases, many individuals have loss of stamina and incoordination on the affected side (hemiparesis). Improvement after stroke occurs over three to six months. Once stabilized, individuals with CVA benefit from rehabilitation evaluation, beginning with an assessment of functional limitations and capabilities, both physical and psychological.

A variety of chemicals and drugs affect the CNS. These substances cause a multiplicity of effects and reactions. Abnormalities include cognitive and behavioral deficits, seizures, and peripheral neuropathies. Predictable effects related to drug (both legal and illegal) intoxication and idiosyncratic reactions to medication are two areas related to drug and chemical effects on the nervous system. Predictable effects are linked to drug dosage. Idiosyncratic reactions are peculiar to an individual and are unpredictable and unrelated to the amount of drug taken. Cocaine, for instance, can cause a CNS vasculitis (inflammation of the vessels) that leads to small strokes. These people generally have diffuse brain involvement, and may have decreased cognition and deteriorated intellectual functioning. Chronic alcohol abuse causes several specific neurological problems such as peripheral neuropathy, cerebellar degeneration, and alcohol-related dementia. With abstinence, improved nutrition, and rehabilitation, these are partially reversible (Ropper et al., 2014)

Degenerative Dementias

Degenerative dementias are caused by the death of neurons essential to the CNS. Alzheimer's disease (AD) is classified within this category. The hippocampus, a structure critical to memory, is often the first impacted by AD, which undergoes marked atrophy. Found first in the hippocampus, neurofibrillary tangles spread throughout the brain as the disease progresses. Senile plaques are also associated with AD, but their correlation with cognitive impairment is weaker than with the neurofibrillary tangles.

There is an early onset of AD (5-10% of cases) affecting people ages 28 to 60 years. People with Down Syndrome are more susceptible to AD due to its relationship with chromosome 21. Dementias are not specifically treatable but medication may slow progression.

The presence of a brain tumor often denotes a poor prognosis with progressive deterioration. Brain tumors include primary tumors (arising directly from brain cells) and metastatic tumors (spreading from a tumor elsewhere in the body). The brain is affected in approximately 20% of cancer cases. Once the brain is affected, prognosis is extremely poor and death follows rapidly, often within several months of diagnosis. Metastatic disease comprises the largest percentage of brain tumors; primary brain tumors are less common. Generally, brain tumors grow and cause local destruction within the brain. The rate of growth is variable, at times very rapidly with death ensuing after several months, or sometimes more slowly with the person living several years. For individuals with brain tumors, attempts at continuing current employment may be appropriate, depending on the symptoms, deficits, and rate of tumor growth. Occasionally, very slow growing tumors are found in younger people. In these cases, the counselor should obtain information from the treating physician regarding prognosis (Longo et al., 2011).

Aphasias

Language function can be associated with focal areas of the cortex; advances in neuroscience suggest that language functioning spreads across a large area of the cortex (Beaumont, 2008). For right-handed people, a significant portion of language functioning is in the left hemisphere. In the case of left-handed people, very few actually have right (contralateral) hemisphere dominance in language; most have the same brain functioning as right-handed people, and a smaller percentage have bilateral representation of language functioning (Carter, Hohenegger, & Satz, 1980). In either case, disorders of the language system are called aphasias. Classification of aphasias is "one of the most hotly contested issues in the history of neuropsychology, and there is yet no firm agreement" (Beaumont, 2008, p. 136). The most widely accepted paradigm divides aphasias into several categories. *Global aphasia* involves massive and severe disturbance in language functioning. Some of these also involve *alexia* (a specific disorder of reading) and *agraphia* (a specific disorder of writing). In almost all aphasias, singing, producing simple automatic phrases, and swearing are often preserved.

Broca's aphasia (expressive aphasia) manifests as impaired ability to express oneself verbally. Speech may omit articles, adverbs, and adjectives, or in more extreme cases muteness occurs. Prompting with sounds or contexts assists people with less severe forms of the disorder; some may not realize their problem. Difficulties occur while language comprehension is unimpaired, where people understand what is being said and can read. Broca's area was described above as one of the language centers of the brain, located typically in the left rear frontal lobe.

Wenicke's aphasia (receptive aphasia) is characterized by a severe deficit in auditory comprehension. Impaired reading and writing often accompany it, and while most individuals are capable of expressive speech, because of the comprehension deficit that impairs self-monitoring of speech production, speech may contain substituted but related words or sounds, resulting in a *word salad* that is not always intelligible. Wernike's area is located in the left temporal lobe.

With **conduction aphasia**, people comprehend both speech and writing and produce nearly-normal speech, but at times substitute one sound for another (*phonemic paraphasia*). For example, one might substitute *fable* for *table*. Severe impairment may be noted when the person is asked to repeat a phrase that is spoken or while reading aloud. It has been hypothesized that this type of aphasia results from problems with communication between Broca's and Wernike's areas.

The most common form of aphasia is **anomic aphasia**, which may exist in residual form while one recovers from other types of aphasia. The key element is difficulty with name finding, especially for nouns. Those recovering from it may substitute related words as a means of coping with the difficulty, so it may go undetected in spontaneous speech.

The last two types of aphasia reviewed here are **transcortical motor** and **sensory aphasias**. In the worst case of combined motor and sensory aphasia (which is very rare), the person cannot understand speech or read, is totally nonfluent in speech, speaks only when spoken to, and usually cannot write. Strangely enough, the person can repeat what is heard, also referred to as *echolalic aphasia* (the person echoes back whatever is said). In *transcortical motor aphasia,* most evident is the impairment of speech output. In *trancortical sensory aphasia,* language reception is usually severely affected, while the ability to repeat is preserved, even though little is understood of what is repeated or read. These aphasias are referred to as transcortical because it is assumed that intact cortical language functions are not connecting with the underlying supporting structures (Brust, 2011).

Parkinson's Disease

Parkinson's disease (PD) is a degenerative disorder that results in the loss of neurons in subcortical structures that serve involuntary movement (e.g., basal ganglia, brain stem). Its major effects include loss of motor control and problems with initiation of motor operations (freezing). Medication and environmental toxins can produce Parkinsonism with symptoms similar to PD, but due to other factors. Symptoms of both involve tremor, slowness (bradykinesia) or rigidity in movement, a shuffling gait, loss of associated movements (e.g., arms moving as one walks), and loss of emotional expression. With PD, there may be specific or general psychological impairment, including difficulties with executive functioning, memory, and visual spatial skills. While the cause is not certain, treatment with dopaminergic drug therapy is helpful, suggesting a lack of dopamine as a cause (Brust, 2011; Pfeiffer, Wszolek, & Ebadi, 2012).

Huntington's Disease

Sometimes referred to as a subcortical dementia, Huntington's disease (HD) affects the integrity of the basal ganglia. Persons having either parent with HD have a 50% chance of inheriting it. HD is a neurodegenerative disorder that begins midlife with the onset of involuntary body movements. Dysarthria, difficulty with upper limb movements, abnormal gait, and progressive loss of mental functioning occurs, including disinhibition, depression, personality change, and even schizophrenia-like symptoms. Ultimately, problems with physical functioning lead to death within 15 to 20 years. There is no cure for HD; medications are used to treat symptoms (Quarrell, 2008).

Motor Neuron Disease

Amyotrophic lateral sclerosis (ALS), also known as Lou Gehrig's disease (a famous New York Yankees' baseball player) occurs on one side of the body and involves one arm and leg. It is a disease of the alpha motor neurons involving specific cells in the brain stem and spinal cord. This disease is degenerative, of unknown etiology, and rapidly progressive. There is loss of strength with hyperflexia and fasciculation (involuntary small movement of muscles). ALS is progressive and individuals eventually require wheelchairs for mobility. At times, the downhill progression is such that the person cannot eat or swallow within a year of initial onset (Papadakis et al., 2014).

Diseases of the Peripheral Nervous System

Peripheral nervous system (PNS) disease involves the nerves and nerve roots (neuropathies) and associated muscles. These diseases may be progressive or nonprogressive.

Diseases of the Muscle

Muscular Dystrophies

Muscular dystrophies are inherited or genetically determined illnesses involving a progressive weakening of muscles. Particular types are described based on the muscle groups involved; etiology is unknown. These diseases usually begin in childhood or in the teen years and are slowly progressive. Individuals with muscular dystrophy usually require sedentary work, either because of current limitations or future anticipated impairments. Because muscular dystrophy progresses, short-term goals need to be established; periodic reevaluation and modification of these goals is necessary. The more sedentary the work activity, the longer the individual will be physically able to maintain employment. Prescribed exercise is recommended as prolonged inactivity leads to worsening of the disease state. Maintaining activities and possible physical therapy during non-work hours is beneficial for most persons.

Primary Myopathies

These are a rare group of diseases with histological abnormalities involving muscle fiber or muscle cell mitochondria. They produce mild diffuse weakness and a decrease in stamina. The abnormalities are slowly progressive, although life expectancy is not significantly affected. No specific treatment is available. Individuals with primary myopathies do best in light and sedentary types of employment.

Neuropathies

Cranial Neuropathies

The 12 cranial nerves manifest their own specific symptomatology when involved in a disease process. Abnormalities involving eye and face movements present significant barriers to employment. Cranial nerves three, four, and six control eye movements. Abnormalities of these cranial nerves cause variations of eye movement, including diplopia (double vision). Often, the physician prescribes an eye patch for this condition, leaving the person monocular as long as the patch is worn. Seventh nerve (the facial nerve) abnormalities cause difficulty moving facial muscles and closing the eyes. Individuals with this problem need protective glasses and must avoid environments where particles of dust can irritate the eyes. Additionally, they may have some degree of dysarthria (difficult and defective speech). Eighth nerve or auditory nerve abnormalities are associated with hearing deficits and vertigo.

Radiculopathy

Radiculopathy refers to an abnormality of a nerve root that produces pain in the affected region of the spine. This is accompanied by limited motion of the spine, muscle spasm, and nerve root pain radiating down an extremity. Sensory and motor losses occur in the affected area. There are various causes for radiculopathy, including degenerative changes in the spine with the formation of bony osteophytes (outgrowths). A ruptured or bulging disc is also a frequent cause. Pain generally is experienced below the knee in lumbar radiculopathy.

Individuals with radiculopathies may require surgery to help alleviate symptoms, depending on pathology and severity of the condition. Work limitations for individuals with radiculopathy frequently involve limitation to light or sedentary work. Since many sedentary jobs involve extended sitting, workers may need accommodation allowing them to alternate positioning between sitting and standing. Frequency of change in position is dependent on an individual's tolerance for discomfort. Generally, it is beneficial to avoid either prolonged sitting or standing.

Back and neck pain are major employment problems in industrialized countries. Workers frequently have chronic back and neck pain complaints without objective findings. Often, there is an initial injury, possibly a strain, with ongoing complaints of severe pain. For rehabilitation purposes, one must distinguish between actual physical limitations and pain complaints. A thorough medication history should be obtained with particular attention to addicting or sedating drugs (Brust, 2011).

Peripheral Neuropathy

Peripheral neuropathy is a disease that can affect any of the nerves within the body. Frequently, peripheral neuropathy affects lower extremity nerves more than the nerves of the upper extremities. Weakness, sensory loss, and incoordination occur. There are multiple causes of peripheral neuropathy. Approximately one-third is due to systemic disease, such as diabetes. Another third of the cases are due to autoimmune inflammation. The final third have multiple causes, both inherited and degenerative.

Despite medical treatment, some mild residual symptoms may persist, with symptoms such as mild incoordination, weakness, diminished stamina, and decreased sensation in the extremities. These individuals require lighter types of employment that do not involve frequent use of fine coordination and manual dexterity. At the time of referral for rehabilitation, the level of dysfunction should be stable and not anticipated to change, thereby permitting the counselor to provide vocational rehabilitation services based on current limitations (Greenberg et al., 2014).

Mononeuropathy

Mononeuropathy involves injury or disease of a single nerve. This usually results from compression of a nerve in a specific area of the body (segmental mononeuropathy). The most frequently seen mononeuropathies involve the medial nerve of the wrist (carpal tunnel syndrome), ulnar nerve at the elbow (cubital tunnel syndrome), and peroneal nerve at the head of the fibula.

Carpal tunnel syndrome. This condition involves compression of the median nerve in the carpal tunnel of the wrist. It causes numbness and pain in the thumb, palm, and second through fourth fingers. The person may experience radiating pain and pain during the night. Repetitive wrist motion, sustained grip and pinch activities, continuous wrist angulation, poor posturing, repetitive vibration, and physical injury cause carpal tunnel syndrome. There is weakness in the affected hand and a loss of grip strength. Individuals with carpal tunnel syndrome need to avoid frequent pronation, supination, and extension of the wrist. Repetitive activities, such as using a screwdriver for long periods of time, operating a typewriter or computer terminal, need to be modified or avoided.

Ulnar neuropathy. Individuals with ulnar neuropathy have decreased strength in the muscles of the hand. There is weakness of grasp and frequently a decreased coordination of the hand. Sensory disturbance occurs in the fourth and fifth fingers. Usually, the nerve is injured at the elbow level; the individual should avoid activities where the elbow rests on a firm surface or in which minor trauma to the elbow occurs repetitively.

Peroneal neuropathy. In the lower extremity, peroneal neuropathy causes a foot drop. Thus, the person is not able to lift the foot against gravity and walks with a peculiar gait termed a steppage gait. Often a brace is used to maintain a $90°$ angle of the foot with the ankle. Individuals with peroneal neuropathies have difficulty walking and climbing stairs; they require sedentary work. Sensory disturbance, if seen, is usually minimal.

Rehabilitation potential for persons with mononeuropathies is generally good. Functional disability is limited to one specific area of the body. These conditions are often stable and improve with treatment; they typically do not worsen over time. Yet, temporary exacerbation frequently is experienced. Rehabilitation counselors working with people who have these conditions need to consider job modification with the current employer, whenever possible (Ropper & Samuels, 2014).

Rehabilitation Case Planning

Knowledge of the history, onset, and course of the disease process is significant in rehabilitation. To maintain employment or return a person to work, the neurological disorder must be stabilized or slowed in its progression. If a patient has had an acute episode that has run its course and reached maximum improvement, the counselor can formulate a rehabilitation plan based on the knowledge that the deficit will not deteriorate further. When an individual is under optimal medical control, but continues to have debilitating neurological symptoms, frequency and intensity of these events help determine the feasibility of providing vocational rehabilitation services (Greenberg et al., 2014).

Case Study

Ms. Nancy Smith is 48-years of age, African-American, and married. The Smith's have three children, two living at home and dependent on their parents' support, and one married and living in the same community. Mr. Ralph Smith works full-time as a computerized numerical control (CNC) machinist. After graduating from high school, Ms. Smith attended a community college and received an Associate of Science degree in nursing. Ms. Smith has been a grocery checker for the past 12 years.

Before this job, Ms. Smith worked for three years as a nursing assistant in a convalescent home, and for four years as a pharmacy technician in a retail drugstore. Her first experience in employment was as a house cleaner, which Nancy performed for two years. The work of a nursing assistant involves lifting of 25 pounds repetitively and up to 50 pounds occasionally. A pharmacy technician lifts up to 15 pounds and stands or walks one half of the work shift. Ms. Smith's job as a house cleaner required lifting and carrying up to 40 pounds on an occasional basis with repetitive lifting and carrying of 20 pounds or less.

For the past year, Ms. Smith has had complaints of pain and numbness in her left nondominant hand, primarily the second through fourth fingers. She has night pain and pain radiating into the left shoulder. There is hand weakness and a slight loss of grip strength. Dr. Elizabeth Kim stated that Ms. Smith has a mononeuropathy involving compression of the median nerve in the wrist. Recently, Nancy has complained of low back pain, and feels she is unable to lift and carry more than 25 pounds without experiencing mild pain.

Currently, Ms. Smith receives physical therapy three times a week at 5:00 p.m. on Monday, Wednesday, and Friday. Work hours for a grocery checker on her shift are 8:00 a.m. to 5:00 p.m. Nancy leaves work early at 4:30 p.m. to attend physical therapy. Her employer has expressed concerns about her missing 1½ hours of work each week.

The physical therapist suggested to Ms. Smith that she see a rehabilitation counselor. She has followed through with this suggestion. You have been assigned this case.

Questions

1. Assign Ms. Nancy Smith a vocational profile, including age category, educational level, and work history (skill and exertional levels).
2. What medical conditions do Nancy's symptoms indicate she may have?
3. Describe Ms. Smith's functional limitations in regard to her job.
4. Should she attempt to continue working as a grocery checker for her current employer? Explain.
5. If you recommend she continue her employment, what advice would you give Nancy and the employer regarding reasonable accommodation?
6. Describe the occupationally significant characteristics (worker traits) and possible transferable skills of Ms. Smith.
7. Suggest rehabilitation possibilities, including use of transferable skills from previous work and possible training programs if Nancy does not continue working for this employer. Please remember that this client has a college degree.

References

Alexander, G. E., DeLong, M. R., & Strick, P. L. (1986). Parallel organization of functionally segregated circuits linking basal ganglia and cortex. *Annual Reviews of Neuroscience, 9*, 357–381.

Beaumont, J. G. (2008). *Introduction to neuropsychology* (2nd ed.). New York, NY: Guilford.

Biller, J., Gruener, G., & Brazis, P. (2011). *DeMyer's the neurological examination: A programmed text* (6th ed.). Columbus, OH: McGraw-Hill.

Brust, J. C. M. (2011). *Current diagnosis and treatment neurology* (2nd ed.). Columbus, OH: McGraw-Hill Professional.

Carter, R. L., Hohenegger, M., & Satz, P. (1980). Handedness and aphasia: An inferential method for determining the mode of cerebral speech specialization. *Neuopsychologia, 18*, 569–574.

Greenberg, D. A., Aminoff, M. J., & Simon, R. (2014). *Clinical neurology* (8th ed.). Columbus, OH: McGraw-Hill.

Grefkes, C., & Fink, G. R. (2011). Reorganization of cerebral networks after stroke: New insights from neuroimaging with connectivity approaches. *Brain, 134*(5), 1264–1276.

Hallett, M. (2000). Transcranial magnetic stimulation and the human brain, *Nature, 406*, 147–150.

Hauser, S. L., & Josephson, S. (2013). *Harrison's neurology in clinical medicine* (3rd ed.). Columbus, OH: McGraw-Hill.

Lezak, M. D., Howieson, D. B., Bigler, E. D., & Tranel, D. (2012). *Neuropsychological assessment* (5th ed.). New York, NY: Oxford University.

Longo, D., Fauci, A., Kasper, D., Hauser, S., Jameson, J., & Loscalzo, J. (2011). *Harrison's principles of internal medicine* (18th ed.). Columbus, OH: McGraw-Hill.

Papadakis, M. A., McPhee, S. J., & Rabow, M. W. (Eds.). (2014). *Current medical diagnosis and treatment*. Columbus, OH: McGraw-Hill.

Pfeiffer, R. F., Wszolek, Z. K., & Ebadi, M. (Eds.). (2012). *Parkinson's disease* (2nd ed.). Boca Raton, FL: CRC.

Quarrell, O. (2008). *Huntington's disease* (2nd ed.). New York, NY: Oxford University.

Ropper, A. H., Samuels, M., & Klein, J. P. (2014). *Adams & Victor's principles of neurology* (10th ed.). New York, NY: McGraw-Hill.

Schmahmann, J. D., & Sherman, J. C. (1998). The cerebellar cognitive affective syndrome. *Brain, 121*(4), 561–579.

About the Authors

David B. Peterson, Ph.D., is a licensed clinical psychologist, Certified Rehabilitation Counselor, and Professor in Rehabilitation Education at California State University, Los Angeles. He has contributed to the development of the World Health Organization's International Classification of Functioning, Disability, and Health, publishing a text addressing psychological aspects of the same. Dr. Peterson is on the Panel of Medical Experts of the Office of Disability Adjudication and Review, Social Security Administration, where he provides psychological expert testimony.

Thomas Van Vleet, Ph.D., is a licensed Clinical Neuropsychologist and Research Neuropsychologist specializing in the development of *neurotherapeutics* – behavioral interventions for the treatment of brain dysfunction following injury, degeneration, or psychiatric illness – at the Veterans Affairs Medical Center, Northern California Health Care System in Martinez, California, and the Brain Plasticity Institute in San Francisco, California. Dr. Van Vleet is also a Visiting Scholar at the University of California, Berkeley and Principle Investigator on several National Institute of Health funded research projects examining the use of various neurotherapeutic treatments in clinical populations.

Chapter 16

SPINAL CORD INJURY

Gonzalo C. Centeno, M.S.
Nancy M. Crewe, Ph.D.
James S. Krause, Ph.D.

Introduction

Compared with many other disabling conditions, spinal cord injury (SCI) affects a relatively small number of people; each year about 12,000 new diagnoses are made to the current United States total of approximately 273,000 people with this condition. Yet it commands the attention of rehabilitation counselors and other health care professionals because SCI causes profound changes in virtually all physical systems and functional abilities. Further, the majority of people who sustain new spinal cord injuries are young adults with a lifetime of experiences ahead of them. Over half these individuals are in the 16-30 year age group; however, as of 2010, the average age at injury is 42.6 years (National Spinal Cord Injury Statistical Center [NSCISC], 2013). Individuals with SCI require multidisciplinary medical and rehabilitation services to rebuild their lives and contemplate the opportunity for an independent and productive future. This chapter provides essential information on physiological, functional, and psychosocial characteristics pertinent to people with SCI, along with important factors contributing to their rehabilitation needs and potentials.

The public views the inability to walk as the primary consequence of SCI. Although walking may be impacted, SCI also affects such areas as arm and hand strength and dexterity, bowel and bladder control, sexual function, temperature regulation, susceptibility to infections, and even the ability to breathe. To understand these consequences, it is necessary to become familiar with the anatomy and physiology of the central nervous system.

Anatomy and Physiology
Spinal Cord Structure

Voluntary motion takes place when nerve impulses travel from the brain down the spinal cord and out to the body through peripheral nerves. Sensory stimuli are carried from the peripheral nerves through the spinal cord to the brain. The full circuit enables tactile perception and coordinated movements. As a result, damage to the spinal cord can result in both loss of voluntary movement (paralysis) and loss of sensation.

The spinal cord extends from the brain stem to a point in the lower back called the conus medularis. Beyond that point, nerve fibers known as the *cauda equina* (horse's tail) fan out. The spinal cord is encased in a protective canal that is formed by the spinal vertebrae. At each vertebral junction, a pair of spinal nerves exit from the spinal cord and innervate specific muscles, and sensory nerve filaments enter the spinal cord. The vertebrae and nerves are classified into several sections beginning at the neck with seven cervical vertebrae, seven pairs of nerve roots that exit above each of those vertebrae, and an eighth pair that exits below the seventh vertebra. Below the cervical vertebrae are 12 thoracic vertebrae and 12 pairs of spinal nerves. In the lower back, there are five lumbar vertebrae and nerve roots and five fused sacral vertebrae with five nerve roots. The lowest part of the spinal column is a single bone called the coccyx. The vertebrae and nerves are numbered from the top with a letter that corresponds to the spinal section. For example, the first vertebra below the skull is C-1, whereas T-1 is the first vertebra in the thoracic section.

Nerves for the voluntary motor system originate in the motor cortex of the brain and extend down through the basal ganglia to the brain stem. Here they cross over to the opposite side and continue to descend in the spinal cord until they synapse at the point where they are about to exit from the spinal cord. The nerves that originate in the motor cortex of the brain's left hemisphere cross over to innervate the right side of the body, and those from the right hemisphere cross over to the left side. These are known as *upper motor neurons*. Beyond the synapse, the *lower motor neurons* exit the cord and extend to their particular muscle destination.

When the spinal cord is damaged, communication is disrupted between the brain and parts of the body that are innervated at or below the lesion. The lesion may be complete (no nerve fibers are functioning below the level of injury) or incomplete (one or more nerve fibers is secure). The cord need not be completely severed to result in a complete injury; the nerve cells may be destroyed as a result of pressure, bruising, or loss of blood supply, and if they die they do not regenerate. The amount of functional loss depends on the level of injury (the higher the damage, the more of the body that is affected) and the neurological completeness of the injury. Individuals with neurologically complete injuries have more severe and more predictable patterns of functional impairment.

The level of SCI damage can be determined in two ways. The first method specifies the level of bony damage as indicated by x-rays. The more useful approach, however, indicates the level of neurological damage, measured by careful testing of an individual's ability to perceive pinprick. Skin surface has been mapped into segments called *dermatomes* (see Figure 1); each dermatome is known to be innervated by sensory nerves at a particular spinal level. Testing the skin, therefore, can reveal the level at which the spinal cord has been damaged.

Spinal Cord Function

Individuals who sustain damage at the cervical level will have impaired function in both their upper and lower extremities, a condition known as tetraplegia (previously classified as quadriplegia). More than half of spinal injuries result in tetraplegia (NSCISC, 2013). Those who are injured at or below the thoracic level will have paraplegia, with function maintained in their upper extremities but some degree of impairment in the trunk and lower extremities

The American Spinal Injury Association (ASIA) developed a system for describing the severity of injury that is widely used in the medical community using letters that pertain to the extent of injury (usually A through D) (Young, 2006). ASIA A injuries are complete, with no motor or sensory function preserved below the neurological level of injury, including the sacral segments S4-S5. ASIA B injuries are incomplete, with sensory but no motor function preserved below the neurological level of injury. ASIA C and D classifications refer to incomplete injuries with increasing degrees of motor function preserved below the neurological level of injury.

Certain incomplete spinal cord injuries produce unusual patterns of deficits. If the damage occurs within the central part of the cervical cord, leaving the outer ring of fibers intact, the individual will have greater weakness in the upper limbs than in the lower limbs, and sacral sensation may be spared. Brown-Sequard syndrome is a lesion that affects only one side of the spinal cord. This causes paralysis on the same side of the body as the lesion, and loss of pain and temperature sensation on the opposite side of the body.

Acute Medical and Rehabilitation Care

Nearly half of spinal cord injuries are the result of motor vehicle accidents; other major causes include falls, violence, and sports accidents (NSCISC, 2013). Recent reports suggested that the number of new injuries due to violence have decreased from 24.8% during the 1990s to 14.3% reported in 2010. However, acts of violence with specific mention of gunshots remain the primary cause of SCI among some minority populations in the 16-30 age category, with African Americans and Hispanics being most affected (Chen, Tang, Vogel, & DeVivo, 2013). The number of spinal injuries stemming from motor vehicle accidents has diminished over the last few decades, probably as a result of air bags and other improvements in automobile safety.

FIGURE 1
Dermatomal Patterns of Spinal Cord Injury

Source: Kirshblum, S. C., Burns, S. P., Biering-Sorensen, F., Donovan, W., Graves, D. E., Jha, B., ... Waring, W. (2011). International standards for neurological classification of spinal cord injury (Revised 2011). *Journal of Spinal Cord Medicine, 34*(6), 535-546.

Medical emergency procedures executed at the scene of an injury have improved over the years, with careful stabilization of the neck and spine from the injury scene to the hospital, the availability of emergency transportation, and an increasing tendency to utilize specialized trauma hospitals. Damage to the spinal cord from trauma, bleeding, swelling, and oxygen deprivation are also crucial factors during injury. The damage is quickly compounded by the body's release of free radicals and other toxic substances, which leads to inflammation and scarring. Neuroprotective agents, such as methylprednisolone, are often administered soon after injury in an attempt to disrupt this cascade of events and prevent further cell death. Although the use of neuroprotective agents may still be controversial, the goals of medications like methylprednisolone are to reduce the possibility of secondary injuries to the nerves resulting from toxic substances. There are two other drugs which are still undergoing clinical trials, but have been showing significant promise. Riluzole has been approved by the United States Food and Drug Administration (FDA) and is currently being used in the treatment of amyotrophic lateral sclerosis (Wilson, Forgione, & Fehlings, 2013; Cifra, Mazzone, & Nistri, 2013). The second drug, Minocycline, is currently being used for the treatment of acnea, rosacea, and rheumatoid arthritis. According to studies, it contributes to functional improvement and recovery of motor function (Sonmez et al., 2013).

During hospitalization, physicians may determine that the spinal column is unstable and further neurological damage could ensue. In this case, surgery may be recommended to fuse the spine at the point of injury or otherwise stabilize it with rods or other surgical hardware. The individual may be fitted with a halo or body cast to enable him or her to maintain immobility of the fracture site without being confined to bed for excessive periods of time. Approximately 75% of these patients have one of the following spinal cord stabilizing procedures: laminectomy, neural canal restoration, open reduction, spinal fusion, or internal fixation of the spine (NSCISC, 2013).

When the need for acute medical services has passed, the individual is usually transferred to a rehabilitation unit for multidisciplinary services to help build strength, redevelop skills in activities of daily living, identify and obtain adaptive equipment, and prepare for a return to home and community. An SCI rehabilitation team typically includes one or more physicians, nurses, physical therapists, psychologists, occupational therapists, rehabilitation counselors, and social workers. A network of comprehensive Model SCI Centers has been established across the country, providing medical services as well as research on medical and psychosocial aspects of SCI. Studies have demonstrated that the post-discharge support system takes into account involvement in social and recreational activities, perceived ability to move about within the community, and the degree of comfort within their family and with other relationships (Hitzig, Romero Escobar, Noreau, & Craven, 2012). This is probably the most important time for the person affected by SCI because the process of assimilation of new body limitations is not only difficult, but it sets the stage for physical and psychological growth.

Changes in the health care system have greatly reduced the length of time needed to complete rehabilitation. Decades ago, a person with SCI would receive most of the rehabilitation as an inpatient before going home and out into the community; it was not unusual for a person to be in hospital and rehabilitation center for six months or more before being discharged. The average length of stay in a hospital for individuals with SCI from 1973-1979 was 142 days, which significantly dropped to 56 days from 1995-2012 (NSCISC, 2013).

Levels of Injury and Functioning

Table 1 summarizes the functions of the nerves at various spinal levels. For individuals with complete lesions, patterns of functional loss and preservation are fairly consistent from person to person. The most dramatic changes in function are apparent between adjacent neurological levels in the cervical area. For example, nerves that innervate the diaphragm are at cervical level 3-4, leading many persons with injuries at or above C-3 to need ventilator assistance to breathe. Most individuals with C-4 injuries regain breathing capacity, but do not have usable function in their arms and hands. As a result, they need assistance with activities of daily living (ADL).

Individuals with injuries at the C-5 level usually have function in the deltoid and bicep muscles, so they can bend the arm at the elbow. Some have the ability to develop a weak pinch by using an automatic motion known as tenodesis (when the wrist is extended, the thumb and index finger come together). This makes it possible to hold a light object (such as a washcloth) and carry out some self-care activities. Most people with C-5 injuries use power wheelchairs for mobility.

Many individuals with C-6 injuries use manual wheelchairs, particularly if the chairs are equipped with plastic wheel rims and projection knobs. Most people with C-6 tetraplegia can move independently with the use of appropriate equipment. Assistive devices (e.g., tableware with built-up handles) make many activities of daily living possible. Individuals who have limited manual dexterity may use hand braces (e.g., ratchet splint) that enable grasping items with their hands, such as a pencil or toothbrush.

People who have C-7 and C-8 levels of injury are almost fully independent in their daily lives. They have the use of triceps muscles (which allow them to straighten and lock their arms for transfers from wheelchair to automobile or chair) and finger extensors (which allow them to open their hands).

At the thoracic levels, the nerves innervate muscles that provide control of the trunk; injuries below this level allow for some balance and trunk stability. Control over hip muscles is maintained at the lumbar level, so individuals with injuries below T-12 are sometimes able to ambulate using crutches and braces. This takes a great amount of effort however, and most people choose to use wheelchairs for mobility, particularly when traveling long distances.

TABLE 1
Muscles Supplied and Functions Served by Spinal Nerve Motor Roots

Root Segment	Representative Muscles	Functions Served
Cervical		
C1 & C2	High neck muscles	Aid in head control
C3 & C4	Diaphragm	Inspiration (breathing in)
C5 & C6	Deltoid Biceps	Shoulder flexion, abduction (arms forward, out to side) Elbow flexion (elbow bent)
C6 & C7	Extensor Carpi Radialis Pronator Teres	Wrist dorsiflexion (back of hand up) Wrist pronation (palm down)
C7 & C8	Triceps Extensor Digitorum Communis	Elbow extension (elbow straight) Finger extension (knuckles straight)
C8 & T1	Flexor Digitorm Superficialis Opponens Pollicis Interossei (intrinsics)	Finger flexion (fist clenched) Thumb opposition (thumb brought to little finger) Spreading and closing the fingers
Thoracic		
T2—T6	Intercostals	Forced inspiration (breathing in) Expiration (breathing out, coughing)
T6—T12	Intercostals—Abdominals	Forced inspiration (breathing in); aid in expiration (coughing); aid in trunk flexion (sitting up)
Lumbar		
L1, L2, & L3	Iliopsoas Adductors	Hip flexion (thigh to chest); hip adduction, thigh to midline (legs together)
L3 & L4	Quadriceps	Knee extension (knee straight)
L4, L5, & S1	Gluteus Medius Tibialis Anterior	Hip abduction (thigh out to side, legs apart) Foot dorsiflexion (foot up, walk on heels)
L5, S1, & S2	Gluteus Maximus Gastrocneumius	Hip extension (thigh in line with trunk, hips straight, e.g., standing); foot plantar flexion (foot down, walk on toes)
Sacral		
S2, S3, & S4	Anal Sphincter Urethral Sphincter	Bowel function (fecal continence) Bladder control (urinary continence)

Source: Stolov, W. C., & Clowers, M. R. (1981). *Handbook of severe disability.* Washington, DC: U.S. Government Printing Office.

Injuries at the lumbar level often result in paraplegia. Persons with L1-L2 injuries may be capable of standing and walking with braces. Yet, this involves a great amount of energy and a wheelchair will be needed for mobility of long distances. Those with an L3-L4 injury also may be able to walk with the assistance of orthotic devices.

Innervation for bowel, bladder, and sexual functioning occur at the sacral level. Persons who have injuries at the cervical or thoracic level have sustained damage to all the upper motor neurons that innervate the body at or below the point of injury. This results in loss of voluntary control of bowel and bladder function. Fortunately, an intact lower motor neuron reflex arc may be retained from these muscles to the synapse in the spinal cord and back. This enables the possibility of *retraining* the body to respond to direct stimulation (for example, tapping on the lower abdomen to trigger voiding), and provides some degree of control over bowel functions. Individuals who have sacral injuries, on the other hand, may have direct injury to the lower motor neurons in this area. Thus, they may not have the ability to develop these reflexive responses.

Following SCI, most individuals lose voluntary control of bowel and bladder function and need to develop ways to manage these functions. The bowel can be trained to empty at regular intervals by using a suppository and/or digital stimulation. For people who are working, the time that is required to complete the bowel program (up to two hours) can affect productivity. People need to carefully monitor the food they eat and avoid items which cause irregularity or intestinal irritation. If bowel management becomes highly problematic, physicians may recommend a colostomy (surgical procedure that provides for emptying fecal contents through an abdominal stoma). This procedure may reduce the amount of time required for bowel care and serve to prevent accidents.

Bladder and kidney functioning is a complex issue following SCI. Persons who retain reflexive function in the bladder may be able to initiate voiding through direct stimulation by tapping on the bladder around the pubic area. This will cause the sphincter muscle to relax and the bladder to drain. However, those who have a flaccid bladder need catheterization or external pressure to void (NSCISC, 2013).

Many people have recurrent episodes of urinary tract infections that cause fever and other symptoms. Infections develop because the bladder does not empty often enough or completely, allowing bacteria to multiply. Without sensation, a person does not receive automatic signals indicating the bladder needs to be emptied. If the bladder becomes overly full, urine backs up into the kidneys (a condition known as reflux) and causes damage. For many years, renal problems were the major cause of premature death among persons with SCI (DeVivo, Black, & Stover, 1993), but antibiotics and better preventive care have reduced this danger.

Functional Complications and Limitations

Sexual Dysfunction

Researchers continue to try to find ways to enhance the sexual lives of individuals with SCI and to diminish the impact of injury on sexual functioning. This area merits additional research and also counseling because of its importance within marriage, and as a component of personal identity and self-esteem. The connection between sexual arousal, which occurs in the brain and genital organs, is usually broken, making it impossible for most men to attain an erection or women to produce lubrication in response to psychological arousal. Yet, if the lower motor neuron reflex arc is intact, a physical response may be produced by direct stimulation. For men with SCI between T6 and L5, sildenafil (Viagra) has been shown to significantly improve the quality of erections and lead to higher levels of satisfaction (Rahimi-Movaghar & Vaccaro, 2012). Other techniques have been developed to enable intercourse, including penile implants and injections.

For men, fertility is a more difficult challenge. Ejaculation typically does not occur after SCI, or semen may be deposited into the bladder rather than being discharged externally. Sperm motility may be low so that pregnancy is unlikely to occur. In recent years, clinicians have successfully used techniques, such as electrical stimulation, to induce ejaculation or artificial insemination.

A woman who has SCI frequently does not have a menstrual period for several months after the trauma. Many women with SCI remain fertile and can become pregnant. A woman will require prenatal and delivery care from a physician knowledgeable in SCI to avoid complications resulting from the pressure that a growing fetus places on her lungs, bladder, skin, and circulatory system. Special issues may arise during childbirth, in part because she may not experience the typical sensations that signal the onset of labor. Care must be taken to manage any occurrence of autonomic hyperreflexia during labor. A woman with tetraplegia needs to plan the way in which she will be able to care for a baby — perhaps with help from a personal care assistant.

Autonomic Hyperreflexia

Autonomic hyperreflexa is potentially life-threatening for persons with injuries above the level of T-6. As a result of the SCI, this is a response to a noxious stimulus (e.g., a urinary tract infection, a blocked catheter, or even wrinkled clothing that is irritating the skin), where blood pressure drastically increases, producing symptoms of a crashing headache, dizziness, and sweating. Unless treated quickly, the individual is at risk of seizures, stroke, or possibly even death (Linskell & Bouamrane, 2012).

Spasticity

Immediately after SCI, the muscles that would be innervated by neurons below the lesion are usually flaccid. The upper motor neurons that were destroyed do not recover, so voluntary motor function will not return. The lower motor neurons some distance below the lesion may not have been directly injured; however, as the initial shock passes, they may begin to conduct signals in a reflex arc from the peripheral nerves to the synapse in the spinal cord and then back to the stimulated muscle. In an intact nervous system, the signal goes to the brain and the brain modulates the body's response. A lesion blocks that pathway and sets up, in effect, a reverberating circuit. Resulting spasticity can be quite disruptive and may cause pain and possible embarrassment for the individual.

A positive side of spasticity is that it can serve to help maintain tone in paralyzed muscles and may be functionally useful in some instances, such as in facilitating wheelchair transfers. Psychoactive medications are now available to control spasticity. Other procedures, such as motor point blocks (to block nerve impulses) and surgery, are tried when other means of control are ineffective. Non-medication treatments for spasticity include stretching and similar activities (Strommen, 2013).

Contractures

Joints and muscles not regularly moved through their full range of motion shorten into permanently flexed positions known as contractures. The reduction of range of motion caused by contractures makes everyday life functions difficult; the use of an elevator or simply turning a light switch on and off can be difficult because of an inability to reach. Hygiene is made difficult by permanent contractures and any functional capacities that the individual may possess become compromised. Rehabilitation nurses and physical therapists make a concerted effort to avoid development of contractures; range of motion exercises need to be a daily routine.

Pressure Sores

Decubitus ulcers, also known as pressure sores, are a frequent and costly problem for individuals with impaired sensation. This condition is a severe medical complication of SCI. Whereas people with intact nervous systems shift their positions at frequent intervals due to signals of discomfort, those with SCI need to train themselves to shift their weight regularly. A recent study reports pressure sores as being "a common medical complication" that affects individuals with an incidence of 15.2% in the first year after injury. Essential to the prevention and management of pressure sores is on-going education to anyone at risk of acquiring them, including patients with acute injuries and individuals aging with SCI (Bogie et al., 2013).

Subsequent Injuries

Subsequent injuries are those that occur in the years and decades after the initial SCI. In one study, 19% of individuals in a sample of 1,391 participants reported at least one other injury during the previous 12 months that required medical attention (Krause, 2004). Of those with one or more injuries, 27% reported at least one injury-related hospitalization during the same timeframe. Sensation seeking, heavy drinking, prescription medication used for pain, spasticity, depression, and lack of sleep were all associated with an elevated risk of subsequent injuries (consistent with the risk factors for the initial SCI). Brotherton, Krause, and Neitert (2007) surveyed 119 participants with ambulatory SCI where 75% reported at least one fall the previous year. Of those who had at least one fall, 18% had fractures and 45% noted decreased participation in community activities as the result of a fall.

Bone Changes

Almost immediately after SCI, osteoporosis begins to develop. Part of the reason for bone loss is the increased bed rest needed and general disuse that follows trauma (Burns, Wilson, & Craven, 2013). The loss occurs throughout the body, but initially directly affects areas below the pelvis, especially the knees. Decreased bone density makes a person vulnerable to future fractures.

Another sequela of trauma is heterotopic ossification, a condition in which the body begins to develop pieces of bone in soft tissue. Heterotopic ossification affects individuals with SCI below the level of neurological injury, often affecting range of motion of knees, shoulders, elbows, and hands. Besides being painful, this phenomenon interferes with functioning, sometimes to the point where joints fuse. Surgery is used to treat severe cases of heterotopic ossification (Burns et al., 2013).

Respiratory Function

Persons with complete SCI above the level of C-4 are likely to need ventilators to help them breathe. Questions have been raised about quality of life experienced by people with tetraplegia who are ventilator dependent. Interestingly, studies have shown that individuals with such conditions consistently rate their lives as more satisfying than health care professionals predicted (Bach & Tilton, 1994). With sufficient support and assistive technology, these individuals may be capable of working, socializing, and living rewarding lives.

Respiratory function is often a matter of concern for people who are not placed on ventilators. Because of weakened chest muscles, people with tetraplegia and those with high thoracic injuries may not be able to cough with sufficient force to clear their lungs of irritants and mucus, and are prone to pneumonia. This is especially dangerous if they have developed immunity to several antibiotics because of frequent use in combating other infections. Pneumonia is the most common cause of death among people with SCI (Burns et al., 2013). Pulmonary embolism is another serious condition that occurs at greatly increased rates for this population.

Cardiac Issues

Among people with SCI, heart problems triggered by neurogenic shock resulting from hypotension and persistent bradycardia causes blood pressure to drop to dangerous levels (Krassioukov, 2013). Furthermore, cardiac insufficiency may contribute to reduced energy and strength and can lead directly or indirectly to the development of other secondary disorders, such as pressure ulcers. Paralysis poses formidable barriers to exercise and the maintenance of cardiovascular fitness.

Chronic Pain

The majority of people with SCI experience neuropathic pain that affects functioning and quality of life (Finnerup, 2012). They may report a sharp, stabbing pain below the level of injury that occurs intermittently, or a dull, aching pain that persists for long periods of time and becomes worse with activity. The cause for pain is not well understood and there may be no means of relief available.

Another source of pain comes from overuse of shoulders and upper extremities needed to propel a wheelchair and transfer from one surface to another. According to Finnerup (2012), pain which did not respond to ordinary therapies was treated and relieved with complimentary treatments such as warm baths, physical activities, and finding a balance between activity and rest.

Psychosocial Aspects of SCI

Adequately describing the psychological and social consequences of SCI is complex. People experiencing objectively similar levels of trauma respond in entirely different ways as a result of differing personalities, social support systems, cultural and ethnic backgrounds, available resources, age, education, and intellect. Every aspect of a person is affected by the injury; thus, rehabilitation efforts should address the whole person.

There are some characteristics of SCI that play a role in the adjustment process, including:

- SCI usually involves sudden and unexpected onset. In a moment's time, life is irretrievably altered. With no opportunity for preparation, the entire adjustment process takes place after onset. In past years, hospital stays were six months to a year after SCI, allowing time for gradual assimilation to the injury and with the support of a rehabilitation team. Currently, SCI patients are discharged much sooner and have less time to comprehend and plan for the future within a supported environment.

- The person with SCI experiences loss in many areas of life, including the inability to participate in valued activities, financial losses related to interruption or discontinuance of work, and the burden of new expenses. Eventually, most people perceive gains stemming from the injury (e.g., deepening of family relationships, personal growth, and new educational or vocational opportunities).

- One of the most profound changes following SCI is the loss of independence in daily living. The individual with tetraplegia needs to rely on another person to provide basic care, including toileting, bathing, and feeding.

- Individuals with SCI must be aware of non-accessibility when in the community. The Americans with Disabilities Act (ADA) and other legislation have helped in increasing the number of public places that are wheelchair accessible.

- The bodies of persons with SCI are a further source of insecurity because of the loss of voluntary control of functions. A bowel or bladder accident or even a bout of spasticity may bring unwanted attention and embarrassment. Some people choose to stay at home rather than risk such occurrences.

- The person with SCI is subject to attitudinal barriers of people who are uncomfortable with or biased against individuals with disabilities. Many persons have reported that pre-injury friends drift away and new acquaintances must be made to avoid isolation. The incidence of marriage is lower and that of divorce is somewhat higher among individuals with SCI compared with the general population (Crewe & Krause, 1992; DeVivo, Hawkins, Richards, & Go, 1995).

- Some individuals with SCI must cope with additional barriers, such as substance abuse. Up to half the people admitted to emergency rooms with severe trauma, including SCI, were intoxicated at the time of injury (Heinemann, Doll, Armstrong, Schnoll, & Yarkony, 1991). Thus, people who abuse substances are more likely to engage in risky behavior that leads to injury. Furthermore, substance abuse may be a coping strategy subsequent to injury.

- The rate of depressive disorders is approximately three times higher among people with SCI than in the general population. Between 20-40% of individuals with this disability suffer from depression (Kemp, Kahan, & Krause, 1999; Weingardt, Hsu, & Dunn, 2001). Depression can interfere with health, psychosocial functioning, and lead to suicide.

- People are resilient in their abilities to cope with the challenges of SCI. Psychological adjustment (as measured by satisfaction with life and involvement in work and social activities) continues to improve for many years after injury. Without denying that SCI is a tragic event, most survivors rate their quality of life as good to excellent years after the event.

Veterans with SCI

In the United States, there are many veterans returning home with spinal cord injuries. Many studies reflecting the challenges experienced by veterans are focusing on highlighting treatment models post-injury to improve satisfaction with life and enhance overall quality of life. According to one study (Fortman et al., 2013), veterans compose 10% of the U.S. population of which 20% of this number are affected by acquired

SCI. Therefore, organizations such as the Wounded Warrior Project are focusing on the needs of this population and searching for better ways of providing support, guidance, and independence.

Challenges affecting veterans with SCI are depression, post-traumatic stress disorder (PTSD), and substance abuse. Psychological ramifications of these contributing conditions significantly hinder quality of life (deRoon-Cassini, Hastings, de St-Aubin, Valvano, & Brasel, 2013). One five-year study is currently underway that will emphasize an intervention type model that consists of specially trained vocational rehabilitation counselors as members of the SCI team (Sinnot, Cheng, Wagner, Goetz, & Ottomanelli, 2011). Among the job counseling and job services provided, the philosophy is that employment is possible regardless of severity of disability.

Employment

The most prominent benefits of employment are financial. However, employment is also related to other favorable outcomes. For example, individuals who are employed after SCI consistently report greater satisfaction with nearly all areas of life (Krause, 2003). Return to gainful employment is associated with a significantly greater likelihood of surviving SCI over an extended period.

Employment Rates

According to the NSCISC (2013), 57.1% of those affected by SCI were working at time of injury, whereas 15.8% were unemployed. Among those who returned to work after SCI, it took an average of about five years to return to the first post-injury job and just over six years to return to the first full time job (Krause, 2003).

Return-to-Work Approaches

There are two separate tracks to employment—a fast track, defined by return to the pre-injury job or having worked as a professional prior to injury, and a slow track, reflecting the absence of these characteristics. Those in the fast track required substantially less time to return to both their first job (2.1 years compared to 5.5 years) and their first full time job (3.3 years compared to 7.1 years). Differences between those with cervical and non-cervical injuries were observed only for the slow track. These findings suggest there is a window of opportunity shortly after SCI onset where there is greater likelihood of return to work if the preinjury employer is willing to rehire or if preinjury education and work skills can be applied to a new position. An assertive approach may maximize employment opportunities when compared with the frequent practice of delaying discussion of employment issues until after the person returns to his or her community and has had time to adapt to the injury (Krause, 2003; Sinnott et al., 2011).

Employment Outcomes

Primary factors associated with post-injury employment are race-ethnicity, age, severity of injury, etiology, duration of SCI, pre-injury employment status, and years of education. The highest employment rates were obtained by participants who had the following characteristics: Caucasian, 25 years of age and younger at time of injury, ASIA D severity, not injured as the result of violence, had been injured 20 years earlier, were working at time of injury, and had completed 16 or more years of education.

Being employed at the time of injury was associated with a greater probability of employment after injury, but only during the first few years following, after which time this factor was unrelated to work status. The employment rate of those working at injury ranged from 18-31% at one, two, and five years post-injury, compared with a range of 6-16% over the same timeframe for those unemployed at injury. However, by ten years post-injury the trends had reversed (33% compared with 40%).

Severity of Disability

Although severity of injury and functional limitations play a role in return to work, the relationship is not simple. For example, if jobs require manual dexterity, but not lower extremity function, a person with paraplegia is more likely than someone with tetraplegia to return to the position. Another reason why people with tetraplegia find it more difficult to return to work is that they are likely to have higher medical costs, including medications, supplies, and especially personal care assistance. Medicaid often covers these costs; eligibility for Medicaid generally is lost when a person begins earning more than about $500 per month. Enactment of Ticket to Work legislation in 1999 represented an effort to change public policy to remove this disincentive to employment.

Education

It is rare for a person with less than 12 years of education to return to work after SCI, and even more uncommon for them to retain employment. For example, the NSCISC (2013) reported that 48.2% of those surveyed had completed high school or GED, and 6.8% completed a bachelor's degree; only 23.7% completed less than 12 years of education at time of injury.

The significance of education is best demonstrated in conjunction with injury. Education mediates the extent to which severity of injury is associated with diminished labor force participation. Among those with 12 years of education, only 8% of participants with C1-C4, ASIA A-C were currently working, compared to 33% for those with motor function injuries (i.e., ASIA D, all levels). However, the differences disappeared among those at the Master's-Ph.D. level. The benefits of further education were most dramatic for those with the most severe SCI, as the employment rate for the C1-C4 group was nearly eight times greater between high school and Master's-Ph.D. level education compared with less than two times the increase for those with ASIA D. In fact, the employment rate for those with ASIA D injuries flattened, starting at an Associate's degree, but continued to increase for those with Cl-C4 ASIA A-C, all the way through the Master's-Ph.D. (increasing from 36% with a four-year degree to 61% with a master's or higher degree). In summary, education is the great equalizer of employment opportunities for people with SCI (Krause, 2003).

Search for a Cure

Writings from ancient Egypt described SCI as a condition that was untreatable. Survival prospects for those injured did not improve significantly until the discovery of antibiotics in the early 1940s. Cells within the central nervous system do not regenerate once they have been destroyed so medical treatment and rehabilitation have always focused on preventing complications and maximizing residual functional capacities. Today, researchers have been working with increased intensity to find ways to stimulate regrowth of nerve cells, to block the processes that serve to inhibit growth, and to promote connections across the site of injury (Jones, Anderson, & Galvin, 2003; Wilson et al., 2013). Aside from drugs that help prevent cellular destruction at the time of injury, there are further advances in stem cell research to aid in the nerve regeneration process (Jia, Kowalski, Sciubba, & Giocadin, 2013). Repair through transplantation of nerve cells is being studied and many believe that a breakthrough may be achieved in the foreseeable future. Until that time, it is important to remember that thousands of people are experiencing fulfilling and productive lives with severe disability.

Conclusion

A spinal cord injury usually begins with a sudden, traumatic impact on the spine that fractures or dislocates vertebrae. An injury to the spinal cord can damage a few to almost all axons in a particular area. There will be almost total recovery from some injuries, while other injuries result in complete paralysis. Improved emergency care for people with spinal cord injuries and aggressive treatment and rehabilitation can minimize damage to the nervous system and restore function. Rehabilitation programs combine physical therapy with skill-building activities and counseling to provide social and emotional support. Spinal cord injuries are classified as either complete or incomplete. People with incomplete injuries retain some motor or sensory function below the injury. Complete injuries cause a total lack of sensory and motor function below the level of injury. People who survive spinal cord injuries will most likely have medical complications such as paralysis, chronic pain, bladder and bowel dysfunction, along with increased susceptibility to respiratory and heart problems. Successful recovery depends upon how well these chronic conditions are handled on a daily basis. Severity of disability and education has a profound impact on resuming employment.

Case Study

Charles Kopecki is 34 years of age. He sustained a C-6 level SCI a year ago in a motorcycle crash. He was returning from a friend's home on a rainy evening when he struck a patch of gravel and failed to negotiate a curve in the road, striking a tree. A passing motorist telephoned for help, and he was airlifted to a regional trauma center where he underwent emergency surgery to stabilize his spinal column. After three weeks on the neurosurgical service, he was transferred to the rehabilitation unit where he received six weeks of comprehensive services prior to returning home. At the time of injury, Charles had been employed for nine years as a long distance truck driver for an agricultural processing company. Occasionally, he served as a dispatcher for the company. Charles dropped out of high school midway through the 12th grade and never returned to school. He held a number of unskilled jobs in construction and food services after he left high school.

The Kopecki's live in a town of about 10,000 people, approximately 25 miles from a small city. Charles and his wife have two children, ages 9 and 10. His wife has been providing personal care services for Charles since his injury, including bathing and bowel and bladder hygiene. She works at a filling station/convenience store to supplement the public assistance income which Charles receives. Between these responsibilities, housework, and parenting, she is feeling increasingly stressed. At her encouragement, Mr. Kopecki scheduled an appointment with a rehabilitation counselor to discuss gainful employment. He told his counselor that he enjoyed being a truck driver, but does not see a future in that career because of his disability.

Questions

1. Provide a vocational profile for Mr. Kopecki, including age category, educational level, and work history (skill and exertional levels).
2. Does Charles possess transferable skills? If so, what are they and what vocational alternatives might provide an opportunity to use them?
3. What kinds of adaptive equipment would you recommend to increase Charles' independence?
4. How would you learn more about Mr. Kopecki's psychological adjustment to his disability? What services would be appropriate for him?
5. Would you involve the family in Charles' rehabilitation counseling? Discuss.
6. Outline a comprehensive rehabilitation plan for this client.

References

Bach, J. R., & Tilton, M. C. (1994). Life satisfaction and well-being measures in ventilator-assisted individuals with traumatic tetraplegia. *Archives of Physical Medicine and Rehabilitation, 75,* 626–632.

Bogie, K., Ho, C., Washington, M., Foster-Geeter, S., Seton, J. C., Mitchell, S. J., . . . White, J. L. (2012). Interdisciplinary essentials in pressure ulcer management. In M. G. Fehlings, A. R. Vaccaro, M. Boakye, S. Rossignol, J. F. Ditunno, Jr., & A. S. Burns (Eds.), *Essentials of spinal cord injury: Basic research to clinical practice* (pp. 158–178). New York, NY: Thieme Medical.

Brotherton, S. S., Krause, J. S., & Nietert, P. J. (2007). Falls in individuals with incomplete spinal cord injury. *Spinal Cord 45,* 37–40.

Burns, A. S., Wilson, J. R., & Craven, B. C. (2012). The management of secondary complications following spinal cord injury. In M. G. Fehlings, A. R. Vaccaro, M. Boakye, S. Rossignol, J. F. Ditunno, Jr., & A. S. Burns (Eds.), *Essentials of spinal cord injury: Basic research to clinical practice* (pp. 244–262). New York, NY: Thieme Medical.

Chen, Y., Tang, Y., Vogel, L. C., & DeVivo, M. J. (2013). Causes of spinal cord injury. *Top Spinal Cord Injury Rehabilitation, 19,* 1–8.

Cifra, A., Mazzone, G., & Nistri, A. (2013). Riluzole: What it does to spinal and brainstem neurons and how it does it. *The Neuroscientist, 19,* 137–144.

Crewe, N. M., & Krause, J. S. (1992). Marital status and adjustment to spinal cord injury. *Journal of the American Paraplegia Society, 15,* 14–18.

deRoon-Cassini, T. A., Hastings, J., de St-Aubin, E., Valvano, A. K., & Brasel, K. J. (2013). Meaning-making appraisals relevant to adjustment for veterans with spinal cord injury. *Psychological Services, 10,* 186–193.

DeVivo, M. J., Black, K. J., & Stover, S. L. (1993). Causes of death during the first 12 years after spinal cord injury. *Archives of Physical Medicine and Rehabilitation, 66,* 501–504.

DeVivo, M. J., Hawkins, L. N., Richards, J. S., & Go, B. K. (1995). Outcomes of post-spinal cord injury marriages. *Archives of Physical Medicine and Rehabilitation, 76,* 130–138.

Finnerup, N. B. (2012). Pain in patients with spinal cord injury. *International Association for the Study of Pain, 12,* 1–6.

Fortmann, A. L., Rutledge, T., McCulloch, R. C., Shivpuri, S., Nisenzon, A. N., & Muse, J. (2013). Satisfaction with life among veterans with spinal cord injuries completing multidisciplinary rehabilitation. *International Spinal Cord Society, 51,* 482–486.

Heinemann, A W., Doll, M. D., Armstrong, K. J., Schnoll, S., & Yarkony, G. M. (1991). Substance use and receipt of treatment by persons with long-term spinal cord injuries. *Archives of Physical Medicine and Rehabilitation, 72,* 482–487.

Hitzig, S. L., Romero Escobar, E. M., Noreau, L., & Craven, B. C. (2012). Validation of the Reintegration to Normal Living Index for community-dwelling persons with chronic spinal cord injury. *Archives of Physical Medicine & Rehabilitation, 93,* 108–114.

Jia, X., Kowalski, R. G., Sciubba, D. M., & Geocadin, R. G. (2013). Critical care of traumatic spinal cord injury. *Journal of Intensive Care Medicine, 28,* 12–23.

Jones, D. G., Anderson, E. R., & Galvin, K. A. (2003). Spinal cord regeneration: Moving tentatively towards new perspectives. *NeuroRehabilitation, 18*(4), 339–351.

Kemp, B., Kahan, J., & Krause, J. S. (1999). The effects of treatment of depression on symptoms, community activities, and life satisfaction in persons with SCI: A controlled study. *Journal of Spinal Cord Medicine, 22,* 58–61.

Kirshblum, S. C., Burns, S. P., Biering-Sorensen, F., Donovan, W., Graves, D. E., Jha, B., . . . Waring, W. (2011). International standards for neurological classification of spinal cord injury (Revised 2011). *Journal of Spinal Cord Medicine, 34*(6), 535–546.

Krassioukov, A. (2012). Autonomic dysreflexia and cardiovascular complications of spinal cord injury. In M. G. Fehlings, A. R. Vaccaro, M. Boakye, S. Rossignol, J. F. Ditunno, Jr., & A. S. Burns (Eds.), *Essentials of spinal cord injury: Basic research to clinical practice* (pp. 181–262). New York, NY: Thieme Medical.

Krause, J. S. (2003). Years to employment after spinal cord injury. *Archives of Physical Medicine and Rehabilitation, 84*(9), 1282–1289.

Krause, J. S. (2004). Factors associated with risk for subsequent injuries after the onset of traumatic spinal cord injury. *Archives of Physical Medicine and Rehabilitation, 85*(9), 1503–1508.

Linskell, J., & Bouamrane, M. (2012). Assisted living spaces for end-users with complex needs: A proposed implementation and delivery model. *Health Informatics Journal, 18,* 159–170.

National Spinal Cord Injury Statistical Center (NSCISC). (2013). *Annual report for the model spinal cord injury care systems.* Birmingham, AL: Author.

Rahimi-Movaghar, V., & Vaccaro A. R. (2012). Management of sexual disorders in spinal cord injured patients. *Acta Medica Iranica, 50,* 295–299.

Sinnott, P. L., Cheng, A., Wagner, T. H., Goetz, L. L., & Ottomanelli, L. (2011). Cost-effectiveness analysis of the spinal cord injury vocational integration program. *Top Spinal Cord Injury Rehabilitation, 16,* 80–88.

Sonmez, E., Kabatas, S., Ozen, O., Karabay, G., Turkoglu, S., Ogus, F., . . . Altinors, N. (2013). Minocycline treatment inhibits lipids peroxidation, preserves spinal cord, ultrastructure, and improves functional outcome after traumatic spinal cord injury in the rat. *Spine, 38,* 1253–1259.

Stolov, W. C., & Clowers, M. R. (Eds.). (1981). *Handbook of severe disability.* Washington, DC: U. S. Government Printing Office.

Strommen, J. (2013). Management of spasticity from spinal cord dysfunction. *Neurologive Clinics, 31,* 269–286.

Weingardt, K. R., Hsu, J., & Dunn, M. E. (2001). Brief screening for psychological and substance abuse disorders in veterans with long-term spinal cord injury. *Rehabilitation Psychology, 46*(3), 271–278.

Wilson, J., Forgione, N., D., & Fehlings, M. G. (2013). Emerging therapies for acute traumatic spinal cord injury. *Canadian Medical Association Journal, 185,* 485–492.

Young, W. (2006). *Spinal cord injury levels and classification.* Retrieved May 23, 2006 from http://www.sci-info-pages.com/levels.html.

About the Authors

Gonzalo C. Centeno, M.S., graduated from California State University, Los Angeles (CSULA) with a Master of Science degree in Counseling, option in Rehabilitation Counseling. He has worked as the Disability Management Specialist in the Office for Students with Disabilities at CSULA since 1995. In 1979 at the age of 13, he acquired a spinal cord injury at the C5/C6 level and was diagnosed with incomplete tetraplegia; he has since been a wheelchair user. Mr. Centeno received one of the California State Department of Rehabilitation's 50 Notable People in 2013, and was featured in their 50th Anniversary webpage honoring all those who have contributed to the disability community.

Nancy M. Crewe, Ph.D., was a Professor in the Department of Physical Medicine and Rehabilitation at Michigan State University in East Lansing, Michigan. She coordinated the Master's Degree Program in Rehabilitation Counseling. Dr. Crewe conducted longitudinal research on psychosocial adjustment to spinal cord injury for more than 25 years.

James S. Krause, Ph.D., was a research scientist with the Medical University of South Carolina. Before embarking on a full-time career in long-term outcomes research combining work as a behavioral scientist and rehabilitation consultant, Dr. Krause spent five years as a rehabilitation psychologist. He served as principal investigator on six federally funded research grants and for two years, he was a visiting scientist at the Centers for Disease Control in Atlanta, Georgia.

Regretfully, both Drs. Crewe and Krause are no longer with us. This chapter is but a small piece of the tremendous contributions both have made in spinal cord injury research and awareness. Their work has inspired many to never cease the search for a cure, and to improve the quality of life for those affected by SCI. We thank you.

Chapter 17

CEREBRAL PALSY

Sherwood J. Best, Ph.D.

Introduction

Most people recognize the words *cerebral palsy* but few are able to describe this heterogeneous and complex disorder. The first descriptions of cerebral palsy were made in 1843 by Dr. William John Little (1810-1894), who described *spastic rigidity* in a group of children who had suffered brain damage at the time of their births (Fairhurst, 2012). Called *Little's Disease* for decades, the term cerebral palsy was first used in 1937. Each individual with cerebral palsy is unique with clinical, educational, rehabilitative, and vocational needs and outcomes that are not easily predictable.

Cerebral palsy (CP) cannot be cured by medical or educational interventions. As children with cerebral palsy grow into adulthood, they will be faced with a variety of challenges related to physical and emotional maturation. Fortunately, breakthroughs in medical and therapeutic treatments and the advent of assistive technology have done much to improve the quality of life of persons with cerebral palsy. The limitations imposed by cerebral palsy no longer define their educational or career aspirations and outcomes.

Definition

Cerebral palsy is defined as:

> A group of permanent disorders of the development of movement and posture, causing activity limitation, which are attributed to non-progressive disturbances that occurred in the developing infant or fetal brain. The motor disorders of cerebral palsy are often accompanied by disturbances of sensation, perception, cognition, communication, and behavior, including epilepsy and secondary musculoskeletal problems (Moreno-De-Luca, Ledbetter, & Martin, 2012, p. 283).

The components of this complex definition contain the following features: (1) permanent movement and posture disorders that reduce activity; (2) early onset; (3) lack of underlying progressive pathology; and (4) numerous co-occurring deficits. Cerebral palsy is not a disease but the result of damage to the developing brain. The disorders of movement and posture are due to damage to areas of the brain that control motor function. The damage is referred to as *static*; it does not worsen. However, the dysfunction that results from muscle imbalance over time, combined with co-occurring characteristics of CP, contributes to more severe disability as the person ages (Hirsh, Gallegos, Gertz, Engel, & Jensen, 2010). Individuals may develop scoliosis (curvature of the spine), hip dislocation, early degenerative arthritis, uneven bone growth, and chronic pain. These all contribute to reduced activity, functionality, and quality of life.

In addition to posture and motor disorders, people may have secondary outcomes of brain damage, including epilepsy, intellectual disability, sensory and cognitive impairments, and orthopedic complications (Best & Bigge, 2010). Communication impairments that include disorders of speech and language occur in individuals with CP. It is estimated that approximately "… 20% of individuals with cerebral palsy have psychosocial and behavioural problems" (Moreno-De-Luca et al., 2012, p. 284). However, not everyone will experience each of these associated impairments.

The prevalence of CP is approximately 2.0-3.0 per 1000 live births (Fairhurst, 2012). Increases in both incidence and prevalence of cerebral palsy have been attributed to improved documentation, advances in obstetrics, and medical interventions that save the lives of infants and children while failing to prevent central nervous system damage. A recent phenomenon has been the occurrence of multiple births resulting from assisted reproduction. Children who are the products of multiple births, or who are very premature, are more likely to have CP than children who do not experience these intrauterine and birth conditions. The incidence of severe forms of cerebral palsy has decreased since the 1990s due to specialized drug treatments for mothers at risk for premature birth (Hvidtjørn et al., 2010).

Etiology

Many factors contribute to diagnosis of cerebral palsy. Cerebral palsy can occur before birth (*prenatal*), during the birth process (*perinatal*), or after birth (*postnatal*). Prematurity, genetic factors, low birthweight, exposure to maternal infection, metabolic disorders, anoxia (lack of oxygen) due to problems with the placenta, and multiple births are all potential prenatal contributors. Although anoxia during the birth process has historically been proposed as the leading contributor to CP, it is now understood that prenatal contributors pose a greater risk (Moreno-De-Luca et al., 2012). Finally, postnatal trauma can include infections, exposure to toxic substances, and trauma such as child abuse. Gladstone (2010) proposed that postnatal causes, especially in relation to diseases such as cerebral malaria and meningitis, are more likely to occur in what he called *resource-poor* settings than would occur in Western countries, where CP is more highly related to premature birth. Impairments that co-occur with CP, including intellectual disability, seizures, and sensory impairments, help explain why this condition is so complex and varied.

Approximately 5,000 infants in the world are born with CP annually. Brain malformation, genetic syndromes, maternal infection, and anoxia are causes during the prenatal (pre-birth) period. Prenatal brain malformation resulting in CP may be due to genetic syndromes, acquired injuries from infections such as cytomegalovirus, and mutations. Premature infants whose birthweights are very low are at risk of injury to the white matter in the brain. Asphyxia (loss of oxygen) during the later prenatal period may damage deep structures in the brain, leading to dyskinetic cerebral palsy. Finally, multiple births place stress on the uterine environment and heighten the possibility of preterm birth, and an increased risk for cerebral palsy (Hvidtjørn et al., 2010).

The birth process itself can result in cerebral palsy. Risk factors such as maternal bleeding, problems with the placenta, maternal infection (such as herpes), and obstetrical complications such as prolonged labor, use of forceps, prolapsed cord, and abnormal presentation of the infant can all result in brain injury, either from direct insult to the brain or from anoxia.

After birth, the brain can be damaged through direct injury due to lack of oxygen (Best & Bigge, 2010). Infections to the central nervous system from encephalitis, poison, near drowning, suffocation, electrocution, and other traumatic events can result in CP. One entirely preventable cause of postnatal CP is physical abuse; infants and young children can suffer severe head injury from shaking and hitting (Squier, 2011). Another preventable cause of brain injury occurs when infants and children are not properly secured in automobiles.

Diagnosis

Due to the complexity of causes and risk factors associated with cerebral palsy, many infants may not be diagnosed for several years. To make a diagnosis, physicians rely on clinical judgment and comparison of infant function to their knowledge of typical infant development (Hamilton, 2006). Most scales of early development are heavily focused on motor skills, which may be absent, delayed, or distorted in infants with cerebral palsy. Weber and Jenni (2012) support increased pediatric screening as a tool for early detection of CP. Physicians and other professionals look for the presence of certain reflexive motor behaviors to assist in diagnosis. These reflexive behaviors, common to all infants, appear and disappear at predictable times during the course of development. They are involuntary and largely mediated through the brain stem. As infants mature, these motor behaviors are subsumed by higher brain development and become controlled by voluntary movement. Since human development is logical and predictable, the presence of these reflexive motor behaviors past the time when they should no longer be predominant is a strong indicator of brain damage and possible cerebral palsy.

Although it is difficult to predict developmental outcomes in young children with CP, understanding the developmental trajectory of infants and young children assists in implementation of services and interventions (Horovitz & Matson, 2011). Professionals need to work collaboratively with parents for information which will assist in providing optimal treatment. A thorough understanding of available treatments and their efficacy for treating symptoms is needed.

Classification

Cerebral palsy has been classified in several ways, including: (1) type of movement disorder (spastic, dyskinetic, ataxic, and mixed); (2) limb involvement (topographical); and (3) motor limitations and functional abilities (Moreno-De-Luca et al., 2012). The most common form of movement disorder is *spasticity*, which is presumed to occur when there is damage to the cerebral cortex and pyramidal tracts (nerve fibers that originate in the nerve cells in the cerebral cortex and descend to the limbs to provide voluntary control of muscles). In spastic CP, limb muscles contract (tighten) abnormally, resulting in movement that is stiff and jerky. Over time, spastic muscles become shorter and exert differential pull around joints. The result is skeletal deformity, as the limbs, pelvis, and spine become misaligned. The movement disorder of *dyskinesia* is associated with damage in the extrapyramidal tracts (cells in the deep structures of the brain called the basal ganglia).

In dyskinetic CP, purposeful movement is distorted and muscles move randomly and involuntarily, especially in the arms, hands, and face. Movement may range from writhing to jerking to tremor, depending on the type of dyskinesia. Muscle tone may be more normal when the individual is asleep. Finally, *ataxia* is associated with damage in the cerebellum (tissue at the base of the brain that controls balance and coordination). Persons with ataxia may have great difficulty stabilizing their gait, and walk with feet wide apart while holding the arms out for balance. Rarely do these types of cerebral palsy exist in *pure* forms. Frequently, for example, persons have both spasticity and dyskinesia, referred to as mixed CP.

In addition to classification by type of movement disorder, CP also is classified by location of limb involvement, as indicated in Table 1.

Classifying CP by location of damage and quality of movement may not help the practitioner to understand the functional capabilities of persons with CP. Three classification sytems defined by function are the Gross Motor Classification System (GMCS), the Manual Ability Classification System (MACS),

TABLE 1
Classification of Cerebral Palsy by Location (Topography)

Limb Involvement	Description
Monoplegia	Single limb involvement. Uncommon in cerebral palsy.
Paraplegia	Legs only are involved.
Hemiplegia	Limbs on one side of the body are involved. The arm is usually more involved than the leg.
Triplegia	Three limbs are involved, usually both legs and one arm.
Quadriplegia or Tetraplegia	All four limbs are involved. The trunk is often involved.
Diplegia	Greater involvement of the lower limbs than the upper limbs.
Double Hemiplegia	More involvement in the upper limbs than the lower limbs. One side of the body may be more involved than the other.

and the Communication Function Classification System (CFCS). Each system is divided into five levels of mobility, hand/arm use, and communication. These systems have been found to be objective, reliable, and useful for practitioners (Fairhurst, 2012). A synopsis of the systems is provided in Table 2.

Treatment

Persons with cerebral palsy have been the recipients of a variety of medical and therapeutic treatments. These treatments do not *cure* this condition, but are primarily employed to manage symptoms. Because symptoms associated with CP range in severity, location, and form among different persons, treatments may be more useful for some persons than for others. Close communication with health providers, as well as patient and caregiver attention to treatments, ensure the best outcomes.

Medications

Medications are used to treat associated conditions, such as epilepsy or more direct treatment of muscle spasticity. Two of the more recent medications are intramuscular botulinum neurotoxin (BoNT) and intrathecal baclofen (Lioresal). Both medications have been used successfully with children and adults (Zdolsek, Olesch, Antolovich, & Reddihough, 2011).

TABLE 2
Classification of Cerebral Palsy Using the GMCS, MACS, and CFCS

Level	Gross Motor	Manual Ability	Communication Function
I	Walks without limitations	Handles objects easily and successfully; some limitations with manual tasks requiring speed & efficiency	Effective sender & receiver with familiar & unfamiliar communication partners
II	Walks with limitations (long distances & balancing)	Handles most objects but with reduced quality & speed; may avoid some tasks or seek alternative ways to perform	Effective but slower paced sender & receiver with unfamiliar & familiar communication partners
III	Walks using a hand-held mobility device; uses wheelchair for community use	Handles objects with difficulty; needs help to prepare or modify activities	Effective sender & receiver with familiar communication partners
IV	Functions while sitting but self-mobility is limited; may use powered mobility	Handles a limited selection of easily managed objects in adapted situations; needs continuous support	Inconsistent sender & receiver with familiar communication partners
V	Severe head/trunk control limitations; transported using a manual wheelchair	Does not handle objects; severely limited to perform simple actions; requires total assistance	Seldom effective sender & receiver even with familiar communication partners

Botulinum neurotoxins (BoNT) reduces muscle spasticity (Fairhurst, 2012). BoNT is injected into spastic muscles to release tension in the feet, upper limbs, pelvis, and back, which assists in more functional walking and sitting. It is also effective in reducing muscle spasms and migraine, back, knee, pelvic, and foot pain, as well as excessive drooling (Hay & Penn, 2011). Although BoNTs act to relax muscles, the effect is temporary.

Baclofen inhibits spinal reflexes and is administered orally or via a pump that is worn externally or inserted under the skin. Oral Baclofen can result in side effects such as drowsiness, confusion, and nausea, so it is more efficiently and effectively delivered from the pump through a catheter to the cerebral spinal fluid in the lower back (intrathecal Baclofen therapy or IBT). Baclofen has been successful in reducing spasticity in the legs and also improving intelligible speech (Pin, McCartney, Lewis, & Waugh, 2011). "The most common negative side effects have been pump malfunction, catheter displacement, and infection at the pump site or within the central nervous system" (Zdolsek et al., 2011, p. 208).

Surgical Treatments

The goals of surgical intervention are to correct defects, reduce deformity, and increase functionality. A variety of surgical procedures are used to treat symptoms. One neurosurgical procedure is selective dorsal rhizotomy (SDR). Selected nerve rootlets in the lumbar and sacral areas of the back are exposed. After electrical stimulation is applied to elicit muscle response, some rootlets are cut (Fairhurst, 2012). The best candidates for SDR are young persons with lower limb spasticity who have ambulation before surgery. Following surgery, the patient receives physical therapy to maintain the reduced spasticity and improved function. SDR is most successful when it is performed early in life, followed up with intensive physical therapy, and restricted to persons with mild to moderate spasticity (Grunt, Becher, & Vermeullen, 2011).

Orthopedic surgery is complementary to surgical treatment such as IBT or SDR. It is frequently performed to *release* contracted muscles and improve standing and walking, as well as reduce pain, stabilize joints, enhance comfort, and ease caregiver issues (Gormley, 2001). Three fairly common orthopedic procedures illustrate the range of problems addressed by orthopedic surgeons.

Tendon Lengthening

Tendon lengthening involves exposing the tendon and dividing it lengthwise into two halves. The two ends of the cut tendon are then rejoined to create a longer, single tendon. The lengthened tendons reduce the tension of the muscle thus reducing muscle tightness.

Tendon Transfer

In this procedure, the tendon is removed from its point of attachment to the bone. It is then secured to a new site with sutures (stitches).

Osteotomy

This procedure is performed on the femur (thigh bone) to correct alignment. A metal plate and screws are inserted to hold the realigned bone in its new position until it heals. Casting after surgery may or may not be necessary. Once the bone is fully healed - usually nine to 12 months later - the metal plate and screws are removed through the original incision, usually as an outpatient operation. Children are able to walk within two days after plate removal and return to their regular activity level.

Multiple Lower Extremity Procedures

Currently, multiple lower extremity procedures may be performed at one or more locations in the legs (hips, knees, ankles, and feet) and may include any of the above procedures. Benefits of multilevel surgery continue into adulthood.

Surgical management of symptoms of cerebral palsy is complex and has short and long-term effects. Many treatments are complimentary, must be goal-oriented and functional, and should be reasonable, based on such factors as family support and severity of disability (Gormley, 2001). Surgical management is supported with a variety of ongoing therapies to optimize functional outcomes.

Occupational Therapy and Physical Therapy

Occupational and physical therapists work with physicians to facilitate motor development and management. Physical therapists (PT) work to normalize the quality of patient movement through program planning for posture and balance, deformity prevention, and gross motor function, including walking. They work to align the spine, legs, and feet, provide postoperative rehabilitation, assist with physical management at home, and are responsible for fitting and monitoring positioning equipment, braces, prostheses, and casts. Occupational therapists (OT) focus on development of functional skills for performance of activities in daily life. They work on eye-hand coordination skills, use of hands and arms for functional activities such as keyboarding, feeding, and writing; assess and remediate perceptual skills; evaluate the ability to organize and respond to incoming sensory information; and perform prevocational assessments (Best & Bigge, 2010). While physical therapists are more focused on motor abilities in the lower extremities, occupational therapists are focused on abilities in the upper extremities; the disciplines complement each other.

Many systems of treatment have developed in physical and occupational therapy, based on different theories of motor learning (Franki et al., 2012). Two of the most widely recognized approaches are neurodevelopment treatment and sensory motor integration. Neurodevelopment treatment is based on the work of Karel and Bertha Bobath from the 1940s. It features the use of positioning to inhibit inappropriate reflexive movements and enhance postural control. Movement potential is maximized while musculoskeletal complications are reduced. Therapy is applied within the context of functional activities that promote motivation and participation.

Sensory integration was developed by Anna Jean Ayres in the 1970s. It is not designed to teach specific skills but "to improve the child's ability to process and integrate sensory information (visual, auditory, tactile, and kinesthetic) … to allow improved functional capabilities in daily life" (Feferman, Harro, Patel, & Merrick., 2011, p. 335). Children may have dysfunction of sensory-motor integration because they lack normal motor control and therefore do not experience what normal movement *feels like*. Occupational therapists engage children in play activities in a sensory-rich environment to enhance body awareness, stimulate the vestibular system, and support perceptual and fine motor skills.

A critical aspect of therapy support is assessment and use of orthotic devices, which include custom-made braces, splints, and other appliances. Orthotic devices are prescribed after surgery to hold muscles in correct positions and avoid contractures. They also support weak muscles and aid the person in walking. Modern orthotic devices are made of lightweight plastic and can often be worn with regular shoes.

Physical and occupational therapists also assess and recommend equipment for positioning and mobility (Best & Bigge, 2010). This equipment is selected for function, comfort, durability, safety, as well as acceptance by individuals with CP and their families. Equipment to assist with sitting, standing, and lying on the side may be prescribed. Physical therapists assess and recommend mobility equipment, including wheelchairs, walkers, canes, and crutches. Wheelchairs are customized individually and include specialized wheelchairs for street mobility, road racing, and beach use.

Exercise is an area of physical activity that is often limited for persons with CP. It is planned and structured, which differentiates it from general energy expenditure which occurs through walking and other movement. Exercise strengthens muscles, supports physical fitness, and provides opportunities for social interaction. Strength training and aquatic exercise are good forms of exercise. Strength training has enhanced outcomes for walking, running, and jumping (Morton, Brownlee, & McFadyen, 2005). Aquatic exercise is especially appealing because water helps eliminate pressure on joints and reduces the influence of gravity. The resistance offered by water promotes improved outcomes in aerobic activity, muscle strengthening, and toning.

Other Therapies

Many therapies have been used to treat symptoms of CP. Some are not commonly used in the United States, but have gained popularity in other countries. These are categorized as examples of complimentary and alternative medicine (CAM), defined as "a group of diverse medical and health care systems, practices, and products that are not presently considered to be part of conventional medicine" (Weisleder, 2010, p. 7). Complimentary therapies add a therapeutic component to activities that children would otherwise normally perform, like riding a horse, swimming, and skiing. Alternative therapies are separate from traditional therapies and are frequently based on different and "at best, anecdotal evidence and at times unusual ideas of the biology of the condition to which they are being applied" (Rosenbaum, 2003, p. s91). Selected examples of CAM include equine therapy, patterning, conductive education, the Adeli suit, hyperbaric oxygen therapy, and stem cell therapy.

Equine Therapy

Hippotherapy (horse-assisted therapy) works to improve balance, posture, and coordination in persons with CP as they adjust to the movement of the horse beneath them. Riders must keep the head and trunk controlled while astride the horse, and horseback riding provides incentive for these tasks. Several studies have found improvements in muscle symmetry and activity, as well as with walking, running, and jumping (Drnach, O'Brien, & Kreger, 2010; Whalen & Case-Smith, 2012).

Patterning

The premise of patterning is to recapitulate the physiological stages of motor development through exercises, by putting the patient through a series of daily repetitive motor sequences. No studies have confirmed the claims of patterning experts regarding the long-term changes in motor ability (Franki et al., 2012).

Conductive Education

The goal of this therapeutic and educational intervention is enhanced independent functioning through repetitive movements supported by specific verbal guidance by a *conductor*. The combinations of motor repetitions and active cognitive participation, coupled with simple adaptive equipment, makes conductive education an appealing therapy.

Hyperbaric Oxygen Therapy

The assertion of hyperbaric oxygen therapy (HBOT) is that regions of the brain near damaged areas can be *re-activated* with oxygen added in increased concentrations via a hyperbaric chamber (Feferman et al., 2011). HBOT has been successfully used to treat carbon monoxide poisoning, decompression sickness, and infections that receive poor blood supply. Scientific evaluations of this therapy have not resulted in any lasting results other than the positive effect of being involved in clinical trials. However, side effects such as inner ear pain and infections, tumpanic membrane perforation, and even seizures have been observed (Bell, Wallace, Chouinard, Shevell, & Racine, 2011).

Stem Cell Therapy

Stem cells "are naturally occurring cellular elements that retain the capacity to differentiate into various cell lines including neural cells" (Bell et al., 2011). The proposed injection of stem cells to replace lost or damaged neurons is an enticing prospect that has resulted in a proliferation of clinics outside the United States. There is no current evidence of the efficacy of this approach for improving motor performance in persons with CP (Fairhurst, 2012; Feferman et al., 2011). Weisleder (2010) noted that many families turn to CAM when "Western medicine fails to address their needs" (p. 8). The combination of testimonial data and appealing web-based advertising result in continued pressure to resort to many CAM treatments.

Educational and Psychosocial Implications

Early Intervention

Whatever medication, surgical, and therapeutic experiences the child encounters is secondary to the fact that the typical experiences of childhood are necessary for growth and development. Early intervention provides many opportunities for development of the young child with cerebral palsy. Supported by federal law since 1986, early intervention is available for families of infants and young children. It provides opportunities for the child to develop in the domains of gross/fine motor skills, self-care, social/emotional, communication, and cognition. In addition to specific structured activities, many skills in early intervention programs are promoted through play.

Play is a crucial activity that enhances learning in children. Many fine and gross motor skills are practiced and refined during play. Children engage in symbolic play when they *practice* adult activities such as cooking and fantasy play. Play fulfills social needs as children learn to take turns, explore roles, and learn to cooperate. Because it is intrinsically motivating, play is a pleasant activity undertaken for its own value rather than for a particular outcome.

Many children with CP cannot play in typical ways. Their motor impairments prevent them from grasping and manipulating toys. If they have visual or auditory deficits, their interactions with toys is even more limited. The intensity of their motor needs may prevent others from engaging them in play activities. The outcomes of reduced play experiences affect not only the child's motor and cognitive development but reduce the potential for social competence.

Play materials and activities can be effectively adapted for young children. Non-slip mats, Velcro® strips, and magnets can be used to stabilize play materials. Foam padding can be attached to handles or knobs to facilitate grasp. Finally, battery-operated toys can be attached to switches for easier activation (Best, Reed, & Bigge, 2010; Hsieh, 2012).

Assistive Technology in Elementary and Secondary School Programs

In recent years, assistive technology (AT) has opened new worlds of exploration and interactions for children and youth. The Individuals with Disabilities Education Improvement Act (IDEIA) defined assistive technology as "any item, piece of equipment, or product system, whether acquired commercially off the shelf, modified, or customized, that is used to increase, maintain, or improve the functional capabilities of a child with a disability" (20 U.S.C., 1401§ 602[1]). This means that assistive technology can be as simple as a pencil with a thicker handle for easier grasp, a book podium to adjust height and angle of reading materials, or as complex as a computer and its peripheral elements.

Children can learn to operate computer software using switch interface to replace the hand-controlled mouse. A *head mouse* is available that is mounted on spectacles. Head movement controls the cursor, and maintaining the head in a steady position (dwelling) acts to *click* the mouse. Voice-controlled software programs are available for the individual whose speech is adequate but hand use is not.

An exciting variation of environmental control for children and adolescents with CP is virtual reality technology (Gordon, Roopchand-Martin, & Gregg, 2012). Virtual reality technology immerses the child in an experience and allows levels of interaction otherwise prevented by the disability. For example, a child engaged in a virtual reality artistic experience can draw, play paintball or sports, and even play a musical instrument. Active video games can replace sedentary screen activities such as television or internet searching as teaching and rehabilitation tools. "Virtual reality applications have the potential of improving life skills, social participation, mobility, and cognitive abilities, while creating a motivating experience for children with disabilities" (p. 624). In their research, children and adolescents who engaged in virtual reality experiences in sports/games, artistic activities, and technology/computer assisted activities reported increased belief in their ability, creativity, and competence (Gordon et al, 2012).

Psychosocial Implications of Cerebral Palsy

Although breakthroughs in technology have liberated people with CP from some of the constraints of their motor and speech impairments, they remain at risk for reduced self-competence leading to impaired task performance and unsatisfactory social interactions with peers. Individuals with CP and other physical disabilities have been found to show reduced beliefs in their ability to succeed, difficulty determining the factors that contribute to task success or failure, poor response to constructive feedback, and lower task persistence (Varsamis & Agaliotis, 2011). These lower self-attributions are reinforced when tasks cannot be deliberately controlled. In addition, a lack of reciprocated friendships and fewer social behaviors/interactions can lead to social isolation and place the individual at risk for bullying and other forms of victimization.

For children and youth, school provides a venue for implementing social support strategies and boosting self-perceived competence. These include structured disability awareness training for peers and school personnel, direct and firm adult responses to bullying, creation of peer support networks, and greater efforts by teachers for curricular and social integration in school environments (Lindsay & McPherson, 2011). A unique approach for adolescents was the creation of an online social support intervention. Youth with cerebral palsy were able to contact adult mentors with disabilities as well as psychologists through message boards and email. Structured meetings in chat rooms addressed topics including health concerns, bullying, making friends, career planning, recreation and leisure, and relationships (Stewart, Barnfather, Magill-Evans, Ray, & Letourneau, 2011). Participants reported enhanced peer contacts, friendships, social acceptance, self-awareness, family interaction, and reduced loneliness.

Rehabilitation and Vocational Outcomes

Rehabilitation

Persons with cerebral palsy do not acquire their disability as a result of disease, accident, or other experience later in life. Cerebral palsy is a developmental disability, a condition that begins before, during, or shortly after birth or during early childhood. Therefore, the concept of rehabilitation is actually one of *habilitation*, with professionals, family members, and the person focused on maximizing potential physically, intellectually, emotionally, and socially from the time of diagnosis. Previous discussion of medical and therapeutic treatments indicates the need for early intensive intervention. Medical and therapeutic interventions can complicate attainment of an appropriate and complete educational experience. Recuperation from surgeries, therapy sessions, and other necessities such as orthotics evaluations and medication regimens all contribute to lost time from school.

In the educational setting, continuation of occupational and physical therapy services, with additional services such as speech/language therapy and adaptive physical education, may distract the student from academic achievement. Poor preparation of teachers to adequately address the needs of students with CP results in underestimation of academic potential and poor application of critical supports, including assistive technology (AT). Reed and Bowser (2012) noted details for providing appropriate consultation, collaboration, and coaching for integrating AT in schools. A critical aspect of involvement in academic curriculum is meaningful physical access to materials (Best, 2010). For conditions as complex as CP, communication, cooperation, and mutual respect among all parties is necessary to achieve a balanced and successful outcome.

Vocational Potential and Outcomes

Vocational potential for individuals with cerebral palsy is broad and varied. Becoming employed and staying employed is a strong indicator of successful rehabilitation and achievement as adults (Mitchell, Adkins, & Kemp, 2006). Lack of adequate school-based vocational preparation represents an additional hurdle to successful employment. Unfortunately, unproportionately fewer adults with CP are employed than their counterparts who do not have disabilities. When individuals with CP are employed, the rate of employment drops when they are in their 40s. Changes in health status associated with age, increased fatigue, need for medical services, and pain may account for workplace loss (Horsman, Suto, Dudgeon, & Harris, 2010). Persons without a college education had the lowest employment rates throughout their life spans. Unfortunately, disability entitlements (Social Security, Medicare) received by non-working persons with disabilities may eclipse the wage rate for unskilled employment. In addition, lower paying jobs are more physical in nature and often not possible for persons with CP. Maintaining people in the workplace should include knowledge about age-related physical changes, anticipation of changes with appropriate accommodations, and improved workplace and job efficiency (Mitchell et al., 2006).

Research on disability and employment strongly suggests that higher education can do much to mediate the factors that result in early employment loss (Mitchell et al., 2006). In addition, continued therapy that focuses on upper extremity function, self-care, and social skills was positively related to higher levels of enrollment in post-secondary programs. Implementation of supported employment programs for individuals with CP and cognitive impairment is a positive addition to school programs (Clark, Bigge, & Best, 2010).

Interactions among educational personnel and adult service delivery systems can assist with transition to work and other aspects of adult living. These interactions often occur in formal meetings such as those to evaluate the Individual Education Program (IEP) and Individual Transition Program (ITP) while the individual is still in school. Connections to Departments of Rehabilitation, post-secondary vocational training programs, and job placement services can be instituted. Carryover of services that aid in daily living, such as transportation, equipment provision and maintenance, leisure activities, and health care, must be maintained even when the person shifts from school to community and state agency support (Clark et al., 2010). In all these service areas, adolescents with CP and their family members state that caring and supportive professionals, clear communication and readily available information, reduced struggle for services, and awareness of the needs created by disability were the strongest indicators of satisfaction with service delivery.

Unfortunately, an individual with cerebral palsy may be judged more on physical appearance and motor limitations than either intellectual potential or vocational motivation. Although cognitive limitations frequently accompany CP, they are not synonymous conditions. Severity of CP is not a predictor of intellectual ability or limitation. While physical barriers can be eliminated through legislation and its enforcement, attitude is more difficult to manage. Tangible benefits can be derived from hiring a person with CP that far outweigh the effort to provide accommodations. The key lies in believing that the individual can make a valuable workplace contribution.

Important re-adjustment in attitude is one that places responsibility for making accommodations within the community, rather than viewing the person with CP as someone who needs to *meet the challenge* of disability. Incorporating concepts such as universal design into living, education, and work spaces is one example of adaptation that meets the physical needs of all persons, including persons with CP. When all people benefit from physical barrier reduction, such as incorporation of ramps, elevators, and other devices into physical structures, or less tangible accommodations such as flexible work schedules and cyber-commuting, the partition between persons with disabilities and those without disabilities is removed. The concept of universal design needs to be accompanied by services that are individualized and flexible to make a best fit between the individual and the work environment (Darrah, Magill-Evans, & Galambos, 2010).

Assistive Technology

The role of AT in providing educational and vocational access is clear. Within the broad arena of AT is a sub-category known as augmentative and alternative communication (AAC). AAC attempts to compensate, either temporarily or permanently, for the impairment and disability patterns of individuals with severe expressive communication disorders. It can augment speech that is present but difficult to understand or be an alternative for speech that is absent. AAC is a revolutionary breakthrough for persons who previously were unable to express their thoughts and feelings. These systems can be simple, such as two-dimensional picture-based communication boards that are accessed by pointing. It can be complex electronic, dedicated communication devices that store and retrieve entire messages and output them through synthesized voice. These high tech devices frequently interface with computers. The current communication possibilities with AAC are significant (Best et al., 2010).

Persons who use AAC face unique issues of employment and co-worker interaction. Discussion with a group of AAC users who were fully employed in competitive job situations included three themes: (1) barriers to employment; (2) necessary supports for employment; and (3) recommendations for improving employment outcomes for persons who use AAC. Barriers to employment activities include negative attitudes of others, poor educational attainment, lack of technological training, policy and funding shortfalls, inadequate personal care/support services, and problems with transportation. Supports for employment include the user's personal characteristics, education, work experience, family assistance for transportation and personal care, ability to use technology, the presence of workplace mentors, and legislative supports, such as the Americans with Disabilities Act (ADA).

Both AT and AAC are specifically legislated rights for children with disabilities through the Technology-Related Assistance for Individuals with Disabilities Act (also called the Tech Act Amendments of 2000) and the Individuals with Disabilities Education Act of 2000. The ADA (1990) and Section 504 of the Rehabilitation Act of 1973 can be used to support AT and AAC equipment and services for adults. Many avenues of funding exist for the assessment and purchase of AAC systems. Children may be eligible through their school, therapy providers, or private insurance, while adults can work with state rehabilitation agencies.

Quality of Life

Quality of life encompasses the opportunity to be an active part of one's community and engage in interactions crucial to personal well-being (Best, 2010). In addition to objective factors such as physical health and material security, it includes subjective factors such as personal satisfaction and feelings of competence and empowerment.

Like anyone else, persons with cerebral palsy have interests in life fulfillment beyond a good education and employment satisfaction. Attainment and maintenance of physical and material well-being, social relations, participation in community and civic activities, personal development and fulfillment, and recreation all indicate good life quality (Best, 2010). These more inclusive outcomes should be the goal for educators, rehabilitation counselors, and other professionals who assist persons with CP to reach their full potential.

Case Study

Justin is a 20 year-old male who graduated from high school last year. At two years of age, he was diagnosed with cerebral palsy. The CP involvement was later diagnosed as quadriplegia (involving all four limbs), and Level IV on the Gross Motor Classification System. In his early years of school, Justin was enrolled in a special class for students with orthopedic impairments. During the four years from kindergarten through third grade, Justin was frequently hospitalized for respiratory problems and other illnesses associated with his physical impairments. This led to him falling increasingly further behind in school. While he was not unhappy in the environment, his parents felt that Justin would be challenged to excel at a higher level, both academically and socially, if he were transferred to general education classes with his non-disabled peers. His teachers agreed.

From the third grade (which he repeated) until graduation from high school, Justin was included in age-appropriate general education classes with support from special education. Primarily, Justin's special education support involved the provision of physical therapy to assist him in increasing his mobility, and speech and language therapy using augmentative communication devices to help in developing communication skills. Special education teachers provided assistance in developing computer skills and helping him learn to use special switches, as well as other assistive technology to access his computer and thus, the academic curriculum.

Despite undergoing numerous surgical procedures (thereby missing school) as part of the orthopedic management of his contractures and deformities related to cerebral palsy, Justin maintained average achievement from elementary through high school. Since elementary school, Justin has been non-ambulatory and has used a motorized wheelchair. The wheelchair has a special tray designed to carry a lap top computer. With support from a paraprofessional assistant who helps him with personal care and eating, Justin is able to perform all the learning activities required in school.

Justin is sure he will be able to succeed in the world of work. His goal is to obtain a job in the computer field and work while attending university classes part-time until he graduates with a degree in computer science. Using several different assistive technology devices, Justin has developed a high level of proficiency with the computer. Throughout school, he was a member of a group of young men and women who frequently met during high school to play computer games. Justin not only excelled at these games but was able to alter many of them to make them more challenging and entertaining.

In the past year, one of Justin's friends from the group found a position with a computer game manufacturer as a programmer in research and development. This friend assured Justin that the company would be interested in hiring him also. The pay is excellent and includes benefits; Justin feels that he is even more knowledgeable than his friend in this particular area. He could not think of a single reason not to seek employment with this company – until he spoke to his parents.

His parents explained that, while they wanted to join in his excitement, they were concerned that Justin complete college before becoming employed. They reminded him that technology is developing at a phenomenal pace and many technology companies are unable to keep pace and have layoffs or declare bankruptcy. Without a college degree, Justin could find himself out of work with no prospects for finding another job. They asked him if he knew the expectations of the company for work output and whether they expect employees to be able to work at a certain pace.

Justin is sure of what he wants to do. The Americans with Disabilities Act provides some workplace protections against discrimination based on disability and Justin is aware of this. Although he respects his parents and knows they have his best interests at heart, he believes this job is an opportunity of a lifetime. Justin reached a compromise with his parents by agreeing to speak to his rehabilitation counselor at the Department of Rehabilitation and seek the counselor's advice. Both Justin and his parents agreed to seriously consider the counselor's ideas.

Questions

1. The vocational rehabilitation counselor needs to have basic information about the client to recommend a realistic vocational goal. Identify this information.
2. As the counselor, identify how you will handle the dilemma regarding Justin's potential job and his completion of college.
3. Are the career goals of Justin and those of his parents realistic and compatible with his capabilities and limitations?
4. Identify other possibilities for Justin as a client of the Department of Rehabilitation.
5. What obstacles to employment may Justin encounter? How limiting is his disability and society's perception of him, including potential employers? Include a discussion of the concept of a *disabling environment*.

References

Bell, E., Wallace, T., Chouinard, I., Shevell, M., & Racine, E. (2011). Responding to requests of families for unproven interventions for neurodevelopmental disorders: Hyperbaric oxygen "treatment" and stem cell "therapy" in cerebral palsy. *Developmental Disabilities Research, 17*, 19–26.

Best, S. J. (2010). Understanding individuals with physical, health, and multiple disabilities. In S. J. Best, K. W. Heller, & J. L. Bigge, *Teaching individuals with physical or multiple disabilities* (6th ed., pp. 3–31). Upper Saddle River, NJ: Pearson.

Best, S. J., & Bigge, J. L. (2010). Cerebral palsy. In S. J. Best, K. W. Heller, & J. L. Bigge. *Teaching individuals with physical or multiple disabilities* (6th ed., pp. 59–81). Upper Saddle River, NJ: Pearson.

Best, S. J., Reed, P., & Bigge, J. L. (2010). Assistive technology. In S. J. Best, K. W. Heller, & J. L. Bigge. *Teaching individuals with physical or multiple disabilities* (6th ed., pp. 175–220). Upper Saddle River, NJ: Pearson.

Clark, G. M., Bigge, J. L., & Best, S. J. (2010). Self-determination and education for transition. In S. J. Best, K. W. Heller, & J. L. Bigge. *Teaching individuals with physical or multiple disabilities* (6th ed., pp. 342–372). Upper Saddle River, NJ: Pearson.

Darrah, J., Magill-Evans, J., & Galambos, N. L. (2010). Community services for young adults with motor disabilities – Paradox. *Disability and Rehabilitation, 32*(3), 223–229.

Drnach, M., O'Brien, P. A., & Kreger, A. (2010). The effects of a 5-week therapeutic horseback riding program on gross motor function in a child with cerebral palsy: A case study. *Journal of Alternative and Complimentary Therapy, 16*(9), 1003–1006.

Fairhurst, C. (2012). Cerebral palsy: The whys and hows. *Archives of Disease in Childhood, 97*(4), 122–131.

Feferman, H., Harro, J., Patel, D. R., & Merrick, J. (2011). Therapeutic interventions in cerebral palsy. *International Journal of Child and Adolescence Health, 4*(4), 333–339.

Franki, I., Desloovere, K., DeCat, J., Feys, H., Molenaers, G., Calders, P., . . . Van den Broeck, C. (2012). The evidence base for conceptual approaches and additional therapies targeting lower limb function in children with cerebral palsy: A systematic review using the International Classification of Functioning, Disability, and Health as a framework. *Journal of Rehabilitation Medicine, 44*, 396–405.

Gladstone, M. (2010). A review of the incidence and prevalence, types, and aetiology of childhood cerebral palsy in resource-poor countries. *Annals of Tropical Paediatrics, 30*, 181–196.

Gordon, C., Roopchand-Martin, S., & Gregg, A. (2012). Potential of the Nintendo Wii™ as a rehabilitation tool for children with cerebral palsy in a developing country: A pilot study. *Physiotherapy, 98*, 238–242.

Gormley, M. E., Jr. (2001). Treatment of neuromuscular and musculoskeletal problems in cerebral palsy. *Pediatric Rehabilitation, 4*(1), 5–16.

Grunt, S., Becher, J. G., & Vermeullen, R. J. (2011). Long-term outcome and adverse effects of selective dorsal rhizotomy in children with cerebral palsy: A systematic review. *Developmental Medicine and Child Neurology, 53*(6), 490–498.

Hamilton, S. (2006). Screening for developmental delay: Reliable, easy-to-use tools. *Journal of Family Practice, 55*(5), 415–422.

Hay, N., & Penn, C. (2011). Botox® to reduce drooling in a paediatric population with neurological impairments: A Phase I study. *International Journal of Language and Communication Disorders, 54*(5), 550–563.

Hirsh, A. T., Gallegos, J. C., Gertz, K. J., Engel, J. M., & Jensen, M. P. (2010). Symptom burden in individuals with cerebral palsy. *Journal of Rehabilitation Research and Development, 47*(9), 863–875.

Horovitz, M., & Matson, J. L. (2011). Developmental milestones in toddlers with atypical development. *Research in Developmental Disabilities, 32*, 2278–2282.

Horsman, M., Suto, M., Dudgeon, B., & Harris, S. R. (2010). Ageing with cerebral palsy: Psychosocial issues. *Age and Aging, 39*, 294–299.

Hsieh, H-C. (2012). Effectiveness of adaptive pretend play on affective expression and imagination of children with cerebral palsy. *Research in Developmental Disabilities, 33*, 1975–1983.

Hvidtjørn, D., Grove, J., Schendel, D., Svaerke, C., Schieve, L. A., Uldall, P., . . . Thorsen, P. (2010). Multiclicity and early gestational age contribute to an increased risk of cerebral palsy from assisted conception: A population-based cohort study. *Human Reproduction, 25*(8), 2115–2123.

Lindsay, S., & McPherson, A. C. (2011). Strategies for improving disability awareness and social inclusion of children and young people with cerebral palsy. *Child: Care, Health, and Development, 38*(6), 809–816.

Mitchell, J. M., Adkins, R. H., & Kemp, B. J. (2006). The effects of aging on employment of people with and without disabilities. *Rehabilitation Counseling Bulletin, 49*(3), 157–165.

Moreno-De-Luca, A., Ledbetter, D. H., & Martin, C. L. (2012). Genetic insights into the causes and classification of the cerebral palsies. *Lancet, 11*, 283–292.

Morton, J. F., Brownlee, M., & McFadyen, A. K. (2005). The effects of progressive resistance training for children with cerebral palsy. *Clinical Rehabilitation, 19*(3), 283–289.

Pin, T. W., McCartney, L., Lewis, J., & Waugh, M. C. (2011). Use of intrathecal baclofen therapy in ambulant children and adolescents with spasticity and dystonia of cerebral origin: A systematic review. *Developmental Medicine and Child Neurology, 53*(10), 885–895.

Reed, P., & Bowser, G. (2012). Consultation, collaboration, and coaching: Essential techniques for integrating assistive technology use in schools and early intervention programs. *Journal of Occupational Therapy, Schools, and Early Intervention, 5*, 15–30.

Rosenbaum, P. L. (2003). Controversial treatment of spasticity: Exploring alternate therapies for motor function in children with cerebral palsy. *Journal of Child Neurology, 18*(9), s89–s94.

Squier, W. (2011). The "Shaken Baby" syndrome: Pathology and mechanisms. *Acta Neuropathology, 122,* 519–542.

Stewart, M., Barnfather, A., Magill-Evans, J., Ray, L., & Letourneau, N. (2011). Brief report: An online support intervention: Perceptions of adolescents with physical disabilities. *Journal of Adolescence, 34,* 795–800.

Varsamis, P., & Agaliotis, I. (2011). Profiles of self-concept, goal orientation, and self-regulation in students with physical, intellectual, and multiple disabilities: Implications for instructional support. *Research in Developmental Disabilities, 32,* 1548–1555.

Weber, P., & Jenni, O. (2012). Screening in child health: Studies of the efficacy and relevance of preventative care practices. *Deutsches Ärzteblatt International, 109*(24), 431–435.

Weisleder, P. (2010). Unethical prescriptions: Alternative therapies for children with cerebral palsy. *Clinical Pediatrics, 49*(1), 7–11.

Whalen, C. N., & Case-Smith, J. (2012). Therapeutic effects of horseback riding therapy on gross motor function in children with cerebral palsy: A systematic review. *Physical and Occupational Therapy in Pediatrics, 32*(3), 229–242.

Zdolsek, H. A., Olesch, C., Antolovich, G., & Reddihough, D. (2011). Intrathecal baclofen therapy: Benefits and complications. *Journal of Intellectual and Developmental Disability, 36*(3), 207–213.

About the Author

Dr. Sherwood J. Best is Professor and Coordinator of the program for Physical and Health Impairments at California State University, Los Angeles. Dr. Best has presented at many local, state, and national professional conferences, and is Past-President of the National Division for Physical and Health Disabilities (DPHD) of the Council for Exceptional Children and the California Association for Physical and Health Impairments (CAPHI). The seventh edition of her textbook for teaching individuals with physical, health, and multiple disabilities was published in 2014.

Chapter 18

MUSCULAR DYSTROPHY

Roy K. Chen, Ph.D., C.R.C.

Introduction

Muscular dystrophy (MD) is a group of over 40 forms of neuromuscular diseases and related myopathies. Persons with MD differ in terms of age of onset, etiology, severity of progression, locations of muscles affected, and mode of inheritance (Bushby, 2011; Shannon, 2004). A common characteristic present in the wide array of neuromuscular disorders is the gradual weakening of the skeletal muscles that control voluntary movements. Despite recent advances in the molecular diagnosis of defective genes and the continuing breakthroughs in curative treatments over the last decade, MD remains an incurable disease. This disabling illness impacts quality of life for people affected by it, along with their families. Ouyang, Grosse, and Kenneson (2008) calculated the average medical expenditures for individuals with MD and found their costs to be 10 to 20 times higher than for individuals without MD. In addition to learning to cope with the functional limitations associated with this progressively deteriorating physical condition, these individuals encounter attitudinal and architectural barriers to living independently and obtaining gainful employment. Collectively, they experience higher unemployment and underemployment rates, as well as a lower acceptance rate for vocational rehabilitation counseling services than those with other disabilities (Fowler et al., 1997). There is an urgent need to improve the effectiveness of rehabilitation services provided for clients with MD.

The purpose of this chapter is to review clinical and psychosocial aspects involving MD and to offer suggestions for developing and implementing rehabilitation plans for adults with MD from a holistic perspective. This holistic approach includes addressing the disability (functional limitations and capabilities), psychological and emotional factors, education, vocational histories, social resources, and belief systems. Through the use of a holistic approach, counselors can help clients maximize their potential for rehabilitation.

Prevalence of Muscular Dystrophy

Although no exact incidence figures for persons with MD are available, based on the 2005 world population (6 billion, 451 million people) and the prevalence of neuromuscular disorders, it is estimated that there are at least 1.26 million children and adults with MD worldwide. In the United States, more than 250,000 Americans have been diagnosed with one of the 40 types of MD (Centers for Disease Control and Prevention [CDC], 2012); about two-thirds of them are children (Siegel, 1999). Premature death among children with Duchenne MD (DMD) is common. These individuals rarely live past their second decade of life due to the irreversible and continuous weakening of involuntary muscles affecting various body systems and organs such as in the cardiovascular system, pulmonary system, and gastrointestinal system.

The American public tends to view MD as a disease affecting only children, in part due to the huge success of the annual Muscular Dystrophy Association (MDA) Jerry Lewis Telethon held on Labor Day. While it is commendable of Jerry's *poster boys and girls* and their parents to come forth on national television in an effort to share their courageous personal stories and to ask viewers for financial support, adults with MD often go unnoticed. There are several reasons why adults with MD as a group fail to generate strong public interest. First, the debilitating physical condition impedes many people with MD from actively participating in and organizing grass roots support groups. Mobility and transportation difficulties present major challenges for persons who do not drive. Children with MD experience a reduced life expectancy; consequently, the number of persons declines as age advances.

Based on the estimate provided by Shannon (2004), the total number of adult Americans with MD is about 83,000 – a number far fewer than the number of people with AIDS, visual impairments, or psychiatric disabilities. Additionally, due to the onset of disability, the education of children with MD is often interrupted by frequent hospitalizations and a decline in general health. Consequently, people with MD do not always have the necessary education and vocational training to assume leadership positions in professional fields. There are no prominent public figures or celebrities with MD to advocate for the cause and rights of this community. Michael J. Fox and Mohammed Ali are high profile spokespersons for Parkinson's Disease. Christopher Reeves was the charismatic ambassador for people with spinal cord injuries. Elton John is a steadfast ally for AIDS/HIV. The Kennedy family has been a long-time crusader for people with developmental disabilities. There is an absence of strong political representation for MD to facilitate advocacy for greater medical research funding.

Major Types of Muscular Dystrophy

The three most common procedures used by physicians to confirm the presence of MD are blood testing, electromyography (EMG), and biopsy (Alexianu & Gooch, 2004). The first two procedures are non-invasive while the third is an invasive procedure. MD is a taxonomy of several types of hereditary, mostly X chromosome-linked, progressive muscular disorders characterized by gradual degeneration and wasting away of the muscle cells and fibers (Siegel, 1999). The subsequent discussion will examine some of the most commonly seen types.

Duchenne Muscular Dystrophy (DMD)

DMD, named after French physician Guillaume Duchenne de Boulogne, is by far the most common and severe form of MD (Shannon, 2004). DMD occurs in about 1 out of every 1,500 to 6,000 male infants (CDC, 2012). The average onset of the disability is between two and five years of age. Most children diagnosed with DMD lose their ambulatory function during elementary school. Early signs of the disease include frequent falls and difficulty running, trouble changing from a squatting or sitting position, and problems climbing stairs. Initial weakness occurs in proximal muscles – particularly in the hips and shoulders. In contrast to the atrophy of muscles, enlargement of the calf muscles, a sign of pseudo hypertrophy, may occur. A significant number of children do not survive into adulthood (age 20) due to the failure of respiratory and cardiac muscles. Like the wide range of intelligence levels exhibited in the general population, people with MD vary in their cognitive abilities. However, researchers have no explanation as to why people with DMD tend to have lower intelligence scores compared to people with other types of MD (McDonald et al., 1995a; Ouyang, Grosse, Fox, & Bolen, 2012). Reading disability due to poor simultaneous and sequential information processing has been observed in children (Hendriksen & Vles, 2006).

Becker Muscular Dystrophy (BMD)

In 1956, Peter Emil Becker, a German physician, was the first person to recognize this mild, variant form of DMD. The clinical presentations of BMD are similar to that of DMD. However, the time of initial diagnosis usually appears much later (as late as 25 years of age) and has a slower rate of muscle deterioration (Shannon, 2004). BMD occurs in about 1 out of every 18,500 male births (CDC, 2012). The absence of a vital protein surrounding muscle fiber called dystrophin distinguishes DMD from BMD. Dystrophin is needed to allow muscle cells to work properly. The dystrophin produced in people with BMD is often inadequate and of poor quality. As with people with DMD, the body simply fails to manufacture this protein. Muscle weakness begins in the lower extremities and gradually includes the upper body. Due to the late onset of the disease, individuals with BMD often ambulate until about age 30. The major risk in BMD is from cardiac, as opposed to pulmonary complications (McDonald et al., 1995b). Death can occur in the 20s or 30s, yet some patients live beyond this age range. Persons with BMD have longer life expectancies than those who have DMD.

Facioscapulohumeral Muscular Dystrophy (FSHMD)

Face, shoulders, and upper arms are the three groups of musculature affected by FSHDM. It is characterized by persons having difficulty raising the arms, closing the eyelids, sucking from a straw, and swallowing food. Speech may become indistinct if facial muscles continue to weaken. FSHMD affects both sexes and its usual onset is between the ages of 20 and 30. Yet, these persons are expected to have near-normal life expectancies. The prevalence of FSHMD is 1 in 20,000 births (U.S. National Library of Medicine, 2009). As one of the least threatening forms of MD, this disease does not affect pulmonary and cardiac functions. Because the severity is mild in comparison to DMD and LGMD, most people do not develop pelvic muscle problems and retain the ability to walk throughout their lives (Chen & Crewe, 2009).

Limb-Girdle Muscular Dystrophy (LGMD)

The prevalence of LGMD is estimated to be 20 to 40 per million people (Shannon, 2004). Shoulder and pelvic girdle muscles are the primary areas affected by LGMD, which occurs in both sexes. These individuals have weakness in their proximal muscles with a moderate rate of deterioration and the onset of disability occurring in late adolescence or early adulthood. The typical pattern of muscle deterioration begins in the hip girdle and moves toward the arms and shoulders. Weakness in the legs advances more rapidly than in the arms because lower extremities bear more stress from their constant involvement in maintaining posture. In all cases, people who contract LGMD will lose their ability to ambulate and require the use of wheelchairs. Life expectancy is somewhat reduced.

Autosomal diseases like LGMD are characterized by gene mutations in any of the first 22 pairs of non-sex-determining autosomal chromosomes (Mathews, 2003). The diagnosis is generally classified as either an autosomal dominant form (LGMD 1) or autosomal recessive form (LGMD 2). A person with an autosomal dominant disorder usually has one parent who carries mutated genes. Someone with an autosomal recessive disorder has two unaffected parents each carrying defective genes.

Myotonic Muscular Dystrophy (MMD)

The most prominent difference between MMD and other types of MD is that the distal muscles instead of the proximal muscles are the first to be affected. A major characteristic symptom is the delay in timed motor performance. Persons with MMD lack strong small muscles in their hands and have difficulty relaxing a handgrip. Due to stiffness in their hands, it takes them longer to let go of an object. The onset of disability ranges from early childhood to adulthood. MMD has an estimated prevalence of 1 in 8,000 people, similarly affecting males and females (Yu, Blankenship, Yang, & Lee, 2006; U.S. National Library of Medicine, 2010). Noticeable muscle deterioration in the neck and face, forearms and lower legs, cardiac dysrhythmias, endocrine problems, frontal baldness, and cataracts of the eyes are common complications. The severity of this condition increases from one generation to the next (Emery, 1994). Children with MMD who inherit genetic defects show far more serious conditions than their affected parents.

Functional Limitations

In 2012, 17.8% of individuals with disabilities were employed compared to 63.9% for persons without disabilities (U.S. Bureau of Labor Statistics, 2013). Rehabilitation counselors may encounter difficulty pinpointing functional limitations associated with MD because there is no uniform symptom presentation and severity experienced (Chen & Crewe, 2009). Depending on the type of MD, its affect on quality of life varies. Counselors need to evaluate each client individually, as these muscular diseases vary greatly in terms of their symptoms, complications, limitations, and progression. Swenson (2000) suggested examining a client's functional capacity in the following areas: cognitive, social, physical, vocational, and emotional.

Cognitive Functioning

There is lack of consensus regarding cognitive deficits in people with DMD. Studies have shown that lower intelligence is a manifestation (McDonald et al., 1995a; Ogasawara, 1989). However, some investigators have argued that the correlation between low intelligence levels and the presence of DMD is a consequence of experiential conditions (insufficient early education due to illness) rather than being an inherent nature of the disorder. Mean intelligence scores of people with LGMD and FSHMD measured by full scale IQ did not significantly differ from the general population (Kilmer et al., 1995; McDonald et al., 1995c).

Social Functioning

Quality of social interaction suggests a person's capability to interact with the environment. People with pleasing physiques often have higher self-esteem and egos because they have been receiving praise since an early age. Freud (1963) believed that body image is formed in conjunction with the development of the ego, and interpersonal relationships are reflections of body attitude. Because people have an inborn urge to establish kinship with others, rejection can inflict major consequences, such as developing feelings of worthiness. Disability alters not only physical functioning but also reciprocity of human actions and reactions (Marini, Chen, Feist, Flores-Torres, & Castillo, 2011). Walkers, wheelchairs, respiratory ventilators, and other assistive devices often evoke discomfort and fear in others. Not wanting to cause embarrassment or not knowing how to respond to the person's altered physical status, friends and associates may be hesitant regarding how to interact appropriately (Brodwin & Chen, 2000). Opportunities for casual friendly gatherings and dating are diminished due to architectural barriers and unavailability of transportation (Miller, Chen, Graf, & Kranz, 2009).

Physical and Vocational Functioning

Limited range of motion in the upper and lower extremities is a common complication with LGMD, FSHMD, and MMD. The occurrence of muscle contractures in the legs and heels, due to the shortening of muscle fibers and fibrosis of connective tissues, limit ambulatory function (Emery, 1994). In most cases, hand function is maintained long after leg function ceases. Raising the arms above shoulder level and lifting the feet off the ground becomes difficult, however. Buttoning shirts, twisting jar tops, and gripping pens pose difficulties as a result of loss of gross and fine motor movements. As muscles grow weaker, personal attendant care may be needed for personal hygiene and dressing. Lifting, carrying, and walking on uneven surfaces may not be possible and can require accommodation at the worksite. Clients with dystrophy affecting their hips and joints tend to find squatting and kneeling positions difficult or impossible. Fatigue and physical exhaustion occasionally interrupt workflow for brief moments, and people with MD often require short rest breaks to replenish their energy levels.

Emotional Functioning

To revert from a self-reliant person to a dependent person needing assistance is traumatic and emotionally painful. Role reversal inflicts emotional distress. Physical inadequacy produces self-doubts as adults with late onset MD try to come to terms with the reality that functional losses are inevitable and progressive. Having MD greatly impacts self-identity. It is not unusual for someone who has been performing a job for years to lose the identity associated with that profession when he or she is no longer able to perform the work. The self-perception of people with MD varies in accordance with the status of their ever-changing physical condition. Positive and negative moods oscillate with the struggle to deal with stresses.

Employment Profiles for Persons with Muscular Dystrophy

Of the 54 million Americans with disabilities, 26 million of them have severe disabilities (Roessler & Rubin, 2006). Evidence has shown that disability has a negative effect on employment prospects and earnings among persons in the disabled community. Between 2008 and 2010, individuals without disabilities were three times more likely to be employed than individuals with disabilities. Individuals with disabilities account for 9.4 million, only 6% of the civilian workforce (U.S. Census Bureau, 2013). The median monthly earnings for nondisabled male workers between the ages of 21 to 64 are $2,724, compared to $1,961 among those with severe disabilities (Brault, 2012). Not surprisingly, people with neuromuscular diseases frequently are near the bottom level of income (Wevers, Brouwer, Padberg, & Nijboer, 1993). There are several reasons for the disproportionate numbers of people with disabilities and why they are unrepresented in the workforce. The ensuing paragraph will discuss those reasons from the perspectives of both clients and rehabilitation providers.

Education has long been regarded as a necessary requisite for entry into the labor force. Chronic medical conditions often create insurmountable obstacles for receiving the quality education needed in today's labor market. The increasing emphasis on strong communication skills and computer literacy will close windows of opportunity for those who are not prepared. Inadequate job preparation due to insufficient education is of great concern to counselors. About 40% of people with disabilities never finish high school and 69% never attend college (Harris, cited in Mackelprang & Salsgiver, 1999). Another factor that affects employment level is the type of MD. In a study of employment status of rehabilitation clients with MD, Fowler and his colleagues (1997) found a significant difference in employment across MD types. Specifically, 49% of individuals with BMD and FSHD were employed at the time of the survey, compared to 26% of LGMD patients, and 31% of people of those with MMD.

A perceived inability to perform tasks engenders a sense of low self-esteem for people with MD. Consequently, such persons may develop unfounded fears regarding failure and either not seek employment or become easily discouraged during their job search. The Supreme Court's rulings in favor of employers in job discrimination trials have discouraged many individuals with disabilities and their advocates from searching for work. Such pessimistic views were corroborated by Chen and Crewe's (2009) study in which they found people with neuromuscular diseases and neurological diseases had little confidence in what legal protection the 1990 Americans with Disabilities Act provides to defend their rights to employment.

The unfamiliarity with MD among rehabilitation service providers decreases the referral and acceptance rates for vocational rehabilitation services. Rehabilitation counselors at state agencies generally do not possess sufficient working knowledge regarding MD, which in turn has led to a higher denial rate for services (Fowler et al., 1997). Due to the unpredictability of the pace of deterioration in MD, counselors may see questionable or little vocational potential. These negative attitudes inevitably produce unsatisfactory rehabilitation outcomes. It is, therefore, understandable that people with MD underutilize rehabilitation services.

Holistic Interventions

To increase rehabilitation efficacy, counselors must distinguish the type of MD when developing vocational plans with their clients. It is a great disservice to clients if rehabilitation counselors lay out generic plans without regard to the nature of MD. Due to shortened life expectancy and progressive deterioration, mapping out a long-term career plan for clients with this dease will not always be realistic or practical. The complex nature of MD makes it difficult for counselors to understand the general well-being of these clients. A multidisciplinary team approach draws on expertise from different professionals, such as occupational therapists, psychologists, neurologists, physical therapists, counselors, and orthopedists. Bartalos (1990) identified key areas of quality of life that are of great concern to people with neuromuscular disorders: physical symptoms, medical complications, functional limitations, emotional symptoms, interpersonal relations, work adjustment, leisure activities, and sexual function. The following section suggests interventions to ameliorate the debilitating effects of MD.

Psychosocial Counseling Considerations

Clinicians have long believed that persons with MD go through stages of emotional distress similar to persons faced with dying, as described by Dr. Elizabeth Kubler-Ross. These stages include denial, anger, bargaining, depression, and eventual acceptance (Emery, 1994). When considering stage theories, one needs to keep in mind that no two people react in the same way to the diagnosis of a severely disabling condition, nor is progression through the stages necessarily linear. Adaptation to disability is not time-limited. Rather, it is an ongoing lifelong developmental process.

Rehabilitation clients with MD face loss of mobility, reduced opportunities for employment, changes in living arrangements, and diminished social interaction. Clients with these conditions are at high risk for mental health issues; depression is a common problem among people with neuromuscular diseases (Fowler et al., 1997). In addition to social stigma, environmental restrictions, such as architectural barriers, unfriendly terrain, and lack of availability of suitable means of transportation further impede persons with MD from establishing meaningful relationships with others (Chen, Miller, Seo, & Mendoza, 2010).

To improve self-esteem and self-concept for people with disabilities, counselors must listen to their clients' problems with empathy and provide encouragement and support. In a multicultural society like the United States, people practice different religions and beliefs to draw upon sources of power to sustain psychological growth. Spiritual well-being is positively correlated with life satisfaction (Chen & Crewe, 2009). Counselors need sensitivity toward unfamiliar religious beliefs. Because the impact of disability influences the lives of clients and their families, counseling outcomes will be more positive if the healing process invites nondisabled family members to share their own views and expectations.

Vocational Counseling

Formulating feasible vocational objectives requires collaborative efforts between clients and counselors. In addition to teaching job search and interviewing skills, counselors need a thorough understanding of their clients' functional capabilities. Without knowing the functional limitations, it is difficult to match clients' physical exertion levels with jobs they can perform. Counselors can take a proactive approach to educating prospective employers about neuromuscular diseases and recommend accommodations. Hicks (1998) suggested several adaptive techniques and mobility devices to help people with MD increase functional capacities. For example, using an elevated seat cushion or a high stool can help a client get on a chair more easily, rather than having to sit on the edge of a chair and rock back and forth, or push up on their thighs or chair arms to stand.

American society measures success by one's earning power and job status. Holding gainful employment is a way to earn peer respect and command social acceptance and high regard. Myths regarding people with disabilities and unwarranted fears of increases in medical insurance costs can dissuade prospective employers from considering hiring qualified job candidates with MD. Self-employment empowers clients by providing financial independence. Another advantage of being one's own boss is the flexibility of arranging convenient work hours. While self-employment presents a viable alternative for some rehabilitation clients to secure financial security and independence, it is by no means a decision to be made casually in light of the high business failure rate of new entrants. Counselors can consult with their local Small Business Administration (SBA) to evaluate a client's prior work experience, level of educational attainment, complexity of business, technical training, and availability of start-up business financing capital before contemplating this challenging vocational route.

As the business world continues to increase the use of telecommunication and computer technology, the traditional work setting of an office environment is no longer the only option. Electronic transmission via the Internet may be a viable alternative. For those clients who prefer to use personal transportation or for whom telecommunication is not feasible, rehabilitation counselors can direct their clients to contact special driving schools for individuals with disabilities and to locate engineers who perform vehicle modifications. In addition, major automobile manufacturers can provide financial assistance for clients with disabilities to modify their new vehicles. Having accessible transportation is crucial for employment.

Medical Counseling Considerations

Obesity is an issue that tends to be overlooked by many people, including clients with MD. Slow metabolism coincides with low levels of physical activity. Due to diminished mobility, people with MD do not always engage in active cardiovascular tasks. A nutritionist can help clients maintain their ideal weight. Excessive weight makes it more difficult to perform physical activities, difficulties that are already compounded by the functional limitations imposed by this disease.

Proper physical therapy and suitable orthopedic footwear can effectively prolong the duration of a client's ability to walk. Being able to ambulate independently is a strong psychological boost for someone with a prognosis that he or she will eventually need to use a wheelchair. To extend productivity in life, clients need to anticipate the inevitability of the disease and find ways to enrich their quality of life as physical functioning diminishes (Chen & Crewe, 2009; Chen et al., 2010).

Decline in daily physical activities as a result of muscle deficiency is a substantial problem in this population. People with sedentary lifestyles are prone to developing adverse medical conditions including coronary artery disease, osteoporosis, obesity, anxiety, depression, and musculoskeletal impairments

(Matthews, 2003). Healthy bodies need regular exercise to maintain toned and conditioned muscles. Paradoxically, people with MD are at greater risk of damaging muscle fibers when they undergo exercise regimens because the dystrophin protein cannot function properly to repair any injured muscles. Hence, it is advised that patients consult neurologists and physiotherapists before beginning an exercise regimen.

Improved pain management serves to enhance quality of life among people with muscular disease. BMD and DMD cause uncomfortable muscle cramps and painful stiffness. Lethargy in the daytime attributed to poor quality of sleep seriously affects concentration and productivity at work. Weakening in the pulmonary muscles in people with neuromuscular failure requires respiratory support. To minimize sleep disruption, suitable ventilators must be chosen to meet the unique needs of individuals with MD to ensure that respiratory mechanics function to maximum capacity.

Leisure and Recreational Issues

Exercise for persons with MD has been somewhat controversial due to dystrophin deficiency and decreased muscle contractile properties (Hicks, 1998). Nonetheless, an appropriate amount and intensity of exercise is recommended depending on the progression of the disease. While there is a benefit in conditioning muscles, precautionary measures need to be taken to avoid excessive muscular tissue damage. Aquatic therapy and hippotherapy (horseback riding) are ideal exercises for persons with neuromuscular diseases. Resistance in water allows the body to harden its flex and reflex movements with minimal risk of injuring muscles. For persons who have weak spinal, thoracic, cervical, and lumbar muscles, hippotherapy helps strengthen and maintain correct postures.

Rehabilitation clients with MD should be encouraged to take trips to visit different places. Due to mobility, toileting, and respiratory difficulties, clients with DMD, BMD, and LGMD may hesitate to travel. Careful planning before taking a trip can alleviate many of these concerns.

Sexual and Reproductive Concerns

For many people with disabilities, rehabilitation counselors are often the first persons they confide in about their anxiety over sexual issues (Vash & Crewe, 2004). Prior to providing counseling on sexual issues, counselors must first examine their own attitudes. If the counselor feels apprehensive about discussing intimate and sensitive questions with clients, appropriate referrals can be made. Rehabilitation professionals can serve as vital information sources to alleviate clients' anxieties and doubts about sexuality (Brodwin & Chen, 2000). The onset of LGMD and MMD often occurs at the time when youth are entering puberty. The severity of disability and its subsequent impact on social interaction deprive young people of the chance to experience sexual intimacy. Dating and courtship can thus be quite stressful and elusive. To project a warm and amicable image, clients with MD should learn about proper social etiquette and maintaining positive attitudes.

Inheritable disorders are a legitimate concern when planning a family. DNA testing and analysis of cell mutations provide information to predict the likelihood of passing on inherited diseases to offspring (Krajewski & Shy, 2004). The desire to have children can be carefully weighed against the possibility of passing mutant genes to offspring.

Genetic counseling can provide a person and his or her spouse with knowledge of the nature of the genetic disorder, its transmission, and the risk of occurrence in potential offspring. Depending on the type of disorder, the probabilities of genetic risks range from one in two people (with a dominant gene) and one in four people (with a recessive gene) (Gustavson, 1999). While the responsibility of explaining family planning rests on rehabilitation and medical professionals, clients and their families are responsible for the decision as to whether or not to have children.

Conclusion

MD is a group of neuromuscular diseases that gradually lead to the deterioration and erosion of muscles. Although there is no cure, people with this condition do not have to hold a bleak view of their future. When preparing a rehabilitation program or plan, it is imperative for counselors to acquire both knowledge of the client's capacity to handle tasks and knowledge of what the client is unable to manage. Because of the wide range of differences, each client needs careful, individualized evaluation. Fear and uncertainty about the future may induce clients to believe they have no control over the progressive weakening process (Chen et al., 2010).

When helping clients implement planning, rehabilitation counselors are wise to consider holistic interventions, such as psychological counseling, vocational advice, medical counseling, leisure and recreation, and sexual and reproductive concerns. Compassion is an imperative aspect in building rapport between client and counselor. Rehabilitation counselors should neither communicate an overly pessimistic outlook nor raise false hopes. By formulating realistic and practical goals with input from clients, counselors will attain improved rehabilitation outcomes.

Case Study

Mindy Lam is a 20-year-old immigrant who came to the United States from Hong Kong a year ago. She lives with her parents in an apartment adjacent to Chinatown in Los Angeles. Before arriving in this country, Mindy finished the 11th grade in her home country, learned basic conversational English, and worked for two years as an apprentice tailor, never returning to finish high school. Mindy is a referral to the Department of Rehabilitation from a Muscular Dystrophy Association support group. Miss Lam has been working at a clothing factory as a children's apparel seamstress since she arrived in this country.

At age 19, Miss Lam was diagnosed with facioscapulohumeral muscular dystrophy (FSHMD) and was treated at a hospital in Hong Kong. Despite the presence of FSHMD, Mindy has been able to care for herself. Since her arrival in Los Angeles, Mindy has been working for the same employer. Job evaluations indicate she is a reliable employee and gets along well with co-workers and supervisors. Four months ago, Mindy noticed her productivity steadily decreasing. Dust from cutting and sewing textiles irritated her eyes. She had difficulty sewing with precision and maintaining productivity. Her arms quickly became tired after working on the sewing machine for a short time. To meet the daily quota, Miss Lam took fewer breaks and a shorter lunch. Mindy often could not finish her lunch in the designated time due to swallowing difficulties; she does not have this problem when she eats slowly.

This client feels she is on the verge of an emotional breakdown. The fast pace of garment factory work is difficult for her, both mentally and physically. She does not want to be a burden to her family and desires to continue working. Mindy is experiencing mild depression because of social isolation. Typically, she spends her time watching television and cooking for her family. Occasionally, they have dinner out. Presently, Mindy is living with her parents and has doubts about dating due to her physical condition. In addition, her father does not approve of interracial dating. At a co-worker's invitation, Mindy attended a local Chinese-speaking church several times. However, her Buddhist parents prefer that Mindy not attend this particular church.

Before taking a few weeks of sick leave because of MD symptoms, Mindy was considered the top candidate for promotion to floor supervisor. Additionally, the company is in the process of computerizing the production lines. Miss Lam has expressed a strong interest in learning the new computer-aided fashion design software to sketch clothing designs, a position available at her employer. Yet, she is pessimistic about the likelihood of being promoted to a designer position due to her lack of education, limited computer experience, and MD. Except for a brief period of sick leave, she has been able to continue working full time. Additional employment interests of Miss Lam include child care, counseling, and working with people who have disabilities. Due to a family business failure, Mindy had to leave high school at the beginning of the 12th grade.

Questions

1. Identify some problems persons with MD encounter in society and in seeking and maintaining employment.
2. As Miss Lam's counselor, what possible physical and emotional limitations would you take into consideration when planning vocational rehabilitation services?
3. If you recommend continued employment with her employer, what advice would you give concerning reasonable accommodation? Would you recommend one of the two positions available, one being a floor supervisor and the other as a computer-aided fashion designer?

4. How would you suggest Mindy expand her social activities without creating tension with her parents? Provide your rationale within a cultural context.
5. As a counselor, provide a career path for this individual. Remember that Los Angeles is a garment-manufacturing center. Take into consideration her particular type of MD

References

Alexianu, M. E., & Gooch, C. L. (2004). Advances in neuromuscular disease in 2003: The year in review. *Journal of Clinical Neuromuscular Disease, 5*(4), 169–175.

Bartalos, M. K. (1990). Muscular dystrophy: Assessing the impact of a diseased state. *Loss, Grief and Cure, 4*(3/4), 63–73.

Brault, M. W. (2012, July). *Americans with disabilities: 2010* (P70-131). Retrieved from http://www.census.gov/prod/2012pubs/p70-131.pdf

Brodwin, M. G., & Chen, R. K. (2000). Marital and sexuality issues in clients with disabilities. In L. VandeCreek & T. L. Jackson (Eds.), *Innovations in clinical practice: A source book* (Vol. 18, pp. 459–470). Sarasota, FL: Professional Resource Press.

Bushby, K. (2011). Neuromuscular diseases: Milestones in development of treatments. *Lancet Neurology, 10*(1), 11–13.

Centers for Disease Control and Prevention (CDC). (2012). *Facts about muscular dystrophy*. Retrieved from http://www.cdc.gov/ncbddd/musculardystrophy/facts.html

Chen, R. K., & Crewe, N. M. (2009). Life satisfaction among people with progressive disabilities. *Journal of Rehabilitation, 75*(2), 50–58.

Chen, R. K., Miller, E., Seo, W. S., & Mendoza, E. (2010). Living with uncertainty: Impacts of a progressive disability on life perspectives. *Australian Journal of Rehabilitation Counseling, 16*(2), 85–98.

Emery, A. E. H. (1994). *Muscular dystrophy: The facts*. Oxford, England: Oxford Medical Publication.

Fowler, W. M., Abresch, R. T., Koch, T. R., Brewer, M. L., Bowden, R. K., & Wanlass, R. L. (1997). Employment profiles in neuromuscular diseases. *American Journal of Physical Medicine and Rehabilitation, 76*(1 Suppl.), S26–S37.

Freud, S. (1963). *General psychological theory: Papers on metapsychology*. New York, NY: Collier Books.

Gustavson, K. H. (1999). Muscular dystrophy: Genetic counseling and family planning. *Scandinavian Journal of Rehabilitation Medicine, 39*(Suppl.), 38–41.

Hendriksen, J. G. M., & Vles, J. S. H. (2006). Are males with Duchenne muscular dystrophy at risk for reading disabilities? *Pediatric Neurology, 34*(4), 296–300.

Hicks, J. E. (1998). Role of rehabilitation in the management of myopathies. *Current Opinion in Rheumatology, 10*(6), 548–555.

Kilmer, D. D., Abresch, R. T., McCrory, M. A., Carter, G. T., Fowler, W. M., Johnson, E. R., & McDonald, C. M. (1995). Profiles of neuromuscular diseases: Facioscapulohumeral muscular dystrophy. *American Journal of Physical Medicine and Rehabilitation, 74*(5 Suppl.), S131–S139.

Krajewski, K. M., & Shy, M. E. (2004). Genetic testing in neuromuscular disease. *Neurologic Clinics, 22*(3), 481–508.

Mackelprang, R. W., & Salsgiver, R. O. (1999). *Disability: A diversity model approach in human service practice*. Pacific Grove, CA: Brooks/Cole.

Mathews, K. D. (2003). Muscular dystrophy overview: Genetics and diagnosis. *Neurologic Clinics, 21*(4), 795–816.

McDonald, C. M., Abresch, R. T., Carter, G. T., Fowler, W. M., Johnson, E. R., Kilmer, D. D., & Sigford, B. J. (1995a). Profiles of neuromuscular diseases: Duchenne muscular dystrophy. *American Journal of Physical Medicine and Rehabilitation, 74*(5 Suppl.), S70–S92.

McDonald, C. M., Abresch, R. T., Carter, G. T., Fowler, W. M., Johnson, E. R., & Kilmer, D. D. (1995b). Profiles of neuromuscular diseases: Becker's muscular dystrophy. *American Journal of Physical Medicine and Rehabilitation, 74*(5 Suppl.), S93–S103.

McDonald, C. M., Johnson, E. R., Abresch, R. T., Carter, G. T., Fowler, W. M., & Kilmer, D. D. (1995c). Profiles of neuromuscular diseases: Limb-girdle syndromes. *American Journal of Physical Medicine and Rehabilitation, 74*(5 Suppl.), S117–S130.

Marini, I., Chen, R. K., Feist, A. M., Flores-Torres, L., & Castillo, A. (2011). Student attitudes toward intimacy with persons who are wheelchair users. *Rehabilitation Research, Policy, & Education, 25*(1), 15–26.

Miller, E., Chen, R. K., Graf, N. M., & Kranz, P. L. (2009). Willingness to engage in personal relationships with persons with disabilities: Examining category and severity of disability. *Rehabilitation Counseling Bulletin, 52*(4), 211–224.

Ogasawara, A. (1989). Downward shift in IQ in persons with Duchenne muscular dystrophy compared to those with spinal muscular atrophy. *American Journal on Mental Retardation, 93*(3), 544–547.

Ouyang, L., Grosse, S. D., Fox, M. H., & Bolen, J. (2012). A national profile of health care and family impacts of children with muscular dystrophy and special health care needs in the United States. *Journal of Child Neurology, 27*(5), 569–576.

Ouyang, L., Grosse, S. D., & Kenneson, A. (2008). Health care utilization and expenditures for children and young adults with muscular dystrophy in a privately insured population. *Journal of Child Neurology, 23*(8), 883–888.

Roessler, R. T., & Rubin, S. E. (2006). *Case management and rehabilitation counseling* (4th ed.). Austin, TX: Pro-ed.

Shannon, J. B. (2004). *Muscular dystrophy sourcebook.* Detroit, MI: Omnigraphics.

Siegel, I. M. (1999). *Muscular dystrophy in children: A guide for families.* New York, NY: Demos Medical.

Swenson, T. S. (2000). Chronic fatigue syndrome. *Journal of Rehabilitation, 66*(1), 37–42.

U.S. Bureau of Labor Statistics. (2013, June 12). *Persons with a disability: Labor force characteristics – 2012* (USDL-13-1141). Retrieved from http://www.bls.gov/news.release/pdf/disabl.pdf

U.S. Census Bureau. (2013, March 14). *Workers with a disability less likely to be employed, more likely to hold jobs with lower earnings, Census Bureau reports (CB13-47).* Retrieved from https://www.census.gov/newsroom/releases/archives/american_community_survey_acs/cb13-47.html

U.S. National Library of Medicine. (2009). *Facioscapulohumeral muscular dystrophy.* Retrieved from http://ghr.nlm.nih.gov/condition/facioscapulohumeral-muscular-dystrophy

U.S. National Library of Medicine. (2010). *Myotonic dystrophy.* Retrieved from http://ghr.nlm.nih.gov/condition/myotonic-dystrophy

Vash, C. L., & Crewe, N. M. (2003). *Psychology of disability* (2nd ed). New York, NY: Springer.

Wevers, C. W. J., Brouwer, O. F., Padberg, G. W., & Nijboer, I. D. (1993). Job perspectives in facioscapulohumeral muscular dystrophy. *Disability and Rehabilitation, 15*(1), 24–28.

Yu, A. J., Blankenship, L. D., Yang, R. Y., & Lee, M. Y. (2006). Myotonic dystrophy. *American Journal of Physical Medicine and Rehabilitation, 85*(6), 551.

About the Author

Roy K. Chen, Ph.D., C.R.C., is an associate professor in the Department of Rehabilitation, College of Health Sciences and Human Services, at the University of Texas-Pan American. He received his doctorate in rehabilitation counseling from Michigan State University, and his Master of Science degree in rehabilitation counseling from California State University, Los Angeles. Dr. Chen's current research interests include disability-related employment issues, psychosocial aspects of disabling conditions, multicultural rehabilitation, neuromuscular and neurological disorders, and sexuality and disability. A prolific researcher and writer, Dr. Chen publishes in national and international journals and presents his findings at state and national conferences.

Chapter 19

MULTIPLE SCLEROSIS

Barbara Barton, Ph.D., M.S.W.
Frances W. Siu, Ph.D., C.R.C.

Introduction

According to the scientists studying the epidemiology of multiple sclerosis (MS), more people are being diagnosed today than in the past decades (National Multiple Sclerosis Society [NMSS], 2013). Most people diagnosed with MS are between the ages of 20 and 50. Worldwide, MS occurs with much greater frequency closer to the equator or above 40° latitude. It is more common among Caucasians (particularly those of northern European ancestry), but is also diagnosed in people of African, Asian, and Hispanic ancestry. Multiple sclerosis is a progressively disabling autoimmune disease of the brain and spinal cord. Some people experience periods of disease remissions followed by relapse in symptom exacerbations; others experience a steady progression of their disease course, and for a few, the disease remains relatively benign over the course of a lifetime (NMSS, 2013). Because of the variability and the broad range of symptoms, rehabilitation counselors need to understand the scope of MS and its impact on vocational rehabilitation from an individualized perspective. This chapter discusses the prevalence, etiology (cause), forms (types) of MS, symptoms, diagnosis and progression, treatment, management of mood symptoms, and employment.

Prevalence

There are approximately 2.5 million people worldwide who have multiple sclerosis. In the United States, an estimated 400,000 people have MS; each week, 200 people are newly diagnosed with the disease (NMSS, 2013). The average lifetime cost of treatment for one person is $1.2 million. MS is an inflammatory disease of the body's T cells that target the myelin that surrounds nerves in the brain and spinal column. This causes sensory and motor problems that produce symptoms such as fatigue, weakness, muscle stiffness, poor coordination and balance, tingling, numbness, slurred speech, cognition problems, and changes in bowel/bladder function (Bren, 2005). Not every person with MS experiences all these symptoms and the degree to which they occur varies distinctly from individual to individual. Symptoms are identifiable when areas of the white matter of the central nervous system (CNS) are inflamed (plaques), leaving multiple scarring (sclerosis) and possible permanent damage through destruction of the myelin sheath that covers and protects axons (Rodriguez, 2008).

Etiology

Scientists believe that the disease is caused by more than one factor, such as individual genetic susceptibility and unknown environmental triggers that targets the immune system (MS Active Source, 2006).

Several factors increase the risk of developing multiple sclerosis, including age, gender, family background history, medical history, ethnicity, and residing geographic region (NMSS, 2013).

Age – Multiple sclerosis can occur to people of all ages, but most commonly affects those between ages 20 and 40.

Gender – Women are twice as likely as men to have MS.

FIGURE 1
Neuron

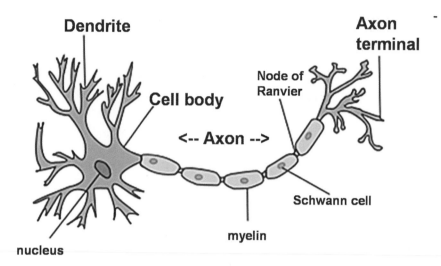

Source: Jones, P. (2013). *All About Sclerosis Information Trust*. Retrieved from http://www.mult-sclerosis.org/howms.html.

FIGURE 2
Insulation of a Nerve Fiber

Neuron with myelin sheath   Neuron with damaged myelin sheath

Source: Wood, D. (2014). *Conditions Indepth: Multiple Sclerosis*. EBSCO. Retrieved from http://web.iadmd.org/PATIENTS/HEALTHLIBRARY/tabid/606/contentid/20382/Default.aspx

Family history – If one of the individual's parents or siblings has multiple sclerosis, the person has a 1% to 3% potential of developing MS. However, the experiences of identical twins show that heredity cannot be the only factor involved. If multiple sclerosis was determined solely by genetics, identical twins would have identical risks. However, an identical twin has only about a 30% chance of developing multiple sclerosis if his or her twin already has the disease.

Ethnicity – Caucasians, particularly those whose families originated in northern Europe, are at highest risk of developing this disease. People of Asian, African, and Native American descent have the lowest risk.

Geographic regions – Multiple sclerosis is far more common in areas such as Europe, southern Canada, northern United States, New Zealand, and southeastern Australia.

Certain infections – A variety of viruses, such as Epstein-Barr virus, appear to be associated with multiple sclerosis. The study of how some infections may be linked to the development of MS is still in progress.

Other autoimmune diseases – Individuals who have thyroid disease, Type I Diabetes, or inflammatory bowel disease are slightly more likely to develop MS.

Forms of Multiple Sclerosis

According to the NMSS (2013), multiple sclerosis is a potentially debilitating disease in which the immune system attacks the protective myelin sheath that covers the nerves. Damage to the myelin causes interference in communication between the brain, spinal cord, and other parts of the body.

This non-reversible process may result in deterioration of the nerves. There are five internationally recognized forms of MS: (a) relapsing-remitting, (b) secondary-progressive, (c) primary-progressive, (d) progressive-relapsing, and (e) benign. **Relapsing-remitting** MS is marked by periods of symptom flare-ups followed by disease stability. The individual may return to full functioning or sustain some disability as a result of the exacerbation. Approximately 55% of people with MS have the relapsing-remitting form of the disease. It is not unusual for these individuals to develop the second form of MS, **secondary-progressive**. This occurs in approximately 50% of people with relapsing-remitting disease within ten years, and in nearly 90% of persons with relapsing-remitting disease after 30 years. In secondary-progressive disease, there is incomplete recovery of function between exacerbations, resulting in progressive disability. Approximately 30% of persons are diagnosed with secondary-progressive MS.

Primary-progressive, another form of MS, is marked by a steady progression of symptoms without remission, resulting in almost complete functional disability. Approximately 10-15% of all people with MS experience this form. The fourth, which many neurologists consider a variant of primary-progressive, is referred to as **progressive-relapsing** and affects 1% of the MS population. This type begins as a progressive form, but has occasional superimposed exacerbations. Although it is called progressive-relapsing, it may be a variant of either secondary-progressive or primary-progressive. There are currently treatments available to slow the progression of the disease for those with relapsing-remitting and secondary-progressive, but no treatment has been found effective against primary-progressive and progressive-relapsing MS. About 10% of persons exhibit a clinical course characterized by relatively few and mild exacerbations, called **benign** MS. It is not possible to predict which individuals will exhibit a particular course (NMSS, 2013). MS is not a life-threatening condition, unless severe complications arise (Blackstone, 2007).

Symptoms

Symptoms of multiple sclerosis arise when an area of the CNS becomes inflamed during the early course of an exacerbation. It can be difficult to diagnose early in the course of the disease because symptoms often come and go, sometimes disappearing for long periods of time (NMSS, 2013). A person may have visible neurological issues, such as gait disturbances, visual problems, or upper extremity weaknesses one day, but return to normal functioning within days, weeks, or months. In relapsing-remitting MS, an exacerbation can last for a day up to several months. Recovery rate and degree of recovery is as unpredictable as the disease course itself. In the secondary-progressive form of the disease, complete resumption of normal neurological status is rare. With the primary-progressive form of the disease, functional neurological status steadily declines. Some people also experience cold sensitivity, especially related to symptoms of spasticity. It is generally recommended that persons with MS who are sensitive to temperature variations avoid exposure to extreme temperature changes in a work environment.

Fatigue related to employment is defined as a state of reduced capacity for work following a period of mental or physical activity (Schwid, Covington, Segal & Goodman, 2002). Fatigue is the most common and difficult symptom of MS and occurs in 80% of cases (Brandes & Willmott, 2002). With some individuals, there is such a high degree of fatigue where accomplishing any physical or mental task becomes impossible. Subjective diaries are used to monitor a person's fatigue triggers and patterns (Krupp, LaRocca, Muir-Nash, & Steinberg, 1989).

Approximately half the people with MS develop some degree of cognitive dysfunction, which affects ability to think, reason, concentrate, and remember (Blackstone, 2007). Cognitive functions most likely to be affected include memory, speed of information processing, executive functioning (planning and prioritizing), visual spatial functions (visual perception and constructional abilities), abstract reasoning and problem-solving, word-finding (aphasia), and attention and concentration. However, only 5%-10% develop problems that are severe enough to interfere significantly with daily life. MRI scans have indicated that the extent of demyelination within the brain is associated with indirect cognitive problems, including depression, anxiety, stress, and fatigue (Rodriguez, 2008).

Neuropsychological examinations can identify areas of deficit so that strategies can be specifically tailored for each individual. Compensatory strategies for dealing with cognitive dysfunction include the consistent use of daily planners or personal data manager devices, limiting multi-tasking, using computers, filing systems, and periodic rest breaks.

Other Potential Symptoms of MS

Multiple sclerosis has the potential to affect every system in the human body. Symptoms are frequently related to the focal area of demyelination or inflammation within the CNS. Possible symptom areas include the following (Brill, 2008; Shannon, 2007):

- Bladder problems - urinary retention problems; stress and urgency incontinence
- Bowel dysfunction - constipation or incontinence
- Dizziness and vertigo
- Depression and emotional lability
- Gait problems - spasticity, poor balance, endurance and coordination, and ataxia
- Numbness and tingling (parasthesia)
- Pain
- Sexual dysfunction - in men, erectile problems; in women, vaginismus (painful intercourse), lubrication difficulties, and anorgasmia (sexual dysfunction)
- Vision problems - diplopia (double vision), optic neuritis (blurred vision), and nystagmus (rapid pupil movement)
- Sensory problems - intense itching, burning, or *rubber band* sensations of the skin
- Tremors
- Speech (dysarthria), word-finding (aphasia); difficulty swallowing (dysphagia)
- Lhermitte's Phenomena - an electric shock-like sensation down the spine to the toes when a person tucks the head to the chest

Diagnosis and Progression

It often takes several years to confirm a diagnosis of MS due to the fluctuating nature of the disease. Diagnosis is often made through a process of elimination of other possible medical conditions. In 2005, revised diagnostic criteria were published, called the McDonald Diagnostic Criteria for MS (Rodriguez, 2008; Shannon, 2007).

- At least two attacks with objective clinical evidence of two or more lesions.
- At least two attacks with objective clinical evidence of one lesion plus dissemination in space shown on MRI, or two or more MRI lesions consistent with MS plus positive cerebrospinal fluid (CSF) finding or second clinical attack.
- One attack with objective clinical evidence of at least two lesions plus dissemination in time on a second MRI or a second clinical attack.
- One attack with objective clinical evidence of one lesion, plus dissemination in space shown on MRI, or two or more MRI lesions consistent with MS, plus positive CSF finding and dissemination in time shown on MRI, or second clinical attack.
- Insidious neurologic progression suggestive of MS plus one year of disease progression determined retrospectively or prospectively and two of the following: positive brain MRI result (nine T2 lesions, or at least four T2 lesions with a positive Visual Evoked Potential), positive spinal cord MRI result with two focal T2 lesions, and positive CSF findings.

Diagrammatically, the progression of disability for each form of MS is indicated in Figure 3 through Figure 6.

Treatment

There is currently no cure for MS, but several treatments are available to manage symptoms and reduce progression of the disease. The most recently approved treatment (Bren, 2005; NMSS, 2013; Rodriguez, 2008), the monoclonal antibody Tysabri, was first used in combination therapy with the interferon Avonex, but was taken off the market due to complications. The Food and Drug Administration (FDA) has approved Tysabri as a stand-alone treatment for relapsing-remitting MS.

Each of the four types of injectable interferon drugs can be self-administered at home. Side effects include flu-like symptoms and potential irritation at the injection site. Copaxone injections may result in a short-term reaction that includes heart palpitations, chest pain, flushing, and shortness of breath. The NMSS recommends patients begin treatment immediately following diagnosis to decrease damage to the nervous system (Shannon, 2007).

FIGURE 3
Relapsing-Remitting MS and Progression of Disability

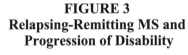

FIGURE 4
Secondary-Progressive MS and Progression of Disability

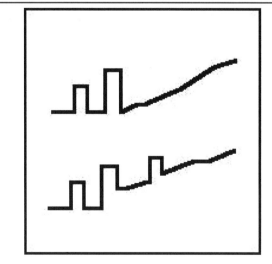

Multiple Sclerosis

FIGURE 5
Primary-Progressive MS and Progression of Disability

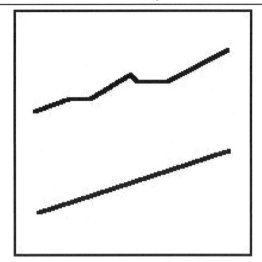

FIGURE 6
Progressive-relapsing MS and progression of disability.

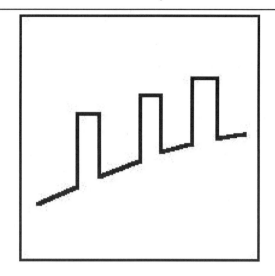

Source for Figures 3-6: Jones, P. (2013). *All About Sclerosis Information Trust*. Retrieved from http://www.mult-sclerosis.org)

Acute exacerbations of the disease are frequently managed with high doses of intravenous (IV) methylprednisolone (Solu-Medrol) which reduces the severity and duration of exacerbations (Brandes & Wilmott, 2002). This steroid, like many others, has multiple effects, including increased blood pressure, hyperexcitability, increased blood glucose levels, and weight gain. Long-term use can lead to loss of bone mass (osteoporosis). Unfortunately, Solu-Medrol is the only known effective treatment for the management of acute relapses. Anecdotal reports indicate that complementary medical interventions such as massage, Reiki, acupuncture, a balanced diet, and nutritional supplements help promote relaxation and relieve stress that accompanies the disease. Scientific data on the benefit of these interventions is sparse, but they may be useful for the overall well-being of the person (Rosner & Ross, 2008).

Contemporary research on MS is focused on further understanding the etiology of disease and identifying safe and effective treatments for all forms (Marrie, 2013). Halting the attacks on the myelin structures, repairing nervous system damage, and identifying effective treatment agents are other focal areas of research (Blackstone, 2007; Rodriguez, 2008).

Management of Mood Symptoms

Research has shown the high prevalence rate of depression among people with MS (Chwastiak, Gibbons, & Sullivan, 2002; Livneh & Antonak, 2012). Contributing factors that induce depression include focal lesions in the brain, the individual's acute response to an exacerbation, and a general fear of the unknown. Treatment with therapy and psychotropic medication provides support to patients experiencing mood instability.

The rehabilitation counselor can positively impact an individual's mood and self-esteem by sharing knowledge and providing encouragement, as well as understanding the value changes occurring in the person with a disability. Emotional support from the counselor provides a hopeful perspective, including (Wright, 1960):

1. *Enlargement of the scope of values* – assist the individual in identifying what is important in his or her life, which may have changed or expanded since the diagnosis.

TABLE 1
FDA-Approved Drugs for the Treatment of Multiple Sclerosis

Brand Name	Generic Name	Manufacturer/Distributor, Year of FDA Approval	Indication (From FDA-Approved Labeling)	Frequency of Injection
Betaseron	interferon beta-1b	Berlex Laboratories Inc., 1993	Relapsing forms of MS	Every other day
Avonex	interferon beta-1a	Biogen Idec, 1996	Relapsing forms of MS	Once a week
Copaxone	glatiramer acetate	TEVA Neuroscience Inc., 1996	Relapsing forms of MS	Every day
Novantrone	mitoxantrone	Serono Inc., 2000	Worsening relapsing-remitting MS and progressive-relapsing or secondary-progressive MS	Four times a year; lifetime limit of 8,12 doses
Rebif	interferon beta-1a	Serono Inc., 2002	Relapsing forms of MS	Three times a week
Tysabri	natalizumab	Biogen Idec and Elan, 2004; marketing suspended Feb. 28, 2005, due to reports of two serious adverse events	Relapsing forms of MS	Every four weeks

Source: National Multiple Sclerosis Society. Retrieved from www.nationalmssociety.org

2. *Subordination of the physique* – since MS is often diagnosed when a person is in the most active period of life, concerns may arise such as: "How will I be able to play with my children?" "Will I have to give up tennis?" "Can I still enjoy hiking with my significant other?" One can provide reassurance while acknowledging that some modifications of physical activity are necessary and, at times, vital to the individual's well-being. A counselor may also explore hobbies, skills, and interests with the client that do not require extensive physical stamina.
3. *Containment of disability effects* – reassuring the individual that although he or she is experiencing a chronic illness, it does not mean that one is less of a parent, partner, or friend. The character traits of caring, compassion, and socialization abilities can still be intact despite the illness.
4. *Shift from comparative to asset values* – a counselor can help identify the client's unique potential and characteristics, rather than comparing her or him with those seen in the media.

Another important framework to embrace when working with clients is the psychosocial adaptation cycle to disability, as explored by Livneh and Antonak (2012). The first of seven stages represents *shock*, a short-term reaction to the diagnosis. The second stage, *anxiety,* is characterized by a panic-like feeling when an individual recognizes the magnitude of the disabling condition. Stage three, *denial,* is regarded as a defense mechanism used to negate the potential severity of the condition. The fourth, *depression,* is a common observance in people diagnosed with chronic illness as they begin to integrate the complexity, severity, and potential future implications of the disease. In the fifth stage, *internalized anger,* clients have feelings and behaviors of resentment, bitterness, deviousness, and self-blame. In contrast, in stage six, *externalized hostility,* an individual puts the blame for the disease or treatment failure on external sources such as friends, family, and the medical profession. The final stage, *adjustment,* occurs when an individual begins to integrate the cognitive, affective, and behavioral components of the diagnosis, and can successfully negotiate disease-related obstacles and positively pursue personal, social, educational, and vocational goals.

Just as the disease is experienced differently by each individual, so are the emotional reactions. This cycle of stages is simply an outline of possible common reactions to a diagnosis of multiple sclerosis. Every new exacerbation after a period of remission can trigger these psychosocial responses (Solan, 2012). The counselor needs an awareness of the diverse nature of the disease to avoid categorizing and stereotyping the person's physical and emotional sequelae.

Multiple Sclerosis and Employment

The average age of onset of MS is 28, often occurring at the time of the height of a career path. Approximately 75% of people are unemployed five years after diagnosis (O'Day, 1998). Unfortunately, this shift can lead to a decreased quality of life, social supports, and financial stability (Schiavolin et al., 2013). As a result, nearly 40% of individuals with MS desire to return to work (LaRocca, Kalb, Scheinberg, & Kendall, 1985).

Vocational Potential

Rehabilitation counselors, with the input of other professionals such as physiatrists and neuropsychologists, can develop employment plans which are both realistic and accommodating to individual strengths and challenges. For example, if fatigue is an issue, the counselor can assess what part of the day the person's fatigue level is at its peak. Accommodations for such fatigue could include breaks during this time, a work schedule modified around the onset of fatigue, or telecommuting (Kieseier & Pozzilli, 2012). Heat sensitivity can be addressed by utilizing indoor work sites, adaptive cooling devices, and employment in an air-conditioned environment. Accommodations for cognitive problems which affect work performance and social relationships with peers are dependent upon severity. A neuropsychological examination can help locate and identify potential workplace accommodations (Rumrill, Hennessey, & Nissen, 2008).

Taking into consideration the recent positive impact of treatments for MS, rehabilitation counselors need to be creative, innovative, and persistent when working with these individuals. Counselors can discuss the higher quality of life that employment provides, variability of symptoms, and the relatively young age of those affected. While working with employers, one can emphasize crafting of jobs that optimize the person's strengths while respecting the limitations of the disease.

Schiavolin et al. (2013) identified six areas to be addressed by counselors, consumers, and employers to promote positive employment rates of individuals with multiple sclerosis. These areas are (a) employer support, (b) program knowledge, (c) external support, (d) service provision, (e) work potential, and (f) health care.

General Attitudinal Barriers

Positive employer relations are crucial to the work atmosphere for people with MS. Title I of the Americans with Disabilities Act (ADA, 2008) provides some protection for employees with disabilities. The National Multiple Sclerosis Society has several free resources on employment and the issue of disclosure. The *win-win* approach for employers and employees suggested by researchers states that an employee should request an appointment with the supervisor or manager and disclose only what is necessary about the disease state, including any needed accommodations (Schiavolin et al., 2013). Barriers such as negative attitudes toward people with MS and lack of knowledge about the disease must also be addressed among fellow employees.

Public opinion about individuals with MS has not kept pace with the disease-modifying treatments that often slow the functional progression of disability. It is still viewed by many as a disease that quickly leads to wheelchair use, communication issues, and cognitive decline. For the majority of people with MS, sporadic exacerbations and limited functional loss of ability are a more realistic appraisal of health. In many, the *invisibility* of the disease is the most frustrating factor since they do not appear to have limitations or disability. People find it difficult to defend fatigue, cognitive problems, bowel and bladder issues, and so forth when their disease is not visible.

The societal response to disability is often a function of the beliefs of the general population toward the disability and individuals with disabilities, in general. These beliefs toward limitations are often negative and affect the interpersonal relationships between persons with disabilities and those without disabilities, as well as society's attempt to rehabilitate persons with disabilities, making rehabilitation a more challenging process (Marini & Stebnicki, 2012; Rumrill et al., 2008).

Conclusion

Multiple sclerosis is a challenging disease, both for the person and the rehabilitation counselor. Management of symptoms is crucial for the person to decrease feelings of hopelessness and allow for normal personal, social, educational, and vocational activities during the course of the disease. Encouraging mood stability and a positive outlook can promote resiliency and appropriate coping. Counselors need to address the role shifts and changes, lack of education about the disease, and pre-conceived negative notions of the future, which can strain even the strongest interpersonal relationships.

A comprehensive resource for professionals and people with MS is the National Multiple Sclerosis Society. This organization maintains chapters in every state. Services such as information, referral to community resources, free literature, support and education groups, and free equipment loans provide an additional support framework.

Case Study

Tracy is a 29 year-old, single, African-American female who lives alone in a suburb on the outskirts of a major Midwestern city. Tracy has been employed for four years as a fund raiser for a statewide non-profit organization which operates federal food banks. As a fund raiser, she meets with individual and corporate donors and coordinates special events throughout the state, setting up agency displays at conferences and other events. This occupation requires long hours, considerable travel, and heavy physical labor, but Tracy enjoys it. Since graduating with her college degree in communications, she has been working for this organization.

Six months ago, Tracy began experiencing episodes of weakness in both arms and dropped a box of brochures on her way to a conference. Tracy experienced balance problems and had to stop wearing high-heeled shoes. She blamed these symptoms on overworking and being tired and did not see her physician. The symptoms disappeared after six weeks.

Recently, Tracy noticed numbness in her right leg; she kept 'stubbing her toe' as she walked (Kieseier & Prozzilli, 2012). In addition, she was exhausted, as if recovering from the flu. This time she decided to see her physician. Tracy told her about the current symptoms, and those she had experienced six months earlier. The physician ordered a complete MRI of her brain and spinal cord, performed a lumbar puncture, and arranged for a visual evoked potential test. The tests confirmed a diagnosis of multiple sclerosis. Tracy had two plaques on her brain and other plaques at C-5 (the 5th cervical vertebrae) and T-11 (the 11th thoracic vertebrae). Her physician immediately referred the case to a neurologist who prescribed one of the immunomodulating MS injection treatments, which have caused additional fatigue and muscle aches.

Between the tests, her symptoms, and the physician appointments, Tracy missed several days of work, which put her behind on several important projects. In the near future, she will be setting up a large display at a golf tournament and reports that she is anxious about the long drive (2½ hours), as she has numbness in her right leg and difficulty feeling the car pedals. Also, there is significant carrying and walking during the event, and she is concerned that she will not be able to physically complete the tasks.

Tracy's boss is very supportive, but travels extensively and does not micro-manage her staff. Tracy does not believe that her boss will have the time to help out at the event. Additionally, she has not disclosed her diagnosis to anyone at the organization, including her boss.

Tracy is concerned about losing her job and wonders if she will require use of a wheelchair for mobility. She is starting to feel anxious as she reads more on the Internet about the symptoms of MS. Tracy's family, except for a brother, lives out of state and she has no close friends. Concern regarding the stability of her job is increasing and she is extremely anxious about her employment options. This individual is a bright, independent person who is having a difficult time adjusting to MS. A nurse gave her the number of the local vocational services office to explore vocational rehabilitation possibilities with a counselor.

Questions

1. As Tracy's counselor, where would you begin?
2. Discuss the positive and negative aspects of Tracy disclosing her MS to her employer.
3. What are some potential accommodations you would recommend to this client? Are these accommodations you are proposing reasonable?
4. Identify mental health issues Tracy is experiencing and how the two of you would develop ways to manage them?
5. Explore several vocational options for this client.
6. Discuss ethnicity/race regarding MS. Does she fit the typical prevalence?

References

ADA Amendments Act of 2008, Public Law 110–325, 122 Stat. 3553.

Blackstone, M. (2007). *The first year – Multiple sclerosis: An essential guide for the newly diagnosed.* New York, NY: Marlowe.

Brandes, D., & Willmott, L. (2002). Multiple sclerosis. In M. G. Brodwin, F. A. Tellez, & S. K. Brodwin (Eds.), *Medical, psychosocial, and vocational aspects of disabilities* (2nd ed., pp. 351–362). Athens, GA: Elliott & Fitzpatrick.

Bren, L. (2005). New treatment, new hope for those with multiple sclerosis. United Stated Food and Drug Administration, *FDA Consumer, 39*(2), 10–17.

Brill, M. T. (2008). *Multiple sclerosis.* Tarrytown, NY: Marshall Cavendish Benchmark.

Chwastiak, L., Gibbons, L., & Sullivan, M. (2002). Depressive symptoms and severity of illness in multiple sclerosis: Epidemiologic study of a large community sample. *American Journal of Psychiatry, 159*(11), 1862–1868.

Kieseier, B. C., & Pozzilli, C. (2012). Assessing walking disability in multiple sclerosis. *Multiple Sclerosis Journal, 18,* 914–924.

Krupp, L., LaRocca, N., Muir-Nash, J., & Steinberg, A. (1989). The Fatigue Severity Scale: Application to patients with multiple sclerosis and systemic lupus erythematosis. *Archives of Neurology, 45,* 435–437.

LaRocca, M., Kalb, R., Scheinberg, L., & Kendall, P. (1985). Factors associated with unemployment of patients with multiple sclerosis. *Journal of Chronic Disabilities, 38,* 203–210.

Livneh, H., & Antonak, R. (2012). Psychological adaptation to chronic illness and disability: A primer for counselors. In I. Marini & M. Stebnicki (Eds.), *The psychological and social impact of illness and disability* (6th ed., pp. 95–107). New York, NY: Springer.

Marini, I., & Stebnicki, M. (Eds.). (2012). *The psychological and social impact of illness and disability.* New York, NY: Springer.

Marrie, R. A. (2013). Observational studies of treatment effectiveness: Useful, useless, or somewhere in between. *Multiple Sclerosis Journal, 19,* 707–708.

MS Active Source. (2006). *What is MS? The complete story.* Retrieved on April 11, 2006 from http://www.msactivesource.com

National Multiple Sclerosis Society (NMSS) (2013, August 20). *What is MS?* Retrieved on August 3, 2013 from http://www.nationalmssociety.org/about-multiple-sclerosis/what-we-know-about-ms/index.aspx

O'Day, B. (1998). Barriers for people with multiple sclerosis who want to work: A qualitative study. *Journal of Neurological Rehabilitation, 12,* 139-146.

Rodriguez, M. (Ed.). (2008). *Advances in MS and experimental demyelinating diseases.* New York, NY: Springer.

Rosner, L. J., & Ross, S. (2008). *Multiple sclerosis: New hope and practical advice for people with MS and their families*. New York, NY: Fireside Book.

Rumrill, P. D., Hennessey, M. L., & Nissen, S. W. (2008). *Employment issues and multiple sclerosis*. New York, NY: New American Library.

Schiavolin, S., Leonardi, M., Giovannetti, A. M., Antozzi, C., Brambilla, L., Confalonieri, P.,...Raggi, A. (2013). Factors related to difficulties with employment in patients with multiple sclerosis: A review of 2002–2011 literature. *International Journal of Rehabilitation Research, 36*(2), 105–111.

Schwid, S., Covington, M., Segal, B., & Goodman, A. (2002). Fatigue in multiple sclerosis: Current understanding and future directions. *Journal of Rehabilitation Research and Development, 39*(2), 211–224.

Shannon, J. B. (Ed.). (2007). *Multiple sclerosis sourcebook*. Westport, CT: Praeger.

Solan, A. (2012). Quality of life reporting in multiple sclerosis clinical trials: Enough quality? *Multiple Sclerosis Journal, 18*, 1668–1669.

Wright, B. (1960). *Physical disability – A psychological approach*. New York, NY: Harper & Row.

About the Authors

Barbara Barton, Ph.D., M.S.W., received her doctorate in Rehabilitation Counseling and Bachelor's and Master's of Social Work from Michigan State University, East Lansing. She is an Associate Professor in the School of Social Work at Western Michigan University, Kalamazoo, and has been involved with the National Multiple Sclerosis Society at the state and local levels for 20 years. Before teaching, she worked in the rehabilitation and health care industries. Dr. Barton teaches interpersonal practice and policy, planning, and administration courses in the undergraduate and graduate programs.

Frances W. Siu, Ph.D., C.R.C., is an Assistant Professor and Coordinator of the undergraduate Rehabilitation Services Program at California State University, Los Angeles (CSULA). She received her Ph.D. in Special Education and Counseling, option in Rehabilitation Counselor Education, from the University of Texas at Austin, her M.S. in rehabilitation counseling and B.S. in psychology, both from CSULA. Research interests of Dr. Siu include medical aspects of disability, multicultural issues, and violence against people with disabilities. She has published over 20 articles and book chapters, and given over 50 professional presentations on violence against people with disabilities, rehabilitation education, and rehabilitation services.

Multiple Sclerosis

Chapter 20

RHEUMATIC DISEASES

Thomas D. Beardmore, M.D.
Penny J. Chong, M.D.

Introduction

Rheumatology is the scientific study and care of rheumatic diseases; a physician who specializes in rheumatic diseases is a rheumatologist. All urban areas in the United States have practicing rheumatologists, and major urban centers have rheumatology training programs within medical schools and major hospitals. The American College of Rheumatology (ACR, 2003) promotes research and education on arthritis and is the professional organization for rheumatologists; the Arthritis Foundation (http://www.arthritis.org/) is the organization that raises funds and conducts arthritis research and patient education throughout this country. Both these organizations have headquarters in Atlanta, Georgia and are comprehensive resources for rehabilitation counselors seeking information about rheumatic disorders (Budd, Gabriel, O'Dell, & McInnes, 2012; Lee & Abramson, 2011).

Definition

Rheumatic diseases are a group of conditions affecting the supporting structures of the body, including the joints and periarticular tissues, connective tissues of the skin, bones, muscles, and diseases of the immune system. They include a group of inflammatory diseases affecting connective tissue that are insidious (develop in a subtle, gradual manner) in onset, characterized by exacerbations and remissions, and resistant to medical therapy (there are no cures, only palliative treatment). Included in this group are arthritis and diseases that cause pain, stiffness, and abnormalities of mobility. Fundamental features of rheumatic diseases are the signs of inflammation: warmth, swelling, redness, pain, and loss of motion. Individuals with rheumatic disease have complaints of pain, loss of energy, easy fatigability, stiffness, and limitations of joint motion. Work endurance and capacity are affected by these symptoms; with severe involvement, activities of daily living and mobility become impaired.

Arthritis and Myositis

The common rheumatic diseases that affect the joints are called *arthritis*, those that affect the muscles are termed *myositis*, and *soft tissue rheumatism* is present when soft tissues (tendons, ligaments, bursa, and muscles) are involved, accompanied by associated stiffness and pain. There are more than 100 rheumatic diseases that result in pain, stiffness, and functional impairment. Some of the more common diseases are osteoarthritis (the most common rheumatic disease), rheumatoid arthritis (the highest rate of disability), gout, bursitis, tendonitis, fibromyalgia, systemic lupus erythematosis, scleroderma, and ankylosing spondylitis. Less common types of rheumatic diseases include myositis (polymyositis and dermatomyositis), scleroderma, and arteritis (Budd et al., 2012; Klippel, Stone, Crofford, & White, 2008).

Arthritis and Rheumatic Disorders

Musculoskeletal diseases, which include arthritis and rheumatic disorders, are the leading causes of disability and absence from work (Budd et al., 2012). They are the second most common reason why people see physicians, affecting 22% of the adult population. Arthritis and the other rheumatic diseases are difficult to diagnosis due to the subtlety of physical signs, the tendency for symptoms to overlap with other medical problems, and the scarcity of diagnostic clinical and laboratory tests. Symptoms tend to develop gradually, respond slowly to treatment, and require long-term care.

Impact and Prevalence

The impact of arthritis in the United States is great. Fifty percent of adults 65 years of age and older reported a diagnosis of arthritis. In 2010, the Centers for Disease Control and Prevention estimated that 49.9 million Americans had an arthritis diagnosis (Cheng, Hootman, Murphy, Langmaid, & Helmick, 2010). Of these, about 300,000 were under age 18; this represents one in every 250 children. Currently, over seven million Americans are disabled by arthritis. Annually, arthritis accounts for 500 million days of restricted activities and 68 million days of lost work. It is the leading cause of absenteeism in business and industry and the second leading cause of disability payments (following heart disease). Rheumatoid arthritis accounts for 2.2 million days of lost work and osteoarthritis accounts for 66 million days of lost work, annually. In the United States, one in every five people or 20% of the population has an arthritic condition (Hootman, Bolen, Helmick, & Langmaid, 2006; Hootman & Helmick, 2006).

Categories of Rheumatic Disease

There are three categories of rheumatic diseases that the rehabilitation professional is most likely to encounter. First, are the **diffuse connective tissue diseases** (rheumatoid arthritis, systemic lupus erythematosis, scleroderma, and polymyositis). This category has the most severe and highest prevalence of disability. Second is **osteoarthritis**, the most common form of arthritis, accounting for the largest number of lost work days. The third category is **ankylosing spondylitis**, which causes severe back pain and often is confused with other causes of back pain.

Rheumatoid Arthritis

Explanation of Disease

Rheumatoid arthritis (RA) is a systemic disorder of the connective tissues of the body, characterized by exacerbations and remissions. Its primary targets are the joints and adjacent supporting structures. The lining of the joint (synovium) is the site of chronic inflammation. Synovial tissues proliferate and lymphocytes (white blood cells) and other chronic inflammatory cells invade its interstices (spaces or gaps in tissues). This inflammatory process produces pain, heat, swelling, and loss of joint motion. The process is locally invasive and rheumatoid tissue erodes cartilage, bone, and ligaments.

The etiology of rheumatoid arthritis is unknown, and was originally characterized as being of insidious onset and slow progression. However, there is substantial data that by the end of the second year from onset of symptoms, 90% of patients show radiographic evidence of damage.

Incidence

RA is a common disorder affecting approximately 1% of the adult population. It has a high disability rate estimated to be 21 per 1,000 people (Cooper, 2000). This disability rate is higher than the next three most common conditions: heart disease, back impairment, and hypertension. In addition, people diagnosed with rheumatoid arthritis utilize more medical services (physicians and hospitals) than patients with osteoarthritis, back pain, or tendonitis. Rheumatoid arthritis is three times more likely to affect women than men and has its peak onset between the ages of 20 and 30, although the incidence of RA has declined over the years. Because of its chronicity and severe consequences, it is a primary focus of arthritis research (Vonkeman & van de Laar, 2013).

Effects

The primary effects of this type of arthritis are pain, swelling, loss of joint motion, joint deformities, and subsequent loss of function. The disease is one of exacerbations and remissions, but the overall course is progressive. Pincus et al. (1984) analyzed a group of individuals diagnosed with rheumatoid arthritis over a period of nine years and found a steady decline in physical functioning; 92% had significantly lower overall functioning. Of those under 65 years of age who were working at the commencement of the study, 85% demonstrated significant work disability. Meenan, Yelin, Nevitt, and Epstein (1981) studied the financial impact of rheumatoid arthritis on wage earning and found that people earned 50% of what was expected based on their earning potential, and average individual income dropped, accounting for a 32% decrease in family income. Most had medical coverage but inadequate disability insurance to cover loss of earnings. Of the 59% of people with insurance coverage for loss of earnings, the coverage provided income for a maximum of six months.

People with RA have a symmetrical arthritis affecting multiple joints. Initially, small joints of the body are affected, but eventually all joints can be impacted. The initial symptoms occur in the small joints of the hands and feet with symptoms of pain, swelling, and joint stiffness. Individuals commonly experience fatigue, morning stiffness, and may have weight loss. As the disease progresses, more joints are affected and the degree of disability increases. Development of characteristic deformities of the hands typically occurs with rheumatoid arthritis. These deformities limit performance of employment and leisure activities. Restriction of range of joint motion frequently accompanies the deformities. Additionally, individuals become self-conscious about the appearance of their hands and feet, restrict their activities, and tend to wear concealing clothing (Klippel et al., 2008; Pincus et al., 1984).

Diagnosis

Diagnosis is established through clinical features and laboratory testing. To establish a diagnosis, the arthritis must be polyarticular (i.e., involve more than one joint) and be at least six weeks in duration. Synovial joints are involved in a symmetrical manner. Initially affected are the small joints of the hands and feet, although any synovial joint may be involved. Rheumatoid arthritis is a systemic condition. Subcutaneous nodules are non-tender nodules varying in size from a few millimeters to several centimeters that may develop at pressure points, most commonly at the elbow. Joints are swollen, tender, with increased synovial fluid. People with more severe disease may have inflammation of the lining of the lungs and heart, lung involvement with fibrosis (scar tissue formation) and nodules, and inflammatory vessel disease of the skin and other organs. Dryness of the eyes and mouth is common, as are compression of peripheral nerves adjacent to joints (e.g., causing carpal tunnel syndrome).

The ACR-EULAR (American College of Rheumatology-European League Against Rheumatism) 2010 classification criteria for RA is based on the size and number of joints with clinical evidence of synovitis; serolgies rheumatoid factor (RF) and anticyclic citrullinated peptide antibody (ACPA); and acute phase reactants C-reactive protein (CRP) and erythrocyte sedimentation rate (ESR). Laboratory results are sparse but persons may have mild anemia, thrombocytosis, elevation of acute phase reactants, but normal urinalysis and uric acid levels, and have a serological abnormality, called rheumatoid factor. RF, an autoantibody, is present in 75% of people with RA; it is associated with extra articular disease and is a poor prognosticator. Anti-cyclic Citrullinated Peptide Antibodies (ACPA) are as sensitive as and more specific than RF, and can predict the development of RA when found in undifferentiated arthritis.

In early disease, x-rays show loss of bone density (osteoporosis) and soft tissue swelling about the joints. X-rays of individuals with more advanced arthritis show loss of articular cartilage, erosion of bone adjacent to joints, and associated deformity (Budd et al., 2012).

Treatment

Currently, there is no cure for RA, although there are good palliative measures that can ameliorate symptoms or induce remission for extended periods. A three-pronged approach to treatment should be considered with 1) non-steroidal anti-inflammatory drugs (NSAIDS) and/or low dose oral and/or intra-articular steroids, 2) disease modifying antirheumatic drugs (DMARDS), and 3) biologic agents (Majithia & Geraci, 2007; Smolen, Landewe, & Breedveld, 2010).

By decreasing inflammation, NSAIDS and steroids reduce pain and swelling and improve range of motion and strength. NSAIDS (e.g., ibuprofen) are generally preferred because they tend to have fewer side effects, although steroids are more potent. NSAIDs and steroids can be taken together.

DMARDS include medications such as Methotrexate, Leflunomide, Hydroxychloroquine, Sulfasalazine, and Azathioprine. Methotrexate is now considered the DMARD of choice to initiate therapy in RA as it has been demonstrated to be very effective alone or in combination with the biologic agents (Smolen et al., 2010). These agents are slow acting and may require up to six months to achieve a therapeutic response. By potentially reducing the inflammatory hyperplastic synovium and reversing erosions of bone and nodules, early use can slow progression of RA and improve overall prognosis.

The biological agents are the newest line of treatment and, like DMARDS, can take weeks to months to have discernible effects. They have very diverse mechanisms of action, including inhibition of tumor necrosis factor (TNF) and depletion of B-lymphocytes. Biological agents are more effective than methotrexate at slowing radiographic progression. The biologic agents, however, do have significant potential side effects, such as increased susceptibility to serious infections. TNF inhibitors are contraindicated in patients with advanced congestive heart failure (Feely, 2010).

Total joint replacement is a standard treatment for advanced joint disease that is progressive, symptomatic, and unresponsive to pharmacologic treatments. Through joint replacement, the diseased joint is surgically replaced with an artificial joint. Surgery relieves pain and frequently improves mobility. Resumption of work and recreational activities may occur after joint replacement (Koopman & Moreland, 2005). Successful joint replacements have been achieved in the hands, wrists, shoulders, hips, and knees with the greatest level of satisfaction with hip and knee replacements.

Functional Limitations

Functional limitations for individuals with rheumatoid arthritis are of primary concern. As the disease progresses and the years pass, functional loss becomes progressive. The American College of Rheumatology established criteria that physicians use to describe functional status. These criteria are illustrated in Table 1 and include Functional Class I (normal function) through Functional Class IV (unable to perform self-care activities). People referred for vocational rehabilitation are usually in Functional Classes II and III. Functional limitations are stated relating to the stage of the disease and areas of the body involved (Hochberg et al., 1992).

TABLE 1
Functional Status in Rheumatoid Arthritis

CLASS I	Able to perform all usual activities of daily living.
CLASS II	Able to perform all usual self-care and vocational activities. Limited in avocational activities.
CLASS III	Able to perform all usual self-care activities. Limited in vocational and avocational activities.
CLASS IV	Unable to perform usual self-care, vocational, and avocational activities.

Source: American College of Rheumatology (ACR) Hotline (2003). The use of anti-cyclic citrullinated pepetide (anti-CCP) antibodies in RA. Retrieved from http:www.rheumatology.org/

Chronic Pain

Individuals diagnosed with rheumatoid arthritis have pain that is chronic in nature and exacerbated by movement of the affected joints. Many people have stiffness of the entire body, which is primarily a morning phenomenon and may last from minutes to hours. Specific functional disabilities occur in each individual, depending on the stage of disease and body areas affected. This disorder causes loss of motion and pain on motion; there is weakness, decreased strength, and diminished endurance. If the hands and upper extremities are involved, pain and loss of motion results in decreased capacity to perform grasping, fine dexterity hand activities, and overhead reaching. With lower extremity involvement, decreased capability to stand and walk for long distances occurs.

Emotional and Intellectual Factors

People with rheumatoid arthritis have no emotional limitations except those imposed by a disorder associated with chronic illness, pain, and loss of motion. There is an increased incidence of depression; however, it is not greater than would be expected for any chronic, progressive disorder. Intellectual capacity is not affected and ability to interact on a social level is unimpaired. Occasionally, because of the deforming nature of the disease, embarrassment is experienced concerning deformities of the hands and feet, as well as use of ambulatory aids such as canes, walkers, and wheelchairs.

Vocational Considerations

If rheumatoid arthritis is not well controlled or of long duration, there may be chronic pain, stiffness, fatigue, and weakness, all of which influence an ability to work. Yet, during the first years of the disease, most people obtain good control with first and second line medications, and vocational limitations are a consequence of the specific area of the body affected. Because of a reduction in strength and involvement of articulations effecting movement, most individuals are unable to perform heavy or very heavy work activities. Employment in the exertional categories of light and sedentary exertion is preferred. If a person, before acquiring rheumatoid arthritis, was performing medium work, it is likely that employment will need to be modified to light work.

Upper Extremity Involvement

Hand and wrist involvement results in decreased power grip; most people with rheumatoid arthritis are assessed below the 5th percentile for grip strength (Cooper, 2000). Additionally, pinch, grasp, and manual dexterity are reduced. If there is involvement of the hands, wrists, elbows, and shoulders, activities involving reaching and rapid movements of the upper extremities are diminished.

Lower Extremity Involvement

Disease in the lower extremities results in impaired ability to rise from a sitting position, stand, and walk for long periods of time. Work activities should accommodate the specific deformities and symptoms of the individual. If the arthritis affects standing and walking, the person may be limited to sedentary work activity.

Other Factors

Some people with rheumatoid arthritis require special considerations because of deformities, weakness, and loss of joint range of motion. Adaptations, such as higher chairs, raised toilet seats, and curb cuts accommodate lower extremity impairments. Occasionally, individuals have other health problems related to rheumatoid arthritis. For example, multisystem involvement from rheumatoid disease usually results in generalized fatigue with decreased strength and endurance.

Rehabilitation Potential

Rheumatoid arthritis does not affect intellectual capabilities. Life expectancy for a person with this disease is shortened by a few years. Therefore, if retraining is required, counselors may consider more extensive training and educational programs. The disease is progressive; however, it is slowly progressive and functional impairments increase at a gradual rate. Most people need accommodation or training for work that requires less exertion, perhaps one or two exertional levels less than prior work activities. Hence, heavy work activities prior to diagnosis will likely need to be restructured to activities involving medium or light work, and performance at the light level will need modification to sedentary work. No matter how severe the disability, the person with rheumatoid arthritis with work modifications should be able to do sedentary work activity. Many can work at the light level, and a few will be able to perform medium work.

Studies on return to work indicated that work disability is related to age, number of involved joints, and a desire to remain gainfully employed. Control of pace and work activities was shown not to be a significant factor (Reisine, McQuillan, & Fifield, 1995). In a report from a state-federal rehabilitation agency, restoration of physical health, amount spent by rehabilitation agencies, and duration the case was open positively correlated with return to work (Straaton, Maisiak, Dortch, & Lopez-Mendez, 1990). Educational level, severity of disability, and financial status had no relationship to the outcome of vocational rehabilitation. As a result, rehabilitation counselors should persist with retraining, re-education, and vocational placement for people with rheumatoid arthritis unable to work at their current or prior positions.

Continued consultation with the physician, allied health professionals (i.e., occupational and physical therapists), and a work environmental specialist can help accommodate needs in the work environment. Prognosis for work is enhanced for individuals who have higher education levels because, in general, work environments for employees with higher levels of education require less physical exertion and mobility. Since intellectual functioning is not affected by RA and the expected lifespan is only a few years less than normal, rehabilitation counselors need to make every effort to return people diagnosed with this condition to the workforce.

Osteoarthritis

Explanation of Disease State

Osteoarthritis (OA) is a degenerative disease affecting the articular cartilage lining the surfaces of joints. It is a localized disease and does not have systemic manifestations. This condition refers to a group of overlapping distinct diseases with different etiologies, but similar biologic and clinical outcomes. OA affects the entire joint, including the subcondral bone, ligaments, capsule, synovial membrane, and periarticular muscles (Brandt, Dieppe, & Radin, 2008). Pathophysiologically, there is degeneration of the articular cartilage with fibrillation, fissures, ulceration, and loss of joint surface. Recently, scientists discovered a decrease in a specific surface protein on joint cartilage leading to the progressive deterioration of the cartilage that constitutes the hallmark of OA (Taniguchi et al., 2009).

Effects

Osteoarthritis is the most common arthritis in the United States, more often affecting women. Virtually everyone over 65 years of age will have x-ray evidence of osteoarthritis; yet, most people do not have symptoms. There is a characteristic wearing away of the surface cartilage at the joint, resulting in pain, swelling, stiffness (particularly with activities), and loss of motion.

The disorder primarily affects the joint cartilage; yet, secondary inflammation involving the joint lining is common. Surface cartilage is disorganized, lost, and adjacent bony growth at the joint margins occurs. Marginal bony spurs are characteristic of osteoarthritis. Diagnosis is primarily based upon symptoms and characteristic x-ray changes, which include loss of cartilage, increased bone density, and bone overgrowth at the joint margin.

Treatment

Nonpharmacologic interventions such as exercise, weight loss, modifying activities of daily living, physiotherapy, braces, and use of a cane and orthotics benefit many people. For hand OA, the ACR recommends topical NSAIDS and topical capsaicin. If these do not work, oral NSAIDS and tramadol are the next steps. In cases of knee OA, ACR recommends acetaminophen, oral and topical NSAIDS, and tramadol. More advanced cases can benefit from intra-articular steroid injections (Hochberg et al., 2012). Other patients require the use of narcotic analgesics for pain relief. Joint prostheses (total artificial joints) are effective for advanced OA when lesser treatments prove ineffective.

Functional Limitations

People with OA do not exhibit systemic features; no other organ systems are involved, and there are no emotional or intellectual consequences. The disorder is localized and may be symptomatic with severe functional problems; more commonly, it does not create major physical limitations. Most people with osteoarthritis are older; many are no longer in the workforce and are not candidates for vocational rehabilitation. Those who are in the workforce have functional limitations that are specific to the areas of the body involved.

If the small digits of the hands are affected, there will be stiffness and loss of motion that interfere with finger dexterity. Pinch and grip may be decreased. Other common areas affected by OA are the cervical and lumbar spine, resulting in pain and loss of motion with rotation of the body and with bending. The weight bearing joints of the lower extremities, especially the hips and knees, are commonly involved and have the highest incidence of disability. People with osteoarthritis of the hips or knees have pain, particularly with standing and walking. Additionally, there is loss of range of motion and stiffness with the initiation of activities (Klippel et al., 2008).

Vocational Considerations

Emotional, intellectual, organ systems, and other health factors do not limit the vocational process. For individuals that have OA of the lumbar spine, ability to bend and lift is reduced by one or more exertional levels. When the knees and hips are involved, tolerance for bending, squatting, ladder or stair climbing, long distance ambulation, and lengthy periods of standing are reduced. With OA of the hands, fine manual dexterity and strength are reduced.

Rehabilitation Potential

Persons with localized osteoarthritis and the lack of systemic features are good candidates for rehabilitation. Both short-term and long-term training and educational programs are realistic. Movement is affected, while strength is preserved. Communication skills, social skills, behavioral abilities, the capacity to learn, comprehend, and other intellectual skills are unchanged. Because of the lack of systemic features of this illness and involvement of only particular joints, rehabilitation potential usually is strong.

Systemic Lupus Erythematosus

Explanation of Disease State

Systemic lupus erythematosus (SLE), commonly called lupus, is a disorder of the immune system, resulting in inflammation of the connective tissue. The disease is characterized by the presence of autoantibodies against the DNA and RNA/protein complexes. Some patients form pathogenic immune complexes (Oelke & Richardson, 2002).

Incidence

This disorder primarily affects women and has an increased incidence in African-Americans, Hispanics, and Asian Americans. In this country, the incidence of SLE is 3.5 per 100,000 per year in whites and 9.2 per 100,000 per year in African-Americans. Prevalence of SLE is 40-50 per 100,000 population with a total of 239,000 Americans affected. African-American females account for the most prevalent group. Eighty-six percent of people with lupus are women. Peak onset of this disease is during the most productive part of a woman's life, between the ages of 20 to 30 (Budd et al., 2012).

Effects

Systemic features of fatigue, fever, weight loss, and joint pain characterize the disease. All individuals have joint pain as a predominant symptom; yet, major disability is not related to the joints, but rather to systemic involvement. The characteristic clinical course is one of exacerbation and remission; remissions may last for many years. Typically, SLE affects multiple organ systems but not all at the same time. Joint pain is the most common symptom with small joints being most affected. When compared to rheumatoid arthritis, there is no morning stiffness and joint deformity is rare. Some people have skin rashes, especially in sun-exposed areas of the body. There may be inflammation of the lining of the heart and lungs, and acute or chronic renal disease that can progress to renal failure. Central nervous system involvement manifests itself as stroke, psychosis, or depression for some individuals. Anemia is a common problem (Lee & Abramson, 2011).

Diagnosis

The diagnosis of SLE requires at least four of the eleven criteria (at any point in time, not necessarily all at once) that the American College of Rheumatology has set forth (Hochberg et al., 2012). These criteria include the presence of a malar rash, discoid rash, photosensitivity (skin rash from the sun), oral ulcers, nonerosive arthritis, serositis, renal disorder, neurological disorder (seizures or psychosis), hematologic disorder (hemolytic anemia, leucopenia, lymphopenia, thrombocytopenia), immunologic disorder, and antinuclear antibody (Koopman & Moreland, 2005). Prognosis depends on the organs involved and is most guarded when there is renal and central nervous system involvement.

Treatment

Treatment is a function of the organ systems involved. Musculoskeletal symptoms (arthralgias, myalgias) are treated with NSAIDS. Corticosteroids are generally reserved as temporary measures when symptoms are resistant to NSAIDS (Dooley & Ginzler, 2006). Leflunomide and Hydroxychloroquine have been shown to improve the musculo-skeletal manifestations of SLE.

In recent years, the biological agents have assumed a prominent role in the treatment of SLE. Beluminab (Benlysta), a biologic agent, inhibits B lymphocyte stimulation and decreases SLE activity. Rituximab, a B cell inhibitor, has been shown to be effective for CNS vasculitis and thrombocytopenia, but has not been successful for *generalized* lupus (Wallace, 2010). The biologics, Epratuzumab and Toclizunab, which have been efficacious in RA, have shown promise in early trials for the treatment of SLE (Chugh, 2012).

Cytoxan and Imuran have been used successfully in the treatment of SLE nephritis. Steroids are often taken concomitantly until other medications take effect. A significant percentage of individuals develop chronic renal failure from the nephritis and require dialysis or kidney transplantation. Because of the variable nature and intensity of this disease, some people experience only minor symptoms while others have major symptoms with increased morbidity and even early death. (Klippel et al., 2008).

Functional Limitations

Fatigue is a major symptom of SLE and a prominent consideration in job placement. It is particularly apparent during periods of exacerbation, but not during remissions. In contrast to other forms of inflammatory arthritis (e.g., rheumatoid arthritis), there are no problems with mobility, motor strength, or control. Limitations are dependent upon the organ systems affected; pulmonary and cardiac involvement causing shortness of breath limits exertional activities. Persons who have central nervous system involvement may be limited by emotional problems and chronic depression. An individual who has had a stroke may have residual problems of hemiparesis (muscle weakness on one side of the body), which interferes with ambulation and motor skills in the involved extremities.

Vocational Considerations

Expected lifespan of people with SLE is good unless there is involvement of the central nervous system or the kidneys; hence, educational and training programs that are longer in duration can be considered. Special environmental factors involve avoidance of cold environments, as vasospasm of fingers and toes may occur when exposed to cold objects and environments. Sun intolerance (excessive ultraviolet light exposure) can worsen the illness; jobs with excessive exposure to sun are inadvisable. Most people are restricted to light or sedentary exertion because of fatigue (Straaton et al., 1990).

Rehabilitation Potential

When SLE is in remission, either naturally occurring or medication induced, the individual will have no physical or emotional impairments. This disorder may have years in which it remains in remission; persons diagnosed with lupus are good candidates for re-training and educational programs. Motor and physical limitations are not a common consequence of this disease.

Scleroderma

Explanation of Disease State

Scleroderma is a chronic disorder of the connective tissue in which there is inflammation of multiple organs of the body, resulting in increased deposits of collagen. Primary target organs are the skin, joints, lungs, gastrointestinal tract, and heart. The etiology is unknown.

Effects

There may be extensive fibrosis and tightening, particularly of the hands, face, chest, and feet. Inflammation may cause sclerosis (scarring) of the lungs, heart, and gastrointestinal tract. People with scleroderma have great intolerance to cold; cold temperatures cause spasm of the peripheral vessels that may result in gangrene in the tips of the fingers and even loss of entire digits. Deformities are not a common part of this disease. General fatigue, weakness, and loss of motion related to fibrosis about the joints and skin are common consequences.

Treatment

Treatment is only palliative and symptomatic; non-steroidal anti-inflammatory drugs are given for inflammation and pain. Second line drugs, such as D-penicillamine, have beneficial effects on interstitial lung disease and renal involvement if given over long periods of time. Recent studies using the B cell stimulation inhibitor Rituximab have shown an improvement in lung function. Skin thickening as evaluated by the modified Rodnan Skin Score, also improved (Caramaschim, Domenico, Scambi, & Adaml, 2011). Pulmonary artery hypertension is the major cause of death in patients with scleroderma (Chang, Wigley, White, & Wise, 2003).

Functional Limitations and Vocational Considerations

Scleroderma causes impairment of fine motor activities of the hands, as well as manipulations requiring hand strength. Grip and pinch are markedly reduced and the ranges of motion of the wrists, elbows, and shoulders may be mildly decreased. There is no intellectual impairment; mobility is usually not a problem. Individuals with pulmonary involvement have fatigue and restricted activity because of shortness of breath upon exertion. Physicians recommend jobs within the light and sedentary exertional categories. Preferred work environments for persons diagnosed with scleroderma are ones that are warm and not subject to extremes or changes in temperature. Job activities should not involve repeated trauma to the hands, since trauma and cold temperatures can result in vasospasm, gangrene, and even loss of fingers. Cognitive functioning is not affected by scleroderma.

Rehabilitation Potential

Many individuals with scleroderma have minimal limitations. In more severe cases, there are problems with manual dexterity, stamina, and working in cold environments. Rehabilitation potential usually is good, with most workers being able to stay on their jobs with possible minor accommodations.

Polymyositis and Dermatomyositis

Explanation of Disease State

Polymyositis and dermatomyositis are uncommon, having an incidence of 0.9 to 9.3 new cases a year per million people. This is an autoimmune disorder of skeletal muscle in which the muscles are inflamed and lose strength. The usual course of polymyositis is a sudden onset of severe weakness and then recovery. Remissions can last for many years with few exacerbations. There is a biomodal distribution of the onset of polymyositis – at ages 10 to 15 and then ages 45 to 60 (Budd et al., 2012). Dermatomyositis is a condition similar to polymyositis, but one in which a skin rash is present in addition to inflammation of the muscles.

Effects

The proximal muscles of the extremities are most involved; hence, patients have major involvement of the muscles about the shoulder and hip regions. Diagnostically, one sees elevation of serum levels of enzymes of skeletal muscle, and abnormalities on an electromyogram (EMG). Symptomatically, there occurs difficulty in raising the arms above the head, arising from sitting, and climbing stairs. For those who do not have full return of strength, there is partial return of strength that can be maintained for years. Only a small percentage of individuals have continued loss of strength.

Treatment

Most individuals diagnosed with polymyositis are treated with high doses of corticosteroids until muscle enzymes normalize. Steroids are tapered slowly over a six month period (Martino & Kagen, 2006). It is estimated that 90% will have a positive response, and 50-75% will go into remission. Those who do not respond well are treated with second line medications, such as azathioprine and methotrexate, either alone or in combination. Alternatively, intravenous immune globulin (IVIg) has been shown to be effective (Dalakas et al., 1993). More recently, it has been demonstrated that Rituximab is an effective treatment in refractory cases, showing an increase in muscle strength (Mahler et al., 2011).

Functional Limitations and Vocational Considerations

When there is not a full recovery, there is either a minor degree of motor weakness (i.e., arising from a chair) or major motor problems (i.e., inability to stand or walk, and capacity to do only activities involving the musculature of the forearms and hands). Individuals in this latter group have functional capacities similar to persons with paraplegia (lower extremity involvement). Those with severe lower and upper extremity limitations have a functional capacity similar to people with quadriplegia. Fortunately, severe extremity complication occurs in only a few individuals with this condition. People with polymyositis who have significant weakness of the lower or upper extremities require jobs with the lowest exertional categories, conducting primarily light and sedentary activities. These persons may require walking aids or wheelchairs; therefore, workstations need modification to accommodate these assistive devices. Once the disability is established, it is usually static. Intellect is not impaired; comprehension and learning are maintained.

Rehabilitation Potential

For the majority of persons with polymyositis, medication effectively controls symptoms. After treatment with various medications, most are able to return to work. Rehabilitation potential, therefore, is positive. For the few who do not respond well to medications, potential for rehabilitation may be poor; alternatively, the individual may have the capacity to do sedentary work activity.

Ankylosing Spondylitis

Explanation of Disease State

Ankylosing spondylitis (AS) is a chronic inflammatory disorder of the synovial joints and entheses (points at which tendons insert into bones) of the spine. Primarily a disorder affecting men, the incidence is nine times greater for men than women. Initial onset occurs during the second and third decades of life and causes pain, stiffness, and loss of motion of the lower back. Frequently, the disorder is mistaken for low back pain of a mechanical or degenerative nature. Prevalence is 197 per 100,000. Other related diseases include Reiter's syndrome, psoriatic arthritis, and enteropathic (i.e., bowel associated) arthritis. These disorders have similar symptomatology and disability patterns. They are known collectively as spondyloarthropathies (Ritchlin, 2006). There is a strong association with HLA B27 antigen in these patients. The mechanism by which inflammation of the back is caused by the B27 antigen is not clear, but it is thought that an aberrant peptide presentation caused by B27 heavy chain misfolding may cause a proinflammatory response (Chakravarty & Paget, 2012).

Effects

This disorder is slowly progressive and, in its full expression, involves the entire spine from the skull to the pelvis. The sacroiliac joints (posterior pelvic joints) are initially involved. Also affected are the synovial joints of the back and ligamentous insertions that join the vertebral bodies. These areas become inflamed resulting in pain, swelling, and loss of motion. Approximately 20% of patients with ankylosing spondylitis have involvement of the peripheral joints, primarily the hips and shoulders. To a lesser extent, there is involvement of the more peripheral joints of the lower extremities and hands.

Symptoms

Pathology of AS involves inflammation of the lining of the posterior joints of the back and ligamentous connections between vertebral bodies. With progression of the disease, there is fibrous ankylosis (fusion) and later, bony ankylosis of the affected joints with consequent loss of all motion in the back. Pain is the main symptom, along with stiffness and gradual progressive loss of motion. When ankylosis is complete, the pain stops but loss of motion in the spine remains.

Treatment

Treatment of AS is symptomatic, primarily with NSAIDS. It is thought that a trial of two or more NSAIDS over a four-week period coupled with physical therapy is the best first-line therapy. Exercise helps retain range of motion. In some cases, sulfasalazine can be useful in reducing the length and severity of morning stiffness and pain. Physical therapy with maintenance of proper posture is encouraged to prevent development of a bent fixed flexion posture of the spine (Klippel et al., 2008). However, the consensus now is that if symptoms last more than four weeks, TNF alpha therapy should be instituted. Currently, there are four FDA approved agents: Remicade, Enbrel, Humira, and Simponi. These agents work on both the spine component and the non-spine inflammatory components. In one study, remission was achieved in 55.6% of patients (Chakravarty & Paget, 2012).

Functional Limitations

Ankylosing spondylitis does not have systemic features; occasionally, patients have involvement of the aortic valve of the heart and pulmonary fibrosis with resultant symptoms. Systemic features are not correlated with loss of work capacity. In the majority of people, functional limitations are related to loss of motion of the spine. Bending, twisting, and rotational motions of the lumbar and cervical spine are impaired. If the hips and shoulders are affected there will be pain, loss of motion, and development of flexion contractures in those areas. Involvement of hips, shoulders, and peripheral joints commonly lead to loss of ability to work.

Vocational Considerations

Intellectual functioning is unimpaired. Aptitudes, interests, and communication skills are similar to the normal population and life expectancy is unchanged, unless there is cardiac or pulmonary involvement. There are no special environmental needs.

Early in the disease, most people with AS have chronic pain, but little impairment in range of motion in the cervical and lumbar spine. Anti-inflammatory medications and analgesics control this; hence, little modification of the work environment is needed. However, most individuals require reduction of exertion in work activities. As the disease progresses, the person becomes unable to perform work that is within the higher exertional categories because of pain and loss of mobility of the lumbar spine, including ability to bend forward. Individuals with the most severe form of ankylosing spondylitis lack motion of the cervical and lumbar spine and must bend from the hips; they need to move their entire body to see to the right or left (Budd et al., 2012). Life expectancy is not affected by ankylosing spondylitis and most people have full, productive lives. Social and behavioral skills are unimpaired, learning comprehension is unchanged and, with the exception of the few who have cardiac involvement, there are no other health problems associated with this condition (Chakravarty & Paget, 2012).

Rehabilitation Potential

Rehabilitation potential for persons with this rheumatic disease generally is strong. With work accommodation for those individuals who have heavier jobs, most maintain productive employment for many years as long as they stay within the lifting and carrying restrictions recommended, usually within the light and sedentary levels. Persons with chronic back pain from ankylosing spondylitis may need jobs that do not involve undue emotional stress. With these factors in mind, the counselor can effectively rehabilitate the majority of people with this disorder.

Case Study

Susan Valdez is 19 years of age and has had juvenile-onset rheumatoid arthritis for 14 years. During this time, she has had long periods of illness where she was confined to her home and, as a result, is still in her last year of high school. Her illness is currently well controlled and Susan has missed no school for the past six months. She takes oral medication three times daily, self-administers subcutaneous injections of etanercept twice a week, and visits her physician on a monthly basis to attempt to maintain her disease in remission.

To maintain ambulation, Ms. Valdez needed surgery for her arthritis. She has had two hip replacements and a knee replacement. Currently, Susan is able to walk about the house unassisted but uses a motorized wheelchair for long distances when in the community. At the current time, Susan experiences morning stiffness and has arranged to take classes at school beginning at 10:00 A.M. or later. Occasionally, she has pain in multiple joints including her feet, shoulders, wrists, and the small joints of her hands. Her physician has prescribed pool exercise and Susan wears a wrist splint when she experiences pain in that area. In addition to her limited ambulation, she requires assistance from her mother to shampoo her hair, has a bilateral grip strength of 20 pounds, and pinch strength of five pounds.

Ms. Valdez is the fifth child of a second generation Hispanic family, and she is bilingual in Spanish and English. Her father passed away and general relief and contributions from the adult children, including Susan's Social Security Insurance (SSI) payments, currently support her mother. Susan's mother does not speak English and has never worked outside the home; she sees her life's role as caretaker for her daughter. The relationship between Susan and her mother is close and has been criticized by the health care team as one that promotes dependence rather than independence.

Psychological testing has shown that Ms. Valdez has high average intelligence, social immaturity, and the absence of depression. The health care team feels that Susan has been an underachiever in school and at home, relying on her mother and siblings rather than taking the initiative. Susan does not drive and has not started dating. Her primary source of emotional support is her family and one girlfriend from school.

The school principal referred Susan for vocational counseling. In six months, she will graduate from high school, and has no plans after graduation. Ms. Valdez has done well in school and has particularly enjoyed the sciences, receiving a senior prize in biology. Unsure about attending college, Susan will be the second in her family to complete high school; however, there are no finances to support a college education. Her sister is currently the head cashier at a grocery store and has assured Susan that she can get her a cashiering job at that store. Susan's mother is against her working and feels that she should stay home and baby-sit for her nieces, nephews, and the neighborhood children.

Questions

1. Is this individual a suitable candidate for vocational rehabilitation counseling services? What additional medical information is needed from her healthcare team?
2. If you feel Ms. Valdez is a suitable candidate for counseling and rehabilitation, what programs would give her the greatest opportunities for long-term employment? Is additional education indicated?
3. Discuss whether the job as grocery cashier with her sister is a good choice for employment.
4. How might her counselor handle Susan's inability to drive and her dependence upon her mother? Is use of public transportation an option? Consider the impact of her motorized wheelchair on further education, training, and work.
5. How will Susan's current illness, physical limitations, and psychological status influence a decision about higher education? Is she a viable candidate for college, or would educational efforts be problematic? Should vocational training, higher education, or on-the-job training be considered?
6. What physical problems need to be considered if job placement is to be conducted? Indicate the impact upon Susan's ability to obtain and maintain employment.
7. List Ms. Valdez' strengths and limitations from a physical and psychosocial perspective that need to be evaluated when formulating vocational planning.
8. Discuss cultural implications regarding this case.

References

American College of Rheumatology (ACR) Hotline (2003). *The use of anti-cyclic citrullinated pepetide (anti-CCP) antibodies in RA.* Retrieved from http:www.rheumatology.org/

Brandt, K., Dieppe, P., & Radin, E. (2008). Etipathogeneis of osteoarthritis. *Rheumatic Disease Clinics of North America, 34*, 531–559.

Budd, R. C, Gabriel, S. E., O'Dell, J. R., & McInnes, R. (Eds.). (2012). *Kelley's textbook of rheumatology* (9th ed). Philadelphia, PA: Elsevier Saunders.

Caramaschim, P., Domenico, B., Scambi, C, & Adaml, S. (2011). Scleroderma lung fibrosis and biologic drugs. *Rheumatology Current Research,. S2*, 1–5.

Chakravarty, S. D, & Paget, S. A. (2012). Ankylosing spondylitis: Pathogenesis, diagnosis, and therapy. *Rheumatology Practice News Special Edition, 3*, 39–43.

Chang, B., Wigley, F. M., White, B., & Wise, R. A. (2003). Scleroderma patients with combined pulmonary hypertension and interstitial lung disease. *Journal of Rheumatology, 30*, 2398–2405.

Cheng, Y. J., Hootman, J. M., Murphy, L. B., Langmaid, G. A., & Helmick, C. G. (2010). Prevalence of doctor-diagnosed arthritis and arthritis-attributable activity limitation – United States, 2007-2009. *Morbidity and Mortality Weekly Report, 59*(39), 1261–1265.

Chugh, P. K. (2012). Lupus: Novel therapies in clinical development. *European Journal of Internal Medicine, 23*, 212–218.

Cooper, N. J. (2000). Economic burden of rheumatoid arthritis: A systematic review. *Rheumatology, 39*, 28–33.

Dalakas, M. C., Illa, I., Dambrosia, J. M., Soueidan, S. A., Stein, D. P., Otero, C.,... McCrosky, S. (1993). A controlled trial of high-dose intravenous immune globulin infusions as treatment for dermatomyositis. *New England Journal of Medicine, 329*, 1993–2000.

Dooley, M. A., & Ginzler, E. M. (2006). Newer therapeutic approaches for systemic lupus erythematosus: Immunosuppressive agents. *Rheumatic Disease Clinics of North America, 32*, 91–102.

Feely, M. G. (2010). New and emerging therapies for the treatment of rheumatoid arthritis. *Open Access Rheumatology: Research and Reviews, 2*, 35–43.

Hochberg, M., Altman, R. D., April, K. T., Benkhalti, M., Guyatt, G., McGowan, J.,... Towheed, T. (2012). American College of Rheumatology 2012 recommendations for the use of nonpharmacologic and pharmacologic therapies in osteoarthritis of the hand, hip, and knee. *Arthritis Care and Research, 64*(4), 465–474.

Hochberg, M., Chang, R., Dwosh, S., Lindsey, T., Pincus, T., & Wolfe, F. (1992). American College of Rheumatology 1991 Revised Criteria for the Classification of Global Functional Status in Rheumatoid Arthritis. *Arthritis and Rheumatism, 35*, 498–502.

Hootman, J. M., Bolen, J., Helmick, C. G., & Langmaid, G. (2006). Prevalence of doctor-diagnosed arthritis and arthritis-attributable activity limitation – United States, 2003-2005. *Morbidity and Mortality Weekly Report, 55*(40), 1089–1092.

Hootman, J. M., & Helmick, C. G. (2006). Projections of United States prevalence of arthritis and associated activity limitations. *Arthritis and Rheumatism, 54*(1), 266–269.

Klippel, J. H., Stone, J. H., Crofford, L. J., & White, P. H. (Eds.). (2008). *Primer on the rheumatic disease* (13th ed.). New York, NY: Springer.

Koopman, W. S., & Moreland, L. W. (Ed.). (2005). *Arthritis and allied conditions: A textbook of rheumatology* (15th ed.). Baltimore, MD: Lippincott Williams and Wilkins.

Lee, S. H., & Abramson, S. B. (2011). Rheumatic diseases. In S. R. Flanagan, H. H. Zaretsky, & A. Moroz (Eds.), *Medical aspects of disability: A handbook for the rehabilitation professional* (4th ed., pp. 511–530). New York, NY: Springer.

Mahler, E. A. M., Blom, M., Voermans, N.C., Van Engelen, B. G. M, van Riel, P. C. M., & Vonk, M. C. (2011). Rituximab treatment in patients with refractory inflammatory myopathies. *Rheumatology, 50*(12), 2206–2213.

Majithia, V, & Geraci, S. A. (2007). Rheumatoid arthritis: Diagnosis and management. *American Journal of Medicine, 120*, 936–939.

Martino, S. J., & Kagen, L. J. (2006). Newer therapeutic approaches: Inflammatory muscle disorders. *Rheumatic Disease Clinics of North America, 32*, 121–128.

Meenan, R., Yelin, E., Nevitt, M., & Epstein, W. (1981). The impact of chronic disease: A sociomedical profile of rheumatoid arthritis. *Arthritis and Rheumatism, 24*(3), 544–549.

Oelke, K., & Richardson, B. (2002). Pathogenesis of lupus. *Arthritis and Rheumatism, 47*(3), 343–345.

Pincus, T., Callahan, L., Sale, W. G., Brooks, A. L., Paynbe, L. E., & Vaughn, W. K. (1984). Severe functional declines, work disability, and increased mortality in seventy-five rheumatoid arthritis patients studied over nine years. *Arthritis and Rheumatism, 27*(8), 864–871.

Reisine, S., McQuillan, J., & Fifield, J. (1995). Predictors of work disability in rheumatoid arthritis patients. *Arthritis and Rheumatism, 38*(11), 1630–1637.

Ritchlin, C. (2006). Newer therapeutic approaches: Spondyloarthritis and uveitis. *Rheumatic Disease Clinics of North America, 32*, 75–90.

Smolen, J. S., Landewe, R., & Breedveld, F. C. (2010). EULAR recommendations for the management of rheumatoid arthritis with synthetic and biologic disease-modifiying antirheumatic drugs. *Annals of Rheumatic Diseases, 69*(6), 964–975.

Straaton, K.V., Maisiak, R., Dortch, M., & Lopez-Mendez, A. (1990). Factors associated with continued employment among arthritis clients served by a state-federal rehabilitation agency. *Arthritis and Rheumatism, 33*(9), Supplement S123.

Taniguchi, N., Carames, B., Ulmer, U., Ronfani, L., Bianchi, M. E., Komiya, S., & Lotz, M. (2009). Aging related loss of chromatin protein HMGB2 in articular cartilage is linked to reduced cellularity and osteoarthritis. *Proceeding of the National Academy of Sciences, 106*(4), 1181–1186.

Vonkeman, H. E., & van de Laar, M. (2013). The new European League against rheumatism. American College of Rheumatology Diagnostic Criteria for Rheumatoid Arthritis: How are they performing? *Current Opinion in Rheumatology, 25*(3), 354–359.

Wallace, D. J. (2010). Advances in drug therapy for systemic lupus erythematosus. *BMC Medicine, 8*(77), 1–5.

About the Authors

Thomas D. Beardmore, M.D. is Professor of Medicine at the Keck School of Medicine, University of Southern California, Los Angeles. He is Chief of Rheumatology and Co-Chief of the Arthritis Service at Rancho Los Amigos National Rehabilitation Center in Downey, California.

Penny J. Chong, M.D. is Medical Director of Cigna Healthcare, Glendale, California. She is a licensed medical practitioner in California and specializes in internal medicine and rheumatology. Prior to joining Cigna, Dr. Chong was Co-Director of Reproductive Immunology Associates in Van Nuys, California, and Assistant Clinical Professor of Medicine at the University of California, Los Angeles.

Chapter 21

PSYCHIATRIC DIAGNOSES

David B. Peterson, Ph.D., C.R.C.
George K. Hong, Ph.D.

Introduction

This chapter begins with the definition of psychiatric diagnosis, followed by a review of the competencies necessary for rehabilitation counselors to work effectively with people presenting with psychiatric diagnoses. It continues with an overview of the prevalence of psychiatric diagnoses and the systems commonly used to classify them, the Diagnostic and Statistical Manual of Mental Disorders, Fifth Edition(DSM-5) (American Psychiatric Association [APA], 2013), and the International Classification of Diseases, Tenth Revision, Clinical Modification(ICD-10-CM) (World Health Organization [WHO], 2014). Next, psychiatric disability is defined using the World Health Organization's model of health (WHO, 2001).

The chapter continues with a discussion of the evolution of the DSM, first with a brief overview of the Diagnostic and Statistical Manual of Mental Disorders, Fourth Edition, Text Revision (DSM-IV-TR) (APA, 2000), as rehabilitation professionals will need to be familiar with it when evaluating medical records generated prior to the release of the DSM-5 (2013). Next, this chapter provides an introduction to the DSM-5, followed by highlights of changes from the IV-TR to the 5th edition. It concludes with a review of general diagnostic categories of psychiatric diagnoses, a discussion on stigma and the recovery model of psychiatric rehabilitation, and a case example illustrating the issues rehabilitation counselors may face in working with someone with the diagnosis of schizophrenia.

Psychiatric Diagnosis Defined

Psychiatric diagnoses are *mental disorders* that manifest certain symptoms or diagnostic criteria that significantly impair psychological functioning. The American Psychiatric Association (2013) defines a *mental disorder* as:

> … a syndrome characterized by clinically significant disturbance in an individual's cognition, emotion regulation, or behavior that reflects a dysfunction in the psychological, biological, or developmental processes underlying mental functioning. Mental disorders are usually associated with significant distress or disability in social, occupational, or other important activities (p. 20).

It goes on to say that a mental disorder is not….

> […] an expectable or culturally approved response to a common stressor or loss, such as the death of a loved one… socially deviant behavior (e.g. political, religious, or sexual) and conflicts that are primarily between the individual and society… unless the deviance or conflict results from a dysfunction in the individual as described above (p. 20).

Advances in science suggest that boundaries between psychiatric diagnoses are less clear than once thought, and that most conditions can be placed on a spectrum with closely related diagnoses that share symptoms, genetic and environmental risk factors, and probable biological bases of behavior (APA, 2013). To understand psychiatric diagnoses, the clinician must be able to distinguish between normal life variations and transient responses to stress, and serious symptomatology manifested as disturbances in behaviors, cognition, personality, physical signs, and syndrome combinations.

Accurate diagnosis of psychiatric conditions lead to appropriate referrals, selection of the most appropriate evidenced-based treatments, and ultimately amelioration or elimination of problematic symptoms that negatively impact health and functioning (Peterson, 2011). Practitioners have learned a great deal about psychiatric diagnoses in the last two decades, and this new information will continue to grow with advances in science and improve the understanding of psychiatric diagnoses, reduce social stigma associated with them, and improve treatment outcomes (APA, 2013).

Competency in Psychiatric Rehabilitation

This section of the chapter provides rehabilitation counselors with an overview of the knowledge, skills, and competencies necessary to understand psychiatric diagnoses, knowledge that is essential to optimize the mental health and functioning of consumers of rehabilitation services. A single book chapter is insufficient to fully train rehabilitation counselors to identify psychiatric diagnoses, but is very useful in highlighting the depth and breadth of knowledge required to do so effectively in practice.

While many consumers of rehabilitation services will begin work with counselors, having already been diagnosed with a psychiatric condition, a rehabilitation counselor may be the first mental health professional to have established any type of therapeutic relationship with them, which may reveal information that had never been a focus of clinical attention. A rehabilitation counselor may be the first allied health professional to accurately identify a psychiatric diagnosis for a consumer, and make appropriate referrals for psychiatric treatment or psychotherapy. After a consumer begins training or job placement, he or she may encounter significant stressors and circumstances that lead to the development of psychiatric symptoms, which rehabilitation counselors may need to identify and plan for in the counseling relationship.

Psychiatric Rehabilitation Defined

The definition of psychiatric rehabilitation as approved by the United States Psychiatric Rehabilitation Association (USPRA) is as follows:

Psychiatric rehabilitation promotes recovery, full community integration, and improved quality of life for persons who have been diagnosed with any mental health condition that seriously impairs their ability to lead meaningful lives. Psychiatric rehabilitation services are collaborative, person directed, and individualized. These services are an essential element of the health care and human services spectrum, and must be evidence-based. They focus on helping individuals develop skills and access resources needed to increase their capacity to be successful and satisfied in the living, working, learning, and social environments of their choice (Anthony & Farkas, 2009, p. 9).

Readers are referred to the Commission on Rehabilitation Counselor Certification (CRCC) and Council on Rehabilitation Education (CORE) websites for detailed criteria that relate directly with the aforementioned definition of psychiatric rehabilitation. Rehabilitation counselors need to be aware of the essentials of the psychiatric rehabilitation process and how to work with it (Anthony & Farkas, 2009).

Competencies Required

Specifically, rehabilitation counselors need training and supervision in several key areas to work effectively with consumers who have psychiatric diagnoses. First, training and supervision in the assessment of psychological functioning is essential to understanding information used in the diagnostic process. Counselors need familiarity with the contemporary classification of diagnoses and related functioning, including the 22 diagnostic categories in the DSM-5 and the WHO's family of classifications; all this is essential to effective and complete case conceptualization, defining disability, and effective intervention targeting. A thorough understanding of the evidenced-based psychotherapeutic and psychopharmacologic treatments is necessary for the elimination or amelioration of functional difficulties and barriers to gainful employment and independent living (CORE, 2013; Peterson, 2011).

It is important to have a conceptual framework from which to draw when conceptualizing a case in rehabilitation counseling. A framework that works very well with psychiatric diagnoses is the World Health Organization's model of health, as operationalized in the International Classification of Functioning,

Disability, and Health (Peterson, 2011; WHO, 2001). This conceptualization of psychiatric disability is presented in this chapter.

Prevalence of Psychiatric Diagnoses

The U.S. Census Bureau's American Community Survey (ACS) of 2008 estimates that over one-third of those seeking rehabilitation services may have a psychiatric diagnosis affecting cognitive functioning (Brault, 2009). The National Comorbidity Survey Replication (NCS-R) conducted by Kessler, Chiu, Demler, & Walters (2005), which surveyed the prevalence, severity, and comorbidity of twelve-month duration DSM-IV disorders, estimated that over one quarter of the population presents with psychiatric diagnoses in any given year, and 57.4 percent will have a psychiatric diagnosis within their lifetime; nearly half of those diagnosed will likely have more than one psychiatric diagnosis.

Diagnostic Systems

DSM-5

The most contemporary diagnostic system available for psychiatric diagnoses is the Diagnostic and Statistical Manual of Mental Disorders, Fifth Edition (DSM-5; APA, 2013). The intent of the latest revision of the DSM was to be useful to mental health professionals, consumers of mental health services and their families, and researchers, by providing clear and concise descriptions of psychiatric diagnoses. Each diagnosis provides explicit diagnostic criteria, dimensional measures that cut across diagnoses, and a concise overview of a given diagnosis, risk factors, associated features, related research, and possible manifestations of the diagnosis (APA, 2013).

ICD-10-CM

The system more commonly used throughout the world than the DSM is the International Statistical Classification of Diseases and Related Health Problems, Tenth Revision (ICD-10; WHO, 1992), recently updated as the International Classification of Diseases, Tenth Revision, Clinical Modification (ICD-10-CM; WHO, 2014). Within the U.S., clinicians use the clinical modification of the 9th revision of the ICD (ICD-9-CM; WHO, 2011).

There have been efforts to *harmonize* the DSM-5 revision with the ICD-11 revision (APA, 2013, p. xli). For now, the DSM-5 references both the ICD-9-CM codes and ICD-10-CM codes as they relate to the DSM's current diagnoses (both codes are listed along with each DSM diagnosis), the former to be used within the U.S. through October 1, 2014, the latter thereafter in coordination with the scheduled adoption of the ICD-10-CM (APA, 2013, pp. xiii & xli).

Psychiatric Disability Defined: The ICF

The most contemporary definition of disability to date can be found within the WHO's conceptualization of health, the International Classification of Functioning, Disability, and Health (ICF) (WHO, 2001). The ICF is the latest addition to the WHO family of classifications. While the ICD provides an etiological classification of health conditions (e.g., diseases, disorders, injuries), the ICF provides information on functioning associated with a broad array of health conditions (Peterson, 2011; Peterson & Elliott, 2008; Peterson, Mpofu, & Oakland, 2010; Peterson & Paul 2009). The ICF is a significant development in healthcare, as it can be used as a standard for defining concepts, building constructs, hypothesizing relationships, and proposing new theories that will further research and practice (WHO, 2001).

The ICF's conceptual framework provides an intuitive model of functioning, disability, and health. The WHO model of health as defined in the ICF conceptual framework describes interrelated, reciprocally interacting factors related to a person in the environment. The framework is comprised of (a) two parts, each with two components. The first part addresses the person, and the two components are body structures and functions and (b) activities and participation. The person is described physically with respect to *body structure*, which in the instance of psychiatric diagnoses involves the brain and nervous system. *Body function* describes a change in function as a result of a change in *body structure*. For example, a lack of a specific neurotransmitter in the brain, serotonin, could result in a change in the brain's neurochemistry, and the related change of function could be unremitting depressive symptoms.

The second component associated with the person as portrayed in the ICF involves one's potential to function, or *activity*, in comparison with one's actual functioning within a current context, or *participation*. In the case of depression, a person's depressive symptoms may include psychomotor slowing that would impact the ability to keep pace in a work environment. If within a specific context the person has access to effective medication in the form of antidepressants, psychomotor slowing could improve. The provision of medication in this *context* can impact a person's ability to *participate* effectively, in this case keep pace in the work environment. Interventions like medication or reasonable accommodations in a work setting target disparities between a person's potential (activity) and actual performance (participation) in a given context.

Psychiatric disability then, according to the WHO model of health, can be defined as a function of how a person's impairment manifests within a context. The contextual or second part of the ICF is comprised of the *environment* and also *personal factors*. The environment addresses the immediate context and more distant but impactful societal contexts. Personal factors address a long list of diversity-related issues that could impact functioning. A mental health professional can target disparities between someone's potential and current functioning because of environmental factors, in order to maximize potential function, and minimize the impact of disability. All interventions should be sensitive to one's individual context as defined in *personal factors* of the framework.

What determines whether a disability is clinically significant? Both the APA and WHO have attempted to separate the constructs of mental disorder from disability (APA, 2013). Mental disorders fall under the ICD WHO classifications of disease. The point has been made that disability does not manifest functional impairment consistently across individuals. An impairment's impact on someone's health and functioning in a specific context is classified using the ICF (WHO, 2001). The WHO Disability Assessment Schedule (WHODAS 2.0) (WHO, 2012) is based upon the ICF, and is proposed for use within the DSM-5 as a standardized measure of disability. However, many psychiatric diagnoses lack reliable measures of severity to inform the use of the WHODAS. The clinical significance of a psychiatric diagnosis remains a matter of clinical judgment as to whether "the disturbance causes clinically significant distress or impairment in social, occupational, or other important areas of functioning" (APA, 2013, p. 21).

Evolution of the DSM

The American Psychiatric Association began classifying *institutionalized mental patients* in 1844 (APA, 2013, p. 6), and the resulting DSM system has been through five revisions since then. To help manage the co-existence of the DSM-IV-TR and the DSM-5 during the two-year trial period and beyond, this chapter reviews the structure of the DSM-IV-TR.

The Multiaxial Assessment Format of the DSM-IV-TR

The DSM-IV-TR consists of five component axes (APA, 2000). The first, Axis I, Clinical disorders and other conditions that may be a focus of clinical attention, involves most psychiatric disorders in the system. Axis II, Personality disorders and mental retardation, may be conceptualized as a group of conditions that are less temporal and more enduring than many Axis I diagnoses.

Axis III, General medical conditions, provides an opportunity to consider how physical condition may affect psychological functioning. Axis IV, Psychosocial and environmental problems, provides a list of possible contextual factors that may impact overall psychological functioning, including interpersonal problems, family discord, death of a family member, and educational, occupational, housing, economic, healthcare, and legal issues. Finally, Axis V, Global Assessment of Functioning or GAF, provides a numeric scale to estimate level of impairment and/or a diagnosis' impact on functioning. The scores on this scale ranged from 1 to 100, with "0" indicating inadequate information. A score in the 1 to 10 range indicates extremely low functioning, and the 90 to 100 range denotes superior functioning. Ultimately, the GAF was eliminated due to inconsistency in its application in practice. The multiaxial system brought attention to a biopsychosocial model of health and functioning comprised not only of physical and mental illness, but also the person within his or her social and environmental context (Peterson, 2011).

The DSM-5

The DSM-5 (APA, 2013) is made up of three sections. Section I reviews the history and developmental process of the latest revision of the DSM, and provides a guide to the basics of DSM-5 clinical diagnosis. Section II contains the diagnostic criteria and codes, classifying psychiatric disorders into 22 major categories, an expansion of the DSM-IV-TR's 17 major categories:

1. Neurodevelopmental Disorders
2. Schizophrenia Spectrum and Other Psychotic Disorders
3. Bipolar and Related Disorders
4. Depressive Disorders
5. Anxiety Disorders
6. Obsessive-Compulsive and Related Disorders
7. Trauma- and Stressor-Related Disorders
8. Dissociative Disorders
9. Somatic-Symptom and Related Disorders
10. Feeding and Eating Disorders
11. Elimination Disorders
12. Sleep-Wake Disorders
13. Sexual Dysfunctions
14. Gender Dysphoria
15. Disruptive, Impulse-Control, and Conduct Disorders
16. Substance-Related and Addictive Disorders
17. Neurocognitive Disorders
18. Personality Disorders
19. Paraphilic Disorders
20. Other Mental Disorders
21. Medication-Induced Movement Disorders and Other Adverse Effects of Medication
22. Other Conditions That May Be a Focus of Clinical Attention

The primary purpose of Section II of the DSM-5 is "to assist trained clinicians in the diagnosis of their patients' mental disorders as part of a case formulation assessment that leads to a fully informed treatment plan" (p. 19). Section III, Emerging Measures and Models, provides new assessment measures, cultural formulations, an alternative model for disorders of personality, and conditions for further study. The contents of Section III are suggested to require further study before full implementation with Section II of the manual, but users are encouraged to use them to enhance clinical decision-making (APA, 2013).

Changes from DSM-IV-TR to DSM-5

Organization of the diagnostic categories in the DSM-5 was changed to harmonize with the most recent version of the Mental and Behavioral Disorders section of the ICD (versions 10 and 11). This was done to minimize the impact of having two different diagnostic systems affecting collection of health statistics and future research replication. Advances in neuroscience are reflected in expanded diagnostic categories and subtypes of neurocognitive disorders.

The DSM-5 has transitioned away from the multiaxial system of diagnosis, to a non-axial system. Axes I and II are combined, and Axis III, physical conditions, if they affect psychological functioning, are to be noted along with the psychiatric diagnoses. Axis IV was eliminated, as the DSM-5 task force decided not to further develop its own psychosocial and environmental problems classification schema (APA, 2013, p. 16). With the elimination of the axial system, the order of diagnoses presented in the DSM-5 reflects a developmental and lifespan perspective.

Axis V, Global Assessment of Functioning or GAF score, has been eliminated. In its place, within section III of the DSM-5, Emerging Measures and Models, and related to the prior ICF discussion, the WHODAS 2.0 (WHO, 2012), a derivative of the ICF, provides a new standard method for assessing global disability levels for mental disorders. The WHODAS conception of disability replaces the GAF, and specifically address *disability* (APA, 2013, p. 16). Also included in section III are 13 symptom domains with dimensional measures of severity proposed for all DSM diagnostic groups.

The frequently used "not otherwise specified" or "NOS" qualifier for DSM-IV-TR, which meant a diagnosis came close to but did not satisfy all the diagnostic criteria required for the formal diagnosis, has been changed to one of two new options. *Other specified disorder* is used to highlight the specific reason why a set of symptoms does not meet diagnostic criteria. *Unspecified disorder* is the qualifier used if the clinician decides not to highlight the specific reason. Clinical judgment is used in determining whether there is sufficient evidence to use *other specified* versus *unspecified disorder*.

The DSM-5 has online supplemental information, including more symptom and functional impairment severity measures that cut across diagnostic categories. To enhance cultural sensitivity of DSM diagnoses, the *Cultural Formulation Interview* is provided with supplements (see www.psychiatry.org/dsm5). Pages 14 and 15 of the DSM-5 provide an overview of the myriad of cultural and gender issues that affect the boundary between normality and pathology, and the systems in which healthcare is provided.

Some of the diagnostic changes in the DSM-5 include the pervasive developmental disorders combined into an *autism spectrum disorder*, and the term mental retardation has been replaced by *intellectual disability* (or intellectual developmental disorder). Severity of these conditions is estimated using measures of adaptive functioning rather than measures of IQ. The various learning disorders have been combined into one *specific learning disorder* diagnosis. Substance abuse and dependence are now described as *substance use disorders*, and the distinction between tolerance and withdrawal (formerly associated with dependence) and addiction is made clear. The subtypes of schizophrenia have been removed due to their lack of clinical utility. The commonly used cognitive disorder not otherwise specified is now *neurocognitive disorder*. There are other detailed changes not covered here; for details, the reader is referred to pages 809-816 of the DSM-5.

Diagnostic Groups

This section of the chapter provides overviews of some of the diagnostic groups within the DSM-5 (and related diagnostic groups in the ICD-9-CM and the ICD-10-CM). This text contains stand-alone chapters that focus on specific diagnostic categories within the DSM, such as alcoholism and addictions, intellectual disability, specific learning disorders, neurological diagnoses, and acquired brain injury (related to neurodevelopmental and neurocognitive disorders).

The brief descriptions of diagnostic groups do not replace the direct use of the DSM-5; readers are encouraged to refer directly to it for specific diagnostic criteria. In contrast, the ICD-10-CM is a free system and available online at the World Health Organization's homepage. The brief descriptions of diagnoses in this chapter can be referenced back to these ICD systems; the most recent versions 10 and 11 have been and are being harmonized with the DSM-5 system (WHO, 2014). Next, are concise reviews of specific diagnostic groups commonly encountered in rehabilitation counseling.

Anxiety Disorders

Second only to substance use disorders that have a lifetime prevalence of 35.3% (National Institute of Mental Health [NIMH], 2007), anxiety disorders are among the most commonly occurring psychiatric diagnoses, with a lifetime prevalence of 31.2%. In a given year, about 40 million American adults age 18 and older, or 18.1% of people in this age group, have anxiety disorders (Kessler et al., 2005). These statistics were calculated while the DSM-IV-TR was in use, and when posttraumatic stress disorder (PTSD) was within this category; it has since been moved to the Trauma-and Stressor-Related Disorders category, reviewed later in this chapter.

Anxiety symptoms include nervousness, trembling, muscular tension, sweating, lightheadedness, palpitations, dizziness, epigastric discomfort, and various forms of worries and forebodings. This diagnostic category includes separation anxiety disorder, selective mutism, specific phobia, social anxiety disorder, panic disorder, agoraphobia, generalized anxiety disorder, and substance/medication-induced anxiety disorder. Specific diagnoses selected within the DSM-5 are a matter of what may have caused the anxiety (e.g., substance or medication-induced, a medical condition), when it occurred, and duration (APA, 2013). For this diagnostic group, features of generalized anxiety disorder, panic disorder, agoraphobia, and social anxiety disorder (social phobia) are highlighted. According to the NIMH study, the comorbidity of anxiety disorders with both depression and substance use is high (Kessler et al., 2005).

Generalized Anxiety Disorder

This condition involves excessive anxiety or worry that is pervasive and chronic, lasting six months or longer. Symptoms include anxiety and worry that is far out of proportion for the context, restlessness, feeling on edge, easily fatigued, concentration problems, irritability, muscle tension, and difficulty with sleep. Some have reported that they struggled with such symptoms for many years before seeking treatment. About 6.8 million American adults or 3.1% of the adult population have generalized anxiety disorder in a given year, with a lifetime prevalence of 5.7% (NIMH, 2007).

Panic Disorders

Panic disorders involve the presence of sudden panic attacks and intense experiences of psychological fear and physiological arousal. A panic attack starts suddenly with a feeling of severe apprehension, fearfulness, or terror associated with feelings of impending doom. During an attack, the individual experiences physiological symptoms like shortness of breath, rapid or skipped heartbeats, chest pain or discomfort, and choking or smothering sensations. There is a fear of losing control or even dying. The lifetime prevalence for panic disorders is 4.7% (NIMH, 2007).

Agoraphobia

In the DSM-IV-TR, panic disorders were classified as with or without agoraphobia, but agoraphobia is no longer associated with panic disorder; it stands on its own as a marked fear of social situations. Individuals fear or avoid social situations because they believe escape might be difficult in the event of an embarrassing situation (e.g., panic attack, falling asleep in public, incontinence).

Social Anxiety Disorder, Specific Phobias

Social anxiety disorder, or social phobia, consists of a marked fear or anxiety about one or more social situations where one might be scrutinized. Approximately 15 million adults in the U.S., or 6.8% have social phobia in a given year (Kessler et al., 2005), with a 12.1% lifetime prevalence (NIMH, 2007). Finally, about 19.2 million of the same population, or 8.7% have some type of specific phobia in a given year, with a 12.5% lifetime prevalence (NIMH, 2007).

Treatment of Anxiety Disorders

Medication, psychotherapy, or combinations of both methods are effective means to treat anxiety disorders. Temporary relief is available from a class of medications called benzodiazepines, which provide rapid relief, but are addictive. Antidepressant medications are a better long-term medical treatment for anxiety, and most effective with psychotherapeutic techniques that provide behavioral and cognitive strategies for managing anxiety (Preston, O'Neal, & Talaga, 2013). Consumers of rehabilitation services may have struggled with anxiety their entire lifetime and coped with it using substance abuse or avoidance of anxiety provoking situations. There is a high comorbidity between anxiety disorders and alcoholism and other substance use (Sadock, Kaplan, & Sadock, 2010). The rehabilitation counselor may need to make appropriate treatment recommendations to minimize debilitating anxiety in the rehabilitation process, and to help teach new and functional coping skills to deal with anxiety.

Mood Disorders

Bipolar and depressive disorders, whose primary impairment is disturbance in mood, are one of the most commonly diagnosed conditions. Depressive disorders involve only depressive episodes, while bipolar disorders involve both manic or hypomanic (elevated mood) and depressive episodes.

According to NCS-R, 20.9 million American adults, or 9.5% of the U.S. population age 18 and older in a given year have a mood disorder, which may include major depressive disorder (the leading cause of disability in the U.S. for ages 15 to 44) (WHO, 2004), dysthymic disorder (affecting 1.5% of the U.S. population age 18 and older in a given year), and bipolar disorder (affecting 2.6% or 5.7 million adults age 18 and older) (Kessler et al., 2005). The NIMH update on lifetime prevalence for any mood disorder is 21.4% (NIMH, 2007).

Depressive Disorders

The DSM-5 reported that the 12-month prevalence of Major Depressive Disorder is 7% in the United States, with higher rates for younger individuals and women (APA, 2013). Depressive disorders often occur comorbidly with anxiety and substance-related disorders (Kessler et al., 2005). The depressive disorders in the DSM-5 and ICD-10 have in common moods that are sad, empty, or irritable, with somatic and cognitive effects on health and functioning. The specific depressive diagnosis selected within the DSM-5 is a matter of what caused the mood disturbance (e.g., substance or medication-induced, a medical condition, bereavement), when it occurred, and for how long (see APA, 2013).

Depression may manifest as anhedonia, or a lack of interest in pleasurable activities. Depression makes it hard to fall asleep, or causes early morning awakening, adversely impacting restorative sleep. It can increase or decrease appetite. The person may demonstrate psychotic features, such as hallucinations or delusions. Depression often is accompanied by anxiety. There is a high prevalence of alcohol and substance abuse with individuals who have mood disorders so it is common to encounter clients with dual diagnoses (Sadock et al., 2010). Persons with mood disorders may use alcohol or other substances as self-medication (i.e., for their sedative, disinhibiting, or stimulating effects).

Severe depression causes difficulty with concentration, the ability to persist on a job, keeping appropriate pace due to psychomotor slowing, or fatigue, resulting in both personal and occupational difficulties. Disturbance in mood adversely impacts social functioning as well, has an impact on where an individual can find employment, and how he or she interacts with the system of social support. Self-esteem and confidence diminishes as a result.

There is a high rate of mortality with more severe forms of depression. According to the Centers for Disease Control and Prevention (CDC, 2010), 33,300 people in the U.S died from suicide in 2006, and historically more than 90% of those who end their life had a diagnosable mental disorder, most often depression or substance-related disorders (Conwell & Brent, 1995).

Treatment of Depression

Major depressive disorder is treated using medication, psychotherapy, or a combination. Response to treatment takes several weeks with antidepressants, symptoms can be unresponsive to medication, dosage or type of medication often needs periodic adjustment, or symptoms remit and return later as a matter of course or in response to stressful life situations. There are adjunctive therapies using atypical antipsychotic medications when antidepressant medications alone are not effective. Longitudinal research suggests that psychotherapy and medication combined are more effective than either treatment alone (Preston et al., 2013).

People experiencing depression often consider their symptoms to be related to physical illness rather than psychiatric illness, so they may seek help from general health care professionals (Sadock et al., 2010). The majority of psychotropic medications are prescribed by non-mental health professionals (Pomerantz et al., 2004). Mental health professionals, including counselors, can provide collaborative support to other health professionals to maximize treatment efficacy.

Bipolar Disorders

The lifetime prevalence of people with any type of bipolar disorder is 4.4% (NIMH, 2007). People with bipolar disorders were historically referred to as being *manic-depressive*. In contrast with depressive disorders, bipolar disorders involve depression and either a manic (elevated mood) or hypomanic (less severe mood elevation) episode. Depression, in this condition, is defined the same as for depressive disorder above. According to the DSM-5, bipolar I disorder manifests both depression and mania. Bipolar II disorder manifests depression and hypomania (APA, 2013).

During mania or a manic episode, a person demonstrates a distinct period of abnormally and persistently elevated, expansive, or irritable mood. Oftentimes, the person feels euphoric, has inflated self-esteem, or becomes extremely gregarious, talkative, and overly active socially or occupationally. They feel that their thoughts are racing, and become very distractible or impulsive. The person appears overly energetic with a decreased need for sleep. Similar to major depressive disorders, individuals with severe cases of bipolar disorders may experience hallucinations and delusions (APA, 2013).

Persons experiencing manic symptoms often do not recognize that something is wrong. They seek help only at the insistence of family members or employers who find their behaviors disturbing. They may be brought in by law enforcement officers for unruly or bizarre behaviors in public, or for engaging in activities that are dangerous to themselves or others. Other features include poor judgment, risky business ventures, disregard for ethical concerns, and engaging in antisocial behaviors. Substance abuse and other risk taking behaviors can accompany a manic or hypomanic episode.

Treatment of Bipolar Disorders

People with bipolar disorders require medication for mood stabilization, which include antidepressants, atypical antipsychotics, anti-seizure medication (which have a mood stabilizing effect), or lithium. Unfortunately, manic and hypomanic episodes may be accompanied by the belief that one is *cured*, and the person stops medication compliance, resulting in exacerbations in mania and depression. Many cases of bipolar disorder require medication management for life. Psychotherapy can be of limited use when someone is in a manic state, but pharmacotherapy can be very useful for overall mental health and functioning (Preston el al., 2013).

Trauma- and Stress-Related Disorders

This category is new to the DSM-5; all disorders share in common the exposure to a traumatic event, and the variable psychological distress that ensues. Within this group are the following diagnoses: reactive attachment disorder, disinhibited social engagement disorder, posttraumatic stress disorder, acute stress disorder, and adjustment disorder (APA, 2013). In this section, the chapter focuses on the three diagnosis.

Posttraumatic Stress Disorder (PTSD)

Formerly one of the anxiety disorders (APA, 2000), NIMH numbers for lifetime prevalence of PTSD is 6.8% (NIMH, 2007). PTSD gained significant attention during the Vietnam War, and the more recent conflicts in Afghanistan and Iraq brought further attention to the diagnosis. A study reported in the *New England Journal of Medicine* (Hoge et al., 2004) indicated that among soldiers and marines deployed to Iraq, the prevalence of PTSD is 9.3% for those who had experienced one to two firefights, 12.7% for those with three to five firefights, and 19.3% for those with more than five firefights. Similar rates were found for those deployed to Afghanistan.

PTSD is a diagnosis associated with a delayed and/or protracted response following exposure to stressful or traumatic events. Traumatic events that lead to the development of PTSD are as varied as the human experience. A famous example of a traumatic event was the terrorist bombing of the World Trade Center, which affected many first responders to the tragedy, as well as many New York City residents who lived through the aftermath (Ganzel, Casey, Glover, Voss, & Temple, 2007). Other such events include natural or man-made disasters, serious accidents, witnessing the violent death of another, being a victim of torture, terrorism, or rape, and other serious crime. Related symptoms include reliving the trauma in intrusive memories (flashbacks) or dreams, feeling detached or emotionally numb, or diminished interest or participation in social or daily activities (WHO, 2014). Other persistent symptoms include increased arousal, insomnia, irritability, emotional outbursts, difficulty concentrating, hypervigilance, and exaggerated startle response. Symptoms can be triggered by events in the environment that remind one of the distressing event.

Acute Stress, Adjustment Disorders

Acute stress disorder is a stress reaction shorter in duration than PTSD, lasting less than one month. The diagnosis is changed to PTSD if symptoms persist beyond a month. Adjustment disorder is a state of distress and emotional disturbance resulting from a significant life change or stressful event, that interferes with personal, social, or occupational functioning (WHO, 2014). Related symptoms can manifest as anxiety, depressed mood, or disturbance in conduct.

Treating Trauma- and Stress-Related Disorders

Psychopharmacological treatment is useful in treating debilitating anxiety associated with stress and trauma. Alpha blockers, blood pressure medications, have been shown to help with night terrors and nightmares in military personnel with PTSD. Antidepressants, antianxiety, and atypical antipsychotic medications are effective in managing mood instability that may be associated with stress and trauma-related symptoms. Behavioral and cognitive approaches in psychotherapy help manage the body's reaction to symptoms, and provide compensatory strategies for troubling thoughts and recollections (Lambert, 2013; Preston et al., 2013).

Schizophrenia Spectrum Disorders

Based on nearly 200 studies from 46 nations, international lifetime prevalence rates for schizophrenia are less than 0.005% (Bhugra, 2005), much lower than the 1% reported in the DSM-IV-TR (APA, 2000). Small numbers notwithstanding, schizophrenia and related spectrum disorders are often chronic and severe conditions that require specific clinical skills of the rehabilitation professional.

Based upon the ICD-10-CM (WHO, 2014), *schizophrenic disorders* are characterized by fundamental and characteristic distortions of thinking and perception, and by inappropriate or blunted (unusually unexpressive) affect. Hallucinations, delusions, and gross behavioral disturbances may be present when people are diagnosed. Noncompliance with medication and subsequent psychotic episodes can lead to irreversible changes in brain structure resulting in cognitive deficits (Preston et al., 2013).

Key Features of Psychotic Disorders

The DSM-5 (APA, 2013) defined five key features of psychotic disorders in general; they include delusions, hallucinations, disorganized thinking (speech), grossly disorganized or abnormal motor behavior (including catatonia), and negative symptoms. *Delusions* are false beliefs and can include the idea that an external force is remotely controlling one's actions or that one's thoughts are being monitored by some kind of transmitter. These ideas are often bizarre and clearly discerned to be without grounds by practically everyone else, including those from the same social and cultural background as the client. *Hallucinations* are sensory perceptions not based on external stimuli. As an example, the person may hear voices when there is clearly no one speaking.

Disorganized thinking is manifest through speech that reveals incoherent or tangential thought processes difficult to understand. *Disorganized or abnormal motor behavior* ranges from silliness to unpredictable agitation and socially inappropriate behavior. An individual may act in an eccentric manner or demonstrate a marked decrease in reactivity to the environment (catatonia). Finally, *negative symptoms* relate primarily to diminished emotional experience, and avolition or a decrease in motivated, self-initiated, purposeful activity. Consumers of rehabilitation services with psychotic or negative symptoms of schizophrenia may appear irrational, incoherent, withdrawn, or engage in inappropriate behavior. The onset of symptoms of schizophrenia typically occurs during young adulthood, and its course differs. Complete recovery is unlikely (Sadock et al., 2010).

Diagnoses within Schizophrenia Spectrum Disorders

The DSM-IV-TR (APA, 2000) identified five major types of schizophrenia: paranoid type, disorganized type, catatonic type, undifferentiated type, and residual type; these categories no longer exist in the DSM-5 (APA, 2013). The first three types are characterized by their most prominent symptoms, namely paranoia, disorganization, and catatonic behavior, respectively. Undifferentiated type refers to a form of schizophrenia that currently does not display the specific criteria for any of these three dominant symptoms. Residual type is diagnosed in individuals who once had an active diagnosis of schizophrenia but currently do not show any major symptoms.

Within the DSM-5, diagnoses in this category are now organized along a gradient of severity of psychopathology (APA, 2013). First, schizotypal personality disorder is mentioned (but defined elsewhere among the personality disorders group) as a condition manifesting social and interpersonal deficits, which may include milder forms of bizarre thinking, behavior, or psychoses. Next, is brief psychotic disorder, symptoms remitting within a month. Schizophreniform disorder may ultimately develop into schizophrenia with sufficient duration of symptoms. Schizophrenia may be diagnosed if lasting at least six months in duration. Finally, schizoaffective disorder shares features of schizophrenia and a major mood episode (depression or mania) (APA, 2013).

Treatment of Schizophrenia Spectrum Disorders

Schizophrenia is typically treated with psychotropic medication; psychotherapy has also proven useful with some promise shown for family systems-based psychotherapy and assertive community-based treatment (Lambert, 2013). Unless they have an adequate support network of family members and helping professionals, individuals with more severe forms of schizophrenia spectrum disorders face chronic unemployment and related financial problems. People with diagnoses of schizophrenia account for a portion of the homeless population in the United States (Sadock et al., 2010).

Medication may be essential in controlling the symptoms of schizophrenia and preventing relapse; and side effects present a major health concern. Typical and atypical antipsychotic medications have neurological and other side effects including involuntary movements of the tongue, jaw, and extremities; muscular rigidity; Parkinsonian tremors; weight gain; new onset Type II diabetes mellitus; and for some patients the risk of sudden cardiac death (Preston et al., 2013; Sadock et al., 2010). The consequences of not taking prescribed medication can be dire.

Personality Disorders

Personality disorders are defined in the ICD-10-CM as clinically significant conditions and behavior patterns that may be a persistent expression of one's lifestyle and mode of relating to self and others. The various types of personality disorders all share deeply engrained and enduring behavior patterns that manifest as inflexible and maladaptive responses to a broad range of personal and social situations. This causes personal distress that results in significant problems in social and occupational functioning (WHO, 2014).

DSM-IV-TR and DSM-5 Clusters

The specific diagnoses of personality disorders do not match perfectly between the DSM and the ICD systems, and in the DSM revision those diagnoses that existed in DSM-IV-TR remain in the 5th revision. The 12 personality disorder diagnoses can be summarized into three clusters. Cluster A diagnoses share odd or eccentric behavior; Cluster B diagnoses share dramatic, emotional, or erratic presentations; and Cluster C diagnoses share in common a fearful or anxious presentation (APA, 2013).

Effect of Personality Disorders

Personality disorders play a role in the potential development of other psychiatric diagnoses, and also as factors affecting the treatment of co-existing conditions. One psychiatric diagnosis can cause exaggeration of a preexisting personality trait, which appears to be a personality disorder, but resolves once the related diagnosis is resolved. Also, many psychiatric diagnoses evolve over time and at first appear to be personality disorders. Certain personality disorders predispose an individual to increased risk of developing another psychiatric diagnosis, or complicate the treatment of a co-occurring condition.

Stigma and Psychiatric Diagnoses

Stigma Manifest

Historically, the public viewed people with severe mental illness more negatively than those with physical illnesses. Individuals with mental illness have been considered by some to be undesirable as friends, co-workers, tenants, and employees. The mass media often misrepresents and demeans people with psychiatric diagnoses, portraying them as unreliable, erratic, irrational, and violent (Corrigan, 1998; Hingsaw & Cicchetti, 2000). While public understanding of mental illness has improved in recent years, stigma continues to be a major social barrier.

Stigma affects people with mental illness in a number of ways. It may discourage them from seeking help for their conditions. It affects their self-esteem and causes additional stress on those in their social support system. Stigma has an adverse impact on social relations and may reduce employment and housing opportunities.

Solutions to Stigma

Rehabilitation counselors can help reduce stigma, using the focal points of WHO's model of health to target different interventions (Peterson, 2011). At the societal level, counselors may address stigma by bringing psychiatric diagnoses out into the open, allowing people to talk about them, and refute harmful stereotypes to reduce social stigma (Carter, Golant, & Cade, 2010). They may seek out opportunities to collaborate with other professionals and client advocacy groups to promote an accurate and sensitive image of people with psychiatric disabilities. For example, while some people with serious psychiatric diagnoses may be violent, the majority are not. There is little risk of harm to a stranger from casual contact with a person with mental illness.

Counselors can help employers and co-workers dispel the myths surrounding psychiatric diagnoses. Some might fear that people with psychiatric disabilities could become disruptive or violent at work. Others are concerned that if they say the wrong thing, it will cause the person to become unstable. While these concerns are relevant in some cases, they are overly generalized to encompass all individuals with mental disorders. Those who have worked in psychiatric rehabilitation realize the value of using counseling skills to help those close to the person with a psychiatric diagnosis to demystify the diagnosis, refute negative stereotypes, offer ideas for reasonable accommodation, and provide an opportunity to change the focus from disability to ability. Rehabilitation counselors providing job follow-up support need to address ostracism by co-workers, or occasional jokes or remarks by insensitive colleagues. Finding supportive ways to proactively address such concerns helps avoid the creation of a hostile and stressful work environment.

At the individual level, the client may or may not want to disclose his or her disability to an employer, depending on the particular job setting, degree of recovery, and personal preferences. Counselors should advise clients about the appropriateness of disclosing or not disclosing psychiatric disability. The decision of whether or not to disclose, and how much information to disclose, is made on an individual basis, and can be informed by good clinical judgment of the rehabilitation counselor. Ultimately, whether there needs to be disclosure depends on a client's desire to request reasonable accommodation. The consumer and counselor can together to weigh the pros and cons of disclosure so that the consumer can make an informed choice.

The Recovery Model in Psychiatric Rehabilitation

A recovery model is being advocated in the public mental health system (Davidson, O'Connell, Tondoora, Styron, & Kangas, 2006; Jacobson & Greenley, 2001). The origin of this model is the recovery approach defined within psychiatric rehabilitation. This is a comprehensive model with many elements, one of which is to help clients manage and live with mental disorders, rather than expecting or waiting for them to be symptom free before returning to full participation in society. This model emphasizes self-determination and input from clients and their family members in the recovery process, and in the design and operation of the mental health service system. Rehabilitation counselors working in public mental health settings with clients who have psychiatric diagnoses may need to be familiar with the recovery model approach for intervention planning and documentation of treatment outcomes (Anthony & Farkas, 2009).

The psychiatric rehabilitation process as defined by the Boston University Center for Psychiatric Rehabilitation is an evidence-based approach with specific job descriptions, record keeping formats, and quality assurance mechanisms that require intensive training and supervision over time to implement. The approach stemmed from the deinstitutionalization movement that began in the 1950s, which discharged large numbers of patients from state hospitals into communities that were ill prepared or unwilling to provide appropriate support. Essential services provided within a recovery-oriented system include treatment for symptom relief, crisis intervention, case management, rehabilitation goals, enrichment activities for self-development, rights protection for equal opportunity, and support for healthy lifestyle, empowerment, and basic support of essential needs (Anthony & Farkas, 2009).

Case Study

Mr. Robert Arsenije is a 23 year-old immigrant from Kosovo with chronic schizophrenia. At age 18, he was diagnosed with this disorder. His specific diagnosis is schizophrenia, paranoid type, episodic with inter-episode residual symptoms. This indicates he has occasional relapses into episodes of active symptoms and has residual or less severe symptoms between these episodes.

Robert is the second of three children of an intact family. Prior to the onset of his mental disorder, he had a stable and impressive school performance record, including being a member of the high school golf team. When his problems first started, he was a 12th grade honor student. As the academic term progressed, he became increasingly reclusive and abruptly quit school. Robert reported paranoid ideation, believing that people were reading his mind for evil purposes; he began to neglect hygiene and self-care, and engaged in angry outbursts toward his family when they confronted him about his poor school performance and issues of self care. When his family felt his condition became unbearable, they brought him in for psychiatric services; Robert was diagnosed with schizophrenia and hospitalized.

After two weeks in the hospital, Robert's condition stabilized and he was discharged for outpatient services, which included daily medication and weekly psychotherapy. While the intensity of his symptoms subsided, he continued to experience residual symptoms. Robert was particularly anxious in the presence of strangers. The idea that people were reading his mind, even though he acknowledged this to be impossible, continued to preoccupy him. After a few months of therapy, Robert re-enrolled in high school, but soon dropped out. He was unable to concentrate in school, always feeling that someone was reading his mind. Feelings of depression and helplessness about his condition and being rejected by his classmates predominated his thoughts. Most of his time was spent at home. During summer, he attended a GED (General Equivalency Diploma) program and obtained a high school diploma.

After obtaining his diploma, Robert began to feel motivated. With the encouragement of his therapist, he attempted various jobs during the following year, but quit each job after a month or two, indicating that they were boring. These jobs included short order cook, automobile detailer, landscape assistant at a golf course, and golf starter (takes golf reservations, collects fees, and assigns golf starting times). Robert decided he wanted to obtain a college education so that he could secure more fulfilling employment. A four-year college within commuting distance from his home accepted him. However, he dropped out in the first semester. He denied experiencing stress as a result of attending school full time. Instead, he claimed that he did not like the college or the courses he was taking. After a few months, he re-enrolled, this time in a junior college. During the next three years, Robert periodically took classes. Most of his free time was spent at home, watching television or reading books; he had no friends.

During this period, Robert had a few relapses into active symptoms, triggered by his refusal to take medication appropriately. On one occasion, Robert simply stopped taking medication, insisting that he had learned to control or ignore his paranoid thoughts. On other occasions, he stopped taking his medication after family arguments. Each time, his symptoms intensified. Fearful that evil people were reading his mind and coming to harm him, he would hide in his room. His family had him involuntarily hospitalized. After resuming his medication, Robert's condition stabilized; he was discharged home and treated with outpatient services.

Through therapy, Robert accepted that his paranoid ideations were irrational, but was still distressed by them. Whether he was in college or home watching television, he would suddenly feel that someone was reading his mind. These thoughts were frightening, even though he kept reminding himself that this could not happen. Recently, after an active episode followed by hospitalization, his family decided it was too stressful for them to have Robert at home. By mutual agreement, Robert was discharged to a supervised housing unit, where he could receive close monitoring. For a few months Robert worked in a sheltered workshop. However, he wanted to continue classes at junior college and was adamant about obtaining a college degree, rather than going through a job training program. While discussing his career goals, Robert alternated between pursuing his high school dream of becoming a famous scientist, or majoring in business.

Questions

1. Based on this chapter review and the WHO's model of health, what does a rehabilitation counselor need to conceptualize for this case?
2. Assign Robert a vocational profile including age category, educational level, and work history.
3. What vocational alternatives can you recommend?
4. How should a rehabilitation counselor help Robert establish and achieve realistic educational goals?
5. What measures would you take to assure that Robert complies with his medication schedule?
6. Discuss prejudice and discrimination toward persons with mental illness and how these can be diminished in the workplace.

References

American Psychiatric Association. (2000). *Diagnostic and statistical manual of mental disorders* (4th ed., text rev.). Washington, DC: Author.

American Psychiatric Association. (2013). *Diagnostic and statistical manual of mental disorders* (5th ed.). *(DSM-5)*. Arlington, VA: Author.

Anthony, W. A., & Farkas, M. D. (2009). *A primer on the psychiatric rehabilitation process*. Boston, MA: Boston University Center for Psychiatric Rehabilitation.

Bhugra, D. (2005). The global prevalence of schizophrenia. *PLoS Medicine, 2*(5), 151.

Brault, M. W. (2009). *Review of changes to the measurement of disability in the 2008 American Community Survey*. Washington, DC: U. S. Census Bureau.

Carter, R., Golant, S. K., & Cade, K. E. (2010). *Within our reach: Ending the mental health crisis*. New York, NY: Rodale.

Centers for Disease Control and Prevention (CDC). (2010). *Web-based injury statistics query and reporting system (WISQARS)*: Retrieved April 1, 2010 from www.cdc.gov/ncipc/wisqars

Conwell, Y., & Brent, D. (1995). Suicide and aging. I: Patterns of psychiatric diagnosis. *International Psychogeriatric, 7,* 149–164.

Corrigan, P. W. (1998). The impact of stigma on severe mental illness. *Cognitive and Behavioral Practice, 5,* 201–222.

Council on Rehabilitation Education (CORE, 2013). *Accreditation manual for masters level rehabilitation counselor education programs*. Schaumburg, IL: Author.

Davidson, L., O'Connell, M., Tondoora, J., Styron, T., & Kangas, K. (2006). The ten top concerns about recovery encountered in mental health system transformation. *Psychiatric Services, 57*(5), 640–645.

Ganzel, B., Casey, B. J., Glover, G., Voss, H. U., & Temple, E. (2007). The aftermath of 9/11: Effect of intensity and recency of trauma on outcome. *Emotion, 7*(2), 227–238.

Hingsaw, S. P., & Cicchetti, D. (2000). Stigma and mental disorder: Conceptions of illness, public attitudes, personal disclosure, and social policy. *Development and Psychopathology, 12*, 555–598.

Hoge, C. W., Castro, A. A., Messer, S. C., McGurk, D., Cotting, D. I., & Koffman, R. L. (2004). Combat duty in Iraq and Afghanistan, mental health problems, and barriers to care. *New England Journal of Medicine, 351*, 13–22.

Jacobson, N., & Greenley, D. (2001). What is recovery? A conceptual model and explication. *Psychiatric Services, 52*(4), 482–485.

Kessler, R. C., Chiu, W. T., Demler, O., & Walters, E. E. (2005). Prevalence, severity, and comorbidity of twelve-month DSM-IV disorders in the National Comorbidigy Survey Replication (NCS-R). *Archives of General Psychiatry, 62*, 617–627.

Lambert, M. J. (Ed.) (2013). *Bergin & Garfield's handbook of psychotherapy and behavior change* (6th ed.). Hoboken, NJ: Wiley.

National Institute of Mental Health. (2007). *Lifetime prevalence of DSM-IV/WMG-CIDI disorders by sex and cohort*. Retrieved from www.nimh.nih.gov

Peterson, D. B. (2011). *Psychological aspects of functioning, disability, and health*. New York, NY: Springer.

Peterson, D. B., & Elliott, T. R. (2008). Advances in conceptualizing and studying disability. In S. Brown and R. W. Lent (Eds.), *Handbook of counseling psychology* (4th ed., pp. 212–230). Hoboken, NJ: Wiley & Sons.

Peterson, D. B., Mpofu, E., & Oakland, T. D. (2010). Concepts and models in disability, functioning, and health. In E. Mpofu & T. Oakland (Eds.), *Rehabilitation and health assessment: Applying ICF Guidelines* (pp. 3–26). New York, NY: Springer.

Peterson, D. B., & Paul, H. (2009). Using the International Classification of Functioning, Disability & Health (ICF) to conceptualize disability and functioning in psychological injury and law. *Psychological Injury and Law, 2*(3-4), 205–214.

Pomerantz, J. M., Finklestein, S. N., Berndt, E. R., Poret, A. W., Walker, L. E., Alber, R. C., . . . Ebert, T. H. (2004). Prescriber intent, off-label usage, and early discontinuation of antidepressants: A retrospective physician survey and data analysis. *Journal of Clinical Psychiatry, 65*(3), 395–404.

Preston, J. D., O'Neal, J. H., & Talaga, M. C. (2013). *Handbook of clinical psychopharmacology for therapists* (7th ed.). Oakland, CA: New Harbinger.

Sadock, B. J., Kaplan, H. I., & Sadock, V. A. (2010). *Kaplan and Sadock's synopsis of psychiatry*. Philadelphia, PA: Lippincott Williams and Wilkins.

World Health Organization. (1992). *International statistical classification of diseases and related health problems* (10th revision) (ICD-10). Geneva, Switzerland: Author.

World Health Organization. (2001). *International classification of functioning, disability, and health: ICF*. Geneva, Switzerland: Author.

World Health Organization. (2004). The World Health Report 2004: Changing history, annex table 3. *Burden of disease in DALYs by cause, sex, and mortality stratum in WHO regions, estimates for 2002*. Geneva, Switzerland: Author.

Word Health Organization. (2011). *International classification of diseases (*9th revision). Clinical Modification (ICD-9-CM). Geneva, Switzerland: Author.

World Health Organization. (2012). *Measuring health and disability: Manual for WHO Disability Assessment Schedule (WHODAS 2.0)*. Geneva, Switzerland: Author.

Word Health Organization. (2014). *International classification of disease* (10th revision). Clinical Modification (ICD-10-CM). Geneva, Switzerland: Author.

About The Authors

David B. Peterson, Ph.D., is a licensed clinical psychologist, Certified Rehabilitation Counselor, and Professor in Rehabilitation Education at California State University, Los Angeles (CSULA). He has contributed to the development of the World Health Organization's International Classification of Functioning, Disability, and Health, publishing a text addressing psychological aspects of the same. Dr. Peterson is on the Panel of Medical Experts of the Office of Disability Adjudication and Review, Social Security Administration, where he provides psychological expert testimony.

George K. Hong, Ph.D., is a Professor in the Division of Special Education and Counseling, Charter College of Education, at CSULA. As a clinical psychologist, Dr. Hong has extensive experience in providing mental health services; he served as President for the Division of Family Psychology, American Psychological Association. Dr. Hong was the recipient of the Distinguished Contribution Award in 2002 presented by the Asian American Psychological Association.

Chapter 22

SEXUAL HEALTH AND DISABILITY

Leo M. Orange, M.S.

"After surviving a battle with cancer and an automobile accident which left me paralyzed with quadriplegia, I wondered if anyone would ever see me as a sexual human being and want to love me again" (L. M. Orange).

Introduction

Sexuality refers to the expression of sexual sensation and related intimacy between human beings and the expression of identity through sex. Sexuality comprises a broad range of behaviors and processes, including those that are biological, psychosocial, emotional, spiritual or religious, cultural, and political. Beginning with how we see ourselves, it extends to influence and encompass our relationships with others (Best, 1993).

Sexuality goes above and beyond intercourse. It is also about feelings and attractions. The most widely recognized labels people use to identify their sexuality are as follows:

Heterosexual: Attracted mostly to people of the opposite sex or gender.

Gay: Attracted mostly to people of the same sex or gender (usually used by males).

Lesbian: Attracted mostly to people of the same sex or gender (usually used by women).

Bisexual: Attracted to both men and women.

Asexual: Not sexually attracted to people of the same or opposite sex or gender.

Transsexual: Identify as a member of the sex opposite to that assigned at birth and desire to live as such.

Same-sex marriage is legally recognized in several states. As of July 2013, thirteen states including California, Connecticut, Delaware, Iowa, Maine, Maryland, Massachusetts, Minnesota, New Hampshire, New York, Rhode Island, Vermont, Washington, as well as the District of Columbia have legalized same-sex marriage. Two Native American tribes also legalized same-sex marriage in 2013.

The recognition of people of non-traditional identities as members of society is a first step in the process of integration or allowing all people to express themselves sexually. Increased access to information and educational material is integral to affirming this process. Because sexuality is both physiological and psychological, so too are the societal obstacles that people with disabilities encounter in regards to sexual expression. From a psychological perspective, sexuality involves expressions of intimacy, affection, caring, and love.

Although recent laws have officially recognized members of non-traditional sexual identities, they do nothing for people with disabilities, who are still largely thought of as non-sexual (Brodwin & Orange, 2014; Brodwin, Orange, & Chen, 2004). In recent years, representations of people with disabilities in the media have improved; people with disabilities are beginning to be portrayed as legitimate beings with desires, needs, and capabilities for success. Either as a consequence or a precursor to this portrayal, the lives of people with disabilities have improved. Hahn (1991) illustrated these changes when he wrote that people with disabilities, despite having experienced isolation, alienation, and rejection, have been able to enjoy the pleasures of intimate relationships, marriage, and child rearing.

Gender and Sexuality

Any discussion about people with disabilities having sex is guaranteed to raise a few eyebrows. An individual in a wheelchair is often viewed as an object of pity, not of desire. In our society, the existence of a physical, mental, or intellectual disability has implications of asexuality. For example, for many men, a spinal cord injury that results in impotence is seen as the end of their sexuality. Often, even less dramatic disabilities cause individuals to shut themselves off sexually due to feelings of inadequacy and a fear of rejection (Gill, 1996).

Women with disabilities face multiple barriers to social inclusion. Some experience what is known as *double discrimination*, or being socially judged based upon both their disability and gender. Women with disabilities marry less often and those who acquire disability during marriage have higher rates of separation and divorce (Brodwin & Frederick, 2010). People with disabilities do not fit the image of beauty in society and, therefore, are thought to be incapable of being supportive partners or parents.

Sexual Functioning

Sexual function is a model developed at the Karolinska Institute in Stockholm, Sweden, which identified different aspects of the assessment of sexual dysfunction (Helgason, 1997). Masters and Johnson (1966) defined the aspects of sexual function as relevant, including sexual desire, erection, orgasm, and ejaculation.

Individuals with disabilities and chronic illnesses may question their ability to function sexually and their capability to have children. According to Best (1993), the age of onset and the nature of the disability (e.g., progressive or static, congenital or acquired, long term or recent onset) impact the adjustment process. Stressors, such as anxiety, depression, grief, and physical limitations all play significant roles in the expression of one's sexuality. Previous sexual experience and disability-related characteristics (including mobility, assistive devices, medications, pain, strength, bodily function, and prosthetic devices) need consideration. Additionally, severity of disability, the presence of multiple disabilities, and the attitudes of the individual and others are factors requiring appropriate assessment. Rehabilitation needs to focus on highlighting the strengths and capabilities of people with disabilities, rather than their limitations.

Human Sexual Response Cycles

Masters, Johnson, and Kolodny (1995) described sexual response as a result of two principal physiological changes: increasing blood flow to various parts of the body (vasocongestion) and increasing muscle tension (myotonia). Specific phases of the human sexual response cycle include excitement, plateau, orgasm, and resolution. These phases correspond to the levels of sexual arousal and describe typical physiological responses. While traditional sexual response cycles may change as the result of disability, injury, or chronic illness, excitement, ejaculation, and orgasm are all possible (Masters et al., 1995).

Immediate signs of sexual excitement include erections of the penis or clitoris and lubrication. As an individual becomes sexually aroused, his or her heart rate and blood pressure increase. Nipple erection and an increase in muscle tension throughout the body occurs; there is often a noticeable *sex flush* in the face, neck, and ears that is associated with increased blood flow or vasocongestion. As the excitement phase moves into the plateau phase, one sees significant increases in blood pressure, sex flush, breast size, respiration rate (heavy breathing), and muscular tension. At orgasm, physiological responses peak and are followed by a rapid release of muscular tension, returning the body to its pre-excitement physiological levels.

With the changes in sexual functioning that may accompany disability and chronic illness, individuals may or may not experience erections or lubrication as signs of sexual excitement. Men with disabilities may not experience erection and ejaculation usually associated with orgasm. Some experience retrograde ejaculation, in which semen is forced into the bladder instead of through the penis. Women with disabilities may or may not experience contractions in the uterus and around the vagina. Members of both genders may or may not experience orgasms. All the above responses, while they may be affected by the presence of disability, injury, or illness, are possible, provided that during the act of intercourse both partners are attentive (Masters et al., 1995).

Monitoring by the Brain

The brain receives signals indicating that arousal and readiness are occurring. At this point, the brain either enhances or inhibits the process by the thoughts and images it receives and processes. While negative thoughts, such as *"I should not be doing this,"* reverse arousal, positive thoughts, such as, *"I really enjoy this person's company,"* initiate or enhance it.

Orgasm and Surrender

Orgasm requires that the individual momentarily surrender and partially give up control. This requires trust. Trust is the process of letting another be a part of one's experience and is especially crucial when experiencing sex for the first time after acquiring a disability or chronic illness. The ability to communicate with one's partner about the physical and mental changes that are occurring during the sexual experience is paramount. A new sexual experience can be positive as well as negative, and how one feels needs to be expressed. Understanding and enjoying the sexual experience without judging oneself is important because like everything else in life, this process is something that should be experienced and modified as needed. Though perfection may not be achieved the first time, the experience can be adapted if the desire exists for a fulfilling sexual life (Masters et al., 1995).

The typical arousal period is usually no longer than a few minutes. As the sympathetic nervous system gains control over the parasympathetic, it begins to set in motion the process leading to orgasm. Cellular products of the sympathetic system that play a role in the flight or fight response increase blood pressure, send blood to the skeletal muscles, and inhibit digestion. Their function during intercourse differs by gender. In men, sympathetic nerve fibers carry chemicals that cause contractions in structures within the pelvic area, moving semen from these areas to the penis. In women, these cellular products stimulate the uterus and vagina, causing them to contract.

Usually, within minutes after sympathetic activation, muscles in the pelvic and genital areas in both sexes contract rhythmically for several seconds. In men, these contractions move semen from the penis to outside the body. In women, they move semen up the canal. Some of the muscles that contract during this phase are involuntary, triggered by the autonomic nervous system rather than by conscious intention in a process that resembles shivering. Similarly, when the body is very cold, the autonomic nervous system activates motor nerves that correspond with muscle movements that increase body temperature.

Psychological Perspectives

People with disabilities may experience reduced sexual functioning and feeling, concerns about body image, and doubts as to how to negotiate the sexual act because of lack of knowledge or physical capacity (Cash & Hrabosky, 2004). People with disabilities may also have reduced sexual opportunities because of lack of privacy necessitated by the disability or illness. Finding ways to express one's sexuality can thus be a vital part of rehabilitation, especially for adults who acquire disability during this stage of life.

The inability to move or perform in the same manner as before the onset of a disability does not imply an inability to please or to receive pleasure. The absence of sensation does not correspond with an absence of feeling. Persons with disabilities still feel desire even though their cognitive abilities, lower or upper body extremities, or genitals function differently. The ability to enjoy intimacy, passion, and closeness persists even with an inability to perform certain sexual activities. Although it may be different from the one shared prior to the disability or chronic illness, individuals with disabilities can still enjoy loving, close, and intimate relationships.

Physical changes occur as a result of disability and chronic illness. Psychological factors such as emotional stress, depression, and grief may diminish interest in sex and create performance anxiety. Pressures of not being able to work or feelings of being a burden affect one's feelings of sexuality. An individual may believe that the disability or illness has changed the way he or she looks and feels causing that person to be less independent with a restricted ability to play the *traditional* role in the relationship. For others, pain can make sexual response unpredictable and make uncomfortable what once felt stimulating. Bladder or bowel incontinence causes embarrassment and anxiety, and an indwelling catheter diminishes sexual interest. In addition, weakness, fatigue, and breathing difficulties become barriers to sexual activity (Thomas, 1992). To enjoy one's sexuality, an individual must have the opportunity to share and communicate feelings with others. The potential to experience and enjoy one's sexuality becomes broadened when one desires to engage with another person sexually.

People with disabilities learn new ways of viewing relationships (Miller, Chen, Glover-Graff, & Kranz, 2009). With the intervention of medicine and sexual aides such as injections, implants, and pharmaceuticals such as Viagra, a man with a disability has greater chances of having an erection and intercourse. Regardless of medical intervention, however, a person cannot enhance a relationship unless he or she surpasses the fears and insecurities that occur with newly acquired physical limitations.

Men rarely discuss sexual difficulties with friends, acquaintances, or physicians (Moore, Davidson, & Fisher, 2009). It is often the case that a man requests treatment from an urologist at the insistence of a partner, perhaps after years of repressed depression, decreased self-esteem, and denial (Nusbaum & Hamilton, 2002). During classic denial, the pain of the perceived loss of *manhood* may be too great to face or express. Perhaps what is at issue is not the male sex drive or sexuality, but the fact that men are raised to believe that there are specific ways to express their emotions. Sexual intercourse may be one of the few permissible ways for a man to be close to someone. Due to cultural values and belief systems, for many men it is the only acceptable place to express feelings of love. This may be the result of deep cultural fears of women's sexual passion, non-traditional roles, culture, and issues of power and status.

Women who have disabilities, on the other hand, are often viewed as unfit to fulfill the traditional roles of mother, wife, homemaker, nurturer, and lover, and are seen as asexual (Fine & Asch, 1988; Miller et al., 2009). Although the traditional image of the mother as the sole caretaker and nurturer of her children is changing, it remains the predominant social conception. Since women with disabilities are seen as helpless, dependent, and in need of being taken care of, it is difficult for many to accept a woman with a disability as a potential mother and provider (Brodwin & Frederick, 2010).

Social Components of Sexuality

One of the major difficulties facing the study of sexuality and disability has been the tendency to view disability strictly from a clinical or biological perspective rather than a social one. Although there has been much discussion about social issues in the literature on disability, most have been limited to exploring the impacts of particular physical impairments on sexuality (Goffman, 1963). Since the concept of disability encompasses social as well as physical components, there is a need to devote increased attention to the social problems that may affect sexual relationships involving people with disabilities.

Beauty and strength are perceived as integral, beneficial components of life in American culture (Esmail, Darry, & Knupp, 2010). At the interpersonal level, persons who are physically attractive are evaluated on the basis of their sexuality. A physical disability thus leads to the categorization of a person as abnormal. When it is used to discredit an individual in this stereotypical manner, it becomes a source of stigmatization (Arokiasamy, Rubin, & Roessler, 2008).

Pervasive social norms reinforce taboos against sexual contact and interaction with people who have disabilities (Brodwin & Orange, 2014). Often, physical attractiveness alone is considered paramount in the development of relationships. This emphasis may reflect traditional values that are attached to physical strength, power, beauty, and grace. There is a coexisting significance to the terms the *whole body*, or the body *beautiful*, and the narcissistic anxiety that is easily aroused in many people who are plagued by doubts about their own supposed physical flaws or defects.

Sexual Identity

Sexual identity is at the core of one's sexuality. As with other aspects of identity, including gender, age, and ability, sexual identity involves self-perception and expression. Like age, sexual identity is not static, but may change over time.

Sexual behaviors, like dating, often involve physical skills that are beyond the capacity of people with major disabilities. As a result, the person with a disability and the non-disabled individual in a relationship may face negative feelings and attitudes from others, including parents and friends who regard the relationship as inappropriate or inadvisable (Miller et al., 2009). Those who are able to overcome the effect of adverse attitudes and taboos against physical contact between persons with and without disabilities must still confront the handicaps resulting from ambiguous social values and dating norms. Social customs, perhaps more than physical differences, are powerful deterrents to these relationships.

Many professionals are implicitly or explicitly aware of the social problems restricting the sexuality of people with disabilities; these problems increase vulnerability. Reduced prospects for forming sexual and marital relationships pose a serious threat to the natural instinct of all human beings to find love, and establish stability (Brodwin & Chen, 2000). Although professionals who work with people with disabilities may be cognizant of the reduced probability that their clients will achieve sexual and marital relationships, they often appear reluctant to acknowledge and discuss these subjects (Kroll & Klein, 1995).

Self-Esteem

One of the most difficult accomplishments in life is being courageous enough to take chances with love, as it requires not only loving oneself but caring for another person. Self-esteem helps people with disabilities maintain positive attitudes. Research indicates that almost every aspect of our lives including personal happiness, success, relationships, achievements, creativity, and sexuality are dependent upon positive self-esteem (Ivey, Ivey, & Zalaquett, 2014; Miller et al., 2009). With positive self-esteem, a person is more effective, productive, and responsive to others in healthy and affirmative ways.

Anxiety due to disability may cause an individual to withdraw and, as a result, lead to depression and loneliness (Trieschmann, 1988; Vash & Crewe, 2004). This loneliness or depression is often a symptom of frustration. If the frustrated individual is unable to socialize, he or she may become anxious and withdrawn. Increased loneliness, anxiety, and depression can make it problematic for people with disabilities to recognize their role in society.

Body-Image

Body image encompasses perceptions and attitudes about one's physical appearance (Wiederman, 2012). The role of body-image and attitudes in human sexual functioning include one's appearance-related thoughts, emotions, and behaviors. Specifically, body dissatisfaction and excessive psychological investment in one's physical appearance may lead to physical self-consciousness and body exposure avoidance during sexual relations, which in turn may impair sexual desire, enjoyment, and performance.

Most body image research has focused on eating disturbances among women (Cash, 2011; Cash & Hrabosky, 2004). Clearly, body image has implications for other facets of psychosocial functioning in both sexes and can influence one's interest in and experiences during sexual activities. Wiederman (2012) has recently found that body dissatisfaction may inhibit sexual behavior and interfere with the quality of sexual experiences.

Western culture has firm ideas on the appearances of men and women. Persons with disabilities may feel unattractive, or even *less worthy* of sexual partnerships, because they cannot live up to the idealized image. If the disability was acquired later in life, the person may remember how they used to look and feel unattractive by comparison. Talking with others who have overcome their body image problems may be helpful (Kroll & Klein, 1995).

Sexual Violence and Abuse

To express and enjoy one's sexuality, one must be able to grow in a healthy, nurturing, and loving environment. Sexual violence and abuse refer to a completed or attempted sexual activity without the willful consent of the victimized individual or involving a victim who is unable to consent or refuse due to age, disability, unconsciousness, or being under the influence of drugs or alcohol. Sexual abuse of individuals with disabilities is a problem of epidemic proportions that is only beginning to attract the attention of researchers, service providers, and funding agencies. People with disabilities are more at risk of abuse and neglect than individuals without disabilities (Siu & Brodwin, 2014). Adults with disabilities who have been sexually assaulted may have experienced the sexual assault or abuse during childhood, as adults, or both.

Factors that place these individuals at higher risk include: societal misconceptions about people with disabilities, especially children (including family members and non-family caregivers); factors that relate to the particular disability itself; and program policies and procedures governing the care of individuals with disabilities (Orange & Brodwin, 2005a).

Spirituality

Research (Havranek, 2003; Vash & Crewe, 2004) suggested that people, in particular those with disabilities, depend on spirituality and religion as an important, if not primary, method of coping with physical health problems and life stressors. Spirituality has been shown to have a positive impact on enhancing people's health and ability to cope with disability or illness (Keonig, 2002). Ironically, however, spirituality is not addressed in the rehabilitation process because many believe that spirituality is equated with religion.

Although research about spirituality in the context of disability is sparse, many thoughtful writers have considered religion and spirituality to be crucial factors in adjustment to disability (Havranek, 2003; Koenig, 2002; Vash & Crewe, 2004). According to Vash and Crewe, high rates of belief in God indicate that spirituality cannot be ignored as a source of power within the individual. This spirituality can help overcome the adversity of living with a disability or chronic illness. Spirituality concerns issues of inner beliefs and feelings, and is closely associated with religion and philosophy. Its various forms hope to shed light on the human experience of reality, purpose, and one's meaning of life.

Multicultural Perspectives

Culture encompasses the socially transmitted behavior patterns characteristic of a community or population (Ivey et al., 2014; Moore et al., 2009). People with disabilities have developed a culture as a result of characteristics that are part of the environment in which they live (Orange, 1995). Counselors may attempt to understand these characteristics, which are often viewed as peculiarities, without seeing their own cultural biases. This is true of sexuality and disability. With regard to sexuality, people with disabilities are seen as needing to be corrected to fit into the dominant, non-disabled culture. Professional services always reflect the dominant culture.

To provide appropriate services when counseling ethnic minorities about issues related to sexuality and disability, counselors need to understand both the meaning of disability in their lives and the cultural context within which they live. Ideas about sexuality are part of a larger culturally-based belief system. All cultures have shared ideas of what makes people sexy, appealing, and helps them maintain health through time (Esmail et al., 2010; Orange & Brodwin, 2005b). These beliefs help people understand their sexuality and make sense of the world around them. All cultures have beliefs about the *appropriate* type of sexuality; cultural and ethnic beliefs describe how people view what is sexually desirable. Defining sexuality from a multicultural perspective is particularly important for people with disabilities. Counselors need the understanding that people are all sexual beings, young or old, married or single, heterosexual, gay, lesbian, bi-sexual, transsexual, or questioning. As people change, their sexuality changes which remains a lifelong process no matter what the disability, culture, ethnic background, or sexual orientation.

Heterosexual relationships are not the sole form of interpersonal attraction. As more people feel comfortable acknowledging their sexual orientation (gay, lesbian, bi-sexual, transgender, and questioning), these relationships have gained wider acknowledgement and acceptance. With the gradual subsidence of homophobia over the last several decades, individuals with disabilities with same sex gender orientations are becoming less intimidated from expressing their true sexuality.

Conclusion

Sexuality is a form of communication, a way of expressing part of one's personality to another individual. The way people present themselves largely depends on how they see and feel about themselves. Sexuality is a very intimate area of an individual's personal life and is usually shared among a few people who care and respect one another. Relationships are developed between people sharing their experience and insights concerning their sexuality and learning to appreciate each other for who they truly are as unique human beings.

Learning to appreciate one's sexuality is a lifelong process that takes courage and understanding, with or without a disability.

> "I feel extremely privileged to wake up each morning knowing that I have the ability to love and be loved. My beautiful wife, Marie, and our two sons, Leo Jr. age 20, and Brandon age 16, fill each day and moment of my life with joy, happiness, and a passion for living. My professional life is filled with many rewarding challenges as Coordinator of Disabled Student Services at Oxnard College in Oxnard, California. One must never lose sight of the ability and opportunity to live and love" (L. M. Orange).

Case Study

Larry Young is a 28-year-old male who sustained an incomplete spinal cord injury three years ago at the C-5 level. While on vacation from work with his fiancée, he was injured in a swimming accident. He was flown to a nearby trauma center where he received six weeks of neurosurgical care before being transferred to a rehabilitation center in his home community. During the next two months, he received interdisciplinary rehabilitation and was then transferred to his parents' home where he has lived until this time. There is permanent and significant decreased function in all four extremities, and Larry must use a wheelchair to ambulate. He has about a 50% loss of function in both upper extremities, with a capability for some gross and fine hand dexterity. Since leaving the rehabilitation center, Mr. Young has spent the majority of his time in his room watching television, using the Internet, and reading while his mother provides his personal care. His fiancée and friends visit infrequently, and although he used to be socially active and well known in his community, he is now alone much of the time. Recently, Larry has become dissatisfied with his life and is seeking rehabilitation counseling services to help him plan for a possible return to college and a career. Prior to his accident, Larry obtained an Associate of Arts degree in liberal arts with an emphasis in library services and history. Before the accident, Mr. Young held various positions in his parents' computer retail store, involving sales, computer repair, stock clerking, and cashiering. He had planned to marry his fiancée and take over the family business someday, but he feels that this is no longer possible due to his physical limitations.

Questions

1. What are some issues that need to be addressed in regard to Larry's sexuality?
2. How would you try to learn about Mr. Young's psychosocial issues and how he feels about his body, sexual activity, and social interaction? If Larry wants counseling in this area, will you, as his rehabilitation counselor, provide it? Discuss.
3. What kind of adaptive equipment and devices would you recommend to increase Mr. Young's independence?
4. Does Larry possess transferable skills? Explain.

5. As his counselor either at a college or state rehabilitation agency, discuss educational and vocational counseling services and planning which you will provide.

References

Arokiasamy, C., Rubin, S. E., & Roessler, R. T. (2008). Sociological aspects of disability. In S. E. Rubin & R. T. Roessler, *Foundations of the vocational rehabilitation process* (6th ed., pp. 167–195). Austin, TX: Pro-ed.

Best. G. A. (1993). Sexuality and disability. In M. G. Brodwin, F. Tellez, & S. K. Brodwin (Eds.), *Medical, psychosocial, and vocational aspects of disability* (pp. 79–90). Athens, GA: Elliott and Fitzpatrick.

Brodwin, M. G., & Chen, R. K. (2000). Marriage and sexuality issues in clients with disabilities. In L.Vandecreek & T. L. Jackson (Eds.), *Innovations in clinical practice: A source book* (Vol. 18) (pp. 459–470). Sarasota, FL: Professional Resource Press.

Brodwin, M. G., & Frederick, P. C. (2010). Sexuality and societal beliefs regarding persons living with disabilities. *Journal of Rehabilitation, 76*(4), 37–41.

Brodwin, M. G., & Orange, L. M. (2014). Attitudes toward disability. In J. D. Andrew & C. W. Faubion (Eds.), *Rehabilitation services: An introduction for the human services professional* (3rd ed., pp. 164–185). Linn Creek, MO: Aspen Professional Services.

Brodwin, M. G., Orange, L. M., & Chen, R. K. (2004). Societal attitudes toward the sexuality of people with disabilities. *Directions in Rehabilitation Counseling, 15*, 45–52.

Cash, T. F. (Ed.). (2011). *Body image: A handbook of theory, research, and clinical practice* (2nd ed.). New York, NY: Guilford.

Cash, T. F., & Hrabosky, J. I. (2004). The treatment of body-image disturbances. In J. K. Thompson (Ed.), *Handbook of eating disorders and obesity* (pp. 515–541). Hoboken, NJ: Wiley.

Esmail, S., Darry, K., & Knupp, H. (2010). Attitudes and perceptions towards disability and sexuality. *Disability and Rehabilitation, 32*, 1148–1155.

Fine, M., & Asch, A. (Eds.). (1988). *Women with disabilities: Essays in psychology, culture, and politics*. Philadelphia, PA: Temple University.

Gill, C. J. (1996). Dating and relationship issues. *Sexuality and Disability, 14*(3), 183–190.

Goffman, E. (1963). *Stigma*. Englewood Cliffs, NJ: Prentice-Hall.

Hahn, H. (1991). The social component of sexuality and disability: Some problems and proposals. *Sexuality and Disability, 4*, 220–233.

Havranek, J. E. (2003). The spirituality exploration guide: A means to facilitate discussion of spiritual issues in the rehabilitation counseling process. *Journal of Applied Rehabilitation Counseling, 34*(1), 38–43 & 55–56.

Helgason, A. R. (1997). *Prostate cancer treatment and quality of life: A three level epidemiological approach*. Stockholm, Sweden: Karolinska Institutet.

Ivey, A. E., Ivey, M. B., & Zalaquett, C. P. (2014). *Intentional interviewing and counseling: Facilitating client development in a multicultural society* (8th ed.). Independence, KY: Cengage Learning.

Koenig, H. G. (2002). *Spirituality in patient care*. Randon, PA: Templeton Foundation.

Kroll, K., & Klein, E. L. (1995). *Enabling romance: A guide to love, sex, and relationships for the disabled (and the people who care about them)*. Bethesda, MD: Woodbine.

Masters, W, & Johnson, V. (1966). *Human sexual response*. Boston, MA: Little, Brown.

Masters W., Johnson, V., & Kolodny, R. (1995). *Human sexuality* (5th ed.). New York, NY: Harper Collins.

Miller, E., Chen, R. K., Glover-Graff, N. M., & Kranz, P. (2009). Willingness to engage in relationships with people with disabilities. *Rehabilitation Counseling Bulletin, 52*, 211–224.

Moore, N. B., Davidson, J. K., & Fisher, T. D. (2009). *Speaking of sexuality: Interdisciplinary readings* (3rd ed.). Oxford, England: Oxford University.

Nusbaum, M.R., & Hamilton, C. (2002). The proactive sexual health inquiry: Key to effective sexual health care. *American Family Physician, 66,* 705–712.

Orange, L. M. (1995). Skills development for multicultural counseling: A quality of life perspective. In S. Walker, K. A. Turner, M. Haile-Michael, A. Vincent, & M. D. Miles (Eds.), *Disability and diversity: New leadership for a new era* (pp. 59–65). Washington, DC: President's Committee on Employment of People with Disabilities.

Orange, L. M., & Brodwin, M. G. (2005a). Assessment and treatment of children with disabilities who have been abused. In L. Vandecreek, & J. B. Allen (Eds.), *Innovations in clinical practice: A source book* (pp. 131–142). Sarasota, FL: Professional Resource Press.

Orange, L. M., & Brodwin, M. G. (2005b). Childhood sexual abuse: What rehabilitation counselors need to know. *Journal of Rehabilitation, 71*(4), 5–11.

Siu, F. W., & Brodwin, M. G. (2014). Abuse and neglect of people with disabilities. In J. D. Andrew & C. W. Faubion (Eds.), *Rehabilitation services: An introduction for the human services professional* (3rd ed., pp. 146–163). Linn Creek, MO: Aspen Professional Services.

Thomas, M. B. (1992). *An introduction to marital and family therapy: Counseling toward healthier family systems across the lifespan.* New York, NY: Merrill.

Trieschmann, R. B. (1988). *Spinal cord injuries: Psychological, social, and vocational rehabilitation* (2nd ed.). New York, NY: Demos.

Vash, C. L., & Crewe, N. (2004). *Psychology of disability* (2nd ed.). New York, NY: Springer.

Wiederman, M.W. (2012). Body image and sexual functioning. In T. F. Cash (Ed.), *Encyclopedia of body image and human appearance* (pp. 148–152). Philadelphia, PA: Elsevier.

About the Author

Leo M. Orange, M. S., is the Coordinator of Disabled Student Services at Oxnard College in Oxnard, California. Mr. Orange has various book chapters and article publications in rehabilitation and counseling journals addressing attitudes towards disability, reasonable accommodation, childhood abuse issues, multicultural counseling, sexuality of people with disabilities, and psychosocial aspects of disability. Additionally, he has presented numerous professional papers and workshops on various topics of disability studies at local, state, regional, and national conferences.

Chapter 23

ADDICTIONS AND RELATED DISORDERS

Fredrick Payo, M.S.
Frances W. Siu, Ph.D., C.R.C.

Introduction

Drugs pervade every aspect of life. For many people, what starts as casual use quickly leads to drug addiction. Drug addiction can have long-term consequences, from problems with physical and mental health, to difficulties maintaining interpersonal relationships or a steady job. Reasons for drug use vary on an individual basis; while some say they use to fit in, others want the enhanced athletic or cognitive performance that some drugs can offer. Still others are seekers of pleasure or thrills. The human psyche is deeply embedded with a tendency to look for coping mechanisms to lessen the fears, frustrations, disappointments, social difficulties of everyday life, as well as to deal with specific traumatic events (Connors, DiClemente, Velasquez, & Donovan, 2013).

Individuals with current substance use and addiction issues may need help from counselors, physicians, family members, friends, and support groups or treatment programs to overcome addiction (Connors et al., 2013). Recovering drug users and addicts benefit from the same resources, and can eventually lead normal and productive lives. The 1990 Americans with Disabilities Act qualifies a person with a history of illegal drug use as having a disability when the individual (a) has successfully completed a supervised rehabilitation program; (b) is participating in such a program and no longer engaged in the illegal use of drugs; or (c) is regarded erroneously as an illegal drug user (U.S. Commission on Civil Rights, 2011). The Rehabilitation Act Amendments of 1992 also protect individuals with addiction issues.

According to the fifth edition of the *Diagnostic and Statistical Manual of Mental Disorder* (DSM-5) (American Psychiatric Association [APA], 2013), there are ten substance-related classes of drugs (some of which are legal): (1) alcohol; (2) caffeine; (3) cannabis (marijuana); (4) hallucinogens; (5) inhalants; (6) opioids; (7) sedatives, hypnotics, and anxiolytics; (8) stimulants; (9) tobacco; and (10) other (unknown) substances. Other behaviors have been linked with mental illness and addiction in recent years, including gambling, shopping, and sex. Because no formal diagnostic criteria or course descriptions have yet to be established, however, these have not yet been officially identified as mental disorders. Furthermore, drugs that are legal, such as alcohol and prescription or over-the-counter medications, can be as dangerous as illegal drugs. This chapter offers a comprehensive overview of the medical aspects of addictions including behavioral addictions and related disorders. It describes the common categories of drugs, signs and symptoms, and discusses current treatment strategies against addictions. Lastly, the chapter presents issues on reasonable accommodation and service delivery models for individuals with addiction issues.

Prevalence

The consequences of drug abuse and addiction are not limited to adults. Infants and young children exposed to illegal drugs may experience delayed intellectual development. Adolescents who use drugs may act out more than others their age, perform poorly in school, or even drop out. Parental addiction and related disorders have profound effects on children. Parents with addiction and related disorders more often engage in child abuse and neglect. Children of parents who abuse drugs are more often seriously injured or die in motor vehicle accidents; they are more likely to become substance dependent or abusers themselves. Combined data from 2002 to 2007 indicated that over eight million children (12%) lived with at least one parent who was dependent on or abused alcohol or an illicit drug in the past year. Of these, six million (9%) lived with a parent who was dependent on or abused alcohol, and about two million (3%) lived with a parent who was dependent on or abused illicit drugs (National Survey on Drug Use and Health [NSDUH], 2007).

The National Institute on Drug Abuse (NIDA, 2012a), published a factsheet indicating that 22.5 million Americans (nearly 9%) over age 12 had used or abused an illegal drug or psychotherapeutic medication within the past month. While the use of some drugs has increased, the use of others has declined. Between 2007 and 2011, for example, the number of current marijuana users rose from 14.4 to 18.1 million. Conversely, the number of current cocaine users declined from 2.4 to 1.4 million between 2006 and 2011. The use of psychotherapeutic drugs for non-medical purposes (without prescription) also declined from 2.7 percent in 2010 to 2.4 percent the following year. Additionally, the following drugs were reported to show declines in current use (used in the past month) (NIDA, 2012a):

- Hallucinogens (includes Ecstasy and LSD): from 0.5 percent in 2010 to 0.4 percent (972,000 Americans) in 2011
- Methamphetamine: from 731,000 current users in 2006 to 439,000 in 2011
- Underage (ages 12-20) drinking: 29% in 2002 to 25% in 2011
    - Binge drinking: from 19% to 16%
    - Heavy drinking: from 6% to 4%
- Tobacco: from 26% in 2002 to 22% in 2011
    - Teen smokers (ages 12 to 17): from 13% in 2002 to 8% in 2011

Despite reports on the decrease of the above drugs of abuse, three million Americans began using drugs in 2011. Of those three million new users, or initiates, more than half were under 18. Moreover, the majority of illicit drug users are between 18 and 20. People in their 50's have also shown a historical increase in drug use when compared to those from previous cohorts. Nonetheless, marijuana appears to be the initial drug of choice for new users, followed by prescription pain-relieving medications and inhalants (most commonly used among teens).

NSDUH continues to report the under-utilization of treatment services for persons in need of substance abuse and addiction treatment. In 2009, about 24 million Americans aged 12 and older reported having problems with alcohol and drugs. Of those, only 2.6 million received treatment services at an inpatient/outpatient treatment facility. The following table provides a breakdown on treatment admissions to publicly funded substance abuse treatment programs (NIDA, 2011).

The illegal drug trade is one of the largest global businesses, estimated at some $322 billion yearly. Each year, drug trafficking costs Americans upwards of half a trillion dollars and claims the lives of more than 100,000 people. Rates of HIV infection, viral hepatitis, and STDs are also substantially higher among persons who use illicit drugs than among those who do not (Belani et al., 2012).

Addiction Defined

According to the American Society of Addiction Medicine (2011), addiction is primarily a chronic disease characterized by dysfunction of the brain circuits involved with reward, motivation, and memory. This dysfunction is manifested biologically, psychologically, socially, and spiritually. Those who are addicted to a substance are not only unable to stop using the substance but suffer from impaired behavioral control, craving, cycles of relapse and remission, diminished recognition of significant problems with one's behaviors and interpersonal relationships, and a dysfunctional emotional response. While the media and the public tend to associate addictions mainly with illicit drugs, the reality of misuse and abuse of legal drugs such as alcohol, medical prescriptions, and over-the-counter substances can be equally dangerous.

The *DSM-5* (APA, 2013) includes two groups of substance-related disorders: (a) substance use disorders and (b) substance-induced disorders. Substance use disorders refers to the collection of cognitive, behavioral, and physiological indicators signifying that the person continues to use the substance regardless of significant substance-related issues. This is indicative of a collective set of pathological behaviors associated with that substance. Conditions associated with substance-induced disorders, or the symptoms

TABLE 1
Hospital Admissions According to Drug, Race/Ethnicity, and Age

BY DRUG (in 2008)

% of Admissions	Substance or Drug
23.1	Alcohol only
18.3	Alcohol and another drug
17.0	Marijuana
14.1	Heroin
8.1	Smoked cocaine (crack)
6.5	Stimulants
5.9	Opiates (not heroin)
3.2	Nonsmoked cocaine (powdered form)
0.6	Tranquilizers
0.2	PCP
0.2	Sedatives
0.1	Hallucinogens
0.1	Inhalants
0.4	Other drugs
2.2	None reported

BY RACE/ETHNICITY (in 2008)

% of Admissions	Race/Ethnicity
59.8	White/Caucasian
20.9	African American/Black
13.7	Hispanic Origin
2.3	American Indian/Alaska Native
1.0	Asian/Pacific Islander
2.3	Other

BY AGE (2008)

% of Admissions	Age Group
14.8	25-29
14.4	20-24
12.6	40-44
11.7	35-39
11.5	45-49
11.3	30-34
10.4	50-59
7.5	12-17
4.1	18-19
1.2	60-64
0.6	65 or older

that arise from continued or excessive use of the substance include intoxication, withdrawal, and other mental disorders caused by prolonged use of the substance. These include psychosis, anxiety, bipolar, depressive, neurocognitive, or obsessive-compulsive disorders, sleep disorders, sexual dysfunctions, and delirium (APA, 2013).

Dual Diagnosis

Persons with dual diagnosis are those who have mental illness and a substance abuse disorder. First identified in the 1980s, dual diagnosis is also referred to as co-occurring disorders. According to NSDUH (2007), an estimated 2.7 million adults aged 18 and older reported a co-occurring major depressive episode and alcohol use disorder in 2007.

Drugs and the Brain

Drugs can alter critical brain areas necessary for life-sustaining functions, and can drive the compulsive drug abuse that marks addiction. When sending a message from one cell to another, the brain releases a chemical called a neurotransmitter into the space separating two cells (the synapse). As the neurotransmitter crosses the synapse, it attaches to proteins called receptors on the receiving brain cell. The changes brought on by this process in the receiving brain cell indicate the message has been delivered. The reason addiction is considered a brain disease is because the drug changes the brain, both structurally and functionally. These changes can be long lasting and lead to harmful behaviors (Connors et al., 2013).

Etiology

Substance-related and addictive disorders are thought to be caused by a combination of environmental (family beliefs, attitudes, and exposure to drug use) and genetic (inherited traits) factors (Mayo Clinic, 2013). Physical addiction appears to occur when repeated use of a drug alters the way the brain feels pleasure. The addicting drug causes physical changes to some nerve cells (neurons) in the brain and consequently changes the messages communicated among the neurotransmitters.

Risk Factors

Certain risk factors can increase the likelihood that an individual will develop an addiction. Some of the more common factors include psychological problems, such as attention-deficit/hyperactivity disorder, post-traumatic stress disorder, behavioral disorders, depression, anxiety, and poor social coping skills.

Symptoms

Most addictions start with casual use of a drug or alcohol. For some people, using the drug or alcohol becomes a habit and frequency of use increases. As an addiction worsens, persons using the substance find that they require larger doses of the drug to experience the symptoms of relief or euphoria that they experienced initially. Soon, the person may feel the need for the drug simply to function. At this point, users may find that when they stop using, they are left with intense cravings and/or experiences of withdrawal, including nausea, uncontrollable shaking, and vomiting (Mayo Clinic, 2013).

Addiction symptoms or behaviors vary among drugs; common addiction symptoms or behaviors include (Mayo Clinic, 2013):

- Desire to use the drug regularly (daily or even several times a day)
- Failure in attempts to stop using the drug
- Having a constant supply of the drug
- Continued spending on the drug (despite negative financial repercussions)
- Obtaining the drug via behaviors previously unexhibited by the individual, such as stealing
- Need of the drug to deal with problems
- Performing risky activities when under the influence of the drug
- Focusing more time and energy on getting and using the drug

Categories of Drugs

Various resources have assigned drugs into specific drug classes. The introduction of this chapter described the ten classes of drugs in the *DSM-5*. The Drug Enforcement Agency (DEA) (2011), however, classified drugs into five categories or classes based on the Controlled Substance Act (CSA): (1) narcotics; (2) depressants; (3) stimulants; (4) hallucinogens; and (5) anabolic steroids. The Drug Recognition Experts (2004) categorized drugs into seven classes: (1) CNS depressants; (2) CNS stimulants; (3) hallucinogens; (4) PCP and its analog types; (5) narcotic analgesics; (6) inhalants; and (7) cannabis.

This section discusses the five drug classes based on the DEA's (2011) standards, but also includes other drugs of concern based on emerging trends. In addition, this section provides a brief definition of each of the five drug classes, and includes a table (see Table 2) that provides background information for each drug class. It should be noted that there are prescription drugs that are classified under certain drug categories such as prescription stimulants, prescription depressants (sedatives, sleeping pills, and anxiolytics), and prescription narcotics (opioids). The DEA identified narcotics as any substance synthesized from opium, opium derivatives, and their semi-synthetic substitutes. Narcotics are generally known to reduce pain or other senses. Depressants, as the name implies, are substances that lower or slow down the functions of the central nervous system (CNS) inducing sleep and decelerating action and reaction responses. Stimulants produce the opposite effects of depressants. Drugs in this category accelerate action and reaction responses of the CNS, producing heightened states of wakefulness and alertness. Hallucinogens are substances that alter or distort perceptions of reality and physical senses. The DEA includes marijuana, steroids, and inhalants under the hallucinogens category. Lastly, anabolic steroids, according to NIDA, are substances whose synthetic compounds affect the male hormone testosterone to increase physical appearance and performance.

TABLE 2
Drug Fact Sheet by Category

	1) NARCOTICS (Opioid)
Drug Types:	Heroin, Hydromorphone, Methadone, Morphine, Opium, Oxycodone, Oxycontin, Vicodin, Codeine, Fentanyl, Meperidine
Street Terms:	Smack, Brown Sugar, OC, Purple Drank, Ox, Black Tar, Chiva, Juice, Dillies, Fizzies, Maria, Dreamer, Unkie, Morpho, Gee, Black Pill, Toxy, Perc
Physical & Psychological Effects:	Euphoria, relaxation and relief of physical pain, drowsiness, inability to concentrate, apathy, general sense of well-being, slowed physical activity, dry mouth, constipation, nausea, slowed breathing, nervousness, rash, changes in blood pressure, mental clouding, restlessness
Overdose Effects:	Constricted pupils, cold clammy skin, confusion, blue fingernails and lips, convulsions, dizziness, slowed and shallow breathing, reduction in blood pressure, extreme drowsiness, coma, death
	2) DEPRESSANTS
Drug Types:	Fiorina, Seconal, Valium, Xanax, Ativan, Amytal, Rohypnol, Gamma-Hydroxybutyric Acid (GHB)
Street Terms:	Barbies, G, Roofies, Tranks, Pinks, Vals, Scoop, Reds, Liquid X, Downers
Physical & Psychological Effects:	Euphoria, relieve anxiety and muscle spasms, alleviate seizures, amnesia, reduced reaction time, impaired mental function and judgment, confusion, slurred speech, loss of motor coordination, weakness, blurred vision, nausea, vomiting, low blood pressure, sleepiness, paranoia, suicidal ideation
Overdose Effects:	Unconsciousness, slowed heart rate and breathing, shallow respiration, clammy skin, dilated pupils, coma, death

Addictions and Related Disorders

3) STIMULANTS

Drug Types:	Adderall, Ritalin, Didrex, Dexedrine, Desoxyn, Methamphetamine, Cocaine, Methcathinone, Khat
Street Terms:	Speed, Cristy, Crystal, Snow, Crank, Ice, Crack, Coke, Kat, Yaba, Shabu, Tweak
Physical & Psychological Effects:	Euphoria, sense of exhilaration, enhanced self-esteem, enhanced mental and physical performance, hyperthermia, suppressed hunger, insomnia, dizziness, restlessness, anxiety, headaches, tremors, flushed skin, excessive sweating, abdominal cramps, paranoia, convulsions, increased blood pressure and pulse rate, physical exhaustion
Overdose Effects:	Agitation, convulsions, increased body temperature, hallucinations, high fever, stroke, heart attack, coma, death

4) HALLUCINOGENS

Drug Types:	MDMA (3,4-methylenedioxy-*N*-methylamphetamine), K2/Spice, Ketamine, LSD (lysergic acid diethylamide), Peyote (mescaline), Psilocybin, PCP (phencyclidine)
Street Terms:	Acid, Shrooms, LSD, Adam, XTC, Spice, Bliss, Special K, Kit Kat, Blotters, Dots, Mesc, Buttons
Physical & Psychological Effects:	Distortion or alterations of the senses, euphoria, confusion, anxiety, depression, paranoia, tremors, involuntary teeth clenching, blurred vision, chills, nausea, giddiness, increased heart rate and blood pressure, involuntary rapid eye movement, dilated pupils, tear secretions, muscle stiffening, illusions, impaired motor coordination, vomiting, psychosis
Overdose Effects:	Hyperthermia, cardiovascular system failure, unconsciousness, dangerously slow breathing, psychosis, coma, death; Coma and death are rare from acute overdose of LSD, psilocybin, mescaline, and K2/Spice, but PCP and ketamine can lead coma or death due to respiratory arrest

4a) ANABOLIC STEROIDS

Drug Types:	Synthetically produced variants of the naturally occurring male hormone testosterone
Street Terms:	Arnolds, Juice, Stackers, Roids
Physical & Psychological Effects:	Dramatic mood swings, feelings of hostility, increased level of aggression, depression
Overdose Effects:	Not applicable…however, prolonged use of anabolic steroids may cause adverse effects such as stunted growth, physiological and physical changes in men and women, increased risk of coronary artery disease, stroke, and heart attack

4b) MARIJUANA

Drug Types:	Cannabis Sativa…over 480 constituents
Street Terms:	Bud, Weed, Ganja, Dope, Pot, Sinsemilla, Kush, Skunk, Chronic, Blunts, Indica, Hash Oil, Hash
Physical & Psychological Effects:	Euphoria, distorted perception, difficulty in thinking and problem-solving, loss of coordination, dizziness, nausea, tachycardia, merriment, relaxation, talkativeness, enhanced sensory perception (giving rise to increased appreciation of music, art, and touch), impaired judgment, ataxia, emotional lability, dysphoria, confusion, paranoia, increased appetite, bloodshot eyes
Overdose Effects:	Headache, shakiness, sweating, stomach pains, paranoia

	4c) INHALANTS
Drug Types:	Any household or other products that produce chemical vapors and can be inhaled such as nitrous oxide, computer cleaners, glue, spray paint, permanent markers, butane, correction fluid, cleaning solvents
Street Terms:	Elmo, Huff, Whippets, Nitrus, NO
Physical & Psychological Effects:	Mild impairment to severe dementia, slight stimulation, loss of consciousness, euphoria, dizziness, slurred speech, or effects similar to alcohol intoxication
Overdose Effects:	Unconsciousness, asphyxiation, "sudden sniffing death"

	5) OTHER DRUGS OF CONCERN
Drug Types:	Bath salts (synthetic stimulants), DXM (dextromethorphan), Salvia Divinorum, Desomorphine, Phenethylamine (LSD synthetic substitute), cough syrup with Codeine and Promethazine, Pure MDMA
Street Terms:	Bath salts: Bliss, Vanilla Sky, Stardust, Meow Meow DXM: Poor Man's PCP, Robo, Skittles, Triple C, Velvet Salvia Divinorum: Sally, Salvia, Maria Pastora, Desomorphine: Krok, Krokodil, Phenethylamine: N-Bomb, Smiles Cough syrup with Codeine and Promethazine: Syrup, Purple Drank, Sizzurp, Lean Pure MDMA: Molly
Physical & Psychological Effects:	Bath salts: similar to stimulant effects DXM: similar to the effects of marijuana and ecstasy Salvia Divinorum: similar to hallucinogenic effects Desomorphine: similar to heroin Phenethylamine: similar to hallucinogenic effects Cough syrup with Codeine and Promethazine: similar to narcotic effects Pure MDMA: similar to stimulant effects
Overdose Effects:	Bath salts: similar to stimulant effects DXM: similar to the effects of marijuana and ecstasy Salvia Divinorum: similar to hallucinogenic effects Desomorphine: similar to heroin Phenethylamine: similar to hallucinogenic effects Cough syrup with Codeine and Promethazine: similar to narcotic effects Pure MDMA: similar to stimulant effects

Source: National Institute on Drug Abuse. (2013). *The science of drug abuse: Fact sheet*. Retrieved September 8, 2013 from http://www.drugabuse.gov/publications/term/31/Fact%20Sheets

Prevention Approaches to Drug Abuse

Before describing the different types of drug abuse services, helping professionals must understand that prevention programs are separate from treatment programs. While prevention professionals help their clients access opportunities for increased education and awareness, treatment services professionals use intensive counseling, with some emphasis on prevention, as part of the therapeutic process. Drug abuse programs and services use one or both of the following models of prevention: the **Public Health Model** or the Substance Abuse and Mental Health Services Administration's **Behavioral Health Continuum of Care Model**.

The **Public Health Model** defines prevention on a scale, with **primary prevention** services defined as delaying or inhibiting the onset of a disease before it occurs through education and awareness programs that illuminate the consequences and complications of drug abuse (Nitzkin & Smith, 2004). **Secondary prevention**, on the other hand, focuses on identifying the symptoms of a disease before more serious complications arise (Nitzkin & Smith, 2004). Drug abuse programs emulate secondary prevention by reducing the symptoms of drug abuse behaviors before they worsen; professionals who work in this area focus their efforts on individuals who are misusing or abusing drugs but have not yet become addicted. Lastly, **tertiary prevention** aims to avert the complications of an illness with different forms of treatment (Nitzkin & Smith, 2004). In the field of drug abuse, drug abuse treatment programs providing tertiary prevention services offer treatment and therapy to treat drug addiction (dependency and withdrawal symptoms) and promote relapse prevention (abstinence) through intensive inpatient, outpatient, and residential treatment programs.

Although the public health model continues to be practiced by many drug abuse prevention programs, others began to use SAMHSA's adaptation of the **Behavioral Health Continuum of Care Model** proposed by the Institute of Medicine (IOM) as an effective approach in providing behavioral prevention and care services to populations affected by drug abuse. Substance Abuse and Mental Health Services Administration's (SAMHSA) Collaborative for the Application of Prevention Technologies developed a set of informational factsheets for drug abuse prevention and behavioral health specialists describing the four service components to SAMHSA's behavioral health continuum of care model: promotion, prevention, treatment, and maintenance. As part of its prevention services component, the SAMHSA model includes universal, selective, and indicated target areas. **Universal prevention** focuses on the general population, those not classified with individual risk factors. Similar to primary prevention, universal prevention provides education and awareness on drug abuse and related issues. **Selective prevention**, however, focuses on persons or subpopulations who are at-risk biologically, psychologically, or socially. Lastly, **indicated prevention** focuses on high-risk persons who display nominal symptoms of drug abuse but have not yet been diagnosed (SAMHSA, 2012).

Treatment Principles and Modalities

Service providers interested in working in the field of drug abuse prevention and rehabilitation must recognize that recovery is a lifelong journey. According to the National Institute on Drug Abuse (2012b), effective treatment includes a combination of services targeting not only the repercussions of addiction but the disease as well. Figure 1: Components of Comprehensive Drug Abuse Treatment illustrates a multitude of services that may be necessary for clients to access during the recovery process.

Additionally, substance abuse counselors must demonstrate competencies in the 13 Principles of Effective Treatment to ensure maximum compliance and efficiency with treatment for clients (NIDA, 2012b):

1. Addiction is a complex but treatable disease that affects brain function and behavior.
2. No single treatment is appropriate for everyone.
3. Treatment needs to be readily available.
4. Effective treatment attends to multiple needs of the individual, not just his or her drug abuse.
5. Remaining in treatment for an adequate period of time is critical.
6. Behavioral therapies, including individual, family, and group counseling are the most commonly used forms of drug abuse treatment.
7. Medications are an important element of treatment for many patients, especially when combined with counseling and other behavioral therapies.
8. An individual's treatment and service plan must be assessed continually and modified as necessary to ensure that it meets his or her changing needs.
9. Many drug-addicted individuals also have other mental disorders.
10. Medically assisted detoxification is only the first stage of addiction treatment and, by itself, does little to change long-term drug abuse.

FIGURE 1
Components of Comprehensive Drug Abuse Treatment

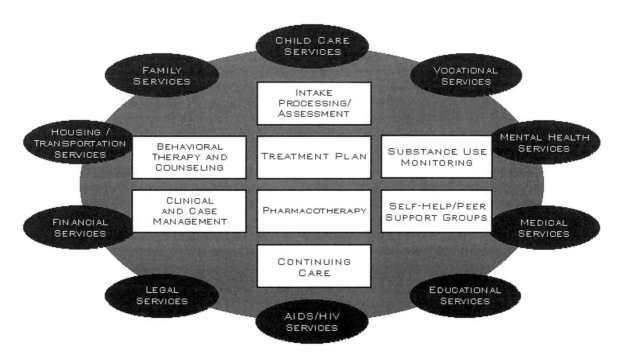

Source: National Institute on Drug Abuse. (2012b). *Principles of drug addiction treatment: A research-based guide* (3rd ed.). Retrieved from http://www.drugabuse.gov/publications/principles-drug-addiction-treatment

11. Treatment does not need to be voluntary to be effective.
12. Drug use during treatment must be monitored continually, as lapses during treatment occur.
13. Treatment programs should test patients for the presence of HIV/AIDS, hepatitis B and C, tuberculosis, and other infectious diseases, as well as provide targeted risk-reduction counseling, linking patients to treatment, if necessary.

John Herman (2013), a licensed psychologist and alcohol and drug counselor, developed a sixth edition of *The Global Criteria: The 12 Core Functions of the Substance Abuse Counselor* that aims to better prepare professionals by increasing their entry-level competencies. This book discussed eight performance domains and required core functions in which applicants must demonstrate proficiency; cumulatively, these cover the standards outlined by the International Certification and Reciprocity Consortium (IC&RC) and the Certified Alcohol and Other Drug Abuse Counselor Job Task Analysis Report of 2008. Derived from SAMHSA's (2011) Technical Assistance Publication, *Addiction Counseling Competencies: The Knowledge, Skills, and Attitudes of Professional Practice*, the eight performance domains include:

1. Clinical Evaluation
2. Treatment Planning
3. Referral
4. Services Coordination
5. Counseling
6. Client, Family, and Community Education
7. Documentation
8. Professional and Ethical Responsibilities

The tasks in each domain may include one or more of 12 core functions: screening, intake, orientation, assessment, treatment planning, counseling, case management, crisis intervention, client education, referral, reports and record keeping, and consultation (Herman, 2013).

The following section underlines the 13 principles of effective treatment, that "No single treatment is appropriate for everyone." Substance abuse counselors must make use of an array of treatment modalities to best fit the client's needs by modifying and/or interchanging treatment approaches when necessary and accommodating to the changing attitudes and behaviors of each client. Although various treatment modalities can be applied during the treatment process, before choosing one form of treatment, professionals need to understand the types of treatment programs that exist. In general, treatment programs are designed to assist persons dealing with dangerous and possibly fatal withdrawal symptoms through detoxification or *medically managed withdrawal therapy* in addition to delivering other comprehensive services based on the client's needs (NIDA, 2012b).

Detoxification is the body's process of cleansing itself from the chemicals of the drug. In medically managed withdrawal therapy (also known as pharmacotherapy), patients are given medications to assist in alleviating unpleasant and potentially fatal effects of withdrawals from opioids, benzodiazepines, alcohol, nicotine, barbiturates, and other sedatives (NIDA, 2012a). An example of medically managed withdrawal therapy is a methadone clinic, where professionals use methodone to treat persons with heroin addiction. Detoxification and medically managed withdrawal therapy are conducted as part of an inpatient or outpatient program.

Depending on the severity of the person's addiction, he or she can be admitted to long-term residential treatment, short-term residential treatment, outpatient treatment, and criminal justice-involved treatment. All treatments involve individualized and group counseling. Table 3 outlines a breakdown of each treatment program and their services; Table 4 illustrates the differences between individualized and group counseling.

Pharmacotherapies for addiction differ depending on the drug abused. While persons withdrawing from opioids are usually prescribed methadone, buprenorphine, or naltrexone, those experiencing withdrawal effects from tobacco addiction are prescribed nicotine replacement therapy, bupropion (zyban), or varenicline (Chantix). Persons experiencing alcohol withdrawal, on the other hand, are given naltrexone, acamprosate (campral), disulfiram (antabuse), or topiramate. It is recommended that persons undergoing pharmacotherapy also receive behavioral treatment (NIDA, 2012b).

Behavioral therapies are effective in modifying attitudes and behaviors associated with drug abuse and addiction. They help increase life skills, making it easier for people in recovery to handle stressful situations and environmental cues that may be triggers for potential relapse (NIDA, 2012b).

Reasonable Accommodations

Workers currently engaging in the illegal use of drugs are not protected by the Americans with Disabilities Act of 1990 (ADA) (U.S. Commission on Civil Rights, 2011). ADA qualifies individuals who (1) have been rehabilitated successfully and are no longer engaging in drug use; (2) are participating in a supervised rehabilitation program and are no longer engaging in such use; or (3) are erroneously regarded as engaging in drug use, but are not engaging. Only these individuals have the employment rights to receive reasonable accommodation. Depending on the individual's needs, the array of accommodations varies greatly and should be individualized. Most employers refer such individuals to their Employee Assistance Programs (EAPs) for counseling and support, if available. The ADA's confidentiality provisions do not permit employers' disclosures of any employee receiving reasonable accommodation.

Service Delivery Models

Many service delivery models are employed to help recovering addicts obtain and retain employment. Four of the most common models utilized among drug rehabilitation agencies are the following:

Work as positive outcome – obtaining employment after completion of treatment.

Work infusion – integrates vocational services within treatment.

TABLE 3
Description of Treatment Programs

Treatment Programs	Description
Long-term Residential	• 24 hours a day of care in nonhospital setting • Uses the Therapeutic Community model • Length of residence: 6 to 12 months • Focuses on "resocialization" of the individual and the entire program's community – other residents, staff, and the social context • Treatment is highly structured and confrontational • Addiction is viewed as a deficit and focuses on the development of personal responsibility and accountability that includes socially productive living • Activities involve residents to examine damaging beliefs, self-concepts, and destructive patterns of behavior • To adopt new, more harmonious and constructive behaviors • Offers comprehensive and other support services
Short-term Residential	• Provides intensive but brief treatment • Based on the modified 12-step approach • Usually designed to treat alcohol problems • After mid-1980s, began to treat other drug-related disorders • Length of treatment: 3-6 week hospital-based treatment, followed by outpatient therapy and participation in a self-help group • Individuals must continue utilizing outpatient and/or aftercare programs to reduce the chances of relapse after leaving residential
Outpatient Treatment	• Varies in types of intensity of services offered • Cost for service is less than that of inpatient or residential • More accommodating for those with jobs or extensive social supports • Low-intensity programs may offer more than drug education • Intensive day treatment may emulate services from residential programs in both services and effectiveness • Group counseling can be a major component • Some programs are also designed to treat patients with medical or other mental health issues in addition to drug disorders
Criminal Justice-involved Treatment	• Applied to those involved with the criminal justice system • Intervention services are provided prior to, during, after, or in lieu of incarceration • Combines criminal justice sanctions with drug treatment (known to reduce drug abuse and related crimes)

Source: National Institute on Drug Abuse. (2012b). *Principles of drug addiction treatment: A research-based guide* (3rd ed.). Retrieved from http://www.drugabuse.gov/publications/principles-drug-addiction-treatment

TABLE 4
Individual vs. Group Counseling

Individual Counseling	Group Counseling
• Focuses on reducing or stopping illicit drug or alcohol use • Addresses related areas of impaired functioning – employment status, illegal activity, and family/social relations • Advisor to the content and structure of the patient's recovery program • Emphasizes short-term behavioral goals • Emphasizes development of coping strategies and tools for relapse prevention and maintenance • Encourages 12-step participation • Provides referrals for supplemental medical, psychiatric, employment, and other services	• Capitalizes on social reinforcement through peer-based discussion and facilitation to promote drug-free lifestyle • Works in conjunction with individualized counseling • Is formatted to reflect the principles of cognitive-behavioral therapy or contingency management for increased positive outcomes

Source: National Institute on Drug Abuse. (2012b). *Principles of drug addiction treatment: A research-based guide* (3rd ed.). Retrieved from http://www.drugabuse.gov/publications/principles-drug-addiction-treatment

Contingent sanctions – has punitive consequences for not obtaining and maintaining employment.

Work as reinforcement – utilizes employment as a positive outcome for remaining abstinent.

Case Study

You are a counselor/case manager working at a community-based organization providing general services. These include mental health counseling and case management, after school programming, community recreational services, and so forth.

Jasmin De Los Reyes is a 29 year-old Filipino female who is married with three children. She and her husband have high school diplomas and certificates from a vocational school. They both completed several community college courses. While her husband was a construction worker, Jasmin was a certified nurse assistant (CNA) for about two years. Before this job, she did other work in the health field.

Jasmin was referred to your organization from friends and family members who can no longer provide help for her and her family. The De Los Reyes family was evicted from their apartment four months ago. With their combined savings from work, Jasmin and her family have been able to stay at inexpensive motels, but their savings is diminishing partially due to her husband's meth addiction. Jasmin admitted to using meth occasionally with her husband, but states she quit once they were evicted. Both Jasmin and her husband lost their jobs several months before the eviction. Two of their children are in elementary school, while the other attends middle school.

Ms. De Los Reyes is upset, frustrated, and expresses anger towards her husband for failing to show initiative to look for a job. She is also angry that her husband continues to abuse meth and is not supporting her efforts to reach out for assistance.

In a session with you, Jasmin tells you that she cannot live this kind of lifestyle any longer, especially when it is affecting her children. Jasmin does not know what steps to take with her husband, but she is willing to make changes to benefit her and her children. She admits to having attempted suicide and still contemplates killing herself.

As a CNA, Jasmin assisted with preparing food trays and feeding patients, and helping them with other activities of daily living including bathing, grooming, and dressing. She also measured and recorded vital signs; administered medication; transported patients; sterilized equipment; and administered catheterizations, irrigated bladders, and gave enemas; used other medical instruments; and cleaned rooms and changed linen. As a CNA, Jasmin was also required to have knowledge in the following areas: customer and personal delivery of services; diagnosis and treatment of injuries and wounds, illnesses, and infections; and use of techniques for rehabilitation of physical and mental conditions. She also possesses the following skills: innovative approaches to helping people; understanding medical and administrative language related to documenting daily activities; being observant of patients' reactions and the reasons for their response; and effectively and competently communicating with others. In summary, CNAs must be able to be creative, autonomous and independent, responsible, and adaptive.

Questions

1. Assign Jasmin De Los Reyes a vocational profile and recommend additional information about her personal, social, educational, and vocational background that may be helpful in rehabilitation planning.
2. As the rehabilitation counselor, what services are appropriate for Jasmin?
3. Develop a support system most beneficial for Ms. De Los Reyes and her family.
4. What factors are important in developing a vocational objective with Jasmin, and how will you assist her in proceeding with a vocational rehabilitation plan?
5. Identify possible job options for Ms. De Los Reyes.

References

American Psychiatric Association. (2013). *Diagnostic and statistical manual of mental disorders (5th ed.)*. Arlington, VA: Author.

American Society of Addiction Medicine. (2011). *Definition of addiction: The voice of addiction*. Retrieved from http://www.asam.org/for-the-public/definition-of-addiction

Belani, H., Choba, T., Fletcher. F., Hennessey, K., Kroeger, K., Lansky, A., . . . Wynn, B. A. (2012). *Integrated prevention services for HIV infection, viral hepatitis, sexually transmitted diseases, and tuberculosis for persons who use drugs illicitly: Summary guidance from CDC and the U.S. Department of Health and Human Services*. Retrieved from http://www.cdc.gov/mmwr/preview/mmwrhtml/rr6105a1.htm?s_cid=rr6105a1_w

Connors, G. J., DiClemente, C. C., Velasquez, M. M., & Donovan, D. M. (2013). *Substance abuse treatment and the stages of change: Selecting and planning interventions*. New York, NY: Guilford.

Drug Enforcement Administration. (2011). *Drugs of Abuse*. U.S. Department of Justice. Retrieved from http://www.justice.gov/dea/pr/multimedia-library/publications/drug_of_abuse.pdf

Herman, J. W. (2013). *Global criteria: The 12 core functions of the substance abuse counselor* (6th ed.). Lincoln, NE: Parallels: Pathways to Change.

Mayo Clinic. (2013). *Drug addiction*. Retrieved from http://www.mayoclinic.com/health/drug-addiction/DS00183

National Institute on Drug Abuse (NIDA). (2011). *InfoFacts: Treatment statistics*. Retrieved from http://www.drugabuse.gov/sites/default/files/treatmentstats.pdf

National Institute on Drug Abuse. (2012a). *Drug facts: Nationwide trends*. Retrieved from http://www.drugabuse.gov/sites/default/files/nationwide_0.pdf

National Institute on Drug Abuse. (2012b). *Principles of drug addiction treatment: A research-based guide* (3rd ed.). Retrieved from http://www.drugabuse.gov/publications/principles-drug-addiction-treatment

National Institute on Drug Abuse. (2013a). *Drugs of abuse: Emerging trends*. Retrieved from http://www.drugabuse.gov/drugs-abuse/emerging-trends

National Institute on Drug Abuse. (2013b). *The science of drug abuse: Fact sheet*. Retrieved from http://www.drugabuse.gov/publications/term/31/Fact%20Sheets

National Survey on Drug Use and Health. (2007). *Co-occurring major depressive episode (MDE) and alcohol use disorder among adults*. The NSDUH report. Retrieved from http://www.samhsa.gov/data/2k7/alcDual/alcDual.pdf

Nitzkin, J., & Smith, S. A. (2004). *Clinical preventive services in substance abuse and mental health update: From science to services*. DHHS Pub. No. (SMA) 04-3906. Rockville, MD: Center for Mental Health Services, Substance Abuse, and Mental Health Services Administration.

Substance Abuse and Mental Health Services Administration (SAMHSA). (2011). *Addiction counseling competencies: The knowledge, skills, and attitudes of professional practice* (Tap Publication No. SMA13-4171). Retrieved from http://store.samhsa.gov/shin/content//SMA12-4171/SMA12-4171.pdf

Substance Abuse and Mental Health Services Administration. (2012). *Prevention and behavioral health*. Retrieved from http://captus.samhsa.gov/sites/default/files/capt_resource/CAPT%20Behavioral%20Health%20Fact%20Sheets%20(2012).pdf

U.S. Commission on Civil Rights. (2011). *Substance abuse under ADA. Sharing the Dream: Is the ADA accommodating all?* Retrieved from http://www.usccr.gov/pubs/ada/ch4.htm

U.S. Department of Justice Drug Enforcement Administration. (2011). *Drugs of abuse 2011 edition: A DEA resource guide*. Retrieved from http://www.justice.gov/dea/docs/drugs_of_abuse_2011.pdf

U.S. Drug Enforcement Administration. (2013). *Drug fact sheets*. Retrieved from http://www.justice.gov/dea/druginfo/factsheets.shtml

United Nations Office on Drugs and Crime. (2007). *Drug Trafficking. World drug report*. Retrieved from https://www.unodc.org/pdf/research/wdr07/WDR_2007.pdf

About the Authors

Frederick Payo, M.S., is a case manager specializing in HIV and substance abuse prevention. He has worked with a diverse HIV and substance abuse at-risk and high-risk population for over 20 years. To date, he has provided over 300 health-related prevention training and presentations to adolescents, parents, young adults, and health care professionals. In addition, Fred has spoken at state and national conferences. Mr. Payo received his B.S. in rehabilitation services and M.S. in rehabilitation counseling from California State University, Los Angeles (CSULA). Research interests of his are in the area of alternative medicines for HIV/AIDS patients, provision of services to high-risk populations, and substance abuse counseling

Frances W. Siu, Ph.D., C.R.C., is an assistant professor at CSULA. She received her Ph.D. in special education and counseling, option in rehabilitation counselor education, from the University of Texas at Austin, her M.S. in rehabilitation counseling and B.S. in psychology from CSULA. Research interests of Dr. Siu include medical and psychosocial aspects of disability and violence against people with disabilities. In addition, she is the principle investigator of a multi-year Substance Abuse Mental Health Service Administration grant.

Chapter 24

ALCOHOL-RELATED DISORDERS

Roman Carlos, M.S., C.R.C.

Introduction

Alcohol addiction is one of the most common addictions worldwide. Because of its legal availability and almost worldwide social acceptance, except in a few cultures (e.g., Muslim), alcohol is relatively easy to abuse. Annually, 2.5 million alcohol-related deaths occur worldwide. However, for most people, regular, even weekly, drinking does not create a dependency on the substance (Carson-DeWitt, 2003).

For the population that develops an addiction, however, alcohol's deleterious effects can be wide ranging. Alcohol addiction affects many people close to the alcoholic, including his or her spouse, children, friends, employers, co-workers, and classmates. In 2001, 15,990 people in the United States died of alcoholic liver disease (Centers for Disease Control and Prevention [CDC], 2013). Today, approximately 18 million Americans abuse alcohol. Every year, more than 100,000 people die of alcohol-related causes. Almost half of all drivers killed in automotive crashes who tested positive for drugs also had alcohol in their system. In 2010, over 1.4 million drivers were arrested for driving under the influence of alcohol (National Institute on Alcohol Abuse and Alcoholism [NIAAA], 2013).

Alcohol-related problems range from mild to fatal. It is a major public health problem intricately connected with other social issues like crime, homelessness, teen pregnancy, and domestic violence. One in every four children grows up in a home where someone drinks alcohol excessively (Acton, 2013).

Alcohol

Alcohol is a sedative-hypnotic drug with anesthetic properties. Twelve ounces of beer, 4 ounces of wine, or 1¼ ounces of distilled alcohol contain about the same amount of alcohol. When a woman consumes one (or a man who consumes two) alcoholic drinks per day, is more than 21 years of age, and is not pregnant, ill, or taking medications that could interact with alcohol, his or her consumption is not classified as problematic (Boyle et al., 2013; O'Brien, 2013).

Blood alcohol content is the concentration of alcohol in a person's blood stream; it is measured by mass per volume. The size and weight of the person drinking is a factor in determining his or her level of drinking and classifying it as alcoholic abuse or not. Larger, heavier people require greater amounts of alcohol to reach the same blood level percentage than smaller, lighter individuals (Schuckit, 2006). As of July 2007, all 50 states in the United States have laws defining driving with a blood alcohol content at or above a level of 0.08% as illegal (Highway Loss Data Institute, 2007).

Alcohol Abuse

The NIAAA of the National Institutes of Health (2013) defined alcohol abuse as a maladaptive pattern of drinking that leads to clinically significant impairment or distress. An individual diagnosed with alcohol abuse drinks despite alcohol-related physical, social, psychological, or occupational problems. Alcohol abuse does not necessarily involve a consistent pattern of heavy drinking, but is defined by the adverse consequences associated with the drinking pattern. These include failure to fulfill major obligations at work, school, or home (e.g., repeated absences or poor work performance related to substance use, substance-related absences, suspensions or expulsions from school, neglect of children or household).

Alcoholism

The American Society of Addiction Medicine (ASAM) and the National Council on Alcoholism and Drug Dependence (NCADD, 2007) defined alcoholism as a primary, chronic disease that is often progressive and can be fatal. In historical use, alcoholism refers to any condition that results in the continued consumption of alcoholic beverages despite negative personal and social consequences. NIAAA (2013) stated that alcoholism is characterized by the following four symptoms: (1) craving, i.e., a strong need or urge to drink; (2) loss of control, i.e., not being able to stop drinking once drinking has begun; (3) physical dependence, i.e., the occurrence of withdrawal symptoms, such as nausea, sweating, shakiness, and anxiety after stopping drinking; and (4) tolerance, i.e., the need to drink greater amounts of alcohol to become intoxicated.

Etiology

There is no single cause of alcoholism. Research has indicated that a genetic component may play a role in the abuse of alcohol (Schuckit, 2006). For example, studies of identical twins show the son of an alcoholic father is four times more likely to become alcoholic than the child of a non-alcoholic father. Female children of alcoholics have an increased incidence of alcoholism and a much higher incidence of severe depression (O'Connor, 2012).

Aside from possible genetic factors, environmental and cultural influences play significant roles in substance abuse (Fletcher, 2013). There is no evidence of an addictive personality, and no valid tests exist to predetermine one's predisposition to addiction. Certain personality characteristics develop during addiction, however (Powers & Dell Orto, 2004). Family history of addiction and prior addiction to other drugs, including tobacco, are strong predictors of alcoholism.

The concurrent use of alcohol and other drugs is an increasing problem (O'Conner, 2012; Schuckit, 2006). Many people who drink use other recreational or prescription drugs including sedatives, stimulants, diet pills, and marijuana. Combining alcohol with such intoxicants can result in synergistic and additive interactions, with a greater incidence of disruptive effects. When multiple substances are used, withdrawal and recovery are complicated, prolonged, and more likely to require professional care in the early period of recovery. Additionally, for people who use alcohol with other drugs, the risk of early relapse is high.

Diagnosis

Frequently, hospital records of the alcoholic include a diagnosis of alcoholism. Such a diagnosis, however, may not have been made or recorded prior to an interview by the rehabilitation counselor. There are many screening devices and questionnaires for this purpose. A skilled interviewer may use any of these instruments to do an assessment. Alcoholics are not accurate in reporting their own alcohol use or its effects. Questions addressing symptoms and experiences rather than quantity consumed are likely to reveal more accurate assessments.

Treatment

Treatments for alcoholism are varied. Those who approach alcoholism as a medical condition or disease recommend different treatments than those who approach the condition as one of social choice. In general, most treatments focus on helping people discontinue their alcohol intake. These treatments include life training and/or social support strategies to help the individual avoid a return to alcohol use. Since alcoholism involves multiple factors that encourage a person to continue drinking, each must be addressed individually to successfully prevent a relapse once drinking is stopped (Acton, 2013).

Detoxification

Alcohol detoxification is only the first step in recovery. Although symptoms of withdrawal are treatable, addiction, which has both physical and mental characteristics, must be treated over an extended period of weeks or months. While some alcoholics can stop drinking for a period of time, alcoholic drinking generally recurs. Rarely are people who show signs of alcoholism capable of maintaining prolonged abstinence without assistance (McDonald, 2013). For most people with alcoholism, it is a life-long problem requiring comprehensive treatment. Because a return to asymptomatic drinking is unlikely, the commitment to long-term abstinence is needed to prevent further alcohol-related problems. Sobriety is achieved by many through regular participation in recovery programs, such as Alcoholics Anonymous (Alcoholics Anonymous, 1981; 2001).

Withdrawal ranges from mild to severe (life threatening) and sedative hypnotics decrease the symptoms of withdrawal. Hangovers are the mildest form of alcohol withdrawal syndrome. They usually consist of nausea, headache, thirst, and dysphoria (exaggerated feelings of depression and unrest). Additionally, tremulousness and irritability may be present. Moderate withdrawal symptoms include severe agitation, tremulousness, irritability, insomnia, difficulty concentrating, anxiety, and increased dysphoria. Symptoms arise as early as two to four hours after the last drink and reach a peak within 12 to 72 hours (Weiss, 2012).

The most severe form of alcohol withdrawal syndrome is delirium tremens (DTs). This consists of delirium, increased pulse rate, elevated blood pressure and body temperature, and severe agitation. Delirium tremens has a mortality rate of about ten percent; early and intense medical intervention is required to prevent death. Cardiac arrhythmias can occur during withdrawal from alcohol. Symptoms of mild withdrawal usually last for two to three days; more severe withdrawal syndromes last much longer (Acton, 2013).

Detoxification treats withdrawal symptoms but does not resolve the illness of alcoholism or alcohol abuse (Carson-DeWitt, 2003). Rapid recovery usually occurs during the first week of abstinence manifesting in physical and cognitive improvements. Recovery is affected by factors such as severity and duration of alcohol dependence, age, concurrent emotional and physical diseases, and intensity of medications used to help the person withdraw from alcohol.

Alcoholics Anonymous

Alcoholics Anonymous (AA) is a fellowship of men and women who share their experiences of strength and hope with each other to resolve their common problem and help others recover from alcoholism. The only requirement for membership is a desire to stop drinking. There are no dues or fees for AA membership; it is self-supporting through voluntary contributions. Our primary purpose is to stay sober and help others achieve sobriety.

– Alcoholics Anonymous (2001)

Of great importance in AA is service to other alcoholics and practicing a program of complete honesty, tolerance, and service in daily living. Recovery in AA is viewed as a life-long process, requiring consistent effort and regular involvement in the organization. Its effectiveness as a recovery program is widely accepted by the helping professions and the judiciary. Hundreds of thousands of sober alcoholics worldwide attribute their lives to AA (*Alcoholics Anonymous*, 2001).

A Chronic Disease

Alcohol dependence is a chronic disease that is subject to relapse (Morsehead, 2013). A relapse should not be viewed as a treatment failure, but rather as a symptom of the illness. Though never desirable, relapses can be therapeutic in that, if properly handled, reinforce the need for sobriety. With prolonged or repeated relapses, however, recovery becomes increasingly difficult. A person who has met the criteria for the illness of alcoholism rarely can return to moderate drinking. Individuals recovering from alcohol dependence must abstain from alcohol entirely to ensure the best recovery outcome.

Dual Diagnosis or Co-Occurring Disorders

Individuals who experience a dual diagnosis often face a wide range of psychosocial issues and may experience multiple interacting illnesses. The term co-occurring disorders refers to dual diagnosis, or co-occurring substance abuse disorders and psychiatric or emotional illnesses.

Dual Recovery Anonymous (an independent, self-help fellowship) defines dual diagnosis as two separate but very interrelated diagnoses (Acton, 2013; Boyle et al., 2013):

1. A psychiatric diagnosis
2. A substance abuse diagnosis, which may include both drugs and alcohol

A dual diagnosis occurs when an individual is affected by both alcoholism and an emotional or psychiatric illness. Each illness has symptoms that interfere with a person's ability to function effectively, and interfere with relating to self. Not only is the person affected by two separate illnesses, but the illnesses interact with one another. Symptoms can overlap and even mask each other, making diagnosis and treatment more difficult. An individual may sincerely try to recover from one illness and not acknowledge the other. As one neglects his or her mental illness, that illness may recur. This recurrence can, in turn, lead a person to feel the need to *self medicate* through the use of alcohol.

Alcoholism as a Family Disease

Living with a person who is alcohol dependent has powerful emotional repercussions. Families and close associates of individuals with this disease should seek support systems that provide information and counseling (Morsehead, 2012). ALANON, a group mutual-help program for adult relatives and friends of alcoholics, enhances such support. Similar 12-step oriented programs exist for children of alcoholics. If an alcoholic is not willing or able to become sober and maintain sobriety, support groups help the family to free themselves of the emotional bonds of guilt, hopelessness, and despair which are often felt by people connected to those with alcoholism (Weiss, 2012).

Assessment for Rehabilitation Services

Generally, individuals in treatment for alcoholism are not referred for vocational rehabilitation during the initial phases of treatment (detoxification period or during the first month of treatment) (Acton, 2013). Persons evaluated for vocational rehabilitation services should undergo an assessment procedure that is similar to that which is provided for other chronic illnesses and disabilities. Attention is given to physical and psychological limitations, work history, training and education, assessment of specific skills acquired, and areas of interest for employment. Many alcoholics have sporadic work histories, with numerous job and career changes. Some have a history of self-employment in the skilled trades or professions, which may have allowed for greater flexibility to accommodate periods of reduced functioning due to heavy drinking.

An assessment includes physical status, medical problems, psychosocial issues, functional limitations, the nature of current treatment, and whether or not the individual is still drinking. If currently sober, questions need to be asked regarding efforts to remain sober. Many people with alcoholism have had experiences in treatment with varying degrees of success. Because alcoholism is a chronic disease, many recovering alcoholics do not achieve or maintain long-term sobriety on their first attempts (Fletcher, 2013). Vocational rehabilitation may have to be deferred for persons who are repeatedly relapsing or unable to maintain sobriety.

During an assessment for rehabilitation services, special attention is given to attitudes toward work and career. Overall, persons in the early stages of recovery may not have the ability to make accurate self-assessments of their capabilities and limitations. Thus, the rehabilitation counselor and others involved with treatment and recovery play a key role in developing an accurate evaluation regarding motivation to return to gainful employment.

Vocational Rehabilitation

In the early stages of recovery, many alcoholics need work levels that are less demanding, minimally stressful, and potentially less rewarding than the employment performed when at maximal functioning. Focusing on the acquisition of appropriate work habits and a more stable employment history are positive initial vocational rehabilitation goals for the recovering alcoholic; the specific job chosen is less crucial. Likewise, job finding and retention skills are an integral part of the rehabilitation program. Changing attitudes toward work and maintaining employment is a considerable challenge for alcoholics during the first year or two of recovery (McDonald, 2013). Because career progress can be initially slow and challenging, several years are often required before a person reaches maximum career success. Alcoholics often display impatience with this slow progress in their careers. Work stability is a primary goal; the counselor needs to stress that work habits and attitudes have more to do with success than any specific experience in an occupation. Overall, maintaining sobriety is considered the first priority (Boyle et al., 2013).

Need for Retraining

Because some individuals lack marketable vocational skills, they have difficulty obtaining work appropriate to their age and educational background. Once stable sobriety is achieved, job retraining is frequently needed. Many recovering alcoholics indicate considerable interest in returning to school to complete education they abandoned at an earlier time. As with anyone in society, the acquisition of marketable skills is essential.

Living and working without alcohol can be an anxiety filled and apprehensive experience. Familiar activities may seem new and difficult. Many alcoholics experience a loss of confidence in their ability to adequately perform past work at any skill level. To help ameliorate this situation, the counselor's office should be a safe place for the person to talk about his or her fears and discuss realistic, attainable goals, from the beginning of the assessment through long term and stable employment at the highest level achievable. Counselors provide assistance by placing prior experiences in the proper context. Honest feedback and encouragement from the counselor is essential.

Vocational Rehabilitation and the Recovering Alcoholic

Vocational rehabilitation counselors occupy a central role during recovery. To be of assistance, they must possess familiarity with the difficulties facing the recovering alcoholic (Boyle et al., 2013). Depending on the setting where recovery takes place, counselors may become involved in assisting recovering alcoholics at any point in the recovery process following initial detoxification. Hospital-based programs, for example, may either have a rehabilitation counselor on staff or refer clients for state-provided vocational rehabilitation services. Similarly, non-medical or social model recovery programs, such as 12-step oriented recovery homes, have staff trained to provide vocational exploration and counseling (Schuckit, 2006).

Functional Limitations

Physicians knowledgeable about addictions can help determine what residual functional limitations, emotional and physical, are present in individuals who are recovering from substance abuse (O'Brien, 2013; Weiss, 2012). The rehabilitation counselor needs to assess a person's (a) ability to work effectively both with others and with supervisors; (b) limitations due to mood or emotional disorders (dual diagnosis); (c) ability to work independently without close supervision; and (d) capacity to tolerate stress.

Some late-stage alcoholics become overly dependent on others and are unable, at least for a time, to work independently. These individuals can benefit from more structured work settings to make the successful transition to gainful employment. The recovering person also faces a decreased tolerance for stress during the first months of return to work, and this may continue for up to two years of sobriety. Employment involving low stress during the early months of a person's sobriety is likely to result in a more successful transition.

Although complete recovery from alcoholism leaves few specific functional limitations, the recovery to maximum functioning is slow and gradual, occurring over several years. A return to productive employment improves one's overall recovery by enhancing self-esteem and beginning the process of resolving financial difficulties. It is for this reason that some recovery programs emphasize an early return to some type of work, generally beginning after one month of participation and sobriety.

Rehabilitation Potential

Assessment of the potential for rehabilitation is a challenging task for counselors. Many factors affect rehabilitation potential including age, educational background, prior work history, functional limitations, and motivation to work. Though not always immediate, most recovering alcoholics are eventually able to return to productive employment. Factors likely to affect the potential for effective participation in vocational rehabilitation include (a) length of sobriety and active participation in a recovery program; (b) history of relapses and their frequency; (c) commitment to maintaining sobriety; and (d) residual functional limitations (physical, cognitive, and emotional) resulting from the alcoholism or other chronic conditions (Carson-DeWitt, 2003). Once sober, the recovering alcoholic needs to demonstrate the same traits as any other person in rehabilitation, including willingness to accept responsibility for behavior, personal well-being, capacity to meet vocational expectations, and personal determination to succeed (Boyle et al., 2013).

Most alcoholics demonstrate moderate rehabilitation potential and eventually return to gainful employment because of financial necessity. Functional limitations diminish over time with continuous sobriety and active participation in an on-going recovery program. Those with repeated arrests for more serious legal charges present special challenges for rehabilitation. Individuals on probation or parole need coordinated efforts with the legal system.

Emotions and Attitudes Affecting Vocational Rehabilitation

Improvement in coping with emotions and negative attitudes is noticeable within the first few months of recovery, though more permanent changes require time (Alcoholics Anonymous, 2001). Although progress is noticeable early in recovery, it is unrealistic to expect a person with many years of alcoholism to be fully recovered in a few weeks or even several months. The counselor must regularly acknowledge the long-term nature of recovery. Additionally, when depression or severe anxiety persists, or other signs of emotional illness evolve, referral to a mental health professional experienced in substance abuse counseling is appropriate.

Conclusion

Alcohol consumption has negative consequences not only for the health and well being of the client, but also the health and well being of those around him or her. Alcohol addiction is common, costly, and imposes a negative impact on all aspects of the individual's life. Alcoholism is a disease in a sense that once an alcoholic drinking pattern is present, if left untreated, the severity and consequences of drinking are generally progressive and sometimes fatal. Although the effects vary widely, detoxification from alcohol is the first step to recovery. The desired goal is to abstain from drinking and maintain sobriety. Rehabilitation counselors need to understand and familiarize themselves with the process, stages, and difficulties facing both recovering alcoholics and clients whose current drinking affects the ability to maintain employment or return to work. Appropriate interventions and holistic supports are the keys to rehabilitation for individuals with alcohol-related disorders.

Case Study

Sally, a 32 year-old woman, is currently undergoing detoxification at a local alcohol treatment center. Two previous attempts to become sober and maintain long-term sobriety failed. She is married, although separated, and has two children, three and six years of age. The present attempt at sobriety was prompted by the departure of her husband as a result of her continued drinking behaviors. The children are living with her mother in a nearby city.

There is a history of alcoholism in Sally's family. Her father was a diagnosed alcoholic and died at age 47, as the result of physical complications resulting from alcoholism. The mother's present husband was previously married to an alcoholic. Sally states that her parents are not sympathetic or supportive of her sobriety. Her parents indicate that they are willing to provide care for the children, but that Sally is not welcome in their home when she is drinking.

Drinking did not become a problem for Sally until she became an adult, although she began drinking secretly from her father's stock of alcohol at age 12, and enjoying the feelings she experienced. Drinking continued in high school. Once she was expelled from a school dance due to drinking. Serious trouble from alcohol consumption began during her freshman year in college; Sally experienced problems in classes due to absences. She had to move from her apartment on three occasions when her roommates refused to put up with her drinking. College life thus became impossible and Sally dropped out after the second term.

At the age of 20, Sally secured employment with a ticket agency, where she met and married a band musician. Six months later, she was divorced, again the result of her drinking and socially unacceptable behavior. She enrolled in an alcohol treatment program at the time of the divorce but left the program after five days. Continuing to drink, she was eventually fired from her job and returned home to live with her parents under the condition that she seeks help for her drinking problem. She attended several meetings at a women's center and enrolled in an outpatient treatment program at a local hospital. She continued participating in the outpatient program for three months, but stopped when she married her current husband, a produce manager at a local supermarket.

Sally controlled her drinking for the next eight years, during which time she gave birth to two children. During these years, she worked part-time at a local printing shop doing general office work. When she was 30, drinking again became a serious problem for Sally. While at home, she would drink secretly, but her practices soon became obvious to all around her. On several occasions, she would leave the children unattended to stay out all night. She lost her job, and the week after her 31st birthday, her husband left after she had destroyed much of the furniture at home in a drunken rage. Sally's parents took her and the children home and again insisted that she enter some type of treatment program.

Alcoholics Anonymous (AA) became Sally's support system; she attended meetings regularly but continued to drink. Her mother and stepfather eventually told Sally that she could no longer reside with them but that they would continue to care for the children until she regained the capacity to care for them. Sally was angry, frustrated, and hurt, but enrolled at a county detoxification center where she is currently seeking help from a counselor.

Questions

1. Identify any factors which might have contributed to Sally becoming an alcoholic.
2. What are the positive factors in this case for rehabilitation?
3. As Sally's counselor, identify the first three measures you would recommend.
4. In your intervention, how would you involve Sally's significant others?
5. What types of intervention would you suggest for this individual?

References

Acton, Q. A. (Ed.). (2013). *Alcoholism: New insights for the healthcare professional*. Atlanta, GA: Scholarly Editions.

Alcoholics Anonymous. (1981). *The twelve steps and twelve traditions*. New York, NY: Author.

Alcoholics Anonymous. (2001). *The story of how many thousands of men and women have recovered from alcoholism* (4th ed.). New York, NY: Author.

Boyle, P., Boffetta, P., Lowenfels, A. B., Burns, H., Brawley, O., Zatonski, W., & Rehm, J. (2013). *Alcohol: Science, policy, and public health*. New York, NY: Oxford University.

Carson-DeWitt, R. (Ed.). (2003). *Drugs, alcohol, and tobacco: Learning about addictive behavior*. New York, NY: Macmillan.

Centers for Disease Control and Prevention (CDC). (2013). *Alcohol use: Fast statistics*. Retrieved on August 25, 2013 from http://www.cdc.gov/nchs/fastats/alcohol.htm

Fletcher, A. M. (2013). *Addiction treatment – and how to get help that works*. New York, NY: Viking.

Highway Loss Data Institute (2007). *Laws and regulations. Alcohol-related laws – DUI/DWI laws*. Retrieved on August 26, 2007 from http://www.iihs.org/laws/state_laws/dui.html

McDonald, F. (2013). *The thirteenth step*. Bloomington, IN: Balboa.

Morsehead, A. (2013). *Blind drunk: Light at the end of the tunnel for anyone living with a loved one's alcohol problem*. Bloomington, IN: Balboa.

National Council on Alcoholism and Drug Dependence (NCADD). (2007). *Overview*. Retrieved on August 26, 2007 from http://www.ncaddnj.org/about/default.asp

National Institute on Alcohol Abuse and Alcoholism (NIAAA). (2013). *MADD – Statistics*. Retrieved on August 25, 2013 from http://www.madd.org/statistics/htm

O'Brien, P. G. (2013). Substance-related disorders. In P. G. O'Brien, W. Z. Kennedy, & K. A. Ballard (Eds.), *Psychiatric mental health nursing* (2nd ed., pp. 342–369). Burlington, MA: Jones & Bartlett.

O'Connor, P. G. (2012). Alcohol abuse and dependence. In L. Goldman & A. I. Schafer (Eds.), *Goldman's Cecil medicine* (24th ed., pp. 146–153). Philadelphia, PA: Elsevier Saunders.

Powers, P. W., & Dell Orto, A. E. (2004). *Families living with chronic illness and disability: Interventions, challenges, and opportunities*. New York, NY: Springer.

Schuckit, M. A. (2006). *Drug and alcohol abuse: A clinical guide to diagnosis and treatment* (6th ed.). New York, NY: Springer.

Weiss, R. D. (2012). Drug abuse and dependence. In L. Goldman & A. I. Schafer (Eds.) *Goldman's Cecil medicine* (24th ed., pp. 153–159). Philadelphia, PA: Elsevier Saunders.

About the Author

Roman Carlos, M.S., C.R.C., received his B.S. Degree in Rehabilitation Services and M.S. Degree in Counseling, with an option in Rehabilitation from California State University, Los Angeles. Currently, he is employed as a Senior Vocational Rehabilitation Counselor for the California State Department of Rehabilitation, and he provides alcohol and drug rehabilitation counseling with an emphasis on return to work. For the past 20 years, Mr. Carlos has been a consultant to many substance abuse treatment agencies in Southern California, volunteering his time to keep people in the recovery process.

Chapter 25

LEARNING DISABILITIES

Diane Haager, Ph.D.
Christine C. Givner, Ph.D.
Martin G. Brodwin, Ph.D., C.R.C.

Introduction

This chapter focuses on the various issues related to the successful habilitation and rehabilitation of persons with specific learning disabilities (LD). Unlike other disabilities, LD can be thought of as an invisible disability in that it may not be physically evident. Defining characteristics are typically evident in cognitive functioning and language processing. There is a common misconception that LD is only a *mild* disability and therefore has little impact on quality of life (Sabornie & deBettencourt, 2004), but a learning disability can occur along a continuum from mild to severe and can have a tremendous impact into adulthood. "Issues of stigma and a lack of awareness and understanding of LD by the general public have contributed to the confusion about their existence and impact" (Cramer & Ellis, 1996, p. xxvii). Despite a lack of consensus in how to define and measure specific learning disabilities, especially in the adult population, there is no question that the learning and life challenges experienced by individuals with this disorder play a significant role in determining their adult outcomes (Kirsch, Jungeblut, Jenkins, & Kolstad, 1993)

Upon completion of this chapter, the reader will have (a) an understanding of the various dynamics and life implications that people with LD face, and (b) the ability to design effective vocational rehabilitation plans for persons with learning disabilities. Topics covered include: prevalence, definition of LD, diagnosis and evaluation, characteristics of LD, reasonable accommodation, rehabilitation potential, and a case study.

Prevalence

LD affects approximately 15% of the United States population; additionally, many people who have learning disabilities are never diagnosed. In 2004, the federal government estimated that there were 2.8 million students with learning disabilities in school. Getzel and Gugerty (2001) noted that it is estimated that 35% of youth with learning disabilities drop out of high school. Of those students who complete high school, 62% are unemployed a year following graduation. Approximately 56% of students with LD who drop out of high school eventually are arrested.

The term *learning disabilities*, by federal definition, is a heterogeneous set of conditions that may manifest differently across individuals (Fletcher, Steubing, Morris & Lyon, 2013). Generally speaking, the term refers to any combination of difficulties in the domains of listening, speaking, reading and writing, mathematics, and reasoning. These disabilities interfere with an individual's ability to store, process, and produce information, and are often hidden by the individual's general level of functioning. Learning disabilities may occur with or be complicated by problems involving inadequate attention and inappropriate social skills (Cramer & Ellis, 1996).

As of yet, no single current database exists to determine the prevalence of learning disabilities in the adult population. Although the actual number of adults with LD in this country has not been determined, the 2004 national estimate of about 2.8 million students in schools, suggests the number of adults with LD is likewise substantial (Rubin & Roessler, 2008). Estimated prevalence discussed below has been derived from various national data sources.

A 2011 report, "The State of Learning Disabilities" published biennially by the National Center for Learning Disabilities (2011) estimates that approximately 5% of the school-age population, or about 2.5 million students, are considered to have LD and receive educational services. Though we would expect a similar proportion in the adult population, estimates rely solely on self-report in populations that are accessible to researchers. Surveys of students in post-secondary institutions estimate 2-3% of students with self-reported LD. Another survey of adult literacy in the general population found 3% of adults reported reading-related LD (Vogel, 1998). Thus, the adult population of individuals with this disorder appears to be under-identified.

The United States Employment and Training Administration (1991) reported that between 15% and 23% of Job Training Partnership Act (JTPA) trainees have learning disabilities, while 50% to 80% of adults reading below the 7th grade level have learning disabilities. Additionally, between 10% and 50% of Adult Basic Education students likely have learning disabilities (Adult Education Amendments, 1988).

Regarding gender-related prevalence, it is a common observation that the school-identified LD ratio of males to females is 4:1. In research and self-identified samples, gender ratio was found to be almost equivalent (1:1), very similar to the self-reported numbers described in the National Adult Literacy Survey (NALS) results (Kirsch et al., 1993; Lyon, 1994). Researchers (Heward, 2012; Sabornie & deBettencourt, 2004) have suggested that the discrepancy between school-identified and self-reported LD gender ratios is related to referral bias in school samples and higher prevalence of attention deficit hyperactivity disorders (ADHD) in males. This increases the likelihood of identification of males in school-age special education programs.

Definitions of Learning Disabilities

The earliest and most widely used definition of LD was integrated into federal legislation as the Education for All Handicapped Children Act of 1975. Each subsequent version was incorporated into the Individuals with Disabilities Education Act (IDEA, 1990) and the Individuals with Disabilities Education Improvement Act of 2004. The earlier definitions included only children. The 2004 definition includes adults with LD, and is written as follows:

> The term "specific learning disability" (SLD) means a disorder in one or more of the basic psychological processes involved in understanding or using language, spoken or written, which disorder may manifest itself in an imperfect ability to listen, think, speak, read, write, spell, or do mathematical calculations. SLD includes such conditions as perceptual disabilities, brain injury, minimal brain dysfunction, dyslexia, and developmental aphasia. It does not include a learning problem that is primarily the result of visual, hearing, or motor disabilities; mental retardation; emotional disturbance; and environmental, cultural, or economic disadvantage (IDEA, 2004).

Adults with LD have legal protection from discrimination under federal statutes, including the Rehabilitation Act of 1973, specifically Section 504; the Americans with Disabilities Act (ADA) of 1990; IDEA (1990); and the Individuals with Disabilities Education Improvement Act of 2004. These statutes acknowledge the lifelong nature of specific learning disabilities. While Section 504 has its greatest impact on educational environments, the ADA concerns employment. These acts protect persons with disabilities from discrimination, provide for equal access to education and employment, and recommend the provision of reasonable accommodation (Heward, 2012; Rubin & Roessler, 2008).

Diagnosis and Evaluation

Diagnostic Criteria

Given the complexity and heterogeneity of learning disabilities, maintaining a database of vocational and other services for adults with LD is essential. The U. S. Department of Education has funded a national longitudinal study since 2001. According to the most recent report, 66.8% of individuals with LD attend some type of post-secondary education up to eight years post high school, with 21% attending a four-year college or university (Newman et al., 2012). Aside from individuals with speech and language impairment (66.9%), this is higher than the percentage of any other disability group.

The diagnostic criteria for vocational and post-secondary education services may vary across institutions (Gregg, Coleman, Davis, Lindstrom, & Hartwig, 2006), but the diagnosis of LD for vocational rehabilitation purposes should directly relate to the criteria established in the Rehabilitation Services Administration (RSA) definition. Major definitional criteria include evidence of a central nervous system processing difficulty and manifest deficits in one or more of the following areas: attention, reasoning, processing, memory, communication, reading, spelling, writing, calculations, coordination, social competence, and emotional maturity. Psychological evaluation must be preceded by a thorough medical examination; the physician needs familiarity with specific learning disabilities to rule out any systemic organic abnormality that may be causal to the symptoms of a learning disability. A qualified professional must conduct a formal evaluation that includes an interview, a cognitive test battery, academic testing, and assessment of information processing skills (Gregg et al., 2006). There are numerous cognitive batteries that are widely used for this purpose. An overall IQ score is used to determine the individual's overall cognitive functioning, and specific subtests or additional measures are used to examine cognitive processing skills such as working memory, attention, processing speed, spatial ability, and others.

A multidisciplinary team consisting of a physician, psychologist, and vocational evaluator may participate in the diagnostic evaluation. The vocational evaluator assesses interests, aptitudes, abilities, and work behaviors through inventories, observation, and work samples. Other professionals, including neuropsychologists, speech and language therapists, audiologists, occupational therapists, and medical specialists may serve on the team, depending on the nature of the person's learning disability.

Assessment Practices

The diagnosis needs to focus on overall cognitive processing to rule out an intellectual disability and examination of achievement and specific processing skills. Having an invisible disability, a person with LD may be labeled as bright but bored by his or her parents, "lazy" or "dumb" by teachers, "strange" by peers, and incapable of work by employers (Fletcher, 2007).

Hawks et al. (1990) suggested that to appropriately assess areas of potential deficit or need, four essential sources of information need to be used, including standardized tests, a record review, behavioral observations, and in-depth clinical interviews. The record review, including the person's school and vocational history, previous assessments and results, and the transition plan from high school (if available) must be comprehensive to yield a complete case history specifying previously identified deficits, past interventions, and treatments. Behavioral observations should focus on the following considerations: the person's appearance, punctuality, social skills, activity level, attention span, impulse control, reaction to praise, memory, emotionality, language, and persistence. Clinical interviews include gathering information regarding an individual's self-perception of educational, social, vocational, and cognitive processing abilities and limitations, as well as information on family and personal adjustment issues.

Characteristics of Learning Disabilities

As stated previously, the population of adults with learning disabilities is heterogeneous (Fletcher et al., 2013). The nature of this disability and its impact on a person's life is influenced by various personal characteristics and external contextual variables including: (a) the unique individual strengths and needs of the individual; (b) cognitive capacity; (c) the precise and unique nature of the specific learning disability; (d) educational history; (e) current contextual cognitive and psychosocial demands; and (f) the historical pattern of successes, frustrations, and failures. The following section discusses the medical aspects of disability, learning characteristics, social skills/adaptive behavior, and job-relevant characteristics.

Medical Aspects

The physiological factors related to this disorder focus mainly on the information processing mechanisms in the brain. Sensory input is obtained through visual, auditory, and tactile stimuli, thus allowing a person to learn through seeing, listening, touching, and moving the body (Carter, Lane, Pierson, & Glaeser, 2006). Information is sent to the brain for processing (i.e., analysis, integration, and storage). To assimilate information, a person must pay close attention to relevant details, classifying new information efficiently for later retrieval. The brain creates schemata, or cognitive organizational files, to classify and store information. Persons with LD may have difficulty recognizing crucial details and associating new information efficiently with what has previously been learned. This results in an inefficient memory system, making later retrieval of information difficult. Persons with learning disabilities may appear unorganized, especially in terms of their time management skills (Levy, 2005). Because of the apparent disorganization, a person is often misperceived as lazy, unmotivated, or forgetful. However, learning disabilities are a heterogeneous set of characteristics and these descriptors may or may not apply to a specific individual identified as having LD.

A learning disability is not synonymous with intellectual disability, a common misperception. Learning disabilities occur in individuals irrespective of intelligence level. The learning difficulties experienced are directly related to information processing difficulties involved in cognitive functioning (Osmon, Smerz, Braun & Plambeck, 2006). The majority of persons with LD have difficulties related to reading, but not all individuals with reading difficulties have LD. Between 15% and 20% of school age individuals are affected by specific reading disabilities (Lyon, 1994), ranging from mild to severe while about 5% of the school-aged population has LD. Adults who read below a fourth grade level should be assessed for other indicators of LD. Additionally, many adults with LD have processing deficits that impact mathematics learning, in addition to reading difficulties (Osmon et al., 2006).

Learning Characteristics

Many adults with LD experience reading and other language-related disabilities as major barriers to learning and life functioning. Vogel (1985) conducted a major review of the literature to synthesize the reported manifestations of LD in adults attending college. This information remains current. A brief summary of the most significant limitations follows.

Language

Adults with LD often have difficulty perceiving sounds, recognizing syllables within words, and understanding rapid conversation. Frequently, they cannot find the right word or mispronounce words with several syllables. Adults often experience various reading disorders, including inaccurate decoding of words and various kinds of comprehension difficulties. In written language, they may have great difficulty with legible penmanship, grammar, spelling, and organizing and developing ideas on paper.

Reading

Individuals with reading-related learning disabilities have a language-based, auditory processing difficulty that persists even after learning to read and comprehend with accuracy. For such people, rapid and accurate decoding of unfamiliar, multisyllabic, and foreign language words remains inaccurate and the rate of decoding is slow. Although people with LD read slowly, with appropriate intervention some become proficient at reading comprehension, especially in their fields of expertise (Fletcher, 2007; Sabornie & deBettencourt, 2004).

Vogel (1998) found that adults with significant reading-related LD are more frequently under-employed, earn significantly diminished wages, and have lower occupational status. These statistics have major implications for vocational rehabilitation. First, young adults with learning disabilities would benefit from staying in school, achieving a diploma, and participating in some type of vocational or career planning. Second, upon graduation, students with LD will benefit from postsecondary education or vocational training. To facilitate this process, education and rehabilitation professionals need to: (a) create more meaningful secondary school programs for youth with LD; (b) improve the implementation and procedures involved when transitioning youth from high school to postsecondary training and employment;

and (c) increase the number of adults with LD who enroll in and complete a variety of adult secondary education programs.

Mathematics

People with LD may exhibit limitations related to mathematics. They have difficulty mastering basic operations of mathematics, remembering the sequence of steps in algorithms, and solving multistep mathematical problems. Significant cognitive processing deficits in the areas of spatial relations and executive function are related to LD mathematics difficulties (Osmon et al., 2006).

Study Skills and Attention

Adults with LD may have trouble organizing their time, note taking, focusing on critical components of any task (i.e., becoming distracted readily), and completing tasks. These various limitations impact effectiveness of daily functioning. Appropriate accommodations help alleviate these obstacles and promote success.

Social Skills Issues and Adaptive Behavior

Friendlessness, social ineptitude, and loneliness are social development patterns that sometimes can result from LD. Having this disorder may significantly impact one's psychological well-being, social functioning, emotional adjustment, achievement, motivation, and self-esteem (Fletcher, 2007; Nelson, 2012; Palmer & Roessler, 2000). Persons with LD often exhibit ineffective adaptive behavior across varying life contexts. If individuals have experienced a history of failure and frustration, they may display patterns of procrastination and lack of initiative, attributing failure to external causes and success to luck. Mithaug and Horiuchi (1983) found that adults are often socially inactive as a result of fear of intimacy. This fear leads to social isolation and loneliness. Loneliness and mild depression may lead to the overuse of prescription mood-altering drugs, alcohol, caffeine, and illegal substances. Medical consultation, individual or group therapy, and support groups are helpful in minimizing such psychosocial symptoms.

Young adults with LD are at greater risk for depression, anxiety, and even potential suicide. A study of social skills problems and issues of adults with LD indicated that they (Lehtinen-Rogan & Hartman, cited in Rubin & Roessler, 2008):

- Feel responsible to form themselves into likeable and successful people but find this difficult.
- Find social relationships trying. They want and need others but lack the confidence that people will like or respect them.
- Tend to move between despondency and euphoria in relationships because of an underlying level of depression which is diminished by social contact.
- Are overly sensitive and easily hurt while, at the same time, being tense and anxious.

Job-Relevant Characteristics

Non-academic problems, like those described above, often relate directly to employment (Carter & Lunsford, 2005). Adult employees with LD experience challenges related to cognitive processing difficulties. As previously stated, many individuals experience significant difficulties in the areas of psychosocial functioning and social adaptability. Deficits in social skills are the most debilitating aspect within the workplace (Interagency Committee on Learning Disabilities, 1987). Adults with LD may find it difficult to recognize subtle social cues and misinterpret interpersonal dynamics; they may be *socially incompetent*.

Reasonable Accommodation

The following list was adapted from Vogel (1998, pp. 10-11) describing aspects of reasonable accommodation. Counselors and educators apply reasonable accommodation in schools and employment when assisting individuals who have learning disabilities. Gregg (2012) cited the lack of comprehensive evidence for accommodations in adult education services regarding testing and educational accommodations. With appropriate supports and accommodations, many individuals can be successful in postsecondary education and employment settings (Newman et al., 2012).

1. **Reasonable accommodations** in educational environments include equal opportunity for acceptance, providing or modifying equipment, and modifying instructional methodology and examination procedures to ensure that individuals with disabilities have equal opportunities to learn and be evaluated on the basis of knowledge and skills, rather than on the basis of disability.
2. **Reasonable** refers to the idea that the suggested accommodations will not create an "undue hardship" on an institution. Undue hardship is defined by the ADA as any action that creates "significant difficulty or expense" for an employer given "the size of the employer, the resources available, and the nature of the operation."
3. A person with a **disability** is an individual who has a "physical or mental impairment which substantially limits one or more major life activities, has a record of such impairment, or is regarded as having such impairment" (ADA, 1990).
4. **Physical or mental impairments** include physical disabilities and mental disabilities (e.g., intellectual disability, organic brain syndrome, emotional or mental illness, and specific learning disabilities [ADA, 1990]).
5. **Learning disabilities** are protected under Section 504 of the Rehabilitation Act of 1973, but the learning disability must be significant enough to substantially limit one or more major life activities.
6. A **substantial limitation** occurs when a person is unable to perform a task or is significantly restricted because of a disability.
7. The concept of an **otherwise qualified person** pertains to adults with LD across various settings, such as literacy environments, job training, adult education, adult secondary education classes, and postsecondary institutions meeting the criteria for admission and participation in education programs and activities.
8. A **program or activity** refers to all education programs that receive federal subsidies or grants. This includes all public elementary and secondary schools; adult educational environments, such as adult education programs; postsecondary vocational, trade, and military schools; and public (and most private) colleges and universities.

Requests for accommodation must be documented and establish the identified disability as interfering with the person's ability to perform the relevant tasks in a manner similar to persons without disabilities. It is incumbent upon the instructor, employer, or accrediting organization to establish whether or not the proposed reasonable accommodation will modify the essential requirements, standards, or functions of the task. If it is found that the accommodation does in fact modify those essential functions, the request for accommodation can be denied.

Rehabilitation Potential

Characteristics for Success

Despite the unique challenges facing adults with learning disabilities, many experience success in employment and other life circumstances (Newman et al., 2012; Vogel & Adelman, 2000). A study conducted by Ginsberg, Gerber, and Reiff (1994) investigated 70 adults with LD who were successful in their professions. This study and previous research by Silver & Hagin (1985) suggested that higher socioeconomic status, greater educational levels, and appropriate intervention maximize the possibilities of successful employment.

Ginsberg et al. (1994) indicated that the overriding factor leading to success with persons who have learning disabilities was *control*. Taking control was categorized into several themes related to internal decisions and external manifestations. Internal decisions included the characteristics of desire, goal orientation, and reframing. External manifestations (i.e., adaptability) were characterized as persistence, goodness-of-fit, learned creativity, and social ecologies. All these characteristics were found to interact with one another to either optimize or reduce a person's potential for success.

Internal Decisions

While desire and motivation to succeed relate to general success, they play an even more vital role in the success of adults with learning disabilities. Through goal orientation, practical and obtainable aspirations can be established. Reframing involves a reinterpretation of the LD experience from negative and dysfunctional to positive and functional, allowing one to recognize that obstacles can be overcome (Trainor, 2005). Steps in the process of reframing include: (a) recognition of the disability; (b) acceptance of the negative and positive ramifications of having LD; (c) understanding the disability and its implications, as well as one's own strengths and weaknesses; and (d) taking productive action.

External Manifestations/Adaptability

Various aspects of external manifestations/adaptability are key to success. *Persistence*, for example, involves consistently working hard, being willing to sacrifice, and delaying personal gratification. *Goodness-of-fit* involves personal adaptation to surroundings and environments which encourage success. *Learned creativity* incorporates various strategies, techniques, and other mechanisms devised to enhance one's ability to perform. *Social ecology* includes ability to utilize supportive and helpful people, and develop and implement a variety of self-improvement processes. By identifying unique and personal ways to accommodate limitations to accomplish tasks, anticipating possible difficulties, and devising various options for problem-solving, adults are provided with a variety of alternative coping strategies (Fletcher, 2007; Heward, 2012).

Interventions and Accommodations

Functional Literacy

Various adult basic education and postsecondary education programs exist to ameliorate functional literacy deficits. Whatever program is chosen, instructional interventions should be individualized to meet area-specific functional literacy needs. Crawford (1998) provided a thorough discussion of the process for developing abilities-based literacy and employment preparation services for adults with learning disabilities.

Assistive Technology (AT)

Another tool utilized to maximize functional literacy skills is assistive technology. Various applications and types of AT afford powerful accommodation/compensatory means to ensure the ability to perform competently and successfully despite reading, writing, and organizational problems. For difficulties in written language, assistive devices include word processors, spell checkers, proofreading programs, speech synthesizers, and speech recognition systems. For reading, optical character recognition systems, screen review systems, and tape recorders are options. With organizational or memory compensation deficits, personal data managers and free-form databases are effective. Difficulties in mathematical computations are compensated with use of calculators and simple spreadsheets. An appropriate and useable fit may determine if a person will continue to use the AT.

The importance of AT for people with disabilities cannot be overemphasized. Its effective use provides opportunities for enhanced self-sufficiency, increased independence, and greater potential for gainful employment. AT extends into the areas of daily living, social functioning, recreation, and work opportunities, thus diminishing a person's functional limitations and helping to *level the playing field* (Brodwin, Siu, & Cardoso, 2012).

AT is an effective and powerful tool to increase functioning, enhance quality of life, and remove physical and attitudinal barriers for persons with LD. With increased access to the environment and enhanced social integration, individuals can more effectively and readily interact in all phases of society. Through use of AT, people with LD can achieve greater productivity within both education and employment, leading to enhanced self-sufficiency, independence, freedom of choice, and social integration (Brodwin, Boland, Lane, & Siu, 2010).

Job Relevant Skills and Employability

There are several skills related to employment that affect adults with LD (Gregg, 2012; Newman et al., 2012; Rubin & Roessler, 2008). Adults with LD often lack adequate job acquisition skills. Because of cognitive processing difficulties, such as organizational skills and short term memory, and general reading, writing, and mathematics difficulties, individuals may have significant problems going through the steps of acquiring employment. Persons with LD may have difficulty accessing information about jobs through newspapers, the Internet, and other media, and may have difficulty completing employment applications.

The high level of credentialing and entrance examinations required by vocational and professional jobs are a barrier for adults with LD. These exist despite the ADA mandate for reasonable testing accommodations. Adults often are hesitant to request testing accommodations prior to employment for fear of discrimination by perspective employers.

The interview process is a challenge for many adults with learning disabilities because a positive interview involves the utilization of complex social skills, and the ability to decide whether or not to disclose information pertinent to the learning disability. Job coaches and job preparation workshops can assist people in successfully navigating these job acquisition skills (Trainor, 2005). Through these programs, vocational strategies are devised to optimize work-related assets and minimize disability-related problems (i.e., development of possible reasonable accommodations for a job).

Krishnaswami (1984) identified the following 15 employability factors needed for persons with severe LD to enter the labor market:

1. Hygiene, grooming, and appropriate dress.
2. Ability to relate to supervisors and co-workers.
3. Skills in communication.
4. Increased frustration tolerance.
5. Appropriate responses to criticism.
6. Proper social behavior at work.
7. Punctuality and attendance.
8. Initiative in carrying out work tasks.
9. Awareness of safety and work rules.
10. ncreasing stamina/energy levels for work.
11. Organizational skills with job tasks.
12. Consistency in the various aspects of work.
13. Improved speed performance on the job.
14. Enhanced independent functioning with work assignments.
15. Attending to and following up with directions.

Rubin and Roessler (2008) summarized job adjustment problems for individuals with LD. These included: slow work pace, arriving late to work, problems with coworkers and supervisors, inefficiency, high error rates, proneness to accidents, deficient academic skills, problems in learning sequences of tasks, and deficiency of social skills.

Social Competency and Adaptive Behavior

Job skills training should involve careful development and refinement of needed job-related social skills. Adequate social competence is necessary for all jobs, especially as the workplace becomes more collaborative. Classes in social skills, support groups, and individual sessions with a rehabilitation counselor are various ways of enhancing social competence (Palmer & Roessler, 2000).

Colleagues can provide social assistance help through on-the-job mentoring (Carter & Lunsford, 2005). Mentors can explain the dynamics of inappropriate behavior, provide tools for overcoming specific problems, and explain unspoken cultural mores. Social skills are inherent for job advancement in higher-level positions, and involve managerial responsibilities that include the ability to work closely with a variety of personnel.

Self-Efficacy

Adults with LD develop self-efficacy as they experience various problem-solving strategies. These perspectives allow individuals to increase means, techniques, and strategies to overcome the challenges presented by learning disabilities (Trainor, 2005). To learn effective coping strategies, persons must cultivate a personal understanding, a process aided by perseverance, creativity, and support. By learning and using effective employment techniques, adults with LD can optimize their potential.

Case Study

Dennis Hoover is a 34 year-old Anglo male with a well-documented learning disability; he is currently unemployed. Because Mr. Hoover has been unable to maintain employment for more than seven months at a time, his job counselor at the employment office has referred him to the Department of Rehabilitation for further job training.

As the youngest of six children, Dennis grew up in a working class family in a small rural town. As an infant, he experienced several serious pneumonia infections and spent much of his first two years of life in and out of the hospital. Eventually, his pediatrician discovered that Dennis had a genetic autoimmune disorder. Medical records obtained from the family physician supported this information.

During elementary school, Dennis experienced serious difficulties socially as well as academically. He had trouble learning to read and write. As a result, he failed first grade and reported that his parents were unsuccessful in having school officials provide additional academic help. Finally, in fourth grade, Dennis was referred, evaluated, and identified as having a specific learning disability and was placed in a self-contained classroom for learning disabilities. He remembers being teased by the neighborhood children and his older brother, occasionally being referred to as "retard." Throughout his school experience, Dennis worked hard to learn to read, write legibly, and master basic mathematics.

Upon entering high school, Dennis was fully mainstreamed. His mother and siblings helped him complete reading assignments and written homework. Since his grades were insufficient to qualify for a vocational program at the high school, Dennis was placed on a non-vocational track. Although proud of Dennis' participation in high school football and wrestling, the football coach often complained that Dennis was "clumsy" and "lacked coordination." Standing 6 foot 4 inches and weighing 220 pounds, his nickname became "the Hulk."

After graduating high school, Dennis obtained a job as a cook in an upscale restaurant and bar in his hometown. Though he enjoys cooking and reported considering going to "chef school," Dennis changed his mind after discovering that the nearest program required passing a competency test involving proficient reading. Through intervention by the Department of Rehabilitation counselor, Dennis was able to maintain his job as a cook. However, after one year, he quit because of the irregular and long hours, without notifying his counselor.

Since that time, Mr. Hoover has had several unskilled, general labor jobs. These include a position as a factory worker in the canned food industry, a seasonal laborer, a non-union construction worker, steel worker, dock worker, and dishwasher. Keeping a job has been difficult; at times, Dennis was fired for arriving at work late or leaving before the end of his shift. Other times, he quit a job because he felt the pay to be insufficient. Dennis also had disagreements with fellow workers and supervisors. Currently, Dennis states he wants to "get his act together" and is thinking about acquiring a career which will help him obtain financial stability.

Mr. Hoover's poor finances and its affect on his family have motivated him to request vocational rehabilitation. As Dennis stated, he is tired of feeling overwhelmed and being unable to provide for his family's financial stability. During the past three years, he has been living with a woman and her three teenagers, children from a prior marriage who are frequently in trouble at school. A local social service agency has threatened to take the 13 year-old girl away unless they are able to provide a more stable home environment. He and his girlfriend spend money excessively and drink alcohol heavily on weekends. Dennis wants to be a good provider and father figure, but does not know how to change his current situation.

Questions

1. What kinds of services are available and relevant to Mr. Hoover's needs?
2. Describe how you, as the rehabilitation counselor, will proceed with this case.
3. Develop two appropriate and feasible vocational goals for Dennis. Outline two vocational plans.
4. Are there additional assessments that need to be conducted to better understand the work-related strengths and needs of this client?
5. What kinds of work-related accommodations would you suggest?
6. Identify other human services you would recommend for Mr. Hoover to assist him in stabilizing his life.

References

Adult Education Amendments of 1988, 20 U.S.C. §1201 *et seq.*

Americans with Disabilities Act of 1990 (ADA), 42 U.S.C. §12101 *et seq.*

Brodwin, M. G., Siu, F. W., & Cardoso, E. (2012). Users of assistive technology: The human component. In I. Marini & M. A. Stebnicki (Eds.), *The psychological and social impact of illness and disability* (6th ed., pp. 331–339). New York, NY: Springer.

Brodwin, M. G., Boland, E. A., Lane, F. J., & Siu, F. W. (2010). Technology in rehabilitation counseling. In R. M. Parker & J. B. Patterson (Eds.), *Rehabilitation counseling: Basics and beyond* (5th ed., pp. 333–367). Austin, TX: Pro-ed.

Carter, E. W., Lane, K. L., Pierson, M. R., & Glaeser, B. (2006). Self-determination skills and opportunities of transition-age youth with emotional disturbance and learning disabilities. *Council for Exceptional Children, 72*(3), 333–346.

Carter, E. W., & Lunsford, L. B. (2005) Meaningful work: Preparing transition-age youth with emotional and behavioral disorders for employment. *Preventing School Failure, 49*(2), 63–69.

Cramer, S. C., & Ellis, W. (Eds.). (1996). *Learning disabilities: Lifelong issues.* Baltimore, MD: Paul H. Brookes.

Crawford, R. (1998). Developing abilities-based literacy and employment services for adults with learning disabilities. In S. A. Vogel & S. Reder (Eds.), *Learning disabilities, literacy, and adult education* (pp. 275–294). Baltimore, MD: Paul H. Brookes.

Education for All Handicapped Children Act of 1975, 20 U.S.C. §1400 *et seq.*

Fletcher, J. M. (2007). *Learning disabilities: From identification to intervention.* New York, NY: Guilford.

Fletcher, J. M., Steubing, K. K., Morris, R. D., & Lyon, G. R. (2013). Classification and definition of learning disabilities: A hybrid model. In H. L. Swanson, K. R. Harris, & S. Graham (Eds.), *Handbook of learning disabilities* (2nd ed., pp. 33–50). New York, NY: Guilford.

Getzel, E. E., & Gugerty, J. J. (2001). Applications for youth with learning disabilities. In P. Wehman (Ed.), *Life beyond the classroom* (pp. 371–398). Baltimore, MD: Brookes.

Ginsberg, R., Gerber, P. J., & Reiff, H. B. (1994). Employment success for adults with learning disabilities. In P. J. Gerber & H. B. Reiff (Eds.), *Learning disabilities in adulthood: Persisting problems and evolving issues* (pp. 204–213). Boston, MA: Andover Medical.

Gregg, N. (2012). Increasing access to learning for the adult basic education learner with learning disabilities: Evidence-based accommodation research. *Journal of Learning Disabilities, 45*(1), 47–63.

Gregg, N., Coleman, C., Davis, M., Lindstrom, W., & Hartwig, J. (2006). Critical issues for the diagnosis of learning disabilities in the adult population. *Psychology in the Schools, 43*(8), 889–899.

Hawks, R., Minskoff, E. H., Sautter, S. W., Sheldon, K. L., Steidle, E. F., & Hoffmann, F. J. (1990). A model diagnostic battery for adults with learning disabilities in vocational rehabilitation. *Learning Disabilities: A Multidisciplinary Journal, 1*(3), 94–101.

Heward, W. (2012). *Exceptional children: An introduction to special education* (10th ed.). Saddle River, NJ: Pearson/Merrill/Prentice Hall.

Individuals with Disabilities Education Act (IDEA) of 1990, 20 U.S.C. §1400 *et seq.*

Individuals with Disabilities Education Improvement Act (IDEIA) of 2004, 118 Stat. 2647.

Interagency Committee on Learning Disabilities. (1987). *Learning disabilities: A report to the U. S. Congress.* Washington, DC: U. S. Department of Health and Human Services.

Kirsch, I. S., Jungeblut, A., Jenkins, L., & Kolstad, A. (1993). *Adult literacy in America: A first look at the results of the National Adult Literacy Survey.* Princeton, NJ: Educational Testing.

Krishnaswami, U. (1984). Learning to achieve: Rehabilitation counseling and the learning disabled adult. *Journal of Applied Rehabilitation Counseling, 15*, 18–22.

Levy, G. (2005). Seeing for ourselves: Producing accessible information for people with learning disabilities and visual impairments. *British Journal of Learning Disabilities, 33*, 77–82.

Lyon, G. R. (Ed.). (1994). *Frames of reference for the assessment of learning disabilities: New views on measurement issues.* Baltimore, MD: Paul H. Brookes.

Mithaug, D. E., & Horiuchi, C. N. (1983). Colorado statewide follow-up survey of special education students. *Exceptional Children, 51*, 397–404.

National Center for Learning Disabilities. (2011). *The state of learning disabilities: Facts, trends, and indicators.* New York, NY: Author.

Nelson, J. M. (2012). General and domain-specific self-concepts of adults with learning disabilities: A meta-analysis. *Learning Disabilities: A Multidisciplinary Journal, 18*(2), 61–70.

Newman, L., Wagner, M., Knokey, A.-M., Marder, C., Nagle, K., Shaver, D., . . . Schwarting, M. (2012). The post-high school outcomes of young adults with disabilities up to 8 years after high school. *A Report From the National Longitudinal Transition Study-2 (NLTS2)* (NCSER 2011-3005). Menlo Park, CA: SRI International.

Osmon, D. C., Smerz, J. M., Braun, M. M., & Plambeck, E. (2006). Processing abilities associated with math skills in adult learning disability. *Journal of Clinical and Experimental Neuropsychology, 28*(1), 84–95.

Palmer, C., & Roessler, R. T. (2000). Requesting classroom accommodations: Self-advocacy and conflict resolution training for college students with disabilities. *Journal of Rehabilitation, 66*(3), 38–43.

Rehabilitation Act of 1973, 29 U.S.C. §701 *et seq.*

Rubin, S. E., & Roessler, R. T. (2008). *Foundations of the vocational rehabilitation process* (6th ed.). Austin, TX: Pro-ed.

Sabornie, E. J., & deBettencourt, L. U. (2004). *Teaching students with mild and high-incidence disabilities at the secondary level.* Upper Saddle River, NJ: Prentice Hall.

Silver, A., & Hagin, R. (1985). Outcomes of learning disabilities in adolescence. In M. Sugar, A. Esman, J. Looney, A. Schwartzberg, & A. Sorosky (Eds.), *Adolescent Psychiatry: Developmental and Clinical Studies, 12*, 197–213.

Trainor, A. A. (2005). Self-determination perceptions and beliefs of diverse students with LD during the transition planning process. *Journal of Learning Disabilities, 38*(3), 233–249.

United States Employment and Training Administration. (1991). *The learning disabled in employment and training programs* (Research and Evaluation Series 91-E). Washington, DC: U. S. Department of Labor.

Vogel, S. A. (1985). Learning disabled college students: Identification, assessment, and outcomes. In D. Duane & C. K. Leong (Eds.), *Understanding learning disabilities: International and multidisciplinary views* (pp. 179-203). New York, NY: Plenum.

Vogel, S. A. (1998). Adults with learning disabilities: What learning disabilities specialists, adult literacy educators, and other service providers want and need to know. In S. A. Vogel & S. Reder (Eds.), *Learning disabilities, literacy, and adult education* (pp. 10–11). Baltimore, MD: Paul H. Brookes.

Vogel, S. A., & Adelman, P. B. (2000). Adults with learning disabilities 8-15 years after college. *Learning Disabilities: A Multidisciplinary Journal, 10*(3), 165–182.

About the Authors

Diane Haager, Ph.D., is a researcher and teacher educator in reading and learning disabilities. She is a professor at California State University, Los Angeles (CSULA), where she instructs special education teachers and graduate students. Dr. Haager has worked in urban schools as a reading specialist and special educator. She is the co-editor of *Learning Disabilities Research and Practice.* Recent publications include a co-authored book, *How to Teach English Language Learners: Effective Strategies from Outstanding Educators,* a textbook, *Differentiating Instruction in Inclusive Classrooms: The Special Educator's Guide*, and a reading intervention handbook, *Interventions for Reading Success,* as well as numerous book chapters and articles. Research interests of Dr. Haager include issues related to effective reading instruction for English language learners, students with learning disabilities, and students at risk for reading failure.

Chris Givner, Ph.D., is Dean for the College of Education at the State University of New York (SUNY), Fredonia. Prior to SUNY, she was Professor and Chair of the Division of Special Education, Charter College of Education, CSULA. Dean Givner specializes in the areas of mild/moderate learning disabilities and emotional/behavioral disorders. Over the past 30 years, she has conducted research and published extensively in the areas of general and special education, and has expertise in teacher competency, inclusive education, and lifespan issues for persons with and without learning disabilities.

Martin G. Brodwin, Ph.D, C.R.C., is Professor and Coordinator of the Rehabilitation Counselor Education Program at CSULA. He is a vocational expert for the Office of Disability Adjudication and Review, Social Security Administration, providing testimony on disability-related issues. As a rehabilitation consultant, Dr. Brodwin provides assessment for long-term disability, case management, and reasonable accommodation. He has published over 100 refereed journal articles, book chapters, and books on the subjects of counseling, disability, rehabilitation, and accommodation in business and industry.

Chapter 26

INTELLECTUAL DEVELOPMENTAL DISORDERS

Julie Ton, Ph.D.
Mary A. Falvey, Ph.D.
Kathryn D. Bishop, Ph.D.
Susann Terry Gage, Ph.D.

Introduction

Evidence of intellectual disability can be traced as far back as 1552 B.C.E., during the time of the therapeutic papyri of Thebes (Luxor), Egypt (Ainsworth & Baker, 2004). Through the ages, persons with intellectual disability have faced challenges relative to the customs and beliefs of their culture. It was not until John Locke (1690) published *An Essay Concerning Human Understanding* that the public began to realize that persons with mental illness still maintain a capacity to learn and acquire meaningful skills. He proposed the idea that humans are born with a blank slate (*tabula rasa*) and learn through experience. Locke suggested that society, rather than an innate mental illness, was the more likely contributing factor to intellectual disability. This turning point in the conceptual world of intellectual disability inspired the development of new treatment approaches and ultimately improved cultural perceptions of intellectual disability.

Changes in policies, services, expectations, and personal values over the past several decades have significantly affected quality of life for persons with intellectual disability. This chapter discusses programs, services, and support systems available for these individuals. The framework of the chapter includes the definition of intellectual disability, prevalence, etiology, normalization, functional limitations, and rehabilitation potential generally observed in people with intellectual disability.

Repeated research has demonstrated that employment has had a positive impact on the lives of those with intellectual disabilities (Heller, Arnold, van Heuman, McBride, & Factor, 2012; Steere & Dipipi, 2013). Such positive impacts are evidenced by reported increased confidence, independence, and community membership. However, Wehmeyer and colleagues (2003) asserted that there continues to be challenges associated with employment. We encourage rehabilitation professionals to consider the information presented in the hope that they may develop improved quality programs, services, and support for their clients.

Definition of Intellectual Disability

Throughout the decades, intellectual disability has been described by the level of mental and functional impairment of an individual's abilities. In recent years, the definition and label of such cognitive impairments have been at the forefront of discussion between advocacy organizations, government agencies, and grassroots family movements (Tassé, Luckasson, & Nygren, 2013; Wehmeyer, 2013). In accordance with Rosa's Law (2010) and the *Diagnostic and Statistical Manual of Mental Disorders* (5th Edition) (American Psychiatric Association, 2013), this chapter uses the term *Intellectual Disability* and *Intellectual Developmental Disorder* versus the previous diagnostic category, *Mental Retardation*. In 2010, the U. S. Congress officially struck the term *Mental Retardation* from current federal laws and governmental agencies and replaced it with the term *Intellectual Disability*. The name change reflects an alignment across agencies and disciplines, including the World Health Organization, the American Association on Intellectual and Developmental Disabilities, and the U. S. Department of Education.

The American Association of Intellectual and Developmental Disabilities (AAIDD, previously called the American Association of Mental Retardation [AAMR], 2002) developed the following widely accepted definition:

> Intellectual disability is a disability characterized by significant limitations both in intellectual functioning and in adaptive behavior, which covers many everyday social and practical skills. This disability originates before the age of 18 (AAIDD, 2010).

Significant limitations in the area of adaptive behavior are identified by sub-average performance in at least two of the following: conceptual, social, and practical applied categories; communication; self-care; home living; social skills; community use; self-direction; health and safety; functional academics; leisure; and employment. Through time, there has been a movement to change the definition of intellectual disability from a person's limitations to the importance of identifying that person's needs. This newer way of thinking places the burden of responsibility on society to meet those needs (Falvey, 2005; Wehmeyer, 2013). Additionally, Marc Gold (1980), who developed the *Try Another Way* system, defined intellectual disability by noting that one should consider the following:

> The level of power needed in the training process required for the individual to learn, and not by limitations in what he or she can learn. The height of a person's level of functioning is determined by the availability of training technology and the amount of resources society is willing to allocate and not by significant limitations in biological potential (p. 5).

After Gold's (1980) work was published, the AAIDD updated their definition of intellectual disability to address the interactions between disability and the environment:

> A complete and accurate understanding of intellectual disability involves realizing that intellectual disability refers to a particular state of functioning that begins in childhood, has many dimensions, and is affected positively by individualized supports. As a model of functioning, it includes the contexts and environment within which the person functions and interacts, and requires a multidimensional and ecological approach that reflects the interaction of the individual with the environment, and the outcomes of that interaction with regards to independence, relationships, societal contributions, participation in school and community, and personal well-being (AAIDD, 2010).

Although intellectual disability is always manifested before age 18, people with intellectual disability are not a homogeneous group. The degree of developmental delay (intellectual disability) ranges from mild to moderate, from severe to profound, although the criteria for these categories continue to be debated; intelligence quotient (IQ) scores remain the primary decisive factor. A person with mild intellectual disability has an IQ score between 50-70, while an individual with moderate intellectual disability has an IQ of 35-49. An individual with severe intellectual disability has an IQ of 20-34; a person with profound intellectual disability has an IQ of below 20 and often has other accompanying physical or sensory disabilities (see Table 1).

The degree of developmental delay manifested is related to the assistance, support, and instructional opportunities available to people who have intellectual disability. These individuals possess interests and strengths that are as varied as persons without disabilities, and display equally diverse personalities and characteristics.

Prevalence of Intellectual Disability

Approximately 4.8% of the school-age population and 4.1% of post-school age populations are identified as having cognitive difficulties (U. S. Census Bureau, 2010). The variations of these percentages are expected and are usually related to the labeling and classifying procedures used in school programs (AAIDD, 2010; Brimer 1990). When intellectual disability is classified within the mild to moderate range, pre-school children and adults may not be labeled or in any way classified with cognitive delays or different

TABLE 1
Developmental Characteristics Related to Level of Intellectual Developmental Disorder (DSM-V Criteria)

Mild	Moderate	Severe	Profound
85% of all cases of intellectual disability	10% of all cases of intellectual disability	3% to 4% of all cases of intellectual disability	1% to 2% of all cases of intellectual disability
Function at one-half to two-thirds of CA (IQ: 50 to 70)	Function at one-third to one-half of CA (IQ: 35 to 49)	Function at one-fifth to one-third of CA (IQ: 20 to 34)	Function at < one-fifth of CA (IQ: < 20)
Slight delays in all areas	Noticeable delays, especially in speech	Marked and obvious delays; may walk late	Marked delays in all areas
May have no unusual physical signs	May have some unusual physical signs	Little or no communication skills, but may have some understanding of speech and show some response	Congenital abnormalities often present, hindering speech and physical growth
Can acquire practical skills	Can develop communication skills, especially with augmentative assistive devices	May be taught daily routines and repetitive but meaningful activities	Need close supervision
Useful reading and math skills up to grades 3 to 6 level; can complete most adaptive skills independently	Can learn elementary health and safety habits; can participate in simple activities and self-care	May be taught simple self-care skills	Often need attendant care
Can conform socially and develop peer relationships with support	With assistance, may learn how to respond to common social cues and basic social rules	Need direction and supervision throughout the majority of the day	May respond to regular physical activity and social stimulation
Can acquire vocational skills for self-maintenance	Can perform tasks in supported conditions	Can perform tasks in supported conditions	Not capable of self-care
Integrated into general society	Can travel alone to familiar places	Need supervision and accommodations during travel to and from places	Need supervision and accommodations during travel to and from places

Note: Additional problems with vision, hearing, speech, congenital abnormalities, seizures, emotional problems, or cerebral palsy may be present. DSM-V = *Diagnostic and Statistical Manual of Mental Disorders* (5th ed.) (American Psychiatric Association, 2013); CA = chronological age; IQ = intelligence quotient. Source: D. K. Daily, H. H. Ardinger, & G. E. Holmes (2000). Identification and evaluation of mental retardation. *American Family Physician, 61*(4).

than the general population. Traditionally, schools have grouped and classified school-age students into distinct ability levels, resulting in the labeling of students with intellectual disability. This classification explains the higher percentage identified within the school-age population.

In the past, race and economic status have been used to identify prevalence. Major litigation and legislation, however, has ruled that the identification of intellectual disability among minority groups based on racial factors is unjust and incorrect (Larry P. v. Riles and Diana v. State Board of Education, Public Law 94-142, 1975). A disproportionate number of school-age students continue to be identified with intellectual disability from certain minority groups, especially among African Americans and Hispanics or Latinos (U. S. Census Bureau, 2000). The primary method of identification has been the use of IQ tests; professionals have criticized these examinations as being culturally and linguistically biased in favor of members of the non-Hispanic White, American, middle-class. Thus, researchers consider the results of IQ tests invalid when given to children who are not members of the White middle class community (Bishop & Falvey, 1989).

Etiology of Intellectual Disability

Although up to 50% of cases of intellectual disability have no known or recognizable etiology (Daily et al., 2000), there are many known causes of the condition. When physicians rule out specific syndromes and causes, they often cite other prenatal, perinatal, and postnatal pregnancy conditions which may result in intellectual disability. Intellectual disability can occur before birth (prenatal), during birth (perinatal), or after the birth (postnatal). These causes are described in the following paragraphs.

Prenatal Causes

Down's Syndrome is the most frequently observed genetic cause. Down's Syndrome, identified in 1866 by Doctor Langdon Down, is commonly known as Trisomy XXI. Persons with Trisomy 21 have an extra 21st chromosome. Factors influencing the prevalence of Down's Syndrome include maternal age. The older the mother, particularly over age 35, the higher the possibility the baby may have Down's Syndrome. Other developmental problems, such as respiratory and heart abnormalities often accompany Down's Syndrome, and the degree of intellectual disability observed in persons with Down's Syndrome ranges from mild to significant (Campbell et al., 2013).

In 1934, Dr. Asbjourn Folling, a Norwegian physician, discovered phenylketonuria (PKU) as a cause of intellectual disability. PKU is a sign of deficiency in the production of phenylalanine hydroxylase, an enzyme necessary in the metabolism of phenylalanine, an essential amino acid. Brain damage occurs with the buildup of phenylalanine in the blood. In 1959, Dr. Robert Guthrie developed a screening test for newborns that physicians routinely use today to detect PKU. When a physician identifies PKU in a newborn, a phenylalanine-restricted diet is started. The degree of intellectual disability is significantly less severe for persons with treated versus untreated PKU; dietary restrictions during the primary years of life are essential to lessening the severity of this condition.

Other biological conditions, such as disease, can result in intellectual disability. Tay-Sachs is one such illness. This disease, a lipid metabolic disorder, is most often found in persons of Jewish descent. Besides intellectual disability, it causes a progressive deterioration of nerve tissue and generally results in death at an early age.

There are several physical factors other than genetic ones that influence the presence and severity of intellectual disability. Beginning with the prenatal stages of development, the mother's general eating habits and physical health are crucial. Chronic maternal illnesses, such as diabetes, may impair fetal development. Maternal use of alcohol, drugs, tobacco, and exposure to environmental pollution during pregnancy along with maternal infections and viruses such as rubella, perinatal cytomegalovirus infection (CMV), meningoencephalitis, syphilis, and toxoplasmosis increase the probability of intellectual disability and other disorders. Fetal exposure to radiation during development can cause genetic mutations that result in intellectual disability.

Perinatal Causes

During childbirth, several factors can increase the possibility of intellectual disability (Ainsworth & Baker, 2004). Cephalopelvic disproportion, for example, a condition in which the size of the birth canal is too narrow for the presenting infant's head, can result in brain damage to the newborn. Other factors include extreme prematurity, accidental physical trauma, asphyxia, hypoglycemia, infection, blood cell or blood type diseases, and Rh factor blood incompatibilities between mother and baby.

Postnatal Causes

Following birth, several other factors can increase the probability of intellectual disability. These include malnutrition, acquired traumatic brain injury, meningitis, encephalitis, other infections, and chemical substances (e.g., pesticides, drug abuse, and metal [lead] poisoning). Additional causes are demyelinating and degenerative disorders, consequences of seizure disorders, toxic-metabolic disorders, and environmental deprivation. Hyperthyroidism, whooping cough, chickenpox, measles, and Hip disease (a bacterial infection) may cause intellectual disability if they are not treated adequately. In children, brain injury can be caused by a blow or a violent shake to the head and result in intellectual disability.

Normalization

During the nineteenth and early part of the twentieth centuries, institutions for persons with intellectual disability were created. In the last four decades, organized coalitions of parents and the *normalization* principle played a significant role in developing community-based services as an alternative to institutionalization.

In the 1950s, parents of children with intellectual disability formed an organization called the National Association for Retarded Children (renamed the National Association for Retarded Citizens). These parents rejected institutionalization for their sons and daughters. They organized alternative programs and services for children with intellectual disability. Until the 1970s, many public schools, along with state and local rehabilitation agencies, excluded individuals with intellectual disability. The parents had to raise money independently for their children to receive community services.

Services and Support – The Principle of Normalization

In 1959, the director of the Danish Mental Retardation Service, Bank-Mikkelsen, helped develop Danish law reflecting the principle of *normalization*. This principle states that persons with intellectual disability must be able to ". . . obtain an existence as close to normal as possible" (Wolfensberger, 1980, p. 7). The first systematic statement of normalization in world literature was published by Nirje (1969). In 1972, Wolfensberger applied this normalization principle to American society. As people with intellectual disability move into the community and obtain employment and housing, a reconceptualization of service delivery models has evolved. Instead of social service agency personnel being responsible for supporting a person with intellectual disability, the individual takes charge, utilizing support from family, friends, neighbors, and co-workers.

Deinstitutionalization

The normalization principle has been a strong driving force in establishing the deinstitutionalization movement. This movement involves integrating institutionalized persons with intellectual disability into the community. Biklen and Knoll (1987) identified the major problems with institutions and other large congregate facilities, as well as the primary reasons for deinstitutionalizing people with intellectual disability:

- Institutions are the most expensive way of providing residential or any other services to people with intellectual disability.
- Institutions do not offer the warm, homelike, individualized environments necessary for full human development.
- Institutions do not provide opportunities for interaction with members of the community.

- Institutions do not allow for positive community living experiences or for development of skills needed for community life.
- Institutions perpetuate and reinforce the image that people with intellectual disability are oddities.
- People residing in institutions do not have opportunities to learn adaptive behavior from functioning non-institutionalized people.
- Institutionalized people model their behavior after other people living in the institution; these behaviors are often maladaptive.
- Institutions provide a minimum of social and recreational activities and interaction; when they do, it is often demeaning and age inappropriate.

Along with the above drawbacks, institutional living does not offer opportunities for vocational development. Typical jobs are not performed within an institutional environment, and opportunities to learn through observation are absent. Most, if not all, people living in institutions are unemployed, as few have ever had the opportunity to become employed. Discussion of work is nonexistent; normal vocational development does not occur.

Homelike Settings

As an alternative, state and local communities and parent organizations developed group homes, board and care homes, and foster homes to create homelike settings for persons with intellectual disability. These settings are less restrictive than institutional residences. During the later part of the 1980s, and with increasing success since the 1990s, people with intellectual disability began living in their own homes, with social service agency support (McConkey, Kelly, Mannan, & Craig, 2011).

Self-Advocacy

A movement toward self-advocacy or "people with disabilities asserting their sworn rights and interests, usually without others' help" developed as a result of the normalization principle (Turnbull, Turnbull, Bronicki, Summers, & Roeder-Gordon, 1989, p. 314). Two self-advocacy international networks, *People First* and *United Together*, have become increasingly influential in the areas of employment advocacy, fair working conditions, and financial compensation.

In recent years, self-advocacy also has been referred to as self-determination. Self-determination is a vital part of the education and vocational rehabilitation of persons with cognitive disabilities. Kilsby and Beyer (2002) and Heller (2012) found that enhancing self-determination in job matching increased the success of persons with cognitive disabilities. Participants in the study increased their accuracy of recalling daily experiences and demonstrated a decrease in the need for job coach assistance.

Legislation and Normalization

Rehabilitation Act of 1973

Professionals often refer to Section 504 of the 1973 Rehabilitation Act as the *civil rights* bill for individuals with disabilities. This legislation requires public and private employers, educators, and service providers to use nondiscriminatory and affirmative action practices.

Education of All Handicapped Children Act of 1975

This act and its amendments ensure a free and appropriate education in the least restrictive environment for people between the ages of 3-21. The least restrictive environment mandates education of students in the presence of their peers without disabilities and within the general education program to the *maximum extent appropriate*. Research has consistently supported maximum integration of all students in *regular* education programs (Falvey, 2005; Steere & DiPipi-Hoy, 2013).

1987 Developmental Disabilities Act

The stated goals for the 1987 Developmental Disabilities Act include:

[to] assure that persons with developmental disabilities receive the care, treatment, and other services necessary to enable them to achieve their maximum potential through increased independence, productivity, and integration into the community,

and

[to] establish and operate a system that coordinates, monitors, plans, and evaluates services which ensure the protection of the legal and human rights of persons with developmental disabilities.

Social Security Act Amendments

In 1987, Congress amended the Social Security Act to provide a work incentive program within the Supplemental Security Income (SSI) program. Before these amendments, regulations encouraged dependency. Medicare coverage (medical insurance) and financial support were removed when individuals acquired jobs. The new program allows the SSI recipient to continue to receive Medicare benefits if an employer does not provide equivalent comprehensive medical coverage. Most persons with intellectual disability qualify for SSI benefits and have been more likely to obtain employment since these changes in the Social Security Act.

Americans with Disabilities Act

In 1990, Congress passed the Americans with Disabilities Act (ADA). This act has broad implications concerning employment, transportation, public accommodations, state and local government, and telecommunications. The most significant area for persons with intellectual disability is employment. Employers may not discriminate against individuals with disabilities in hiring or promotion; they need to provide reasonable accommodation to the known physical or mental limitations of employees with disabilities, including job modification and job restructuring. All large employers with 15 or more employees need to comply. Enactment of the ADA has helped rehabilitation counselors facilitate obtaining competitive employment for their clients.

Functional Limitations

The most salient learning characteristics of persons with intellectual disability are slower rates of learning than their typical peers, and difficulty generalizing or transferring information learned from one situation to another. Though the rate of learning is slower in persons with intellectual disability, these individuals maintain the ability to learn and acquire new skills. However, they must be taught specific skills in environments in which they will perform these skills. For example, teaching public transportation skills needs to include using the public transportation system in the person's community; one needs to teach job-related skills in *real work* environments (Magnuson, 2013).

Other functional limitations include behavioral challenges, lack of self-management skills, and inappropriate social skills. Behavioral challenges can be expressed through short attention span, impulsivity, and difficulty in making judgments. Often, persons with developmental disabilities need to be directly taught self-management skills. Although persons with developmental disabilities may be sociable, they are often unaware of social pragmatics or other rules governing social behavior (Boston, Edwards, Jr., Duncan, Edwards, & Mendez, 2014; Heller et al., 2012). In the workplace, persons with intellectual disability will inevitably build interpersonal relationships with their co-workers. With limited ability to process pragmatic cues in social situations, employees with intellectual disability may inadvertently ostracize themselves.

Along with these challenges, persons with intellectual disability face another hurdle – communication. Communication impairment is often associated with intellectual disability. When designing a vocational rehabilitation program, an individual's reading ability, slower rates of information processing (especially instructions given only verbally), and slower rates of information output (vocal expression or performance) must be considered. Some individuals have limited vocal expressive skills (e.g., speech impediment, sing-song rhythm of speech, and difficulty regulating volume). For the rehabilitation professional, it is important to consider using visual tools (e.g., visual schedules and instructions) and/or augmentative adaptive communication tools.

At times, persons with intellectual disability have been characterized as no longer capable of learning or as having reached a plateau (Falvey, 1989, 1995). When an individual's learning has reached such a plateau, it may simply be an indication that different services and support are necessary (Libal, 2004). The learning possibilities and potential of persons with intellectual disability are directly dependent upon the commitment of services and support society is willing to provide, as opposed to limitations inherent in the disability itself.

Learned Helplessness

A phenomenon repeatedly observed in institutions and segregated schools, workshops, and activity centers is *learned helplessness*. This involves a pattern of submissiveness developing when individuals repeatedly discover that their actions are of no consequence and that outcomes are beyond their control (Falvey, 1989). Individuals learn to not demonstrate skill proficiency, independence, or an awareness of their surroundings. This phenomenon has a similar effect to that of the *self-fulfilling prophecy* which states that most people's opinions and expectations about themselves are influenced in significant ways by those around them. If teachers, social workers, rehabilitation counselors, and job coaches believe an individual student or client is unable to learn, that person will be discouraged from learning. If the same group of supportive professionals expect the individual to learn and be successful, the chances for a successful outcome are greatly enhanced (Falvey, 2005).

Environmental Factors

The environment plays a significant role in influencing the success and employability of individuals with intellectual disability. The traditional model provided by adult service agencies has been vocational training in a *train and place model*, such as that which occurs in a sheltered workshop. In such a situation, a client is trained in a simulated job setting and then employed. Because clients with intellectual disability do not generalize well across different settings, this model generally does not result in successful employment in integrated community jobs. The *place and train* model, a reverse method of employment, has resulted in a significantly greater number of employed clients within integrated community job settings (Moore, Flowers, & Taylor, 2000). These two models are discussed in greater detail later in this chapter.

Societal Discrimination

Over the years, society has discriminated against people with intellectual disability, primarily due to ignorance, stereotyping, and incorrect information. Until recently, most employers had no prior interaction with persons with intellectual disability (Magnuson, 2013). Much work is currently being done to change the attitudes and expectations of employers by allowing them to observe other employers who have hired individuals with intellectual disability. This observation often results in raised expectations of what a person is capable of performing and more positive attitudes. Although ignorance and discrimination in the workforce still exists, these attitudes are slowly changing.

Rehabilitation Potential

The Supported Employment Model

Research over the past several decades has influenced changes in the delivery of services. In 1972, Gold demonstrated that persons with severe intellectual disability who were deaf and blind could assemble complex electronic circuit boards. Hunter and Bellamy (1977) taught persons with profound intellectual disability to assemble harnesses. Such discoveries led to the realization that people with intellectual disability could successfully learn work skills for competitive, gainful employment. This form of employment, in which an employee receives support or assistance, is called *supported employment*. Rehabilitation counselors throughout the country are currently using the principles of supported employment. The concept and implementation of supported employment have been expanded through research and legislation (Wehman, 2012; Wehman, Revell, & Brooks, 2003).

The traditional service options available to most adults with intellectual disability before 1980 were developmental centers, work activity centers, and sheltered workshops. Professionals have criticized these settings because they generally do not provide *real* work (work in actual work environments). The purpose of sheltered work environments is to prepare people for employment in the real world. However, after a national survey was conducted by Bellamy in 1985 (Bishop & Falvey, 1989), it was concluded that too much time was spent training people for competitive employment. According to his research, people with intellectual disability spent an average of 37 years in adult developmental centers, ten years in work activity centers, and nine years in sheltered workshops. Since most persons with intellectual disability *graduate* from school at approximately age 21, a person would be, on the average, 77 years old before entering the work force. According to Bellamy, the supported employment model has been extremely successful in placing persons with severe disabilities in gainful work environments. There are several anti-habilitative characteristics of sheltered workshops that do not exist in supported employment (Falvey, 2005):

- Work performed often requires minimal learning on the part of the workers.
- Sheltered workshops often retain the best workers for more demanding work, instead of training them for non-sheltered vocational environments.
- Adequate time is not available for training workers in non-sheltered environments.
- Personnel often lack training in critical areas, such as effective teaching methods, work production, and providing real job training.
- *Down time* or *dead time* is frequent.
- Practitioners often base formal vocational evaluations on inferences, not on actual observations of clients in real community jobs.
- All the students/clients receiving training have disabilities and, therefore, there is no contact with workers without disabilities.
- Tasks vary according to the contracts secured, not according to the client's training needs.
- Equipment is often outdated and in poor condition, resulting in worthless training.
- Frequently, the workshop does not follow normal workdays or workweeks.
- Persons in workshops or activity centers do not have sufficient opportunities to build endurance.
- Workshop personnel do not develop systematic strategies to assist clients in making the transition to less restrictive work settings.
- Irrelevant exit requirements or prerequisite skill requirements are often greater than requirements in real community jobs.

Characteristics of Supported Employment

Supported employment is an alternative to sheltered workshop training. The characteristics of supported employment services are as follows:

Place and Train

This model refers to developing services that reverse the traditional method of *train and place*. *Place and train* involves placing a person on the job, regardless of job readiness and immediately training that person to perform the job. To ensure success, a job coach is available to support the person in the job (Boston et al., 2014).

Integrated Job Settings

Job settings used for training are the same as used for employees without disabilities (Wehman, 2012). Additionally, integrated job settings should not create a disproportionate number of employees with disabilities. Integrated job settings should reflect the natural proportion of persons who do not have disabilities within the community. The rehabilitation counselor needs to make every effort to encourage healthy interactions and relationships among the trainee with intellectual disability and co-workers.

Self-Determination and Individual Placements

Successful supported employment models foster self-determination by empowering employees with disabilities to make their own choices and to take control of their career paths (Boston et al., 2014; Wehman, 2012). Job placements should be based on accessibility along with, most important, the trainee's preferences and strengths.

Meaningful Work

This characteristic implies that rehabilitation counselors need to avoid providing makeshift work or otherwise made-up jobs that persons who do not have disabilities would not perform. Wehman (2012) explained that indicators of meaningful employment occurs when an employee with a disability is hired, supervised, and paid directly by the business where the job setting is located and receives wages/benefits commensurate with coworkers without disabilities.

Job Development and Marketing

This service involves systematically accessing existing jobs, modifying existing jobs, and creating new ones. Job development and marketing are essential to the delivery of supported employment and should be provided by individuals who have knowledge of the local job market and have credibility with employers (Falvey, 2005; Magnuson, 2013).

Job Coaching

Job coaching provides instruction on the job and teaches job-related skills, including social skills. In addition, job coaches provide job-related skills instruction in the client's home and community setting. These skills include preparing for work, using public transportation, depositing and budgeting paychecks, and developing social networks and friendships within the community. The job coach provides salient yet subtle instruction to allow the client to successfully develop skills while not embarrassing or discouraging the person. If the client is not performing correctly, the job coach provides additional instruction. If the individual fails to arrive for work, the job coach will act as a substitute worker and perform the necessary tasks of the absentee. Also, the job coach facilitates natural supports from co-workers and supervisors within the work environment.

Job coaches enhance rehabilitation potential by providing the support needed to access and maintain employment, housing, and other community services and activities (McConkey et al., 2011). Self-determination and autonomy are positively influenced in a supported employment model while a segregated vocational day program is generally less successful. Supported employment services across the United States and within other countries (e.g., Canada and Italy) have successfully employed millions of people with intellectual disability. Nationwide, however, individuals with mild intellectual disability are more likely to be placed in competitive supported employment than individuals with more severe levels (Boston et al., 2014). Overall, many persons have been provided with the support needed to live where they wish and with whom they want while accessing their neighborhoods and communities, while simultaneously receiving sufficient support to ensure success.

Attitudes of people in the community have changed over the years, leading to greater acceptance of their neighbors with intellectual disability (Hampton & Xiao, 2007; McConkey et al., 2011). Technology also has influenced successful integration within the community. Simple adaptations such as calculators and other technological devices, including voice synthesizers and other electronic communication aides, have greatly enhanced the participation of persons with intellectual disability.

Conclusion

This chapter provides rehabilitation counselors with an overview of the issues related to intellectual disability. The most critical concept is that the degree of participation and potential of persons with intellectual disability is dependent upon society's commitment and willingness to support people who have intellectual disability in work, housing, and within the community. The supported employment model has proven to be the most effective service delivery system. The level of fidelity of the supported employment model greatly influences the success of an individual's work experience (Bond et al., 2008).

Case Study

James is a 23 year-old African-American man who has spent the last ten years of his life in an institution. While in the institution, his day consisted of being lifted from his bed, having his clothes changed, being fed pureed foods, and sitting in front of a television set for hours. Five days a week, he attended a classroom on the institutional ground that was referred to as *school*, where he listened to pre-school level music and played games, like placing pegs into a board. There was little interaction with others, unless he was receiving directions or instructions. James never left the institution and had no friends as a result of his limited interaction with others. One day, a social worker came to his room and asked if he wanted to share an apartment with two other men in the neighboring town about ten miles away. Although James had very little reaction to anything that went on around him, he smiled and made direct eye contact with the social worker. A month later, James moved into the apartment and began to learn about living and working in the community.

This individual has multiple disabilities, including severe intellectual disability, cerebral palsy, and significant vision loss. He uses a wheelchair with the support of an attendant for transportation. The attendant assists him with basic self-care skills. After James lived within the community for a few months, the social worker referred him to a supported employment agency in the area. A job developer and job coach visited him in his apartment to begin preparation for possible employment. James used a new picture communication aid which was provided through state rehabilitation services to interact with the job developer and job coach.

The job coach and job developer spent an hour in the apartment observing James participate in various tasks with the support of his attendant. They went into the neighborhood with James to observe his reactions to various stimuli and determine potential job possibilities within the area. Two blocks away, a hardware store supervisor indicated they needed someone to sort the incoming inventory into bins and place the bins on shelves. The job developer suggested to the supervisor that he consider employing two people with developmental disabilities who have complementing strengths to do the job. Together, with the support of a job coach, they could be very successful on the job. The supervisor was reluctant because he lacked experience hiring and working with people with developmental disabilities. The job developer gave him the names, telephone numbers, and email addresses of other employers who had hired employees with developmental disabilities and encouraged him to contact them.

A week later, the hardware store supervisor contacted the job developer and stated that he would like to hire James and Rick (the other person identified in the original conversation). The supported employment agency provided a job coach to support both men.

A year later, both James and Rick were still working at the hardware store; the supervisor was very enthusiastic about their employment. With the support of a job coach, James and Rick share the job tasks of sorting and organizing the inventory of the hardware store. Additionally, they have become friends and have developed good relationships with their co-workers, both at work and away from the job. The quality of life for James has been significantly enhanced. He shows greater interest in life and his surroundings; James smiles and laughs often.

Questions

1. What are the possible causes of James' intellectual disability?
2. Identify the major problems with institutional living and the primary reasons for deinstitutionalizing people such as James.
3. Describe the advantages of supported employment over sheltered workshop employment.
4. Discuss the roles and functions of the job coach in supported employment. If James and Rick were not performing the work correctly or did not show up for work, how would the job coach proceed?
5. Outline the six characteristics of the supported employment services model.

References

Ainsworth, P., & Baker, P. C. (2004). *Understanding mental retardation: A resource for parents, caregivers, and counselors.* Jackson, MS: University Press of Mississippi.

American Association of Intellectual and Developmental Disabilities (AAIDD) (2010). *Intellectual disability: Definition, classification, and systems of support* (11th ed.). Washington, DC: Author.

American Association of Mental Retardation (AAMR). (2002). *Mental retardation: Definition, classification, and systems of support* (10th ed.). Washington, DC: Author.

American Psychiatric Association. (2013). *Diagnostic and statistical manual of mental disorders* (DSM-V) (5th ed.). Washington, DC: Author.

Biklen, D., & Knoll, J. (1987). The disabled minority. In S. Taylor, D. Biklen, & J. Knoll (Eds.), *Community integration for people with severe disabilities* (pp. 3–24). New York, NY: Teachers' College.

Bishop, K. D., & Falvey, M. A. (1989). Employment skills. In M. A. Falvey (Ed.), *Community-based curriculum: Instructional strategies for students with severe handicaps* (pp. 165–188). Baltimore, MD: Paul H. Brookes.

Bond, G. R., McHugo, G. J., Becker, D. R., Rapp, C. A., & Whitley, R. (2008). Fidelity of supported employment: Lessons learned from the National Evidence-Based Practice Project. *Psychiatric Rehabilitation Journal, 31*(4), 300–305.

Boston, Q., Edwards, Jr., D. W., Duncan, J. C., Edwards, Y. V., & Mendez, E. (2014). Supported employment. In J. D. Andrew & C. W. Faubion (Eds.), *Rehabilitation services: An introduction for the human services professional* (3rd ed., pp. 308–325). Linn Creek, MO: Aspen.

Brimer, R. W. (1990). *Students with severe disabilities: Current perspectives and practices.* Mountain View, CA: Mayfield.

Campbell, C., Landry, O., Russo, N., Flores, H., Jacques, S., & Burack, J. A. (2013). Cognitive flexibility among individuals with Down Syndrome: Addressing the influence of verbal and non verbal abilities. *American Journal on Intellectual and Developmental Disabilities, 118*(3), 193–200.

Daily, D. K., Ardinger, H. H., & Holmes, G. E. (2000). Identification and evaluation of mental retardation. *American Family Physician, 61*(4), 1059–1067.

Falvey, M. A. (Ed.). (1989). *Community-based curriculum: Instructional strategies for students with severe handicaps* (2nd ed.). Baltimore, MD: Paul H. Brookes.

Falvey, M. A. (Ed.). (1995). *Inclusive and heterogeneous schooling: Assessment, curriculum, and instruction.* Baltimore, MD: Paul H. Brookes.

Falvey, M. A. (2005). *Believe in my child with special needs.* Baltimore, MD: Paul H. Brookes.

Gold, M. W. (1980). *Try another way training manual.* Champaign, IL: U.S. Department of Education: ERIC.

Hampton, N. Z., & Xiao, F. (2007). Attitudes toward people with developmental disabilities in Chinese and American students: The role of cultural values, contact, and knowledge. *Journal of Rehabilitation, 73*(4), 23–32.

Heller, T., Arnold, C. K., van Heuman, L. McBride, E. L., & Factor, A. (2012). Self-directed support: Impact of hiring practices on adults with intellectual and developmental disability and families. *American Journal on Intellectual and Developmental Disabilities, 117*(6), 464–477.

Hunter, J., & Bellamy, G. T. (1977). Cable harness construction for severely retarded adults: A demonstration of training techniques. *American Association for the Education of Severely and Profoundly Handicapped Review, 1*(7), 2–13.

Kilsby, M. S., & Beyer, S. (2002). Enhancing self-determination in job matching in supported employment for people with learning disabilities: An intervention study. *Journal of Vocational Rehabilitation, 17*(2), 125–135.

Libal, A. (2004). *My name is not slow: Youth with mental retardation.* Broomall, PA: Mason Crest.

Locke, J. (1690). *An essay concerning human understanding* (Republished in 2006 by Adamant Media Corporation, London, England).

Magnuson, L. (2013). Families and uncertainty: Using problematic integration theory in transition services. *Journal of Applied Rehabilitation Counseling, 44*(1), 12–17.

McConkey, R., Kelly, F., Mannan, H., & Craig, S. (2011). Moving from family care to residential and supported accommodation: National, longitudinal study of people with intellectual disabilities. *American Journal on Intellectual and Developmental Disabilities, 117*(6), 305–314.

Moore, C. L., Flowers, C. R., & Taylor, D. (2000). Vocational rehabilitation services: Indicators of successful rehabilitation for persons with mental retardation. *Journal of Applied Rehabilitation Counseling, 31*(2), 36–40.

Nirje, B. (1969). The normalization principle and its management implications. In R. Kugel & W. Wolfensberger (Eds), *Changing patterns in residential services for the mentally retarded* (pp. 51–57). Washington, DC: U. S. Government Printing Office.

Rosa's Law. Pub. L. 111-256.

Steere, D., & DiPipi-Hoy, C. (2013). Coordination in transition planning: The IEP/IPE interface. *Journal of Applied Rehabilitation Counseling, 44*(1), 4–11.

Tassé, M., J., Luckasson, R., & Nygren, M. (2013). AAIDD proposed recommendations for ICD-11 and the condition previously known as mental retardation. *Intellectual and Developmental Disabilities, 51*(2), 127–131.

Turnbull, H. R., Turnbull, A. P., Bronicki, G. J., Summers, J. A., & Roeder-Gordon, C. (1989). *Disability and the family: A guide to decisions for adulthood.* Baltimore, MD: Paul H. Brookes.

United States Census Bureau. (2000). Racial and ethnic classifications used in Census 2000 and beyond. Retrieved from http://www.census.gov/population/www/socdemo/race/racefactcb.html.

United States Census Bureau. (2010). Disability among the working age population: 2008 and 2009. *American Community Survey Briefs.* U. S. Department of Commerce.

Wehman, P. (2012.). *Life beyond the classroom: Transition strategies for young people with disabilities* (5th ed.). Baltimore, MD: Paul H. Brookes.

Wehman, P., Revell, G. W., & Brooke, V. (2003). Competitive employment: Has it become the "first choice" yet? *Journal of Disability Policy Studies, 14*(3), 163–173.

Wehmeyer, M. L., Lattimore, J., Jorgensen, J. D., Palmer, S. B., Thompson, E., & Schumaker, K. M. (2003). The self-determined career development model: A pilot study. *Journal of Vocational Rehabilitation, 19*(2), 79–87.

Wehmeyer, M. L. (2013). Disability, disorder, and identity. *Intellectual and Developmental Disabilities, 51*(2), 122–126.

Wolfensberger, W. (1980). A brief overview of the principle of normalization. In R. J. Flynn & K. E. Kitsch (Eds.), *Normalization, social integration, and community services* (pp. 7–30). Baltimore, MD: University Park.

About the Authors

Julie Ton, Ph.D., BCBA-D., is an Autism and Behavior Program Specialist with Downey Unified School District in Downey, California. She has worked in several capacities in the field of developmental disabilities, in particular as a behavior analyst, special education teacher, teacher trainer, and research team coordinator.

Mary A. Falvey, Ph.D., is Professor of Special Education and the former Dean of the Charter College of Education at California State University, Los Angeles. She has authored several books on community-based intervention and inclusive education, and has consulted with school districts throughout the country.

Kathryn D. Bishop, Ph.D., is Professor of Special Education at the University of San Diego in San Diego, California. She has worked in the area of supported employment as a direct service provider and national trainer. Dr. Bishop also provides consultation in the area of inclusive education issues.

Susann Terry Gage, Ph.D., is a graduate of the Joint Doctoral Program at California State University, Los Angeles and the University of California, Los Angeles. Currently, Dr. Gage is the Special Education Coordinator in Sedona, Arizona.

Chapter 27

AUTISM SPECTRUM DISORDER

Frances W. Siu, Ph.D., C.R.C.
Jessica H. Franco, Ph.D., CCC-SLP, BCBA-D

Introduction

Autism spectrum disorder (ASD) is a group of neurodevelopmental disorders characterized by impairment of social reciprocity, such as limitations in social motivation and emotional recognition. In addition, deficiencies in communication and restricted behaviors like repetitive behaviors (e.g., finger flicking, hand flapping), limited interests, and rituals or stereotypes are typically present. First identification or diagnosis usually occurs between the ages of two and four (American Psychiatric Association [APA], 2013). Approximately, one in 68 children has been diagnosed with an autism spectrum disorder in the United States, while close to 1% of the world population has ASD (Centers for Disease Control and Prevention [CDC], 2014). In 2005, the average annual medical cost for a Medicaid-enrolled child with an ASD was $10,710, six times higher than the medical costs for a child without ASD ($1,810) (Autism Speaks, 2013). In addition, intensive behavioral interventions for each child with ASD cost $40,000 to $60,000 per year. According to the *Diagnostic and Statistical Manual of Mental Disorders*, 5th Edition (DSM-5), ASD covers a group of disorders previously known as *early infantile autism, childhood autism, Kanner's autism, high-functioning autism, atypical autism, pervasive developmental disorder not otherwise specified, childhood disintegrative disorder, and Asperger's disorder.* The *spectrum* of ASD refers to the wide variation of manifestations contingent upon the severity of the autistic condition, developmental level, and chronological age (APA, 2013).

The following sections will focus on (a) etiology, (b) characteristics of ASD, (c) prevalence and incidence, (d) diagnosis, (e) treatment, and (f) rehabilitation potential.

Etiology

According to the *DSM-5* (APA, 2013), there is strong evidence from twin concordance studies that heritability rates for ASD range from 37% to 90%. As many as 15% of the current ASD cases seem to be associated with a known genetic mutation. However, genetic factors alone are very unlikely to be the only factor involved in the development of this disorder. Along with genetic factors, environmental factors are involved and interact with ASD susceptibility genes. For example, the womb is an environment for a fetus; prenatal and perinatal factors such as maternal nutrition, maternal infections, and premature birth contribute to the increase of risk factors beyond genetic mutation.

Many suggestions have been made concerning other possible causes, including diet, environmental pollutants, antibiotics, allergies, mumps/measles/rubella (MMR) vaccines, and traces of neurotoxins, such as mercury in preservatives. None has been scientifically validated. With the MMR vaccine, there were public concerns that the vaccine was responsible for the observed increase in autistic conditions (Wakefield & Montgomery, 2000). After years of research, scientists have concluded that vaccines do not cause autism (CDC, 2014).

Characteristics

ASD is a lifelong condition. Characteristics vary greatly and are unique to each individual. Common signs and symptoms reported are impaired social interaction skills, avoidance of eye contact, rigid adherence to daily routines, unusual or obsessive behaviors and unusual interests, and high sensitivity or under responsiveness to light, touch, and sound (CDC, 2014). The life course of individuals with ASDs varies; some individuals lose skills over time, others reach a plateau in adolescence, while some display patterns of continued development into adulthood (LeBlanc, Riley, & Goldsmith, 2008).

Developmental changes during adolescence and adulthood may resemble changes in key ASD symptoms. The core symptoms of autism often decrease during adolescence and young adulthood, particularly for individuals without intellectual disabilities. As a result, children who have been diagnosed with ASD in childhood may lose this label by the time they reach adulthood. For example, Seltzer, Shattuck, Abbeduto, and Greenberg (2004) found that out of a group of adults who met criteria for ASD diagnosis in childhood, only 55% meet the criteria for autism in adulthood. Language skills were found to be the most improved, while friendship development had the least symptom improvement in adults.

Some persons experience improvements that are limited to certain core features of ASD with variable timing of improvements across behaviors. Shattuck et al. (2007) found that adult participants had fewer maladaptive behaviors (i.e., self-injury, noncompliance, aggression) and experienced more improvement in these behaviors over time when compared to adolescents.

Social Interaction

Individuals with ASD, especially adults with autistic disorder, may be eccentric intellectuals who speak their minds and make insensitive remarks in social situations. Some adults with autistic disorder have delayed use and understanding of speech (Shea & Mesibov, 2005). These individuals tend to have long-standing difficulties in non-verbal expressions, avoid mutual gaze, lack gestures, and have diminished facial expressions. They may misunderstand the reactions of others and lack empathy (Tantam, 2000). People with ASD prefer solitary activities and lack spontaneous desire to share enjoyment, interests, and achievements with others.

Similarly, individuals with high functioning ASD exhibit problems with social interactions. Some isolate themselves from others, taking refuge in a world of idiosyncratic interests, routines, and private preoccupations. For those who cope in this way, close friendships and sexual relationships hold little attraction (Autism Speaks, 2013). Other people with high functioning ASD, formerly known as Asperger's syndrome, have a desire for closeness, and may succeed in making friendships with people of their own gender, but encounter social interaction difficulties (Tantam, 2000).

Generally, even when persons with ASDs develop friendships, there is often more reported loneliness compared to their typically developing counterparts. Although high-functioning individuals are more likely to report having friendships than those with less developed skills, their relationships often focus on common restricted interests rather than social interactions. Besides a low prevalence of friendships, there is minimal presence of participation in social and recreational activities. Also, there is little planning or direction about the future, and a reluctance to accept responsibility (LeBlanc et al., 2008).

Victimization

Throughout their lives, people with ASD are at risk for victimization. For adolescents with ASD, gang attacks, bullying, and peer victimization is common, while robbery is linked with adulthood. Adolescents are at a high risk for emotional bullying by siblings and peers (LeBlanc et al., 2008).

People with ASD who have experienced victimization may ruminate about the trauma for many years; this may lead to oversensitivity to slights, which can accelerate to aggression and lead to social avoidance (Autism Speaks, 2013). When antisocial and conduct problems are part of the repertoire of a person with high functioning ASD, it negatively impacts interactions with his or her environment. A serious offense may lead to long term hospital care or even incarceration.

Work-Related Problems

Individuals with ASD have difficulty with work-related activities and employment (Fleisher, 2006). For example, these individual resist changes in daily routines and take prolonged periods of time to adjust after a long holiday, or refuse adaptation to a new or unfamiliar environment. Adolescents with high functioning ASD are likely to have increasingly conspicuous difficulties with planning and organizational skills, as well as completing assignments in time (Johnson, 2005). Although not due to deterioration in intellectual abilities, there may be a decline in work outcomes. They often become exasperated by stress and change.

Health Problems

As children progress toward adolescence, there is a high likelihood of developing various health problems that co-occur with ASD (Odom, Horner, Snell, & Blacher, 2007). Difficulties with social tasks can continue throughout life and be a constant source of distress. Individuals with ASD exhibit many behavioral difficulties including hyperactivity, attention problems, obsessive-compulsive phenomena, self-injury, tics, and affective symptoms. Problems with impulse control, disorganized behavior, aggression, and disruptions are prevalent (LeBlanc et al., 2008).

Generalized anxiety and depression are more common in high-functioning ASD groups than in individuals of the same age, and typically continue to worsen throughout adolescence and into adulthood (Tantam, 2000). Anxiety disorders are common expressions of distress; long-standing anxiety may lead to depression and substance misuse. Depression may cause increased social withdrawal and self-neglect, leading to social breakdowns (Kim, Szatmari, Bryson, Streiner, & Wilson, 2000).

Generally, causes of emotional disorder are due to (a) vulnerability of affective disorder (e.g., high *trait* anxiety), (b) family tension or breakdown, (c) higher than usual rate of adverse life events, (d) victimization, (e) awareness of difference, (f) over-sensitivity to slight ruminations about past injustice, and (g) broken relationships (Ghaziuddin, Weldmer-Mikhail, & Ghaziuddin, 1998).

Sexuality

Individuals with ASD have less sexual knowledge and experience than their peers. Sexual knowledge is positively correlated with cognitive functioning. Consequently, those with higher cognitive impairments display more inappropriate sexual behaviors, engage in fewer privacy-seeking behaviors, and have less sex education than typically developing peers. Of particular concern is the likelihood that interests on the part of greater functioning individuals might be misinterpreted as threatening or predatory behavior (Stokes, Newton, & Kaur, 2007).

As a result, only a small proportion of individuals with ASD develop intimate relationships in adolescence or adulthood (Mehzabin & Stokes, 2011). As mentioned, the centrality of social impairments in ASD may cause difficulties in initiating and maintaining relationships, making them challenging or unappealing for potential partners. Sexual relationships are more difficult to achieve and many find their self-esteem further eroded by rejections. Sometimes, when relationships do develop, it is on the basis of exploitation of the person with Asperger syndrome, and the effect is undermining rather than rewarding (Jordan, 2013).

Prevalence and Incidence

As noted, about one in 68 children in the United States has been identified with an ASD according to estimates from the CDC Autism and Developmental Disabilities Monitoring Network in 2008 (CDC, 2014); this is a significant rise from one in 150 children in 2000. ASD is five times more prevalent among males than females, and occurs in all racial/ethnic groups and socioeconomic levels.

Possible reasons for the increase in prevalence and incidence include: (a) changes in diagnostic criteria; (b) variations in methods used in research studies; (c) increased awareness among professionals, parents, and the general public of the existence of autistic spectrum disorders; (d) the growth of specialist services; (e) probable causes and relation to age of onset; (f) the association of autism conditions with intellectual disability, other developmental or physical disorders, besides psychiatric disorders of any type; and (g) true increase in these population (APA, 2013; Nebel-Schwalm & Matson, 2008). Nevertheless, most, if not all, of the reported rise in prevalence and incidence is because of changes in diagnostic criteria and greater awareness among professionals and parents.

Diagnosis

Diagnosis for ASD is composed of standardized behavioral diagnostic and clinical observation measures, questionnaires, caregiver interviews, and self-reports, when appropriate. A diagnosis can be made by many different professionals, including developmental pediatricians, neurologists, psychologists, and speech-language pathologists. According to the *DSM-5* (APA, 2013), ASD should be considered only when all four diagnostic criteria are met.

Criterion A: Persistent impairment in social interaction and social communication.

Criterion B: Restricted and repetitive patterns of odd behavior, interests, and activities.

Criterion C: Signs and indicators must surface during early developmental stages.

Criterion D: Symptoms must cause clinically significant impairment in daily functioning (APA, 2013).

In clinical recording for ASD, severities are recorded as the level of support needed for each of the two psychopathological domains: (a) social communication and (b) restricted repetitive behaviors. Severity levels include Level 1: Requiring support; Level 2: Requiring substantial support; and Level 3: Requiring very substantial support (APA, 2013).

Comorbidity

It is not unusual for someone with ASD to be diagnosed with a known medical condition, a genetic condition, an environment factor, or with another neurodevelopmental, mental, intellectual, or behavioral disorder. For example, approximately 50% of children with ASD have at least one of the three co-occurring conditions: attention-deficit/hyperactivity disorder, intellectual disability, or epilepsy. Psychiatric disorders, especially social anxiety disorder and oppositional defiant disorder, are common and frequently co-occur in these children (Jordan, 2013).

Functional Limitations

Table 1 presents a summary of functional limitations of individuals with ASD.

Treatment

Autism is a lifetime condition that, to a vast degree, is controlled with proper care and attention (Fleisher, 2006). In general, individualized and intensive behavioral interventions are used to help individuals with ASD, especially during childhood. The goals of intervention are to (a) optimize the functional independence of the individual by minimizing the symptoms; (b) facilitate development and learning, including social skills of the individual; (c) reduce restricted interests and stereotypical behavior; and (d) eliminate the person's maladaptive behavior. A good plan of treatment is needed for each individual (APA, 2013).

Rehabilitation Potential

Social Skills

Individuals with ASD experience countless challenges in daily living. People with high-functioning ASD often learn the social rules and skills, but do not apply them in social situations. They frequently lack the ability to recognize social cues, understand reciprocal conversation, and use humor appropriately. Social skills are a prominent part of employment success. While employers place great importance on functional aspects of a job, socialization and integration in the workplace also are crucial. As a result, social impairment

TABLE 1
Summary of Functional Limitations of Adolescents and Adults with ASD

Areas	Limitations
Cognitive	• Difficulty with planning and organizational skills • May be eccentric intellectuals who speak their minds
Social/sexual	• Insensitivity • Limited nonverbal skills • Difficulty forming friendships • Delayed use and understanding of speech • Conversations limited to their topics of interest • Low participation in social and recreational activities • Steer away from romantic relationships • Changes in nature of friendship, body shape, and so forth • Social/sexual problems may cause depression and anger • Suffer victimization of different types
Behavior	• Impulsive, disorganized, and disruptive behavior; aggression • Hyperactivity and attention problems • Engage in self-injury • Low empathy • Adherence to rituals
Health problems	• Mood disorders • Depression, generalized anxiety disorders, obsessive compulsive disorders, conduct disorders • Use of illegal substances to cope with daily challenges
Employment	• Inflexibility • Difficulty adapting to new environments • Trouble completing assignments • Interest in only a few types of activities • May not discern the reason for rejection at job interviews • Seldom plan for the future • Hesitant to take up adult responsibilities

of individuals with ASD causes difficulties in employment and job retention. For those qualified individuals in the workplace, employment levels and occupational statuses are typically low; often they are underemployed. As a great majority of this population remains highly dependent, family members are habitually involved in job seeking, while providing other supports (Hiller, Fish, Clopper, & Beversdorf, 2007).

The majority of adults with ASD need lifelong care such as ongoing supervision, work and self-care training, and reinforcement of skills. The public school (K-12) systems provide these services, which terminate when the person exceeds school age. In some cases, adults with ASD continue to live at home, provided that necessary support, such as constant supervision, is available. Otherwise, a variety of residential care facilities in both the private and public sectors providing 24-hour care can be used. Private for-profit residential care facilities are increasing. Unlike many of the older institutions, facilities today view residents as people with human needs, and offer opportunities for recreation and simple but meaningful work. Unfortunately, some facilities are still separating people with autism from the rest of the world.

People with severe or profound autism may work in sheltered workshops or other placements with high levels of support and structured work requirements. Individuals with mild or moderate autism are often successful with supported employment. People with ASD working in an environment utilizing a supported employment model were found to achieve significantly more than those in a non-supported employment (Wehman et al., 2012). Supported employment as an approach to hiring and retaining people with developmental disabilities has a mission to provide stable and predictable work environments where individuals with ASD can become contributing members of the productive workforce. A job coach or employment specialist is usually hired to provide individualized training for the *supported employee* (Villamisar & Huges, 2006). The chapter on intellectual developmental disabilities provides a discussion on supported employment.

Work is a significant aspect of life. Having employment is a source of pride and accomplishment in American society. People with high-functioning ASD have many positive qualities to offer employers. Typically, they are punctual, detail-oriented, appreciate routine and repetitive work, and become loyal employees. However, overshadowing difficulties such as employment issues associated with social skills, problem solving, and on-the-job bullying may mask their positive qualities (Wehman, Targett, & Young, 2007). These difficulties bring the individual with ASD to the attention of rehabilitation professionals.

Job advancement is often a slow, challenging process. Job loss is more common than job advancement. Often, the reason for being terminated is poorly understood by the person with autism (Wehman et al., 2012). Reasons that individuals usually understand, such as harassing coworkers of the opposite sex, could mean nothing to someone with ASD. Finding new jobs becomes increasingly difficult with each job loss, as periods of unemployment have to be explained to prospective employers. When helping a person select training and educational programs, rehabilitation counselors need to be particularly cautious. It is a disservice when individuals with ASD enter programs that do not facilitate employment (Paxton & Estay, 2007).

Basic employment and adaptive skills are often lacking among individuals with ASD. For example, handling of feedback, incorporating requested changes in performance, and adapting to new job routines are challenging. Vocational-related social skills that are crucial for an individual with ASD to learn include: organization of tasks, transitioning, task completion, asking for help, and social greetings/salutations.

Individuals with ASD need to be individually educated and assisted. Besides on-the-job-training, structured teaching with written expectations of job responsibilities and in-depth work procedures are vital to overall success. At the workplace, employees with ASD need to know whom to go to for help (Wehman et al., 2007). Specific training strategies found to be effective in training these individuals include: (1) the use of cognitive aids, particularly technology, to assist with organization and planning, (2) clear differential reinforcement contingencies to provide motivation for task completion and accuracy, and (3) corrective feedback that is specific and multifaceted (Palmen, Didden, & Lang, 2012). The use of aids such as written schedules, checklists, as well as a focus on teaching self-monitoring, have been effective in supporting people with ASD (Rao & Gagie, 2006; Southall & Gast, 2011).

Disclosure

Counselors must assess the potential ramifications of disclosure or non-disclosure with their clients. Younger workers are more likely to disclose their disabilities. Recent support in the education system has taught young employees with ASD to maximize their strengths and ask for accommodation. They frequently have the support of career planning and have greater access to governmental supports than their predecessors. Early intervention has resulted in higher self-esteem among those individuals who have entered the work force in recent years. ASD in high functioning people is *usually invisible*. Many think of low functioning or nonverbal individuals when they hear of autism and do not believe that a high functioning person can have ASD. Although only 10% of people with ASD are considered savants (a rare condition in which persons with developmental disorders have one or more areas of expertise, ability, or brilliance which are in contrast with their overall limitations), many people on the autism spectrum are extremely intelligent and excel in art, math, music, and visual skills (Autism Speaks, 2013). Nonetheless, decision-making on disclosure of disability needs to be individualized.

Conclusion

Each individual living with ASD has his or her unique strengths and weaknesses. Some may be of average to below-average intelligence, while others are above average. Despite the common beliefs and media portrayals of the ingenious abilities of people with ASD, only 10% of the population with ASD have been tested and are considered to be savants. Academic and training goals and objectives need to be tailored to each person's intellectual capability and level of functioning. With the proper services and supports, people with autism can live full, healthy, and meaningful lives.

Case Study

Jorge Garcia is a 19-year old, high school student who has autism; he is in your assigned Transitional Partnership Program (TPP). As long as he follows his routines and is well-informed of possible changes, Jorge is a good student who performs well in school; he enjoys the challenge of video games. Recently, Jorge's mother called and conveyed concerns about her son because he became totally absorbed in computer games and often stayed up all night playing video games. His homeroom teacher informed Mrs. Garcia that Jorge has stopped turning in his homework assignments. When asked, Jorge mumbled without giving any response.

Recently, Jorge has stopped accepting and returning telephone calls from his only friend and is reluctant to go to school. Frequently, he withdraws into his room after school, refusing to come out even for meals. Last night, Jorge expressed no interest in living. Jorge's file indicates a sudden decline in academic performance, along with frequent absences from class during the past six months.

Knowing the urgency of Jorge's situation, you, as his TPP rehabilitation counselor, made a home visit. While you were at the Garcia's residence, Jorge did not respond to his mother's call to come to the living room. You entered his bedroom where he was playing a video game. When he eventually looked up, his eyes were blood-shot and he seemed to have neglected personal hygiene. Jorge reported failing most of his classes. When asked why, he ignored the question and disclosed he recently was terminated from his part-time job at a fast-food restaurant for a reason that he could not understand.

Jorge's job responsibilities included cleaning tables, taking out trash, refilling condiments, and assisting in the kitchen. This was Jorge's first job and he had been working at the restaurant twice a week for the past year and a half. The store manager who has been there since Jorge started the job, recently left the company. Jorge commented that *people are evil* before putting himself in a rocking position. As he covered his head with his hands, you saw both new and older bruise marks on his forearms.

Questions

1. Provide a vocational profile for Jorge. Identify additional information you need to best help this client from a multidisciplinary approach and discuss how you will obtain the information.
2. Besides ASD, do you suspect any additional disorders that Jorge might have? Explain.
3. Has *abuse* crossed your mind? If yes, what are the steps to properly handle the situation?
4. Would a career in computer technology be realistic for this client? Discuss.
5. What services will help Jorge get back on track? Describe these possible services and the potential benefits for Jorge.

References

American Psychiatric Association (APA). (2013). *Diagnostic and statistical manual of mental disorders: DSM-5* (5th ed.). Washington, DC: Author.

Autism Speaks. (2013). *What is Autism?* Retrieved from http://www.autismspeaks.org/what-autism.

Centers for Disease Control and Prevention (CDC). (2014). *Autism spectrum disorders (ASDs): Data and statistics*. Retrieved from http://www.cdc.gov/ncbddd/autism/data.html

Fleisher, M. (2006). *Survival strategies for people on the autism spectrum*. London, England: Jessica Kinsley.

Ghaziuddin, M., Weldmer-Mikhail, E., & Ghaziuddin, N. (1998). Comorbidity of Asperger syndrome: A preliminary report. *Journal of Intellectual Disability Research, 42*, 279–283.

Hiller, A., Fish, T., Clopper, P., & Beversdorf, D. Q. (2007). Outcome of a social and vocational skills support group for adolescents and young adults on the autism spectrum. *Focus on Autism and Other Developmental Disabilities, 22*(2), 107–115.

Johnson, M. (2005). *Managing with Asperger syndrome*. London, England: Jessica Kinsley.

Jordan, R. (2013). *Autistic spectrum disorders: An introductory handbook for practitioners*. Oxon, England: David Fulton.

Kim, J. A., Szatmari, P., Bryson, S. E., Streiner, D. L., & Wilson, F. J. (2000). The prevalence of anxiety and mood problems among children with autism and Asperger syndrome. *Autism, 4*, 117–132.

LeBlanc, L. A., Riley, A. R., & Goldsmith, T. R. (2008). Autism spectrum disorders: A lifespan perspective. In J. Matson (Ed.), *Clinical assessment and intervention for autism spectrum disorders* (pp. 65–87). Burlington, MA: Elsevier.

Mehzabin, P., & Stokes, M. (2011). Self-assessed sexuality in young adults with high-functioning autism. *Research in Autism Spectrum Disorders, 5*(1), 614–621.

Nebel-Schwalm, M. S., & Matson, J. L. (2008). Differential diagnosis. In J. Matson (Ed.), *Clinical assessment and intervention for autism spectrum disorders* (pp. 91–129). Burlington, MA: Elsevier.

Odom, S. L., Horner, R. H., Snell, M. E., & Blacher, J. (2007). *Handbook of developmental disorders*. New York, NY: Guilford.

Palmen, A., Didden, R., & Russell, L. (2012). A systematic review of behavioral intervention research on adaptive skill building in high-functioning young adults with autism spectrum disorder. *Research in Autism Spectrum Disorders, 6*(2), 602–617.

Paxton K., & Estay, I. A. (2007). *Counseling people on the autism spectrum: A practical manual*. London, England: Jessica Kinsley.

Rao, S. M., & Gagie, B. (2006). Learning through seeing and doing: Visual supports for children with autism. *Teaching Exceptional Children, 38*(6), 26–33.

Seltzer, M. M., Shattuck, P., Abbeduto, L., & Greenberg, J. S. (2004). Trajectory of development in adolescents and adults with autism. *Mental Retardation and Developmental Disabilities Research Reviews, 10*, 234–247.

Shattuck, P., Seltzer, M. M., Greenberg, J. S., Orsmond, G. I., Bolt, D., Kring, S., & Lord, C. (2007). Change in autism symptoms and maladaptive behaviors in adolescents and adults with an autism spectrum disorder. *Journal of Autism and Developmental Disorders, 37*, 1735–1747.

Shea, V., & Mesibov. G. B. (2005). Adolescents and adults with autism. In F. R. Volkmar, R. Paul, A. Klin, & D. J. Cohen (Eds.), *Handbook of autism and pervasive developmental disorders, assessment, interventions, and policy* (3rd ed., pp. 288–311). Hoboken, NJ: John Wiley & Sons.

Southall, C. M., & Gast, D. L. (2011). Self-management procedures: A comparison across the autism spectrum. *Education and Training in Autism and Developmental Disabilities, 46*(2), 155–171.

Stokes, M., Newton, N., & Kaur, A. (2007). Stalking and social and romantic functioning among adolescents and adults with autism spectrum disorders. *Journal of Autism and Developmental Disorders, 37*, 1969–1986.

Tantam, D. (2000). Psychological disorders in adolescents and adults with Asperger syndrome. *Autism, 4*(1), 47–62.

Villamisar, D. G., & Huges, C. (2006). Supported employment improves cognitive performance in adults with autism. *Journal of Intellectual Disability Research, 51*(2), 142–150.

Wakefield, A. J., & Montgomery, S. (2000). Measles mumps rubella vaccine: Through a glass darkly. *Adverse Drug Reactions Toxicol Reviews, 19*, 265–283.

Wehman, P. Lau, S., Molinelli, A., Brookes, V., Thompson, K., Moore, C., & West, M. (2012). Supported employment for young adults with autism spectrum disorder: Preliminary data. *Research and People with Severe Disabilities, 37*(3), 160–169.

Wehman, P., Targett, P., & Young, C. (2007). Off to work for an individual with autism: A supported approach. *Autism Advocate, 46*(1), 54–57.

About the Authors

Frances W. Siu, Ph.D., C.R.C., is an Assistant Professor and Coordinator of the undergraduate Rehabilitation Services Program at California State University, Los Angeles (CSULA). She received her Ph.D. in Special Education and Counseling, option in Rehabilitation Counselor Education, from the University of Texas at Austin, her M.S. in rehabilitation counseling and B.S. in psychology, both from CSULA. Research interests of Dr. Siu include medical aspects of disability, multicultural issues, and violence against people with disabilities. She has published over 20 articles and book chapters, and given over 50 professional presentations on violence against people with disabilities, rehabilitation education, and rehabilitation services.

Jessica H. Franco, Ph.D., CCC-SLP, BCBA-D, is a Clinical Assistant Professor in the Department of Communication Sciences and Disorders at the University of Texas at Austin. Dr. Franco has focused her clinical practice and research on assessment and treatment of children with autism spectrum disorders (ASD). She has experience with a variety of evidenced-based approaches for teaching communication skills and methods for reducing severe challenging behaviors. Dr. Franco was the founding Executive Director of Autism Community Network (ACN) in San Antonio, Texas. In addition to remaining active on the ACN board, she is involved in many other autism-related committees and boards, including the Texas Autism Resource and Research Center, Texas Autism Council Advisory Task Force, and Autism Speaks U Longhorn Chapter.

Chapter 28

ORTHOTICS, AMPUTATION, AND PROSTHETICS

Lance R. Clawson, B.S., C.P.O.
Martin G. Brodwin, Ph.D., C.R.C.

Introduction

The fields of orthotics and prosthetics are unique disciplines in the health science field. Orthoses (orthotics), commonly referred to as braces, are devices designed to support, stabilize, and assist compromised segments of the body. Prostheses (prosthetics), most often referred to as artificial limbs, are devices designed to replace the function of missing segments of the body. Amputation involves the loss of all or a portion of a body part; a prothesis is an artificial replacement of that missing part of the body.

Professionals providing braces (orthoses) and artificial limbs (prostheses) are referred to as orthotists and prosthetists. Upon receipt of a prescription from a physician, the orthotist or prosthetist is responsible for evaluating the patient's needs and then designing, fabricating, and fitting a device to meet the prescription criteria that will restore the weak or missing function or part to the greatest extent possible.

This chapter is divided into five sections. Section one briefly describes the history of orthotics and prosthetics. The second, orthotics, discusses lower and upper extremity orthotics, spinal orthotics, other assistive devices, as well as physical and psychological limitations. Amputation, the third section, includes levels of amputation, complications, psychological issues, family involvement, and employment. Section four explores prosthetics and covers treatment, types of lower and upper extremity prostheses, and Medicare Functional Levels. Assistive technology, the workplace, and a case study conclude this chapter.

History of Orthotics and Prosthetics

The study of orthotics began as blacksmiths designing armour. As warriors were injured creating weak, damaged, or missing parts of the body, the blacksmith/armourer would change the design of the armour to accommodate the injured portion of the body while still allowing the soldier to function. This continued to evolve into the ancient art of splint and brace making. Bonesetters and brace makers eventually developed into what we now call orthopedic surgeons and orthotists (Kirkup, 2010). The study of prosthetics has been closely associated with amputation surgery performed as a lifesaving measure from the aftermath of war. Injured soldiers who returned home from battle with traumatic amputations utilized primitive wooden prostheses. Each major war has been a stimulus for the improvement of amputation surgical techniques, and for the development of improved prostheses (May & Lockard, 2011). This continues to be true today with a great deal of money spent by the Department of Defense for specialty projects, once again just like in ancient times with the intent to return warriors to battle.

It was not until the twentieth century when the most significant contributions to prosthetic/orthotic sciences were made; these contributions were stimulated by the aftermath of the first and second world wars and the polio epidemics of the late 1940s and early 1950s. Injured veterans who acquired musculoskeletal and neuromuscular impairments or traumatic amputation and polio survivors with diminished neuromuscular function increased the demand for orthotic and prosthetic services. To improve the quality and performance of assistive devices at the end of World War II, particularly for veterans with amputations, the United States government sponsored a series of research and development projects under the auspices of the National Academy of Sciences that would forever change the manner in which orthotics and prosthetics would be performed (Fishman, 2001).

In the early 1960s, the National Academy of Sciences National Research Council began to promote multidisciplinary scientific research efforts into human locomotion, biomechanics, and the development of new materials and devices (Lusardi, Jorge, & Nielsen, 2012). By the 1980s, the continuing introduction of new materials and methods spurred the profession of prosthetics and orthotics to rapidly evolve as a changing discipline. The 1990s saw significant advances in development of educational programs with the establishment of national education accreditation through a subsection of the American Medical Association (Fishman, 2001). Today, prosthetics and orthotics has developed into a burgeoning multifaceted profession. Continued technological advancements in engineering and medicine have led to advanced prosthetics technology including lighter, more intimately fitting and computer-assisted prostheses.

Orthotics

Each year, thousands of individuals in this country are affected by injuries and diseases that result in failed or weakened parts of the body. A person who has a fractured finger may see a physician who tapes the finger to a tongue depressor; by definition, this splint constitutes a simple orthosis. Physicians, hospitals, and therapists provide many simple orthoses. Other types of simple braces are found at local pharmacies and sporting goods stores. When a simple support is not sufficient and the physician believes a more complex device is needed, he or she prescribes an orthosis and directs the patient to an orthotist.

Orthoses (orthotic devices) are divided into four categories: lower extremity, upper extremity, spinal, and other assistive devices. These are further divided into the categories of acute, chronic, and assistive orthoses. Orthoses are named after the joint areas of the body the particular orthosis stabilizes or affects (see Table 1). A simple brace for the foot and ankle is referred to as an AFO (ankle-foot orthosis); one for the hand and wrist is called a WHO (wrist-hand orthosis). In the prescription for the orthosis, the physician indicates the type of motion to be limited, stabilized, or assisted, and the purpose of the device or goal to be achieved (e.g., greater strength, improved range of motion) (Lusardi et al., 2012).

TABLE 1
Categories of Orthoses

Ankle-Foot Orthosis	AFO
Knee-Ankle-Foot Orthosis	KAFO
Hip-Knee-Ankle-Foot Orthosis	HKAFO
Wrist-Hand Orthosis	WHO
Wrist-Driven Wrist-Hand Orthosis	WDWHO
Shoulder-Elbow Orthosis	SEO
Lumbosacral Orthosis	LSO
Thoraco-Lumbo-Sacral Orthosis	TLSO
Cervico-Thoraco-Lumbo-Sacral Orthosis	CTLSO

External Powered Orthoses

During the last several years, external powered orthoses have become a regular part of the treatment scheme in protocol management of lower and upper extremity weakness, often in conjunction with the management of tone. Bioness and Walk-Aid are two systems that utilize a superficial electrical stimulus to cause muscular contracture at or about the time that the stimulated muscle should function. An interface, much like the leads used for an EKG or EEG, is placed over the muscle and connected to the stimulus system. The intent of this system is to allow an existing muscle within the body to perform its appropriate function, despite there being some defect in the body's ability to transmit stimuli through the normal neural pathways. Stroke, peripheral nerve injuries, traumatic brain injury, and many other conditions have the potential for benefit from these externally powered devices.

Externally powered orthoses, like their non-powered counterparts, improve/restore function, protect the affected part of the body, and contribute to the notion of neuroplasticization. Neuroplasticity also known as *brain plasticity*, refers to changes in neural pathways and synapses which are due to changes in behavior, environment, and neural processes, as well as changes resulting from bodily injury (Pascual-Leones et al., 2011).

Lower Extremity Orthoses

Following the acute episode of a stroke, the physician may prescribe a static or functional (dynamic) AFO (ankle-foot orthosis) or KAFO (knee-ankle-foot orthosis). The ankle-foot orthosis supports lower extremities that have instability in the ankle and foot. This orthosis can be designed to simply compensate for paralytic dropfoot, preventing the foot from dragging during the swing phase of gait and to control the rate at which the forefoot contacts the ground. If more stability is needed, the AFO has a rigid ankle (at 90 degrees), thereby preventing the tibia and knee from collapsing forward in mid to late stance during walking. The same device may be designed with movement, such as with an articulating joint. If the knee also has significant weakness or instability, the orthosis may span another joint (the knee) proximally, becoming a KAFO.

Upper Extremity Orthoses

The arm, hand, and fingers are significantly more complicated to design and fit with orthotic devices than the lower extremities. Sensation, dexterity, and function of the fingers and hand are crucial to activities of daily living and independence. Similar to the lower extremity, the hand and arm may be fit with a static or functional orthosis; a static orthosis is designed to maintain as functional a position as possible. With patients who have had stroke, there is typically less return of function in the upper extremity, and what motion does return is less than the return in the lower extremity. When muscle function begins to return, both static and functional devices are used and continually modified as the muscles slowly regain improved or normal function.

A person with quadriplegia (paralysis involving the four extremities), injured at the C-6 (sixth cervical) level, loses an ability to close the hands. This loss of pinch and grasp is accommodated by use of a wrist driven wrist-hand orthosis (Lusardi et al., 2012). Specialized upper extremity orthotic devices, such as the wrist-driven wrist-hand orthosis (WDWHO), are used for specific levels of quadriplegia. With training from an experienced physical therapist, the individual with C-6 quadriplegia is able to perform many functions otherwise thought impossible (Hamill, Carson, & Dorahy, 2010).

Spinal Orthoses

Spinal orthotic systems are used to decrease pain, provide support, and prevent or reduce unwanted motion in the spine. Simple designs are commonly found in sporting goods and hardware stores where an elastic waist belt with suspenders is used for abdominal/low back support during lifting and moving of heavy objects. While soft orthotic devices provide compression and support, rigid devices are designed to prevent or control unwanted motion; they are typically used after injury or following surgery. For example, after a spinal fusion, spinal orthoses allow the spine to heal or fuse in an optimal position (Seymour, 2002). Spinal braces are designated by the segment of the vertebral spine that needs to be stabilized and supported, such as lumbosacral orthosis (LSO) or thoraco-lumbosacral orthosis (TLSO).

Cervical vertebrae are difficult to stabilize because there is little supportive structure. The human head is quite heavy and rests on top of the spine (the seven cervical vertebrae). The junction between the head and first vertebrae, C-1 (first cervical vertebrae), provides the flexion and extension (up and down tilt) of the head. At the C-1 and C-2 articulation, a majority of the overall rotation is afforded with C-3 through T-1 (first thoracic vertebrae) contributing to flexion, extension, rotation, and lateral bending of the neck in smaller but proportional amounts.

FIGURE 1
Halo Fixture

Source: University of Wisconsin Health. *Health facts for you: Using your halo orthotics at home.* (2011). University of Wisconsin Hospitals and Clinics Authority. Retrieved from http://www.uwhealth.org/ healthfacts/b_extranet_health_information-flexmember-show_public_hffy_1126651619530.html

Whiplash (a snapping backward of the head) is a common automobile accident injury to the cervical spine, often requiring an orthosis. A soft collar is used for comfort and to reduce motion of the head. Cervical orthoses (collars) can be more extensive and rigid to further stabilize the head. With severe injury, or when maximum cervical immobilization is needed, a halo fixation device is used (See Figure 1).

Dr. Jacqueline Perry developed the halo fixation device at Rancho Los Amigos National Medical Center in Downey, California, for use on polio patients. In certain cases, the polio virus renders the muscles of the neck so weak that the head cannot be held erect. The halo holds the head in a functional position while protecting the spine until sufficient strength returns to the muscles of the neck and shoulders. Currently, the halo is used to stabilize the cervical region of the spinal cord (post injury/surgery) while skeletal healing occurs (Lusardi et al., 2012).

Other Assistive Devices

Assistive devices or aids are as basic as canes, crutches, and walkers which assist in ambulation while an injury is healing or used on a permanent basis for support. Assistive devices include adaptive equipment such as self-help aids; included, are devices fabricated to increase a person's daily activities such as dressing and grooming, eating, writing, and operating a computer keyboard. Examples of assistive devices include reachers, long-handled grippers, thickened writing implements, and adapted computer keyboards.

Modifications are made to automobiles such as relocating the brake and gas pedals and providing hand controls, more extensive rear-view mirrors, and easy-to-open door handles. Minivans are modified to accommodate the needs of an individual, making it possible for a person with quadriplegia to drive. Extensive modifications and van conversions for almost any kind of disability can be provided.

Orthotists and prosthetists, being well acquainted with manufacturing and fabricating custom devices, are called upon to design and provide special assistive systems (Falvo, 2014). Mouth sticks are used by individuals with high-level paralysis (quadriplegia). The mouth stick is a device with a portion made to fit into the mouth with a rod extending out to a point where a rubber tip is affixed. The person uses this device to push the buttons of a telephone, type on a keyboard, and perform other tasks. Special equipment is manufactured by certified orthotists that are only limited by the imagination and assessment skills of those involved (Clark, 1993).

There are hundreds of designs for wheelchairs, both power and manual. The orthotist can offer suggestions for modification so the individual can more readily use a wheelchair. The type of power chair is identified through evaluating the person's goals (sensory, cognitive, and anatomical areas of functioning) and level of transfer to get into and out of the chair.

Physical Limitations

A major purpose of orthotic devices is to improve function and thereby decrease physical limitations. Weak muscles are provided support both in the lower and upper extremities as well as the spine. An individual with leg weakness has increased support with orthotic devices, enabling that person to transfer with greater ease, stand longer, and walk greater distances. Adaptive devices for upper extremities support weak and inactive muscles, helping the person perform activities of daily living. Orthotic devices help the employee perform work tasks; they can be custom designed for particular work functions, thereby improving vocational potential. Orthoses assist people who want to drive, consequently enhancing independence (Brodwin, Siu, & Cardoso, 2012). This may allow a person the transportation needed for greater independence and to secure and maintain employment. Orthotic devices for upper extremities increase gross and fine manual dexterity, coordination, and manipulation. For lower extremities, they enhance ambulation and overall physical mobility and may help increase bone density through weight bearing. The goal for assistive devices is to have them help individuals function independently at home, work, and in leisure activities.

Psychological Limitations

Orthotic devices help minimize functional limitations, thus assisting people to overcome physical limitations; as a consequence, emotional concerns may diminish. Use of orthotic devices helps people obtain and maintain employment; one sees a positive impact on a person's emotional state. Provision of orthotic devices helps with activities of daily living and independence, thus impacting self-esteem and confidence. Positive emotions can replace anxiety and depression, and help in adaptation to disability and loss (Marini & Stebnicki, 2012).

Amputation

Amputation is the general term for loss of all or a portion of a body part. The loss can be congenital, the result of injury, or the outcome of a surgical procedure to treat disease (e.g., cancer). The loss of a limb is devastating to both the person and the family. An amputation causes changes in body image and functional capacity; much of this relates to a person's interpretation of the loss. Adaptation depends on the circumstances involving the amputation, usefulness of a prosthetic device, and the person's perception of the resulting disability (Edelstein & Moroz, 2010). In cases of traumatic amputation, such as in a vehicular accident or armed conflict, there is no time for the person to prepare; adjustment and adaptation becomes more difficult than for individuals who have had time to prepare for amputation, such as may occur with systemic illnesses (e.g., cancer, diabetes). A prosthesis can be perceived in a negative way by signifying loss, or in a more positive and productive manner as a means of restoring function, thereby diminishing limitations imposed by the resulting disability.

The majority of amputations within the United States are a result of poor arterial circulation caused by complications of diabetes. Diabetes involves an inability of the body to produce sufficient insulin for glucose metabolism. One long term adverse health effect caused by diabetes is a vasculopathy (poor blood circulation to peripheral tissues), especially in the lower extremities, but also to the nerves, retina, heart, kidneys, bone, connective tissues, muscle, and the vascular system itself. As a result, over time, the tissues become malnourished and die. Commonly, the person who has diabetes loses sensation in a lower extremity at the most distal segment first, such as in the toes. Because of a potential unrecognized injury, the person is also prone to infection (Kirkup, 2010).

Individuals in good control of their diabetes are less likely to have complications and, if they do, to a lesser degree. It is not likely that the person who has diabetes was healthy one day and requires an amputation the next. Diabetes is a chronic condition and a simple accident, such as a stubbed toe, may be all that is needed to cause an injury from which the body of a person with diabetes has difficulty healing. Infection may set in and complicate already diminished circulation; the wound becomes more extensive and, in spite of the best medical care, lacks sufficient blood circulation and cellular metabolism to heal. Infection may become so severe that surgical amputation becomes necessary (Cohen & Edelstein, 2011; Edelstein & Moroz, 2010). If circulation continues to be impaired at a higher level, further surgery may be required.

Levels of Amputation

Lower Extremity

Amputations are classified according to their location relative to the nearest joint (see Figure 2). The lowest level is called a partial foot; as the name implies, it goes through a part of the foot. The next level up is referred to as a Syme and occurs through the ankle joint. Other levels include below the knee (BK), knee disarticulation (KD), above the knee (AK), and hip disarticulation (HD).

Upper Extremity

Amputations involving the upper extremities are likewise categorized relative to the nearest joint (see Figure 2). The lowest level involves removal of part of the hand or fingers and is called a partial hand amputation. If the amputation occurs at the wrist level, it is referred to as a wrist disarticulation (WD). Other levels include below the elbow (BE), elbow disarticulation (ED), above the elbow (AE), and shoulder disarticulation (SD).

FIGURE 2
Levels of Typical Amputations

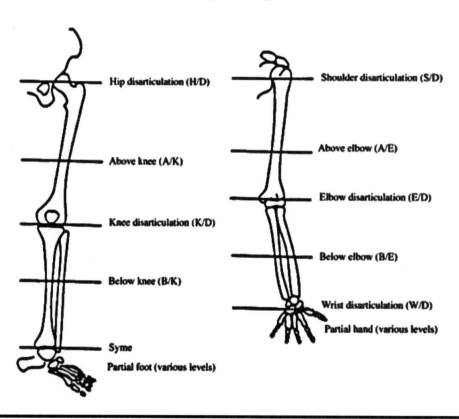

Source: Friedmann, L. W. (1981). Amputation. In W. C. Stolov & M. R. Clowers (Eds.), *Handbook of severe disability*. Washington, DC: U. S. Government Printing Office.

Complications of Amputation

Complications may occur at the site of a recent amputation. These include edema, ulceration, contracture, infection, and pain (Seymour, 2002). Normally, a certain amount of edema (swelling of tissues) of the residual limb occurs following surgery; it has been found that immediate or early fitting of a prosthesis minimizes edema. If abnormal or excessive edema occurs, immediate medical attention is necessary; otherwise, ulceration of the skin can occur. Skin ulcerations also are caused by infection, a poor fitting prosthesis, or excessive pressure where the prosthesis contacts the skin. Medical attention and a new prosthetic socket with an appropriate fit are essential to resolve this problem. Hot, humid environments can lead to breakdown of the skin; dirt and lack of cleanliness in the area can cause a serious problem and lead to potential infection of the amputation area. Treatment involves the use of antibiotics and possible surgical excision of a deeply infected area (Malthijs & Sidransky, 2011). Increased incidence of heterotopic ossification have been found in people with amputations whose limbs were lost as a result of bomb blasts or IED's in armed conflict.

Muscular contractures can occur and may be caused by lack of use of the extremity either before the limb was surgically removed or after removal when the prosthesis was not used. They may occur because of bone blockage within or disuse of a joint; exercise or surgery usually resolves this problem.

Phantom-Limb Pain

Phantom-limb sensation is a feeling following an amputation that the amputated limb still is present, including an awareness or kinesthetic sense of where the missing portion of the body is in space. Phantom-limb sensation is a normal occurrence for most people who have had amputation; it is neither painful nor limiting. A sensation of pain in a removed part is abnormal and known as *phantom-limb pain*. Unlike phantom-limb sensation, phantom-limb pain can be disabling, and cannot always be relieved even through surgical intervention (Knotkova, Crucian, Tronnier, & Rasche, 2012). Phantom-limb pain, if severe, may disable a person from most activities, including work. If a person experiences chronic pain, referral to a medical specialist is appropriate. There are surgical and non-surgical procedures that help alleviate chronic pain. Fortunately, there is a tendency for chronic phantom-limb pain to diminish over time (Edelstein & Moroz, 2010).

A clinician should not tell a patient that his or her phantom-limb pain is not real, such as stating that "Your pain is in your head." Truthfully, all pain is in the head as the brain decodes an electrochemical stimulus through nerves as tickle, itch, pressure, hot, cold, or pain. Whether phantom or real limb pain (pain within an existing portion of the body), the patient hurts. Pain left unaddressed can lead to emotional and interpersonal complications. Patients will commonly claim that their phantom-limb pain is worse at night. At nighttime, there are no distractions of television, construction, traffic, work, and the like. Patients who have phantom-limb pain are then left with the pain alone as the only stimulus.

Lower Extremity Prostheses

Physical implications of amputation are dependent both on the loss itself and on the person's adaptation to that loss. The more proximal the amputation, the more difficult and challenging the adjustment; functional loss is greater and fitting of a prosthesis is more formidable. A lower extremity prosthesis enables a person to stand and walk. As a result of increasing ability to ambulate, an individual is capable of more extensive work than just seated activity. Walking on uneven surfaces, rough terrain, and inclines/declines as well as pushing, pulling, and climbing are difficult with a lower extremity prosthesis.

Microprocessor controlled ankle and knee joints have proliferated in lower extremity prosthetics. The C-Leg provides the ability to have an adjustable high yield knee flexion resistance when the foot contacts the ground and then reverses during the upswing to allow the foot and shin to flex as easily as a ball on a string. This also reduces the energy demands of walking. It allows a patient to walk down stairs, ramps, and other previously difficult terrains without the risk of knee flexion collapse, which previously would cause the patient to fall. Since 1997, several manufacturers have developed microprocessor controlled knees that address the same goals as the C-Leg (Edelstein & Moroz, 2011).

There are several varieties of microprocessor controlled ankles as a prosthetic option. These technologies allow the patient to walk on inclines and declines with the ankle accommodating for the terrain such that the wearer perceives the same forces as though walking on level ground. An individual with two lower extremity prostheses has a more difficult time walking and standing and may use a wheelchair for extended periods or distances of mobility. Many persons become proficient with two lower extremity prostheses and are able to ambulate with use of a cane or other assistive devices (Murphy, 2013). Light or sedentary work not involving significant amounts of standing and walking is appropriate for a worker with bilateral lower extremity limb loss. Some individuals may pursue physically active jobs despite the added effort needed.

Upper Extremity Prostheses

An upper extremity prosthesis increases a person's manual dexterity, bilateral dexterity, and allows for more complex tasks requiring both hands. Some people become quite proficient when using a prosthetic upper extremity. A hook terminal device allows for grasping, gripping, lifting, and carrying. Terminal devices can be specially designed and fabricated to meet specific needs within the workplace. Specialized devices may be fabricated and used solely for particular job functions.

Electronic hand technology has progressed a great deal in the past 15 years with respect to upper extremity systems commercially available. Simultaneous function became available where combinations of motions can be done at the same time. Previous control systems employed skin surface sensors (electrodes) that are placed over the muscle belly of the controlling muscle. More recently, surgeons can implant the sensors into the controlling muscle avoiding the need for specific skin surface contact. More rare but available are surgeries where the electrode sensor can be implanted into the brain so that the thought of (flexing or extending an elbow, opening or closing a hand or finger) result in that very motion. The intent is to make the movement so intuitive that thought causes the body motion (Murphy, 2013). Fingers can be programmed to function independently. The thumb is positionable and functional with an ability to close independent of the fingers.

Psychological Considerations

The emotional impact of amputation of any body part is devastating; the person may experience anger, depression, resentment, fear, and withdrawal. People with amputation need to make permanent behavioral, social, and emotional adjustments to cope with the various problems presented with loss of a limb (Falvo, 2014). Yet, the human mind is flexible and most individuals learn, after a period of grieving over loss, to cope and adapt. After struggling with the loss for months, people hopefully reach a realization that they can work, play, and enjoy companionship and family relationships despite their losses. Early fitting of a prosthesis hastens adjustment; prompt intervention by a rehabilitation counselor makes the adjustment and adaptation less traumatic, and the focus is shifted from loss to the efforts required to be able to return to work. A prosthesis is a tool. It increases capabilities and helps minimize limitations, thereby making emotional adjustment easier; it provides a feeling of *wholeness*. Regardless of the reason for the amputation, one needs to acknowledge and assess the individual's interpretation of the loss.

There are a plethora of emotional affects associated with amputation, and they are founded on factual occurrence and involve cultural perceptions. There is a naturally occurring grieving process involving loss of a part of the body, similar to the stages of death and dying identified by Dr. Elizabeth Kübler-Ross (1969). These stages include: (a) denial and isolation, (b) anger (rage, envy, and resentment), (c) bargaining, (d) depression, and finally, (e) acceptance or adaptation. Not all people go through these stages in the order listed, nor does everyone experience each stage. Some never reach the final stage. Feelings of hope often persist through all these stages and are a positive indication of emotional recovery. A gradual transition takes place from the first four negative stages to the final positive stage – acceptance or adaptation. Time is needed to resolve feelings of loss and adaptation to an altered body image.

An individual who is presented with a recommendation for amputation after months of possible loss of mobility, infection, pain, and failed medical treatment may agree that an amputation will improve the current quality of life. Quite differently, the person who is diagnosed with osteosarcoma (bone cancer) and requires immediate amputation has little time to begin the emotional adjustment process to the impending loss. A person who loses a limb in an accident likewise has no time to adjust. These individuals may need additional time to grieve and adjust to these traumatic losses (Hamill et al., 2010).

Family Involvement

Family counseling usually is made available so that each member of the family understands how best to fill the role of loved one and learn to help with the process of adaptation to a newly acquired disability and the process of rehabilitation. The family can help the person with the grieving process by assisting in adaptation to loss and changed body image. Capability of the family to provide emotional support is invaluable (Hamill et al., 2010). Yet, one must be aware that excessive attention can be dysfunctional to the person's full recovery. Psychological health improves as one adjusts and again begins to enjoy activities and social relationships.

Employment Issues

Lower Extremity

Physical demands of work (walking, standing, lifting, and carrying) may need modification. For an employee with a lower extremity amputation, use of a wheeled cart for transporting material, a backpack for smaller items, powered carts or scooters for greater mobility, and minimizing the need for reaching up, reaching behind, bending down, and squatting is helpful because these actions are difficult to perform with a prosthesis and also involve energy expenditure (Brodwin, Parker, & De La Garza, 2010). Overall amounts of standing and walking need to be decreased; ambulation with a prosthesis requires substantially greater consumption of energy. Climbing, squatting, and kneeling are difficult or impossible to perform (Clark, 1993; Mueller, 1990).

Upper Extremity

With an upper extremity amputation, even with use of a prothesis, the person will lose a significant amount of manual dexterity. Because of the absence of feeling and sensation in the prosthetic device, function is further limited. A prosthetic hook is a tool often with a grasp surface similar to needle nose pliers. Having only one style hook limits the activities that can proficiently be performed. Hooks, hands, and other terminal devices only partially substitute for the wide variety of movements and functions of a normal hand. At work, an individual's use of an upper extremity prosthesis increases manual dexterity, bilateral dexterity, eye-hand coordination, gripping, grasping, lifting, and carrying. Although a prosthesis does not replace a fully functional arm and hand, it allows a worker to perform many essential tasks. A workstation, with appropriate accommodation and modification, can be designed to make possible and efficient the work duties of a person with an upper extremity amputation.

Workplace Accommodation

If a person has chronic pain (i.e., phantom-limb pain) but is able to work, workplace accommodation is beneficial. Employers who understand chronic pain are more willing to consider possible accommodations. Workplace accommodation for chronic pain is as variable as chronic pain itself. Each person with chronic pain needs individualized attention and case management (Brodwin et al., 2010).

Through careful evaluation of needs, limitations, strengths, and an awareness of functioning and the kinds of accommodations and assistive devices available, rehabilitation counselors can enhance the employability of clients who have amputations. Counselors should always remember the psychological trauma that has occurred and its impact on the total functioning of the individual within the home environment, at the workplace, in school, as well as socially.

Prosthetics

Prosthetic Treatment

Immediate post-operative fitting of a lower limb prosthesis hastens the healing process. Emotional benefits of this procedure are well documented (Murphy, 2013). An immediate postoperative prosthesis

(IPOP) is arranged by the surgeon or treating physician. It is a sterile, rigid dressing applied in the operating room immediately after surgery while the patient is still under anesthetic. A soft, sterile dressing is applied, followed by placing a rigid Plaster of Paris cast over the leg; a prosthetic pylon and foot are then added. An IPOP (Esquenazi, 1994; Wilson, 1998):

- provides a sterile environment for healing
- prevents flexion contractures
- protects the limb from external trauma
- allows partial weight-bearing (never greater than 30 pounds)
- maintains proprioception and a kinesthetic position of the limb
- accelerates healing by preventing edema and assisting in venous blood return
- gives an emotional perception and feeling of wholeness

Temporary Prostheses

Generally speaking, after the surgical site has healed, the patient is sent to a prosthetist to have a temporary prosthesis fabricated. The person should have been seen by a licensed physical therapist with which the prosthetist and physician will consult to determine functional levels (see *Medicare Functional Levels* later in this chapter).

Upon completion of a temporary prosthesis, the patient begins functional use that includes gait training. A physical therapist begins the training process. Weight bearing and weight shifting capabilities precede attempts at ambulation. A person with a below knee amputation acquires all the skills needed for ambulation within six weeks. Yet, that same person needs six months for the residual limb and skin to toughen to the point where the tissues and bones tolerate the forces involved with activities the individual chooses to perform.

Adjustments to maintain an intimately fitting socket (interface) are routinely made by the prosthetist during the months the patient is in the temporary prosthesis. Time needed for the limb to mature is typically four to eight months for below knee amputations and four to 18 months for those above the knee. The process of maturation includes reduction caused by muscle atrophy, decreased edema, and loss of adipose (fat) content. Each person has a somewhat different adjustment period (Edelstein & Moroz, 2010).

Permanent or Definitive Prostheses

Fitting with a permanent prosthesis is generally begun when the patient's limb has matured, the majority of tissue volume reduction has occurred, and the patient is competent in the ability to operate the prosthesis. It may be initiated when the prosthetist has exhausted all adjustments to the temporary socket, and there is a need to replace the socket or upgrade the component parts. Sophisticated components may be selected for the permanent prosthesis, as appropriate, to increase function and longevity.

Factors Considered for Permanent Prostheses

The prosthetist takes the following factors into consideration when fitting and designing a permanent prosthesis (Bussell, 2000; Edelstein & Moroz, 2010):

- types of terrain commonly traversed
- velocity of ambulation
- variance in ambulation velocity
- styles of shoes worn
- physical activities, including work
- body weight
- patient variances, such as limb volume due to dialysis

Purchase of Prosthesis

Based on these factors, the prosthetist and patient select a group of components to be used in fabrication of the prosthesis. Most component manufacturers want their components to be used and allow them to be tried in the prosthetist's office, helping ensure the selection that best meets the person's needs (Murphy, 2013). Reimbursement issues require consideration. Third-party payers are increasingly dictating levels of reimbursement and hence the sophistication of prosthetic systems being provided. The individual needs an awareness of what is available and necessary for desired functions. People with limb loss usually have the legal right to purchase components or technology used in the prosthesis that may not be covered by insurance, by paying the difference in cost.

Lower Extremity Prosthetic Components

Components of a lower limb prosthesis include the limb interface, socket, mechanical joints, and foot assembly (Bussell, 2000). An individual with a new amputation will have several changes in limb volume (due to post-amputation swelling and changes in weight) and will require periodic adjustment of the socket. A tight, yet intimate fit is needed for maximum comfort, control, and stability. The person must learn appropriate gait through instruction and practice. Stair climbing and walking on uneven surfaces requires additional practice. Driving is sometimes possible but requires adaptive equipment (hand controls). Most sporting activities can be done with a special prosthetic limb design.

Activities are easier to perform with an amputation below-the-knee as only the ankle joint is missing. An individual with a BK amputation generally expends 10% to 37% more energy for walking (Murphy, 2013; Wilson, 1998). With an above-the-knee amputation, both the ankle and knee joints are artificial making standing and walking more challenging and energy consuming. Since a person with an AK amputation expends 60% more energy walking, some people choose to use wheelchairs for ambulation to save energy for work and other activities (Seymour, 2002; Wilson, 1998). The less excess standing and walking a job involves, the more energy the worker retains for other job functions.

Advanced prosthetics technology has led to the development of lighter, more comfortably fitting, and technologically efficient lower extremity prostheses. As stated, the C-leg system is the first completely microprocessor-controlled prosthetic knee/shin system with hydraulic swing and stance phase control (Holmes, 2005). This product is so revolutionary that individuals who have been fitted with the device often state that the most obvious benefit is that they do not have to think consciously about walking. This occurs because the advanced microprocessor control does the thinking for them (Lusardi et al., 2012; Murphy, 2013).

Upper Extremity Prosthetic Components

Components of upper limb prostheses include the limb interface, socket, mechanical joints, terminal device, and suspension system. A harness system using the shoulder muscles on the opposite side allows the person to operate a body powered terminal device (hook). Normal functioning of a hand and arm cannot be replaced with a prosthetic device. Movements made by the hand are intricate; the hand has an ability to move in various directions and can perform complex motions and tasks, from gross manipulation to fine dexterity. The terminal device of a prosthetic upper extremity is a hook-type device that can grasp, pinch, and hold objects. It cannot feel, do fine dexterity, or manipulate; lifting and carrying are limited to lighter weights.

Functional or cosmetic hands can be used instead of hook devices. The functional hand has a three-finger pinch, grasp, and hold action, but lacks the power and stability of a hook. Cosmetic hands are used primarily for social purposes, as they resemble a natural hand in color, tones, and texture. A more sophisticated device is the external power myoelectric arm and hand. The *myoelectric arm* is computerized and contains electrodes that are placed on the skin over muscles. Electrical impulses from the muscles allow the person to open and close the hand simply by tensing the particular muscles normally involved. Although the myoelectric arm has the appearance of an actual arm and hand, it is not usually prescribed due to the expense (Edelstein & Moroz, 2010).

Medicare Functional Levels

Medicare has established definitions for functional levels of lower extremity amputation. These five levels are described below.
- Level 0 - Patient does not have the ability or potential to benefit from a prosthesis.

- Level I - Person has the ability or potential to use a prosthesis for transfers or ambulation on level surfaces at a fixed cadence. This level is typical of the limited and unlimited household ambulator.
- Level II - Individual has the ability or potential for ambulation with the ability to traverse low-level environmental barriers such as curbs, stairs, and uneven surfaces. Level II is appropriate for the limited community ambulator.
- Level III - Patient has the ability or potential for ambulation with variable cadence. This level is used for the community ambulator who has the capability to traverse most environmental barriers and may have vocational, therapeutic, and exercise activity that demands prosthetic utilization beyond simple ambulation.
- Level IV - Person has the ability or potential for prosthetic ambulation that exceeds basic ambulation skills, exhibiting high impact, stress, or energy levels. Level IV is appropriate for the prosthetic demands of a child, active adult, or athlete.

According to Medicare, the reason for these levels is to set a standard for which types of component parts are appropriate, based on the individual's projected needs.

Conclusion – Assistive Technology and the Workplace

Assistive technology (AT) is defined in the Technology-Related Assistance for Individuals with Disabilities Act of 1988 (popularly referred to as *The Tech Act*) as "any item, piece of equipment, or product system, whether acquired commercially off the shelf, modified, or customized, that is used to increase, maintain, or improve functional capabilities of individuals with disabilities." The goal of AT is to increase the functional independence for people who have disabilities. It is having a profound impact on improving the lives and employment opportunities of many individuals (Young & O'Young, 2011). AT is an effective and powerful device to help restore functioning, enhance quality of life, and remove physical and attitudinal barriers. Rehabilitation counselors are attempting to maximize this independence at the workplace (Brodwin et al., 2010). Through the use of modern-day orthotics and prosthetics, AT enables workers with upper or lower extremity limitations to reduce and perhaps minimize their functional limitations.

Through orthotic and prosthetic devices, rehabilitation counselors have seen their clients achieve greater productivity within education and employment, leading to enhanced self-sufficiency, independence, freedom to choose, and social re-integration. Many workers can continue working, return to work, or secure alternative employment following a disabling event. With the provision of orthotic and prosthetic devices, they are able to participate more fully and actively in all aspects of life. Technology helps equalize the capacities of employees with disabilities when compared to workers without limitations. Greater independence and satisfaction in daily life, including both work and leisure, become enhanced (Edelstein & Moroz, 2010). With daily use of orthotic and prosthetic devices, a person's emotional outlook is improved, as is the capability to interact more readily and comfortably at work and within the social arena (Brodwin et al., 2012).

Case Study

Amy Nguyen, a Vietnamese-born 22-year old, has been residing in the United States for the previous ten years; she has a Bachelor of Arts degree from a local university. At the present time, Amy is living with her parents in a large city. Several months ago, she was in an automobile versus bicycle accident. A serious right leg injury resulted in an AK amputation. Understandably, Amy has had great difficulty accepting the loss of her leg, although recently she has asked to work with her treating physician and prosthetist for fitting of a prosthesis. Currently, she experiences *phantom-limb* and a moderate amount of *phantom-limb pain* (Knotkova et al., 2012).

Having recently graduated from college with a degree in liberal arts, Ms. Nguyen would like to become an elementary school teacher. She needs to attend one more year of college, including student teaching and passing a teaching certification examination. Her parents strongly suggested that she return to college and major in business accounting. At this time, Amy strongly believes she must follow her parents' advise, even though she does not agree with them about majoring in business accounting.

Amy's only employment has been on a temporary or part-time basis. She has worked as a sales person during several Christmas seasons, a cashier and hostess in a restaurant, and a part-time cashier/ticket taker for a movie theater. These jobs took place during several summer and Christmas vacations and occasionally during the school year.

Questions

1. Discuss Dr. Elizabeth Kübler-Ross' stages of death and dying from the standpoint of adjustment to disability. Relate this discussion to the case study and the role of the rehabilitation counselor.
2. Describe the various levels of amputation, the functional limitations at each level, and psychosocial implications. Relate these limitations to school, work, and social activities.
3. What are Ms. Nguyen's functional limitations as related to future employment? Will she be able to drive an automobile? Discuss the psychosocial factors relevant to this case.
4. How would you handle her parents' strong guidance that Amy return to college and major in business accounting rather than becoming an elementary school teacher, and Amy's belief that she needs to fulfill her parents' wishes? From a cultural perspective, how would the two opposing vocational goals affect this client and the provision of vocational rehabilitation services?
5. Amy is having great difficulty with adjustment to her disability. She is also experiencing phantom pain. As her counselor, offer recommendations in regard to these two conditions. Discuss both phantom-limb sensation and phantom-limb pain.

References

Brodwin, M. G., Parker, R. M., & DeLaGarza, D. (2010). Disability and reasonable accommodation. In E. M. Szymanski & R. M. Parker (Eds.), *Work and disability: Contexts, issues, and strategies for enhancing employment opportunities for people with disabilities* (3rd ed., pp. 281–323). Austin, TX: Pro-ed.

Brodwin, M. G., Siu, F. W., & Cardoso, E. (2012) Users of assistive technology: The human component. In I. Marini & M. Stebnicki (Eds.), *The psychological and social impact of disability* (6th ed., pp. 331–339). New York, NY: Springer.

Bussell, M. H. (Ed.). (2000). *New developments in prosthetics and orthotics*. Philadelphia, PA: W. B. Saunders.

Clark, D. R. (1993). Orthotics and prosthetics. In M. G. Brodwin, F. A. Tellez, & S. K. Brodwin (Eds.), *Medical, psychosocial, and vocational aspects of disability* (pp. 407–420). Athens, GA: Elliott and Fitzpatrick.

Cohen, J. M., & Edelstein, J. E. (2011). Limb deficiency. In S. R. Flanagan, H. H. Zaretsky, & A. Moroz (Eds.), *Medical aspects of disability: A handbook for the rehabilitation professional* (4th ed., pp. 381–408). New York, NY: Springer.

Edelstein, J. E., & Moroz, A. (2010). *Lower-limb prosthetics and orthotics: Clinical concepts*. Thorofare, NJ: Slack.

Esquenazi, A. (Ed.). (1994). *Prosthetics*. Philadelphia, PA: Hanley and Belfus.

Falvo, D. R. (2014). *Medical and psychosocial aspects of chronic illness and disability* (5th ed.). Burlington, MD: Jones and Bartlett Learning.

Fishman, S. (2001).The professionalization of orthotics and prosthetics. *Orthotics and Prosthetics Business News, 10*, 24–30.

Hamill, R., Carson, S., & Dorahy, M. (2010). Experiences of psychosocial adjustment within 18 months of amputation: An interpretive phenomenological approach. *Disability Rehabilitation, 32*(9), 729–740.

Holmes, L. (2005). The computer revolution and assistive technology. In. H. H. Zaretsky, E. F. Richter, III., & M. G. Eisenberg (Eds.), *Medical aspects of disability: A handbook for the rehabilitation professional* (3rd ed., pp. 783–795). New York, NY: Springer.

Kirkup, J. R. (2010). *A history of limb amputation*. London, England: Springer.

Knotkova, H., Crucian, R. A., Tronnier, V. M., & Rasche, D. (2012). Current and future options for the management of phantom limb pain. *Journal of Pain Research, 5*, 39–49.

Kübler-Ross, E. (1969). *On death and dying*. New York, NY: McMillan.

Lusardi, M. M., Jorge, M., & Nielsen, C. C. (2012). *Orthotics and prosthetics in rehabilitation* (3rd ed.). Philadelphia, PA: Saunders Elsevier.

Malthijs, S., & Sidransky, R. (Eds.). (2011). *Amputations: Types, procedures, and risks*. Waltham, MA: Nova Biomedical.

Marini, I., & Stebnicki, M. (Eds.). (2012). *The psychological and social impact of disability* (6th ed.). New York, NY: Springer.

May, B. J., & Lockard, M. A. (2011). *Prosthetics and orthotics in clinical practice*. Philadelphia, PA: F. A. Davis.

Mueller, J. (1990). *The workplace workbook: An illustrated guide to job accommodation and assistive technology*. Washington, DC: Dole Foundation.

Murphy, D. E., (2013). *Fundamentals of amputation care and prosthetics*. New York, NY: Demos Medical.

Pascual-Leones, A., Freitas, C., Oberman, L., Horvath, J. C., Hailko, M., Eldaief, M., . . . Rotenberg, A. (2011). Characterizing brain cortical plasticity and network dynamics across the age-span in health and disease with TMS-EEG and TMS-MRI. *Brain Topography, 24*, 302–315.

Seymour, R. (2002). *Prosthetics and orthotics: Lower limb and spinal*. Philadelphia, PA: Lippincott Williams & Wilkins.

Technology-Related Assistance for Individuals with Disabilities Act of 1988, 29 U. S. C. § 2201 *et seq.*

University of Wisconsin Health. *Health facts for you: Using your halo orthotics at home.* (2011). University of Wisconsin Hospitals and Clinics Authority. Retrieved from http://www.uwhealth.org/healthfacts/b_extranet_health_information-flexmember-show_public_hffy_1126651619530.html

Wilson, B. A., Jr. (1998). *A primer on limb prosthetics*. Springfield, IL: Charles C. Thomas.

Young, M. A., & O'Young, B. (2011). The computer revolution, disability, and assistive technology. In S. R. Flanagan, H. H. Zaretsky, & A. Moroz (Eds.), *Medical aspects of disability: A handbook for the rehabilitation professional* (4th ed., pp. 635–646). New York, NY: Springer.

About the Authors

Lance R. Clawson, B.S., C. P. O., received his prosthetics and orthotics education at California State University, Dominguez Hills. In 1987, he completed a prosthetics residency at Rancho Los Amigos National Medical Center in Downey, California, and an orthotics residency at San Bernardino County Hospital. Mr. Clawson is an American Board Certified Prosthetist/Orthotist, and President and CEO of J & K Orthopedics, Inc., in Pomona and Covina, California.

Martin G. Brodwin, Ph.D, C.R.C., is Professor and Coordinator of the graduate Rehabilitation Counselor Education Program at California State University, Los Angeles. As a vocational expert for the Office of Disability Adjudication and Review, Social Security Administration, he provides testimony on disability-related issues. Dr. Brodwin has published over 100 refereed journal articles, book chapters, and books on the subjects of medical aspects of disability, counseling, disability, rehabilitation, and reasonable accommodation in business and industry.

Chapter 29

SOCIETAL REINTEGRATION FOLLOWING A BURN INJURY

Cindy Rutter, R.N., B.S.N.
Ann Malo, R.N.

MY SKIN

Nobody sees what I see
For back of my eyes there is only me
And nobody knows how my thoughts begin
For there's only myself inside my skin
Isn't it strange how everyone owns
Just enough skin to cover their bones
The scars that I wear seem a little unfair
Because there's nobody like me anywhere

Author Unknown

Introduction

Each year, over two million Americans suffer from burn injuries (American Burn Association [ABA], 2012). Of these, 450,000 receive medical treatment, either in a hospital or emergency room. These injuries are the result of fires in homes, vehicle crash fires, and other events, such as smoke inhalation, contact with electricity, scalding liquids, or hot objects. Between 2002 and 2011, 96% of people admitted to burn centers survived. More than two-thirds of these burns occurred in the home. Less than 10% occurred on the job, while 7% happened on the highway. Another 5% were the result of recreational accidents; 10% have other or unknown causes. Almost two-thirds of hospital admitted burn patients were White. Another 12% were Black, while 15% were Latino (ABA, 2012).

Risk factors associated with burn injuries are gender, age, minority race/ethnicity, and lower socio-economic status. While some burns are accidental, others result from child abuse, self-inflicted injuries, and assault. This chapter discusses burn classifications, complications, treatment, challenges, and recovery. Also described are reintegration to life and society, sexuality and intimacy, and information on the Phoenix Society for Burn Injury Survivors.

Caring for a patient who has suffered a burn injury requires a multi-disciplinary team approach, and can require months and sometimes years of surgeries, recovery, and rehabilitation. It is a continuum of care that needs active therapy from surgery for skin grafting, pain management, nutritional care, physical therapy, occupation therapy, and psychological intervention.

Classification of Burns

Skin consists of multiple layers as seen Figure 1.

FIGURE 1
Layers of the Skin

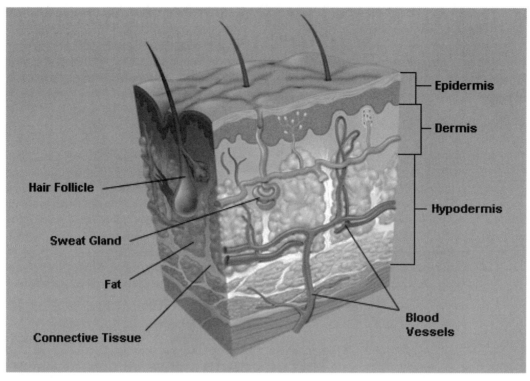

Source: WebMD. (2013). *An overview of the skin.* Retrieved from http://www.webmd.com/beauty/wrinkles/cosmetic-procedures-overview-skin

Burns are classified according to the depth of the burn within the tissue. A first degree, or superficial burn, such as sunburn, affects only the epidermis (top layer) of the skin. Second degree, or partial thickness burns, damages both the epidermis and dermis layers. Third degree, or full thickness burns, involves damage to the epidermis, dermis, hypodermis, hair follicles, sweat glands, fat, connective tissue, and blood vessels. The most severe burn is a fourth degree burn, in which a burn is so deep that organs are damaged as well. An inhalation burn, for example, causes damage to the lung tissue due to the inhalation of smoke or damaging chemicals. Fourth degree burns can necessitate amputations or even lead to organ failure.

Burn injuries are not only classified by their depth; percentage of the body burned is also relevant. This is referred to as a total body surface area (TBSA). Generally, for every 1% of body burned, a patient will require one day of hospitalization. While first degree burns do not require hospitalization, second degree burns may need skin grafting; third and fourth degree burns always require skin grafts (Young, Dewey, & Wolf, 2011). A medical device called a dermatone is used to take skin, a procedure in which an area where the patient has not been burned (called a donor site) is placed over the burn area and sutured or stapled in place.

Complications

The skin is our largest organ; it serves to protect the body in multiple ways. After a severe burn, the ultimate prognosis for the burn patient is determined by a multitude of factors: the extent of the burn and loss of skin, mechanism of injury, patient's age, and presence and severity of other medical issues.

When burns heal, hypertrophic scars may form. This is characterized by raised erythematous (red) borders with significant distinctions from normal texture (Young et al., 2011). Hypertrophic scars occur

FIGURE 2
Body Burn Percentage

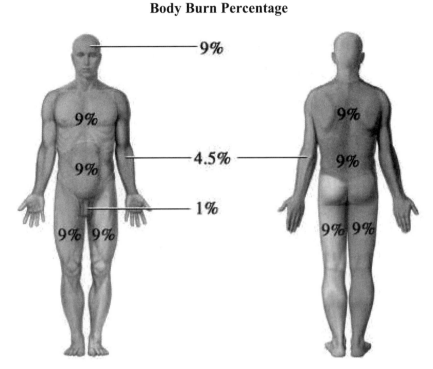

Source: WebMD. (2011). *First aid and emergences: Rules of Nines.* Retrieved from http://www.webmd.com/first-aid/rule-of-nines

when the body overproduces collagen, causing the skin to be raised above the surrounding skin. The occurrence of hypertropic scars ranges between 4% and 75% of all burn scars. There is no clear medical explanation of why this occurs in some people and not in others (Spurr & Shakespeare, 1990). During scarring, the skin can become thick, dry, and discolored. In hypertrophic scarring, patients develop thick, red, raised, and sometimes ropelike scars that remain within the boundary of the injury. *Keloids* occur when the body continues to produce tough, fibrous protein known as collagen after a wound has healed. Keloid scarring involves thick, raised, itchy clusters of scar tissue that grow beyond the edges of the wound or incision, very often red or darker in color than the surrounding skin. Burns can also cause changes in the shape of body parts depending on the damage done to the underlying tissue or body parts.

Burns may cause other physical problems as well. These include contractures, when a scar is located over a joint. Consequences of contractures include severe acute or chronic pain, nerve damage, and loss of the ability to regulate heat and cold in that area. Other problems include the inability to sweat in the affected area, as well as chronic itching.

Treatment

Many burn patients are required to wear pressure garments for up to a year after their injuries. These garments help control scarring by compressing the scar tissue, allowing it to heal faster. The garment pictured below is used on the hand and part of the lower arm.

When the survival rate for burn patients was much lower, physicians focused on the physical and rehabilitative stages of care. Today, when individuals with burns covering as much as 95% of the body are able to survive, physicians and caregivers can focus not only on physical care, but also on the psychological aspects. In addition to physical pain, burn patients may experience depression, anxiety, and post-traumatic

FIGURE 3
Pressure Garment

stress disorder (PTSD). They may also have negative body image, lower self- esteem, guilt, grief, and issues encompassing sexuality and intimacy.

Severe acute or chronic pain can interfere with a patient's physical and psychological healing. Depending on the patient, pain can cause depression and feelings of hopelessness (pain is different for each individual). As a result, it requires continuous assessment. Medication is only one treatment modality to alleviate pain. Alternative methods for pain relief include relaxation techniques, meditation, yoga, and music therapy. In conjunction with pain medication, the following methods can improve a patient's quality of life.

Immediately after suffering a burn, a patent may need multiple surgeries. In addition, some patients require multiple reconstructive surgeries, a process which may span years. Some also require years of physical and occupational therapy, and others may never return to their pre-injury functioning. In the case of amputations, still more complications arise. "A burn injury is a lifelong process" (Jill Sproul [nurse manager], personal communication, August 15, 2013).

Persons with severe burn injuries are generally cared for in hospital burn units. The ABA establishes guidelines for treatment and determines when a burn patient will be transferred depending on the field assessment by Emergency Medical Services. In providing care to burn patients, health care providers must consider the person's existing psychosocial support, insurance, and financial resources. Issues that are faced include concern over family, especially children, insurance, employment, housing, and coping with the losses that accompany burn injuries.

Once a patient is discharged from the hospital, family members may have to take on additional responsibilities to care for the family member, such as changing dressings. This is difficult as the procedure continues to be painful and personal. While healthcare providers can help teach family members how to change a patient's dressings, it may not alleviate the loved one's discomfort.

Psychological Challenges

Many burn survivors ask caregivers if they will ever be like they were before. The reality is that survivors will have to adjust to a new image given all the changes they have had and will face in the future. They must reassess priorities and learn to establish new ones. Patients recovering from burns are often concerned with maintaining relationships with family and friends (Gilboa, 2001). It takes determination, perseverance, and courage for an individual to journey through and recover from a severe burn injury.

Today, patients have an abundance of potential resources to aid in the recovery process (Acton, Mounsey, & Gilyard, 2007). One can view the stages of recovery (sometimes referred to as the *journey through the burn injury*) as (a) the acute in-hospital care and physical recovery, (b) rehabilitation after discharge from the hospital, and (c) reintegration to life and society.

When a loved one has been injured, family members are affected. They too go through stages or phases of recovery or adjustment. Watkins, Cook, May, and Ehleben (1998) outlined what a *normal* psychological healing process might look like for burn survivors in the *Journal of Burn Care and Rehabilitation*. These seven stages include (1) Survival Anxiety, (2) The Problem of Pain, (3) The Search for Meaning, (4) Investment in Recuperation, (5) Acceptance of Losses, (6) Investment in Rehabilitation, and (7) Reintegration into Society.

A second model, described by Herman (1997), outlined the psychological recovery and reclaiming of personal power following a burn injury. The three phases are (a) Recovering a Sense of Safety, (b) Remembering, Telling One's Story, and Mourning, and (c) Reconnecting with Life. Patients and family members may go through these stages and phases at different times and in no particular order.

Survivors Offering Assistance to Recovery (SOAR)

Survivors Offering Assistance to Recovery is a program designed by the Phoenix Society (2013) for survivors and family members so they may offer one-on-one support to burn survivors and loved ones affected by burn injuries. This program is beneficial for the patient, as well as the family. Oftentimes, it is a family member who needs help first; the patient may be too involved with struggling to survive.

The Phoenix Society and the American Burn Association have formed a committee to help develop standards accessible for all burn survivors to have help with their reintegration into life. The Aftercare Reintegration Committee (ARC) includes burn survivors, family members, nurses, physicians, occupational and physical therapists, counselors, and social workers. Together, members of ARC help survivors and family members move forward.

Reintegration to Life and Society

Once burn survivors begin the process of reintegrating into the public sphere, they face a variety of challenges (Blakeney, Rosenberg, Rosenberg, & Faber, 2008). Many survivors experience negative feelings from the public, including staring, question asking, teasing, bullying, avoiding, name-calling, and discrimination. This can be overwhelming. Survivors may feel anxious and unsure of how to react. The Behavioral & Enhancement Skills Tools (BEST) developed by Quayle helps survivors develop skills to address some of the issues noted above; the program is located on the Phoenix Society website (Phoenix Society for Burn Survivors, 2013).

Image enhancement, including the use of corrective cosmetics, is another tool for burn survivors during the reintegration process. The STEPS techniques (Kammer-Quayle, 2002) can help a person feel more comfortable entering new social situations. Steps include **S**elf-Talk, **T**one of Voice, **E**ye Contact, **P**osture, and **S**mile (STEPS). The more burn survivors can create a positive image of themselves, the easier it is for those individuals to help others be more comfortable around them.

Returning to school or work after a burn injury, while challenging, is an important part of recovery because it helps an individual return to a routine (Livneh, 2012; Livneh & Antonak, 2012). Returning to work gives a burn survivor a sense of purpose and can be a confidence builder. At times, a burn survivor needs to be retrained for a new occupation. This can cause confusion and anxiety or excitement. Vocational rehabilitation is a resource for people able to return to work. There are *Re-Entry to Work* programs that help ease the transition back to the workplace (Phoenix Society for Burn Survivors, 2013).

Loving and Relationships Following a Burn Injury

Burn injuries change how a body looks and impacts body image and self-esteem. There are many questions regarding relationships, love, sexuality, and intimacy that need to be addressed for burn survivors. Emotional healing, though infrequently addressed, is just as important as physical healing (Kammerer-Quayle, 2002).

Burn survivors recognize it is important to have relationships in supporting their role in healing after their injuries (Blakeney et al., 2008). Talking about ways to be more comfortable in one's new skin is beneficial. German photographer Rasso Bruckert (www.rasso-bruckert.de) said an important part of experiencing love, partnership, and sexuality is self-acceptance. Seldom does any person fulfill the ideal of beauty in our time, and even less so the person with a physical difference. Bruckert's perfect-imperfect illustrates photographs of people with disabilities posing nude.

Loss of relationships, as well as change in body image and self-concept are all common following a burn injury (Livneh & Antonak, 2012). The physical appearance of the burn survivor's body has undergone change which most likely is permanent. A survivor reconnecting to others after beginning to recover is essential. He or she must learn to take risks, as well as reach out and take on challenges. Survivors have fought a battle to stay alive and now must try to live life to the fullest in spite of what has happened (Blakeney & Meyer, 1994).

Burn survivors must have a relationship with themselves and know who they are and what they want. People need to feel that they are in control of themselves and how they feel about themselves. It takes courage to accept a new image and take pride in one's new image. Our relationship with ourselves includes how we feel about who we are as people, as sexual beings, as men or women, and how we feel about our bodies and behaviors.

Sexuality is integral and inseparable from body image and self-esteem. It is a form of communication, a way of expressing part of one's personality to another. Sexuality spans the biological, psychological, emotional, spiritual, cultural, and social dimensions of our lives; it begins with us and extends to others.

Intimacy and Sexuality

An issue that burn survivors face regarding sexuality and intimacy is altered skin integrity. Skin can be overly hypersensitive or hyposensitive (less sensitive than usual). Survivors will experience changes in the texture, color, and appearance of their skin. They may also experience pain, issues with mobility, and variations in energy level.

With disruption in skin sensitivity, touch may be experienced in a completely different way. The burn survivor must know how to communicate what feels good (as well as what does not) to his or her partner. Initially, survivors may feel hampered by a lack of energy. As a result, one must plan time for intimacy and sex.

Depending on where the burns have impacted the body, mobility and positioning issues may need to be addressed. New positions can be learned that are more comfortable for survivors. In the beginning, being touched may cause pain. Survivors may need their partners to go slow, take baby steps, make it as fun as possible, and try to find some humor in this trying time. Open, honest communication is essential during this period.

To appreciate one's sexuality is a lifelong process that takes courage and understanding, with or without a physical difference. Survivors begin to identify how they view themselves independent of negative interactions with others. Relationships are developed slowly between individuals sharing their experiences and learning to appreciate each other for who they are.

The following is a man's intimate letter to his girlfriend, a burn survivor.

Dear Ann:

This is a letter to you, to tell you how I feel. As you know, I had some familiarity with burns when we first met. Your scars from the burns on your face and hands were quite visible, the ones on the rest of your body were not. Burns over 2/3rds of your body "take a long time to heal." I saw the burns first, because they were there...just as when I meet a very tall or short person for the first time, I notice the most obvious features first... and then as I get to know them, I learn more about their likes, dislikes, job, intelligence, fears, loves and dreams...so they grow (in my mind) to be complete people...and so I grew to know and be attracted to you. We were attracted to each other from the first although you guarded yourself from letting me know you, for a while. I'm the same way about my feelings. Perhaps most of us are. We, I, fear rejection so we keep our distance until we are sure.... and of course, there are no guarantees... so we went ahead and let down the battle defenses. At the party that night, we were feeling "happy" and went home together and got to know each other... we woke up feeling closer. It took a couple of years to learn a lot more about each other since only intimacy really lets out a lot of feelings.

But, this letter wants to talk about burns, love, relationships and sex. Let me put it bluntly. You turned me on...the way you talked, moved and reacted to others and especially to me. One of the most attractive things about others is that they are attracted to us. I was attracted to you, physically at first and as that continued, I learned more about you. We meshed great physically. We could hold on to each other, wrestle, tickle each other and love it.

I know you. Let me tell you about scars and how I feel about yours. I love their texture. I figure I'm lucky. Most people have one or two textures to touch on their partner. I have ten or more. There is the soft smooth part below your hips, on your legs, which weren't burned. There is a soft, slightly rougher part on your thighs from whence came some of your grafts. There's the tough but smoother part under your arms, which wasn't released and so is still tight when you raise your arm. There's the checkerboard pattern on your grafted upper arms, which feels like I'm running my hand over goose bumps. There's the area on your shoulder, which didn't heal to well and is soft but has little hills and valleys. And there's the cheekbone area where the fat was left out and so the skin is closer to the bone. And, there's a dozen more. But I don't think about it quite the way I've described. I just think about each part as part of you. As the saying goes, we're the sum of our parts, good and bad.

Now, if I had known you before the burn, knowing you would be a relearning process. I'd have to change the parts of you, in my mind, but if I knew you then as I know you now, the greatest part of you would be what you are...honest, tender, sensual, caring and a great cook, etc. If I would have known you only in a physical sense and not in a close emotional sense, then yes, I would have to relearn "everything" about you.

But this isn't only for burns. All the ads, stories, movies, and television programs emphasize only the superficial: "Ooh, I'm two pounds over..." "Porcelana gets rid of those age spots...", "Which hands are mine and which are my daughter's?" Part of what the rock generation of the 60's and 70's and the punk rockers of the 80's were trying to say is, "Know me as a person, first, last and always." The punkers make their outward appearance so bizarre that people are forced to look at them as a person. Unfortunately, very few people can get past outward appearance. They say, "Hey there are so many normal regular looking kids, I don't think you are worth the effort." Well, that's their problem.... It's part of our problem too.

The next part of this letter is about questions that go through your mind—-some that you tell me about and some that you don't.

Myth #1*: "Because I have scars, you hit on me because you thought other's won't want me because others have hit on me and tried to pick me up for that reason." Well, there are boys and men like that, but you and I were attracted to each other for the right reasons. The men and boys who "Think they are going for easy pickings", have a low opinion of themselves number one, and number two, they're not much as people.*

Myth #2*: "You like me, but you are only staying with me out of pity." Well, that might be part of some people's makeup, but what a waste that would be of my life and yours. Relationships based on pity are doomed and full of resentment. Our relationship has none of that. I can see where it would be easy to fall in that pattern and I don't know if it's true for others who are burned or have some handicap. The problem with those relationships is that there is no value...no give and receive...no values exchanged by each partner. We exchange values, besides physical contact, which we both dearly love (as if we exchange electricities), but we, you in particular, listen to my dreams, ideas, and bad jokes. You can read my mind, which is helpful, and most important, you let me be myself. You are interested in my work and are willing to cheer me on in my artistic and sports endeavors, etc. On the other side, I feel I support you in your work and play (Though we should go out more)...I listen, though not as well as you.... I let you be yourself.... and I have developed an understanding of the thoughts and fears that go with being burned and having visible scars. There are other things I do, but that is another letter.*

Myth #3: *"When we love or argue or fight or enjoy, the burn plays a large part in what you say or do." Well only in as much as you can't raise your arm to full extension (because of a tight band of tissue) to slug me, and because of how it makes you feel sometimes.*

By and large, when we are together, I don't notice people staring unless they are obvious, and if so I just stare back at them. I know that most of their intentions are benign and not hateful, so it's only a sense of proportion and taste that I am trying to instill in them.

You know that all the things you are is what I know about you. I fell in love with your scars, your shorter nose, your skin, and your sense of life.... your smiles, your frowns, your ups, your downs. They are all part of you and part of who you are. And I like and love who you are. This is not to say you are perfect, but nine out of ten ain't bad!

As to being unsure of our relationship, relationships are built from scratch, and the more we share together the stronger the relationship becomes. That's true for everyone. The burn doesn't have anything to do with the survival of our relationship. That's determined by how we care for each other.

Love always,

William

Burn Traumas United Journal Fall 1983
Sexuality and Burns-Part I: Appearance, Body Image & Relationships

The Phoenix Society for Burn Survivors

For over 30 years, the Phoenix Society for Burn Survivors (2013) has been connecting burn survivors, their loved ones, and burn care professionals with valuable resources and a network of support.

A burn injury not only affects patients but also the people who love and support them. The recovery process is ongoing after one's release from the hospital. For these reasons, groups like the Phoenix Society have created resources for survivors, spouses, significant others, children, siblings, healthcare professionals, first responders, and others who are involved in the recovery process.

World Burn Congress (WBC) is an annual international conference that brings together thousands of burn survivors, their families, caregivers, burn care professionals, and firefighters. It is a forum to share stories, provide support, and increase one's knowledge of burn recovery. For many, it is the first opportunity to meet and share with others who have experienced burn traumas. The three days of the WBC are filled with inspirational stories of survival, courage, and personal growth. Many have described their experience at WBC as both a powerful and life changing experience.

The conference also serves as a productive learning experience for burn care professionals to better understand the issues that impact the lives of burn survivors. Many firefighters that attend talk about the closure it brings for them as they witness burn survivors and their families living meaningful lives. For individuals who are active in the burn support community at a local level, WBC serves as a wonderful networking opportunity.

The Phoenix Society for Burn Survivors serves as a National Resource Center for all survivors. They can direct a person to children's burn camps, adult retreats, and young adult summits throughout the nation. This is the leading national nonprofit organization dedicated to empowering any person affected by a burn injury through peer support, education, and advocacy. For over 30 years, the Phoenix Society has partnered with survivors, families, health care professionals, burn centers, and the fire industry to support recovery, improve the quality of burn care, and prevent burn injury. They promote and support a positive return to life and living (www.phoenix-society.org).

Phoenix Society Resources:

SOAR (Survivors Offering Assistance to Recovery)

World Burn Congress

On-line Learning

On-line Support Community (Chat)

The Journey Back (School Re-Entry)

Burn Support News

BEST Image Enhancement Program

STEPS Social Skills Training

Phoenix Educational Grants

Prevention and Advocacy

Speakers Bureau.

For further information, visit www.phoenix-society.org (800-888-2876).

The process of psychosocially adapting to a severe burn is complex (Corry, Pruzinsky, & Rumsey, 2009). Common issues faced by burn survivors include traumatic stress, depression, body image disturbance, social anxiety, grief, pain, itching, sleep disturbance, substance abuse, adapting to physical limitations, and coping with permanent burn scarring. In addition, burns often interfere with a person's ability to work and perform familial responsibilities (Blakeley et al., 2008). At times, the survivor's family is also traumatized, and the family's material and social resources can be greatly taxed during the course of burn recovery. Despite the sudden life-altering nature of burn injuries, studies of the psychological morbidity for burn survivors suggest that most burn survivors are resilient and adjust well over time.

References

Acton, A., Mounsey, E., & Gilyard, C. (2007). The burn survivor perspective. *Journal of Burn Care and Research, 281*(4), 1–6.

American Burn Association (ABA). (2012). *Burn incidence and treatment in the United States: 2012 fact sheet.* Chicago, IL: Author.

Blakeney, P., & Meyer, W. (1994). Psychological aspects of burn care. *Trauma Quarterly, 11*(2), 166–179.

Blakeney, P., Rosenberg, L., Rosenberg, M., & Faber, A. W. (2008). Psychosocial care of persons with severe burns. *Burns, 34*(4), 433–440.

Corry, N., Pruzinsky, T., & Rumsey, N. (2009). Quality of life and psychosocial adjustment to burn injury: Social functioning, body image, and health policy perspectives. *International Review of Psychiatry, 21*(6), 539–548.

Gilboa, D. (2001). Long term psychosocial adjustment after burn injury. *Burns, 27*, 335–341.

Herman, J. (1997). *Trauma and recovery.* New York, NY: Basic Books.

Kammerer-Quayle, B. (2002). Image and behavioral skills training for people with facial difference and disability. In M. G. Brodwin, F. A. Tellez, & S. K. Brodwin (Eds.), *Medical, psychosocial, and vocational aspects of disability* (2nd ed., pp. 95–106). Athens, GA: Elliott & Fitzpatrick.

Livneh, H. (2012). On the origins of negative attitudes toward people with disabilities. In I. Marini & M. A. Stebnicki (Eds.), *The psychological and social impact of illness and disability* (6th ed., pp. 13–25). New York, NY: Springer.

Livneh, H., & Antonak, R. F. (2012). Psychological adaptation to chronic illness and disability. In I. Marini & M. A. Stebnicki (Eds.), *The psychological and social impact of illness and disability* (6th ed., pp. 95–107). New York, NY: Springer.

Phoenix Society for Burn Survivors. (2013). Retrieved from http://www.phoenix-society.org

Spurr, E. D., & Shakespeare, P. G. (1990). Incidence of hypertropic scarring in burn-injured children. *Burn, 16*, 179–181.

Watkins, P. N., Cook, E. L., May, S. R., & Ehleben, C. M. (1998). Psychological stages in adaptation following burn injury: A method for facilitating psychological recovery of burn victims. *Journal of Burn Care and Rehabilitation, 9*(4), 420–424.

WebMD. (2011). *First aid and emergences: Rules of Nines*. Retrieved from http://www.webmd.com/first-aid/rule-of-nines

WebMD. (2013). *An overview of the skin*. Cleveland, OH: Cleveland Clinic. Retrieved from http://www.webmd.com/beauty/wrinkles/cosmetic-procedures-overview-skin

Young, A. W., Dewey, S., & Wolf, S. E. (2011). Rehabilitation in burns. In S. R. Flanagan, H. H. Zaretsky, & A. Moroz, *Medical aspects of disability: A handbook for the rehabilitation professional* (4th ed., pp. 89–101). New York, NY: Springer.

About the Authors

Cindy Rutter, R.N., B.S.N., is a burn survivor beginning over 55 years ago when she was six years old. After more than 100 surgeries before her 18th birthday, she has devoted her life advocating for burn survivors with the Phoenix Society. Ms. Rutter is a burn recovery nurse and the nurse manager of the University of California, San Diego (UCSD) Regional Burn Center. She is a member of the Phoenix Society's Aftercare Committee, a joint project with the American Burn Association that establishes standards for aftercare in the areas of rehabilitation and reintegration for those who have been affected by burn trauma. In 2011, Cindy received the Alan Breslau Award for her continued commitment to the burn community.

Ann Malo, R.N., has 25 years of nursing experience, including 20 years in burn critical care. Her career in nursing in the area of burns began in 1994 as a nurse for the UCSD Regional Burn Center. She has been active in pediatric burn camp and burn survivor support. Burn prevention education and patient care are her passions. Currently, Ms. Malo is an assistant nurse manager, Department of Surgery, UCSD Regional Burn Center.

Chapter 30

EVALUATING UPPER EXTREMITY FUNCTION AND IMPAIRMENT

George W. Balfour, M.D.
Martin G. Brodwin, Ph.D., C.R.C.
Ashley T. Du, M.S.

Introduction

While the occurrence of upper extremity injuries has become increasingly common, treatment of these types of disabilities has been developing for centuries. As early as 1717, an Italian physician wrote about "the harvest of diseases reaped by certain workers" caused by "certain violent and irregular motions and unnatural postures of the body that impair the natural structure of the vital machine." In the early 20th century, maladies that we call upper extremity disabilities were seen as distinct problems. These disabilities were named individually after the specific blue-collar occupation in which they developed. *Stitcher's wrist*, *bricklayer's shoulder*, *cottontwister's hand*, *writer's cramp*, and *telegraphist's cramp*, are examples of documented upper extremity disabilities. More recently, upper extremity disabilities have been documented within populations of *white collar* workers. Telegraphers were once noted to get *telegraphist's cramp*, for instance, while workers with clerical occupations got *writer's cramp*. Today, upper extremity disabilities are found in all populations of workers, including high-technology fields, such as software engineering, online brokering, and customer service. According to the American Medical Association's (AMA) *Guides to the Evaluation of Permanent Impairment,* 60% percent of the function of a *whole person* is assigned to a single upper extremity, 90% of which is defined to be in the hand (American Medical Association, 2009). Hand function represents more than half (54%) of one's total body functioning. From this medical definition of impairment, the rehabilitation counselor can more readily understand the impact of a hand injury on an individual's ability to function in the workplace. This chapter addresses the etiology of upper extremity injuries, function of the hand, anatomy and physiology of the upper extremity, assessment of impairment, and evaluation and treatment of injuries. Additionally, the chapter covers work and physical capacity, evaluation, functional limitations, work limitations, rehabilitation potential, and assistive technology. Lastly, the chapter concludes with a case study on a veteran who sustained an upper extremity injury during the service.

Etiology

Impairment is the loss of function in the physical sense, while disability is an inability to overcome or compensate for that impairment. Oskamp (1988) defined impairment and disability as follows: **Impairment** describes an abnormality or a loss of a physiological structure or function. **Disability** refers to the consequences of impairment – a restriction or lack of ability to perform some activity that is considered appropriate. Injuries resulting in upper extremity disabilities occur in many different ways and in a variety of different settings such as in the home, highway, sports field, battlefield, and workplace. Internationally, injuries to the hand and upper extremity represent approximately one-third of all work-related injuries. In 2011, approximately 357,000 people working in business and industry in the United States lost time from work due to a hand injury (Bureau of Labor Statistics, 2011). Upper extremity injuries are additionally characterized by long periods of recovery. The better these injuries are understood, the more that can be contributed to the economic, personal, social, and vocational rehabilitation of those injured.

Function of the Hand

A variety of functions rely on the movement of the hands, including sensory, fine manipulation, gripping, cosmetic appearances, and use in social interactions. The hand is a sensory organ; a high concentration of nerve endings in the palms and fingers provide information about one's environment. Imagine picking up an object, feeling it, and discerning its weight, hardness, surface texture, temperature, size, and shape. The somasensory surface of the brain receives signals from touch. Figure 1 is a schematic picture of the somasensory area of the brain that depicts the proportion of brain tissue devoted to the sense of touch. Note that only the lips and face are given more area than the hand. Other areas of the body, like the face or thigh, are not able to read objects with the same accuracy or detail identification as the fingers. The amount of brain surface devoted to a body part is proportional to the sensitivity of that body part. The hand's high sensitivity to touch, for example, is a result of the high concentration of nerve endings in this area, particularly the palmar skin.

Besides providing sensory input, the hands function as the primary instrument of the upper extremities for functions like grasping, lifting, and carrying. Hands also perform fine and gross manipulative tasks such as turning a key, holding a glass, crafting, writing, using tools, and operating office equipment. Hands are also important in social situations: shaking, holding hands, and gesturing of this part of the body signals characteristics such as feelings, emotions, greetings, and enthusiasm. The hands also serve cosmetic purposes, such as painting fingernails, wearing rings, and putting on gloves. Hands also function during activities requiring gross strength (i.e., in lifting, carrying, pushing, pulling, and while using large tools). When working with shovels, hammers, or saws, the function of the hand is to grip and hold the equipment; the principal force and motion occurs at the wrist, forearm, elbow, and shoulder. During the assessment of impairment and rehabilitation potential, each of these multi-faceted functions and any associated limitations needs to be assessed (Strickland & Graham, 2005).

FIGURE 1
Mannequin Illustration of Sensory Distribution of the Central Gyrus of the Cerebral Cortex

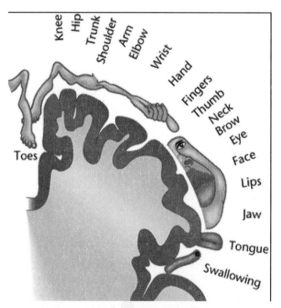

Source: Trux, R. C., & M. B., Carpenter. (1969). *Human anatomy* (6th ed., p. 559). Baltimore, MD: Williams & Wilkins.

Anatomy and Physiology of the Upper Extremity

Neurological

Median Nerve

This nerve supplies sensation to the palm and palmar aspects of the thumb, index, long, and radial half of the ring finger. It is the most important sensory nerve to the hand and is the motor nerve for most of the muscles of the ventral forearm (forearm flexors), the muscles that bend and flex the wrist and flex or close the fingers and thumb. These median nerve controlled flexors provide power for gripping, lifting, and flexing the wrist (Wolfe, Hotchkiss, Pederson, & Kozin, 2010). Below the wrist, the median nerve supplies motor and muscle innervation to the small, intrinsic muscles of the thumb (the thenar muscles) which aid in rowing the thumb out of the plane of the palm into opposition, and contribute to the power of pinch. Median nerve injuries are classified as either *high* or *low* (Strickland & Graham, 2005). A *high* median nerve injury results in an inability to flex the wrist, fingers, and thumb. This type of injury makes gripping of objects impossible and causes numbness of the thumb, index, center fingers, and half of the ring finger. Contrastingly, a *low* median nerve injury causes numbness and weakness of the intrinsic muscles of the thumb, preventing actions relying on these muscles, such as pinching, turning a key, or in touching the tip of the thumb to the tip of the little finger.

Ulnar Nerve

In the hand, the ulnar nerve provides sensation to the little finger, the ulna half of the ring finger, and muscle innervation and control to the small intrinsic muscles of the hand. Intrinsic muscles provide balance to the fingers and fine manipulative control of the hand. Injury to the ulnar nerve principally impairs dexterity and fine manipulation, including functions like pinch and manipulation of small objects, such as screws, coins, and buttons.

Radial Nerve

The radial nerve is the sensory nerve for the back (dorsum) of the hand and thumb. In the forearm, it supplies muscle innervation to the extensor muscle group. These muscles extend the wrist, fingers, and thumb. Radial palsy leads to wrist drop, a condition in which the hand drops toward the ground because the person is unable to raise the hand or fingers against gravity. A lower radial nerve injury causes numbness (Trumble & Buddoff, 2007).

Muscular

Forearm

There are two sets of extrinsic muscles (those located outside the hand itself) in the forearm, the ventral (flexion group) and the dorsal (extensor group). Ventral extrinsic forearm muscles (flexors), reach the hand through tendons and act to flex or bend the wrist and fingers. An extensor group of extrinsic muscles functions principally to extend the wrist, fingers, and thumb; they are innervated by the ulnar nerve (except those of the thumb) and balance finger motion, add strength to grip, and abduct and adduct the fingers (Wolfe et al., 2010). To examine radial nerve function, the physician looks for wrist extension. To test median nerve function, thumb flexion is evaluated. In the case of ulnar nerve function, the physician assesses isolated abduction of the index finger.

Vascular

Most arterial injuries are due to direct laceration, blunt trauma, or thrombosis. Lacerations compromise the blood supply to the affected part (Trumble & Buddoff, 2007). If there is no collateral circulation to a body part, it will become ischemic (deficient in blood) and die. Collateral circulation means that two vessels supply the same part or area. If only one vessel is damaged, collateral circulation (the alternative blood pathway) may be adequate to keep the part alive and functional. Completely divided vessels usually retract, rapidly clot, and then bleeding ceases. Partially divided vessels cannot retract and, therefore, may allow serious blood loss to occur. If an intact vessel clots off because of blunt trauma, an embolism, or arteriosclerosis, the result is loss of blood supply through that particular vessel (Wolfe et al., 2010). Upper extremity hand injuries impacting the blood flow to the hand may result in cold intolerance.

Kinesiology

Combined function of the shoulder, elbow, and wrist allows the hand to move anywhere within a large circular area. The shoulder girdle consists of the arm, scapula, and clavicle. The elbow is a complex set of three joints that control the simple extension and flexion of the elbow and supination (palm up) or pronation (palm down). The wrist involves a complex set of joints that function in supination and pronation, the turning of the hand palm up and palm down. It functions in dorsiflexion and palmar flexion movement of the hand upward and downward (as in the hand motion of saying good-bye), and in radial and ulnar deviation (motion of the hand from side to side) (Baratz, Rosenwasser, Adams, & Kozin, 2006; Geissler, 2005).

The Dermis

Palmar Skin

Skin serves as an outer covering of the body, protecting it from the external environment. Palmar skin is specialized in that it is thicker than the rest of the skin. The early healing phase typically takes three months to resolve, an important characteristic for the rehabilitation counselor to know when providing vocational services for workers with injuries involving the palms. Defects in palmar skin caused by injury such as tears, lacerations, or burns can be covered or replaced with grafted skin or skin flaps. Skin graft is a thin layer of healthy skin removed from one site and placed in an area needing skin coverage. Transferred skin, as compared to palmar skin, is thinner, more mobile, and less adherent to deep structures. Full thickness graft may involve skin with hair follicles. In persons with dark skin, the skin often becomes hyperpigmented (increased pigmentation). A physician may utilize a variety of flaps to provide thicker more durable skin (Jebson & Kasdan, 2006; Trumble & Allan, 2000).

Nails

The nails are specialized structures that act as protective covering for the tips of the fingers. An open wound near or under the nail is a source of pain and a viable route for infection. Nail injuries can heal abnormally with ridges or splits, also known as bifid nails (Jebson & Kasdan, 2006).

Functional Limitations in Commonly Occurring Hand Injuries

Finger Injuries

Fingertip injuries are the most common industrial accidents and the most frequent reason for amputation (Burke, 2005). As a guide, the entire thumb contributes to 40% of hand function, while the long and ring fingers contribute 20% each. The border digits (the index and little fingers) account for 10% each. The loss of several digits increases impairment more than the sum of the parts lost. Multiple digit injuries require longer recovery time, more hand therapy to regain motion and strength, and result in greater residual impairment (American Medical Association, 2009; Beasley, 2003). Variables involved include level of amputation, amount of soft tissue coverage on the remaining part, presence or absence of tender neuromas or bone prominence, and nail deformities. Involvement of flexor tendons influences the person's strength, active motion, and range of motion.

Hand Fractures

Fractures are another common hand injury in industry, with each kind of fracture having a different treatment and prognosis. Physicians can splint simple non-displaced, non-angulation, and non-articular fractures; usually, these fractures heal within three weeks. Employees can typically return to work within six to eight weeks. If the fracture is displaced, angulated, intra-articular, and therefore requires reduction or surgery, the time for healing to resolve stiffness, regain strength, and return to work is much longer. Some of the residual effects may be permanent. Residuals such as tendon adherence (scar between the tendon and bone) can prevent returning to customary work. Common sites for tendon adhesions following surgery are the extensor tendons over the middle and proximal phalanges. For an individual with tendon adherence, the only way to regain motion may be through surgical intervention. Full range of motion is rarely regained after surgery, and manipulative tasks are often impaired as a result (American Occupational Therapy Association, 2013).

Wrist Fractures

The most frequent wrist fractures involve the waist of the scaphoid, one of the eight small bones of the wrist (Baratz et al., 2006). Median time to union in non-displaced fractures is 15 weeks, and the non-union (non-healing) rate is high (in some research reports as high as 40%). Following injury, stiffness and weakness are common; return to heavy labor takes an extensive period of time.

Carpal Tunnel Syndrome

The carpel tunnel is the final common pathway of multiple conditions, all of which increase pressure within the wrist (Katz & Simmons, 2002). Symptoms include tingling, numbness, weakness, and pain (WebMD, 2010). Carpal tunnel syndrome is the most common nerve compression syndrome. Thyroid disease, masses, extra muscles (congenital), rheumatoid arthritis, amyloidosis, repetitive trauma, vibration disease syndrome, synovial hypertrophy, and prior wrist fractures are some of the causes of carpal tunnel. Repetitive use of the hand, as in a cashier's use of an optical scanner throughout the work shift, or activities like typing, packing, and assembling, frequently are the basis of claims of an industrial etiology. Young workers may also develop carpal tunnel as the result of vibrator tools such as pneumatic tools, jackhammers, and power wrenches. Factors which increase the occurrences of carpal tunnel syndrome in women include gender, age, generalized mild synovitis, and physique. Those at or near the age of 40, and women with thin or fragile physiques are more prone to carpal tunnel. Initial conservative treatment consists of decreased use of the wrist, splints, non-steroidal anti-inflammatory medication, and diuretics. Test results indicating carpal tunnel include an abnormal nerve conduction time and an irregular vibratory sense test. If the diagnosis is confirmed, steroid injections into the wrist are given; if this fails and the symptoms are severe and prolonged, surgical decompression may be necessary (Mosier & Hughes, 2013). Following surgery, the individual is splinted in dorsiflexion for a month and the scar can remain tender for up to six months. Return to work will take two to twelve weeks, depending upon the physical demands of the job. Clerical or professional occupations take less recovery time than more physically demanding occupations.

Assessment of Impairment

Assessment of impairment is accomplished using a scoring system which assigns specific values to various functions (Mink Van Der Molen, Ettema, & Hovius, 2003). Within the hand, evaluated functions include loss of parts (amputation), cosmetic defects, pain, tenderness, diminished sensation, limited range of motion, and loss of strength. An assessment must describe subjective pain, including intensity and frequency, along with the appearance of the hand, together with the presence of dirt or calluses, and condition of the nails. An evaluator describes sensation using a variety of testing methods; the report measures loss of parts, presence of scars, ranges of motion, and strength of grip, pinch, lifting, and resistance. In the first part of the evaluation of the upper extremity, the individual reports his or her functional history and present activities. It is best to ask about a variety of activities rather than simply having patients list their functional limitations. The history needs to illustrate the patient's functional capabilities by describing duration and frequency of performed activities. Similarly, the report should explain activities that cannot be performed. Questions concerning lifting, carrying, pushing, pulling, gripping, pinching, manipulating, and sensing are all relevant to the physician's overall assessment of injury (Meyer, 2003).

Range of Motion

The American Academy of Orthopaedic Surgeons has published standards for measuring joint motion. Each joint has a normal or typical range of motion and for any individual, the extremity on the opposite side is used as a normal standard (Wolfe et al., 2010).

Grip Loss

Atrophy can be caused by injury, disease, and disuse. Forearm circumference is measured as an estimation of atrophy; the physician compares the uninvolved extremity as a control to the involved side. Grip strength is measured with a calibrated dynamometer. The ratio between the involved and uninvolved hand determines grip loss.

Radiological Assessment

An examination requires radiological evaluation to define the status of the skeletal system and the degree of joint injury, disorganization, and degeneration (Weiss & Falkerstein, 2013). Bone shortening and angulation is reported in degrees. Density changes, for example, from disuse (osteopenia) are seen on x-rays as thinner, less dense, and more radiolucent bone tissue. The examiner notes joint surface changes, narrowing, sclerosis, fractures, osteophytes, arthritic changes, joint displacements (subluxations), and any additional x-ray findings (Strickland & Graham, 2005).

Medical Reporting

Medical reports begin with subjective complaints and extend to the history of the medical problem or injury in which the individual's past occupational record and social functioning are addressed, followed by the physical examination. The physical exam contains inspection, palpation, range of motion, muscle testing, neurological examination, and results of special tests including x-rays, MRIs, and CAT scans. Recently, there has been emphasis on patient self-reporting tests in the form of examinations, such as patient completed hand diagrams. In such a diagram, the patient is asked to draw his or her symptoms, pain, and numbness on a drawing of a hand. Another form of patient reporting is the DASH (Disability Arm Shoulder Hand) score or a similar patient completed report (Kennedy, Beaton, Solway, Mconnel, & Bombardier, 2011).

Pain and Sensory Deterioration

Pain

Pain is a unique and subjective experience which varies among individuals. *Nosocomia* is defined as a physically unpleasant experience; pain is the individual's perception of that experience. If you take a standardized needle and stick it an equal depth at an equal rate into a dozen individuals, each experiences an equal amount of nosocomia (unpleasant stimulation). Yet, each person describes a different degree and sensation of pain. Swanson, Goran-Hagert, and Swanson (1987) defined pain as "a disagreeable sensation that has as its basis a highly variable complex made up of afferent nerve stimuli interacting with the emotional state of the individual and modified by past experience, motivation, and state of mind" (p. 896). Readers can refer to the Chronic Pain Management chapter for more information on the impact of pain on individuals with upper extremity disabilities.

Sensory Deficits

Subjective complaints of sensory deficits are measurable and, in some patients, quantifiable. Testing for sensory deficits includes distinguishing sharp from dull, static two-point discrimination, moving two-point discrimination, Von Frey hair testing, hot versus cold discrimination, propioception, coin discrimination, and vibration. *Propioception* is the sense that indicates body position. It tells physicians if our hands are open or closed, if they are below our waists or over our heads, and allows us to perform activities such as typing without looking at the keyboard. Propioception can be tested by placing the hand behind a screen to hide it from visual feedback (Geissler, 2005). Stereoagnosis is the sense that allows a person to read or see objects by feel; it is how one tells a dime from a quarter in a pocket without visual feedback, and how Braille is read. Patients with nerve lacerations and poor recovery, or following stroke or spinal cord injury often have severe sensory impairments, and may simply ignore the severely impaired hand; the hand then becomes nonfunctional solely on a sensory basis.

Nerve Compression

Individuals with nerve compression syndromes, such as herniated disks (causing pressure on nerve roots), thoracic outlet syndrome, cubital tunnel syndrome, and carpal tunnel syndrome, also experience decreased sensibility (capability to feel or perceive). Individuals experiencing these losses lose the sense of vibration more than the ability to perceive two-point discrimination. Anyone can experience the sensation of a compression syndrome by crossing the legs until one leg *falls asleep*. *Pins and needles* sensations, deep aching, a loss of the sense of position, and spontaneously dropping objects are associated with compression syndrome (Skirven, Osterman, Fedorczyk, & Amadio, 2011; Wolfe et al., 2010).

Evaluation and Treatment of Injury

Evaluation

Evaluation of upper extremity injuries follows a consistent procedure and order of priorities. The first step includes obtaining a detailed history and physical. During the physical, any abnormalities are noted and each injury is categorized in relation to the skin, color, and overall condition of the hand. Specific examinations will be administered for particular injuries. For example, palpation demonstrates losses of tendon continuity, fractures, dislocations, and torn ligaments. Loss of sensation is tested by touch or pinprick. Radiologic examination (x-rays) provides detail of bone injury and indicates the presence of metal and other foreign bodies.

Treatment

Once the surgeon understands the injury, he or she formulates a treatment plan. If the injury being treated involves an open wound, the first priority is to clean the exposed tissues and remove any bacterial contamination. Individuals with vascular injuries may need arterial and occasionally venous repair. If, however, the vascular injury is categorized as vascular insufficiency, emergency care is necessary. In the case of venous insufficiency, muscle tissue not receiving an adequate blood supply dies within six hours while other tissues of the hand become necrotic less quickly. The patient must undergo repair of tendons, nerves, and skin, though this procedure can be delayed. Skin coverage is done immediately and before any deeper structures are reconstructed to avoid infection and problems due to scaring. The simplest skin replacement is performed with a skin graft in which an extremely thin layer of skin is taken from a healthy place on the body and sewn over a defect or open wound (Trumble & Allan, 2000; Weiss & Falkerstein, 2013).

Stabilization

When a patient has a deformity that cannot be corrected by non-operative methods, he or she undergoes a fracture stabilization procedure. The usual reason for instability is that an unopposed muscle or ligament force creates and maintains a deformity. Another indication for fracture fixation is when the fracture involves a joint surface. Joints are like machine parts; if their smooth surfaces heal unevenly, joint wear is accelerated, eventually leading to painful arthritis. The simplest method of internal fixation includes straight smooth pins which are drilled across the fracture to stabilize the area until it is healed. Many different types of fixation devices can be used (Cohen & Edelstein, 2011).

Ligaments

Many ligament injuries heal spontaneously, while others require casting or surgery. Incomplete tears heal independently with time, but complete tears need surgical repair. Torn ligaments that are not repaired become sources of chronic instability and impairment and, if neglected, will lead to arthritis.

Tendons

Tendon injuries include acute laceration, rupture, avulsion from the bony sites of attachment, erosion (such as in rheumatoid arthritis), attrition, and tendonitis. Tendonitis is a series of very small tears in the tissue or surrounding tendon (WebMD, 2010). Tendons are repaired end-to-end, replaced by tendon graft, or substituted by tendon transfer. Other conditions causing pain can be acute or result in chronic inflammation, such as those which occur in cases of tendonitis of an elbow or knee joint (Burke, 2005). Tendon graft operations are used to avoid problems of scarring by placing tendon suture lines outside of tight areas, lessening the risk of adhesion. These tendon transfer procedures involve rerouting of a muscle tendon complex to a new site of action to replace a lost motor function.

Newer Developments

Like all medical specialties, the discipline of hand surgery continues to evolve (Jebson & Kasdan, 2006). In the past few decades, microsurgery has developed from a research tool into a viable technique commonly performed throughout the country. Free tissue transfers have become common practice and are widely accepted. Arthroscopic surgery, initially developed for the knee, has become an accepted approach for the shoulder, elbow, and wrist (McBeath & Osterman, 2012). Arthoscopic procedures are being performed on small joints, such as metacarpal/carpal joints and metacarpal/phalangeal joints. Similarly, fracture treatment has continued to improve with newer, smaller, and stronger implants and progressively less invasive methods. Surgical treatment plans that only a few years ago would have been considered too risky to attempt have now become accepted surgical practice (Strickland & Graham, 2005).

Work and Physical Capacity Evaluation

Work capacity evaluation measures the capability of a person to function over time. Under the direction of a physician, occupational therapists and work evaluation specialists observe the individual performing tasks over several days to provide an accurate assessment. Specific capacity testing enables the evaluator to quantify the capacity to perform work-related actions. Physical capacity evaluation documents a person's hand function, including strength and range of motion (Skirven et al., 2011). The three components to physical capacity evaluation include administration of hand function tasks, standardized tests, and observation of the person performing the physical demands of the job. An accurate and detailed job description tailored to the specific worker's impairments helps a physician determine if the individual is capable of returning to the previous job, with or without accommodation.

Work Limitations

Injuries to the upper extremities cause limitations in eye-hand coordination, range of motion in one or both hands, manual dexterity, strength for lifting and carrying, as well as pushing and pulling activities (Meyer, 2003). Accommodating such an employee at the workplace may involve dividing heavier weights or large items into lighter or smaller units. Use of mechanical lifts and movable carts decrease lifting and carrying (Mueller, 1990). The most effective way to meet the accommodation needs of the client is to complete a detailed job analysis, paying particular attention to job functions requiring use of the injured hand(s). A step-by-step analysis allows the counselor and injured employee to work with the employer in suggesting reasonable accommodation which benefits both the employee and employer (Brodwin, Parker, & DeLaGarza, 2010). Many people who have serious hand injuries are unable to return to their previous employment because of residual impairments. As a result, some employers offer lighter duty work or a different position within the company. Rehabilitation counselors additionally can provide suggestions concerning alterations to the work environment that will accommodate impairments. In addition to possessing an enhanced awareness of their environment, persons with severe upper extremity injuries, including amputation, face attitudinal, psychosocial, and emotional adjustments. Limitations in activities which can be performed and changes in body image may require an adaptation period. Many individuals also benefit from short-term counseling or in-depth psychological intervention (Livneh & Antonek, 2012). Factors such as a person's interpretation of loss of function, circumstances involved with the injury, premorbid personality (personality before the loss), and extent of loss help the counselor analyze needed rehabilitation and psychological services. Emotionally, everyone reacts differently to injury and impairment. Psychological counseling is an important aspect of rehabilitation for many individuals. Some persons with disfigured hands may engage in various activities and do not feel self-conscious while in public. Others, with even minor injuries, attempt to hide their hand(s) from sight (Vash & Crewe, 2004). The counselor needs to evaluate the impairment considering individual needs.

Assistive Technology

The goal of assistive technology is to increase the functional independence for people who have disabilities. The focus is not on the disability but on the remaining functional (residual) abilities that individuals use to accomplish their chosen objectives and daily tasks. Because the vast majority of jobs require use of the hands and fingers, counselors must be adept at providing accommodation for workers with upper extremity injuries. There are a variety of orthotic and prosthetic hand devices that provide improved function. Prostheses are artificial devices used to replace a missing body part, and orthoses are specialized mechanical devices used to support or supplement weak or damaged joints and limbs (Cohen & Edelstein, 2011). Individuals who use prosthetic and orthotic devices should cultivate an increased awareness of their environment to assure proper functioning of the devices. These devices can be modified to accommodate specific job duties. For example, an adaptive device allowed a filling station attendant, who had lost two fingers from his dominant hand, to pump gasoline. The device was worn only for this job duty and, in essence, was a custom tool that was put away when the worker performed other job functions. Orthotists and prosthetists custom design a variety of devices to help workers perform job duties. The following orthoses may improve an employee's function of the upper extremities: a wrist-hand orthoses, a wrist-driven wrist-hand orthoses, and a shoulder-elbow orthoses. Upper limb orthoses can substitute for the absence of muscle power, assist or support weak areas of the upper extremity, or be used for the attachment of specialized assistive devices (Clawson, 2009). Ability to use the hand involves sensibility, dexterity, and mobility. Rehabilitation of hand injuries often requires time and effort; maximum return of function is the goal of the hand surgeon, hand therapist, work evaluator, and rehabilitation counselor. Counselors must work closely with other professionals to return the person to employment. At the workplace, use of upper extremity prostheses enhances manual dexterity, bilateral dexterity, eye-hand coordination, grabbing, grasping, lifting, and carrying. Although a prosthesis does not replace a fully functioning arm and hand, it may allow an employee to perform necessary work tasks (Clawson, 2009). A workstation, with accommodation and job modification, can help the worker with an upper extremity limitation to efficiently perform required work functions. For additional information, the reader is referred to the Orthotics, Amputation, and Prosthetics chapter.

Rehabilitation Potential

Potential for rehabilitation depends on multiple factors, including whether the injury involves the dominant or non-dominant hand. When the dominant hand is severely injured, training to improve use of the opposite hand is appropriate (American Occupational Therapy Association, 2013). A plan of physical rehabilitation includes:

- Strengthening exercises.
- Exercises to develop skills in activities of daily living.
- Writing exercises.
- Activities to improve manual dexterity.

Hand injuries cause different functional limitations and thus have varying rehabilitation potential. Attitude and motivation play a significant role in the potential for rehabilitation and success in returning to work (Brodwin et al., 2010). When serious injuries result in major impairment, the motivation and attitude of a person may mean the difference between successful medical and vocational rehabilitation and failure. Highly motivated individuals with severe impairment enjoy greater success rates than people who are not as motivated, even if they have significantly less impairment.

Other factors contributing to rehabilitation potential include age, educational level, and work history. Younger, more educated persons with skilled or professional work backgrounds can more readily adjust to impairment and disability, while older workers are more tolerant of residual discomfort. The role of the counselor is to go beyond the injury to include the entire person and his or her functional needs and roles. A comprehensive plan may include therapeutic activities, joint protection, energy modification, sensory re-education, scar management, pain management, work conditioning, and training in activities of daily living. Counselors need knowledge in the following adjunct areas of treatment: wound care, design and fabrication of orthotics, ergonomic principles, diagnostic and post-surgical protocols, manual therapy, biofeedback techniques, and compression therapy (American Occupational Therapy Association, 2013).

Conclusion

Approximately 4.3 million people in the United States have some form of limitation involving impairments of manual dexterity, range of motion, strength, and endurance of the hands and arms. Of this number, almost 357,000 employees are unable to fully use their upper extremities in a significant way. This figure includes people with paralysis or absence of part or all of one or both upper extremities. Many industrial injuries involve the hands and fingers, causing different degrees of impairment depending upon the extent of injury, loss of function, and the dominancy of the hand. Rehabilitation counselors must possess knowledge of hand function and impairment so that they may recommend rehabilitation plans and reasonable accommodations for workers with these disabilities (Brodwin et al., 2010).

Case Study

Jeremy Moore is 34 years of age, married, father of two elementary-aged children, and right-hand dominant. Currently, Jeremy is a Ph.D. candidate in biomedical engineering and has a Master's degree in both Mechanical Engineering and Industrial Design. Before being deployed to Iraq, Jeremy worked in the research and development of tools for biomedical robotic cardiac surgery for a major company. Much of his work involved the use of computers. In Iraq, insurgents ambushed Jeremy's patrol, detonating a device packed with shrapnel and explosives. Jeremy was wounded in the initial explosion, sustaining a massive crush-type injury to his right forearm and hand. The injury included an open proximal radius fracture, skin loss, a long finger metacarpal fracture, and a major muscle injury requiring debridement of non-viable tissue. Initial surgical treatment consisted of wound debridement, internal fixation of the fractures, an intrinsic muscle compartment fasciotomy (surgical incision and division), and split thickness skin grafts. Within two months after his surgery, Mr. Moore's scars were healed and he could fully open and close his hand. Yet, range of motion in his wrist was diminished by 40% and his grip was classified as 50% decreased. Jeremy is interested in assistive technology (AT) as it relates to assisting him with his graduate studies and return to work options.

Questions

1. Define *impairment* and *disability*. Distinguish between these concepts in this case.
2. Discuss attorney involvement with this case and how it would impact your services.
3. As Jeremy Moore's rehabilitation counselor, identify several rehabilitation plans for assisting him in returning to gainful employment.
4. Can Mr. Moore return to his prior job based on his physical limitations? Is the job realistic for this individual?
5. Given Jeremy's education and interests, what AT can you identify that would assist him in his academic goal od completing his Ph.D. program and for returning to gainful employment?

References

American Medical Association. (2009). *Guides to the evaluation of permanent impairment* (6th ed.). Chicago, IL: Author.

American Occupational Therapy Association. (2013). *The role of occupational therapy for rehabilitation of the upper extremity* (Fact sheet). Retrieved from http://www.aota.org/~/media/Corporate/Files/AboutOT/Professionals/WhatIsOT/RDP/Facts/Hand%20Therapy%20fact%20sheet.ashx

Baratz, M. E., Rosenwasser, M. P., Adams, B. D., & Kozin, S. H. (2006). *Wrist surgery: Tricks of the trade.* New York, NY: Thieme.

Beasley, R. W. (2003). *Beasley's surgery of the hand.* New York, NY: Thieme.

Brodwin, M. G., Parker, R. M., & DeLaGarza, D. (2010). Disability and reasonable accommodation. In E. M. Szymanski & R. M. Parker (Eds.), *Work and disability: Contexts, issues, and strategies in career development and job placement* (3rd ed., pp. 281–323). Austin, TX: Pro-ed.

Bureau of Labor Statistics. (2011). *Number of nonfatal occupational injuries & illnesses involving days away from work.* Retrieved from http://www.bls.gov.iif/oshwc/osh

Burke, S. L. (2005). *Hand and upper extremity rehabilitation: A practical guide* (3rd ed.). St. Louis, MO: Elsevier Churchill Livingston.

Clawson, L. R. (2009). Orthotics, amputation, and prosthetics. In M. G. Brodwin, F. W. Siu, J. Howard, & E. R. Brodwin (Eds.), *Medical, psychosocial, and vocational aspects of disability* (3rd ed., pp. 389–401). Athens, GA: Elliott and Fitzpatrick.

Cohen, J. M., & Edelstein, J. E. (2011). Joint deficiency. In S. Flanagan, H. H. Zaretsky, & A. Moroz (Eds.)., *Medical aspects of disability: A handbook for the rehabilitation professional* (4th ed., pp. 381–408). New York, NY: Springer.

Geissler, W. (Ed.). (2005). *Wrist hand arthroscopy.* New York, NY: Springer.

Jebson, P., & Kasdan, M. (Eds.). (2006). *Hand secrets* (3rd ed.). Philadelphia, PA: Hanley and Belfus.

Katz, J. N., & Simmons, B. P. (2002). Carpal tunnel syndrome. *New England Journal of Medicine, 346*(23), 1807–1812.

Kennedy, C. A., Beaton, D. E., Solway, S., McConnell, S., & Bombardier, C. (2011). *The DASH and Quickdash Outcome Measure User's Manual* (3rd ed.). Toronto, Canada: Institute for Work and Health.

Livneh, H., & Antonek, R. F. (2012). Psychological adaption to chronic illness and disability: A primer for counselors. In I. Marini & M. Stebnicki (Eds.), *The psychological and social impact of illness and disability* (6th ed., pp. 95–107). New York, NY: Springer.

McBeath, R., & Osterman, A. L. (2012). Total wrist arthroplasty. *Hand Clinics, 28*(4), 595–609.

Meyer, T. M. (2003). Psychological aspects of mutilating hand injuries. *Hand Clinics, 19*(1), 41–49.

Mink Van Der Molen, A. R., Ettema, A. M., & Hovius, S. E. R. (2003). Outcome of hand trauma: The Hand Injury Severity Scoring System (HISS) and subsequent impairment and disability. *Journal of Hand Surgery, 28*(4), 295–299.

Mosier, B. A., & Hughes, T. B. (2013). Recurrent carpal tunnel syndrome. *Hand Clinics, 29*(3), 427–434.

Mueller, J. (1990). *The workplace workbook: An illustrated guide to job accommodation and assistive technology.* Washington, DC: Dole Foundation.

Oskamp, S. (1988). The editor's page. *Journal of Social Issues, 44.*

Skirven, T. M., Osterman, A. L., Fedorczyk, J., & Amadio, P. C. (2011). *Rehabilitation of the hand and upper extremity* (6th ed.). St. Louis, MO: Mosby.

Strickland, J. W., & Graham, T. (Eds.). (2005). *Master techniques in orthopaedc surgery: The hand.* Philadelphia, PA: Lippincott, Williams, and Wilkins.

Swanson, A. B., Goran-Hagert, C., & Swanson, G. D. (1987). Evaluation of impairment in the upper extremity. *Journal of Hand Surgery - Part 2, 12a*(5), 896–925.

Trumble, T. E., & Allan, C. H. (Eds.). (2000). *Nerve repair and reconstruction.* Philadelphia, PA: W. B. Saunders.

Trumble, T. E., & Buddoff, J. E. (Ed.). (2007). *Hand surgery update IV.* Rosemont, IL: American Academy of Orthopaedic Surgeons.

Trux, R. C., & Carpenter, M. B. (1969). *Human anatomy* (6th ed.). Baltimore, MD: Williams & Wilkins.

Vash, C. L., & Crewe, N. M. (2004). *Psychology of disability* (2nd ed.). New York, NY: Springer.

WebMD. (2010). *Finger, hand, and wrist injuries.* Retrieved from http://www.webmd.com/a-to-z-guides/finger-hand-and-wrist-injuries-topic-overview

Weiss, S., & Falkerstein, N. (Eds.) (2013). *Hand rehabilitation: A quick reference guide and review* (3rd ed.). St. Louis, MO: Mosby.

Wolfe, S. W., Hotchkiss, R. N., Pederson, W. C., & Kozin, S. H. (2010). *Green's operative hand surgery* (6th ed.). New York, NY: Churchill Livingstone.

About the Authors

George W. Balfour, M. D., is an orthopedic surgeon specializing in surgery of the hand. He is in private practice in Van Nuys, California, and is Assistant Professor of Surgery and Director of the Hand Clinic at the Charles R. Drew School of Medicine - Martin Luther King, Jr. Medical Center in Los Angeles. Active in the American Association for Hand Surgery and the American Society for Surgery of the Hand, Dr. Balfour has a special interest and expertise in microvascular surgery.

Martin G. Brodwin, Ph.D, C.R.C., is Professor and Coordinator of the Rehabilitation Counselor Education Program at California State University, Los Angeles. He is a vocational expert for the Office of Disability Adjudication and Review, Social Security Administration, providing testimony on disability-related issues. As a rehabilitation consultant, Dr. Brodwin provides assessment for long-term disability, case management, and reasonable accommodation. He has published over 100 refereed journal articles, book chapters, and books on the subjects of counseling, disability, rehabilitation, and accommodation in business and industry.

Ashley Du, M.S., received her Master of Science degree in Counseling, with options in rehabilitation and school counseling leadership. Her interests are in the areas of chronic pain management and in providing the most effective counseling and rehabilitation services for students. Ms. Du specializes in transitional counseling with an emphasis in college and career.

Chapter 31

ASSISTIVE TECHNOLOGY AND UNIVERSAL DESIGN

R. David Black, Ed.D., C.R.C.
Martin G. Brodwin, Ph.D., C.R.C.

Introduction

People with chronic illness and disability are seeing the benefits of assistive technology (AT), and are increasingly using it to join mainstream society. This development, in turn, benefits society as people with disabilities become more independent and less reliant on public services. As people with disabilities' income increases, so too does their purchasing power to buy goods, services, and products. The field of AT is helping people with disabilities increase or restore functioning, enhance their quality of life, and integrate into society, both physically and emotionally.

Assistive Technology

Definitions

Assistive technology is defined in the Technology-Related Assistance for Individuals with Disabilities Act of 1988 as "any item, piece of equipment, or product system, whether acquired commercially off the shelf, modified, or customized, that is used to increase, maintain, or improve functional capabilities of people with disabilities." Technology service is "any service that directly assists an individual with a disability in the selection, acquisition, or use of an assistive technology device" (Assistive Technology Act, 1998). More than 20 million Americans with disabilities are using assistive devices, equipment, computers, and other apparatus. People benefit from assistive technology at work, in school, at home, and in leisure time activities.

Use of Technology

Practitioners using AT will be able to provide more meaningful, practical, and realistic clinical counseling and services for their clients. As noted by Scherer (2007), technology is radically changing the lives of individuals who have disabilities. AT has helped enhance the quality of life and extend the lifespan of persons with congenital and developmental disabilities, as well as those who have acquired disabilities and chronic medical conditions.

Devices and equipment may be low-tech (mechanical) or high-tech (electromechanical or computer-related) and can help compensate for sensory and functional loss. AT provides the means to move (e.g., adaptive equipment on vehicles, wheelchairs [including power wheelchairs], scooters, lifts), speak (e.g., augmentative and alternative communication devices), read (e.g., Braille input, voice recognition devices), hear (telecommunication devices for the deaf [TDD], hearing aides, audio loops), and manage self-care tasks (e.g., remote environmental control systems, prosthetic and orthotic devices, devices to aid a person in grooming, eating, and other activities of daily life).

Examples of Technology

Computer Assisted Technology

Computer assisted technology includes software that allows individuals with disabilities to adapt to their surroundings and increase their independence. Eye-gaze technology is one example of such technology. Eye-gaze technology works by tracking the movement of one's eye, which in turn activates a computer, provided an individual has sufficient head control and the ability to gaze directly at a camera. Derived from military eye control systems, the camera is typically attached to the head; however, the weight of the camera requires the head to be positioned and supported. Current scientific research promises enhanced eyeglass systems. Researchers are working on innovative gaze technology featuring virtual reality goggles that include an integrated camera and viewing screen to provide communication through icon choice. The user chooses targets by gazing at the icons on the computer screen; the camera, integrated within the goggles, tracks eye gaze motion and relays information for instant processing (Brodwin, Boland, Lane, & Siu, 2012a; Cook, Polgar, & Hussey, 2008; Scherer, 2007).

People with disabilities can benefit from a number of software programs, including screen reading software that helps users with no vision use computers, magnification programs for those with low vision, and voice command software that helps people with hand or arm limitations. Mobile smartphone technology has made great improvements in the field of assistive technology. Products that were once stand alone and very expensive are now more readily available via an application download. Optical character recognition (OCR) scanning programs (for people with visual impairment), for example, once required a computer, screen reading software, and a scanner to convert print documents into characters with text-to-speech output. Now, one needs only a camera-equipped smartphone and the OCR application.

GPS applications on smart phones also help people with visual impairment travel independently. Some connect via Bluetooth to shoes with vibration sensing, which tells users when to make a right or left turn. This technology also tells users about objects in their vicinity and guides them through slow moving traffic. The ability to sense fast traffic, stairs, and sharp drop-offs are now being developed. Some smartphones come with built-in assistive technology, such as screen readers, touch assist for individuals with mobility impairment, and flash alerts and TDD for deaf and hearing impaired. Smart phone technology has made assistive technology less costly and accessible to more individuals.

Sensory Technology

Accommodations for people with visual impairments include both optical and non-optical devices for low vision. Examples of optical devices are magnifiers, specially coated lenses, and telescopes. Non-optical visual aides include talking clocks and watches, talking calculators, closed-circuit televisions that enlarge print electronically, and personal computers and peripherals with the capacity of print magnification, speech output, and optical scanning (Brodwin, Siu, & Cardoso, 2012b). Other assistive devices that aid in navigation include white canes with laser or ultrasonic technology. These devices enhance the reach of a white cane in that it informs users when objects are approaching, if objects are at head level, and the presence of stairs and drop offs.

Additionally, hearing aids, telecommunication devices for the deaf (TDD), electronic ears, amplified telephones, phones or alarms that use flashing lights for alerts, and audio loops are helpful technology devices for persons who are deaf or hard-of-hearing. Currently, a wide variety of AT is available. Technologies used by hearing people are useful to people with hearing loss, such as web-based chat, e-mail, and text messaging. Additional communication technologies have been developed for people who are Deaf or hard of hearing, including text-based telephone relay systems and video relay systems.

A more complicated system is the infrared system. This system transmits sound into light which is sent to a receiver worn by an individual; the light is decoded and converted back to a magnetic signal which is picked up by the person's telecoil. Because the system does not penetrate walls, it is useful in confidential situations. Sound is transmitted to the listener clearly and free of distracting noise in the environment (National Institute on Deafness and Other Communication Disorders [NIDCD], 2011).

Robotics

Technology includes the science of robotic controls. Robotics are able to accommodate for manipulative tasks, perform functions through prosthetic (e.g., artificial extremity) applications, render movement in spinal cord injuries (e.g., paralysis), and perform task operations in fixed workstation (at the work site) technologies (Cook et al., 2008). Someone needing the assistance of a robotic arm can attach it to a powered wheelchair, from which he or she can control it using a selection and toggle interface. Robotic devices provide assistance with such functions as drinking, retrieving items from shelves, manipulating objects, and participating in games or leisure activities. People with disabilities can use fixed workstation (desktop) robots to manipulate objects. Similarly, someone using a desktop vocational robot can use it to perform daily activities such as preparing and eating meals, writing, reading, operating a keyboard, using a telephone, and grooming.

Neuroprosthetics

Neuroprosthetic devices can be used to compensate for a damaged or missing motor or sensory function. The cochlear implant is a well-known example. This technology has been further refined and become more sophisticated with the use of robotics. Based on military technology, neuroprosthetic devices are connected to an individual's nerves and controlled through nerve impulses. These devices help to restore function of a missing or injured limb, and they can also help restore one's sense of touch (Berg et al., 2013). Neuroprostheses are especially helpful for individuals with tetraplegia; by restoring control of movement of one's limbs via a direct connection to the brain, a neuropresthetic device helps someone become more independent (Collinger et al., 2013). Neuroprosthetic technology has been developed to improve sight in people with visual disabilities; by using retina implants or artificial retinas, individuals with macular degeneration (Humayun et al., 2012) can regain some elements of sight. Neuroprosthetics promises to go beyond assistive technology and rehabilitation by actually restoring function.

Prosthetics and Orthotics

In the last 15 years, upper extremity prosthetic systems have become more widely available commercially. People using hand motion control systems can now execute multiple functions at the same time. While previous control systems employed skin surface sensors (electrodes) placed over the controlling muscle, new systems include muscle implants, avoiding the need for skin surface contact. Another type of more rare surgery involves an electrode sensor being implanted into the brain so that the thought of flexing or extending an elbow, opening or closing a hand or finger results in the intended motion. The intent is to make the movement so intuitive that thought causes the motion (Berg et al., 2013).

The field of lower extremity prosthetics has developed in recent years as well. Microprocessor controlled orthotic ankle and knee joints are now more common. The C-Leg, for example, allows the wearer to flex his or her foot and shin. This also reduces the energy demands of walking, allowing a user to navigate stairs, ramps, and other previously difficult terrains without the risk of falling (Edelstein & Moroz, 2010).

Benefits of Technology

Increased educational and employment opportunities and a greater sense of personal well being has lead to greater upward social mobility. Technological devices, equipment, and services have allowed many people with disabilities to: (a) exert greater control over their own lives; (b) participate in and contribute more fully and readily to activities in their homes, schools, employment, and communities; (c) interact to a far greater extent with people without disabilities; and (d) benefit from opportunities taken for granted by people without disabilities (Brodwin et al., 2012b; Scherer, 2007). In the early 2000s, the main reason people with disabilities stopped using computers was because of difficulties they encountered using the product. To diminish discontinuance, the user needs to be involved throughout the process (Riemer-Reiss & Wacker, 2000). AT aims to enhance functional independence for people with disabilities. The focus, therefore, is not on what a person cannot do, but instead on what he or she can do. By exploring a person's capabilities, functional limitations, and feelings about technological devices, rehabilitation practitioners can help people with disabilities achieve their goals.

Universal Design

History and Background of Universal Design

Universal design is the name of a design approach that incorporates inclusive design features while minimizing the need for individual accommodations (Burgstahler, 2012; Hoff, Varney, Enein-Donovn, Thomas, & Fesko, 2009; Mace, 1985; McGuire, Scott, & Shaw, 2006; Roberts, Park, Brown, & Cook, 2011; Sanford, 2012). Universal design can enhance access to higher education and employment for people with disabilities and those with chronic medical conditions. In the 1960s, Ronald Mace, an architect and wheelchair user, said physical environments should be designed to meet the needs of the "broadly diverse individuals who access these areas." Mace formed the Center for Universal Design at North Carolina State University in 1989. The National Institute on Disability and Rehabilitation Research, U. S. Department of Education supported the initiative from 1994 to 1997 (Story, Mueller, & Mace, 1998). While the principles of universal design were originally intended for architecture, they were later applied to product and environment design as well.

Many advocates of barrier-free design and architectural accessibility recognized the legal, economic, and social power of a concept that addressed the common needs of people with and without disabilities (Heylighen & Bianchin, 2013; Mackelprang & Clute, 2009; Story et al., 1998). For example, in architecture, segregated accessible features were not only special, they were also more expensive and usually unsightly. Architects and advocates found that many of the environmental changes needed to accommodate people with disabilities actually benefited everyone, thus laying the groundwork for universal design. These examples may be as simple as having wide doorways and ramp inclines rather than stairs at entrances so that people using wheelchairs or families with strollers may easily pass through. Assisistive technology can aid in universal design, where universal design strives to integrate people with disabilities into the mainstream, and assistive technology attempts to meet the specific needs of an individual (Story et al., 1998). The Blackberry, for example, was originally intended for members of the Deaf community. The *qwerty* keyboard design made texting easier, not just for individuals with disabilities but for everyone else as well. Apple Inc. designs everything from their desktop computers to their mobile devices with universal design in mind. Its products are accessible to people with disabilities right out of the box without requiring the purchase of additional software or equipment.

Realizing its potential, many educators have applied the concept of universal design to education. Silver, Bourke, and Strehorn (1998) used the concept in elementary and secondary education as a new paradigm for making instruction more readily accessible. Teachers who provide electronic copies of lecture notes or handouts are using the principles of universal design.

Workplace designers have begun applying universal design to work environments (Hoff et al., 2009; Mackelprang & Clute, 2009; Wehmeyer et al., 2006). Workstations with adjustable desks are an example of universal design. While these workstations benefit people who use wheelchairs most directly, they also help employees with substantial height differences, or those for whom standing is more effective for certain work functions.

What is Universal Design?

Universal design makes accessibility issues a *proactive and integral focus* of instructional planning and creates an environment that a wide range of individuals can use (Silver et al., 1998). Organizations such as the Center for Applied Special Technology (CAST) are leading the field in applying universal design to teaching and learning environments. CAST (2012) defined universal design as a set of principles for curriculum development that give all individuals equal opportunities to learn. Universal design provides a blueprint for creating instructional goals, methods, materials, and assessments that can work for everyone. It also includes flexible approaches that can be customized and adjusted for individuals.

Universal design incorporates various technologies, both assistive and mainstream. In education, computer-based testing with read aloud capability has demonstrated effectiveness for students with learning disabilities to increase test question comprehension and improve test scores (Pace & Schwartz, 2008). Educators who have embraced universal design have also used it to improve reading comprehension in students with intellectual disabilities. In employment, technologies used to improve function include audio prompting devices, video-assisted training, computers, and augmentative and alternate communication for people with developmental disabilities.

Principles of Universal Design

When originally developed, universal design included seven principles (Center for Universal Design, 1997). When applied to education, designers added two additional principles that can also be used in the workplace (Burgstahler, 2012):

1. Equitable use: design where any groups of individuals can use it. For example, a website that is accessible to all users, including people who use screen readers.
2. Flexibility in use: the design accommodates a wide range of individual abilities and preferences; that is, it provides a choice in methods of use. An example of this principle is reading technology where the software allows the option of reading a textbook aloud so that students with learning disabilities can read along for improved comprehension of the material.
3. Simple and intuitive: use of the design is straightforward eliminating unnecessary complexity, regardless of the user's knowledge, experience, language skills, and concentration level. For example, the controls of safety equipment or telecommunication devices can have alarm signals (light/sound) clearly identified and controls which are accessible and in high contrast.
4. Perceptible information: necessary information is communicated effectively to the individual regardless of ambient conditions or sensory abilities. For example, a closed-circuit television (CCTV) is available for recorded educational materials or employment orientation videos.
5. Tolerance for error: the design minimizes hazards and the adverse consequences of accidental or unintended actions; it anticipates variation in the individual's pace and prerequisite skill. An example is allowing students to turn in individual components of a project for feedback.
6. Low physical effort: designed to eliminate nonessential physical effort, which is a design that can be used efficiently, comfortably, and with a minimum of fatigue. Examples of this are ergonomic chairs that decrease work-related back injuries, or doors that open automatically, beneficial for people who lack strength or physical ability to open a door, someone who uses a wheelchair, or individuals who have their hands occupied while carrying equipment.
7. Size and space for approach and use: appropriate size and space is provided for approach, reach, manipulation, and use regardless of the user's body size, posture, or mobility. An example of this principle is a work station that accommodates persons of different sizes.
8. Community of learners: the environment promotes interaction and communication. For example, an information desk at a business or library that is open and accessible from different angles to encourage engagement of people seeking information.
9. Climate: the instructional or workplace environment is designed to be welcoming and inclusive. An example is where input or suggestions from students or employees are invited.

Legislation and Definition

Section 504 of the 1973 Rehabilitation Act (amended in 1998) prohibited discrimination against an otherwise qualified person with a disability from education, employment, transportation, and architectural access. The Carl D. Perkins Vocational and Applied Technology Education Act (1984) and its amendments addressed the responsibility of postsecondary schools to provide aids and services for individuals with disabilities equal to students without disabilities. In 1990, the Americans with Disabilities Act (ADA) was passed, which extended the Rehabilitation Act of 1973, and prohibited discrimination in key areas, including educational employment settings.

Legislation that first discussed the term universal design was the Assistive Technology Act (1998). This Act provided funding for assistive technology (a device or service used to increase, maintain, or improve functional capabilities of individuals with disabilities) projects to improve quality of life of people with disabilities. Assistive technology allows people with disabilities to more fully participate in education, employment, and daily activities. Universal design was referred to as the concept for designing and delivering products and services that are usable by people with the widest possible range of functional capabilities. It included products and services that are directly accessible (without requiring assistive technologies) and products and services that are interoperable with assistive technologies. An example includes CCTV or screen reading software built into the operating system of a computer.

Recognizing that universal design can be applied to and has the potential to improve practice in classrooms and provide opportunities for students to succeed, the Higher Education Opportunity Act (HEOA) was passed and reauthorized in 2008. It became the first legislation to establish a statutory definition for the term universal design for learning (principles include representation, expression, and engagement). The term means a scientifically valid framework for guiding educational practice that provides flexibility in the ways information is presented, in the ways students respond or demonstrate knowledge and skills, and in the ways students are engaged, with the intent of reducing barriers in instruction, providing appropriate accommodations, supports, and challenges, and maintaining high achievement expectations for all students (Higher Education Opportunity Act, 2008). Universal design promotes the social responsibility of all persons in creating an environment that is usable by the highest number of people possible—whether it is a physical, informational, curricular, or social environment. "The focus moves away from accessible and minimum code requirements to usability" (Block, Loewen, & Kroeger, 2006, p.117).

Accessible Versus Usable

There is a significant difference between accessible and usable. Quite often, these concepts are interchanged it being assumed that if something is accessible, it is also usable. Yet, this is not always the case. Accessible in regard to access by individuals with disabilities means that they can access items such as instructional materials or websites. Usable means that an individual can use the instructional materials or websites efficiently, effectively, and with satisfaction (Bevan, 1995). This idea of usability in design is applied in many concepts and study of design, such as universal design and human factors psychology. Human factors psychology aims to design effective and user-friendly tools, machines, and systems to better match the capabilities, limitations, and needs of people (Carkenord, 1994). Application of universal design principles along with various modalities as human factors psychology, ergonomics, technologies such as assistive technologies, and best instructional practices can all help create an inclusive environment, while taking into account the functional needs of individuals with disabilities, as well as usability.

The following is a study conducted that exemplifies accessibility versus usability. Sapp (2007) evaluated two scheduling systems, Myschooldayonline system compared to Microsoft Outlook in secondary education. Participants included 12 students who were blind (with some or no light perception) who used a screen reader to access the computer, and two students with low vision (who met the definition of legal blindness) who used screen enlargement programs to access the computer. There were eight computer dyads total. Students who are blind worked in groups of two paired by computer skill on each computer, totaling six computers, while the two students with low vision worked on one computer each, totaling two computers. The study revealed student preference for Myschooldayonline. Only one dyad was able to complete all tasks using Outlook. Students were more successful using Myschooldayonline than Microsoft Outlook which they had difficulty using and completing tasks, indicating that Outlook was accessible, but not usable. Students with low vision who accessed Outlook visually demonstrated as many problems and performed equivalently to students who were blind and used JAWS (Job Access With Speech screen reading software) to access Outlook. This study showed that technology also needs to be usable for it to be successful.

Other examples of accessibility versus usability are programs such as Microsoft Power Point. An individual with a visual impairment who uses a screen reader may be able to access these programs with his or her computer. However, navigation and use of the program can be difficult and thus not meet the definition of *usable*, depending on the screen reading software. With Power Point, the screen reader can read what is on the screen when the program is opened. However, when a person who uses a screen reader tries to move to a different slide or make edits, this process can become time consuming since the process may not be intuitive, thus lacking efficiency and effectiveness. Hence, it may be accessible but not usable. Websites are examples of another platform where usability and accessibility concerns can arise (Riley-Huff, 2012).

Schools and businesses have library or intranet websites for their students, staff, and employees. However, not all websites may be both accessible and usable, particularly where websites may have images or Flash where text is not imbedded for a screen reader. Screen readers may access the websites; however, some functionality may be limited and thus not usable. This shows how important usability is along with accessibility.

Application of Universal Design

There are many positive aspects to implementing universal design. Often, applying the principles of universal design and supporting the student or employee with a disability or chronic illness is accomplished through assistive technology, accommodations, changing job requirements, or modifications of the work environment or classroom instruction. These approaches also benefit other students or employees without disabilities (Zolna, Sanford, Sabata, & Goldthwaite, 2007). Applying ergonomic practices can be a strategy of universal design as this benefits other employees by improving the work environment and reducing work-related injuries. Another strategy is changing the physical environment to accommodate individuals with disabilities. An example is the widening of bathroom stalls to accommodate people who use wheelchairs. Sensor equipped sinks and toilets benefit individuals who are unable to reach the sink handles due to height and individuals with visual impairment making operation more convenient.

Other examples in applying the principles of universal design are technologies, such as computers and smart phones with accessibility software built into the operating systems, enhancing access for people with disabilities and decreasing the need for third party applications, which can be expensive and challenging to obtain. Websites of schools and businesses also need to be accessible and usable. Standards and recommendations are available for making them usable and accessible using the principles of universal design (Riley-Huff, 2012). Universal design has been successfully applied to writing centers in education, computer labs, and communication (Brizee, Sousa, & Driscoll, 2012; Campbell, 2004; Wandke, Sengpiel, & Sönkse, 2012).

Researchers noted that neglecting universal design results in a cost to businesses, schools, and society (Björk, 2009). There is a loss of potential sales if companies do not make their places of business and products readily accessible to consumers. There is also a social cost where people with disabilities experience frustration from feeling excluded in the workplace or in education when these areas are not designed to be flexible through the principles of universal design.

Training of staff, faculty, administrators, and employers is necessary to apply universal design principles in educational institutions and within the workplace (McGuire & Scott, 2006; McGuire, Scott, & Shaw, 2003; Mitra, 2006; Zolna et al., 2007). Universal design principles should be incorporated into policies and procedures to ensure universal access to education and employment. Access needs to be usable, flexible, and improve learning in the educational environment, as well as enhance productivity and job satisfaction within the workplace. Although the concept of universal design has been around for over five decades in architecture and product design, the concept is still relatively recent in education and the workplace. Many in the fields of education and business are not used to designing curricula or workplace environments to meet the needs of all individuals. Currently, modifications are placed after an individual with disability requests accommodations rather than during the design process. This mind set or lack of familiarity with universal design serves as a barrier to its implementation. Rehabilitation counselors can educate and assist schools and employers in strategies to accommodate, assist, and include individuals with disabilities by using principles of universal design.

Role of the Rehabilitation Professional

In applying the principles of universal design, the rehabilitation professional must take into account the functional needs of the individual and ensure that accommodations match those needs. This includes use of assistive or adaptive technology, devices, equipment, and changes in work tasks. For example, the use of a CCTV to magnify hard copy material, such as during exams for a student with low vision or for employees while working. In many instances, the CCTV is slow as it takes time for the individual to magnify each section of the text which can cause fatigue. Extended use may cause eye strain, and may not improve understanding of the text. In some situations, use of a CCTV may be more appropriate for short periods of time for materials that may not have been converted to electronic format. In other situations or for some individuals, screen readers or Braille may be more appropriate.

Additionally, rehabilitation professionals must also remember that usability of equipment, technologies, and software is just as significant as accessibility. It is important to keep this in mind in order to limit additional barriers or constraints to individuals with disabilities. Rehabilitation professionals are valuable resources to schools and employers to provide education and evaluation for accommodations and inclusion. There are also resources on universal design principles and how to apply these principles to make school curricula and work environments accessible and usable for individuals of all abilities.

References

Americans with Disabilities Act of 1990 (ADA), PL 101-336, 42 U.S.C. § 12101 *et seq.*

Assistive Technology Act. (1998). 29 U.S.C. § 3002 *et seq.*

Berg, J. A., Dammann, J. F., III, Tenore, F. V., Tabot, G. A., Boback, J. L., Manfredi, L. R., & Peterson, M. L. (2013). Behavioral demonstration of a somatosensory neuroprosthesis. *IEEE Trans Neural Systems Rehabilitation Engineering, 21*(3), 500–507.

Bevan, N. (1995). Measuring usability as quality of use. *Software Quality Journal, 4*, 115–150.

Björk, E. (2009). Many become losers when the Universal Design perspective is neglected: Exploring the true cost of ignoring Universal Design principles. *Technology & Disability, 21*(4), 117–125.

Block, L. S., Loewen, G., & Kroeger, S. (2006). Acknowledging and transforming disabling environments in higher education: AHEAD's role. *Journal of Postsecondary Education and Disability, 19*(2), 117–123.

Brizee, A., Sousa, M., & Driscoll, D. L. (2012). Writing centers and students with disabilities: The user-centered approach, participatory design, and empirical research as collaborative methodologies. *Computers & Composition, 29*(4), 341–366.

Brodwin, M. G., Boland, E. A., Lane, F. J., & Siu, F. W. (2012a). Technology in rehabilitation counseling. In R. M. Parker & J. B. Patterson (Eds.), *Rehabilitation counseling: Basics and beyond* (5th ed., pp. 333–367). Austin, TX: Pro-ed.

Brodwin, M. G., Siu, F. W., & Cardoso, E. (2012b). Users of assistive technology: The human component. In I. Marini & M. A. Stebnicki (Eds.), *The psychological and social impact of illness and disability* (6th ed., pp. 331–339). New York, NY: Springer.

Burgstahler, S. (2012). Universal design: Process, principles, and applications. *DO-IT (Disabilities, Opportunities, Internetworking, and Technology)*. Retrieved from http://www.washington.edu/doit/Brochures/PDF/ud.pdf

Campbell, D. (2004). Assistive technology and universal instructional design: A postsecondary perspective. *Equity & Excellence in Education, 37*(2), 167–173.

Carkenord, D. M. (1994). Promoting human factors psychology thinking through design assignments. *Teaching of Psychology, 21*(4), 235–237.

Center for Applied Special Technology (CAST). (2012). *About UDL*. Retrieved from http://www.cast.org/udl/index.html

Center for Universal Design. (1997). *The principles of universal design, Version 2.0*. Raleigh, NC: North Carolina State University.

Collinger, J. L., Wodlinger, B., Downey, J. E., Wang, W., Tyler-Kabara, E. C., Weber, D. J., & McMorland, A. J. C. (2013). High-performance neuroprosthetic control by an individual with tetraplegia. *Lancet, 381*(9866), 557–564.

Cook, A. M., Polgar, J. M., & Hussey, S. M. (2008). *Cook and Hussey's assistive technologies: Principles and practices*. St. Louis, MO: Mosby Elsevier.

Edelstein, J. E., & Moroz, A. (2010). *Lower-limb prosthetics and orthotics: Clinical concepts*. Thorofare, NJ: Slack.

Heylighen, A., & Bianchin, M. (2013). How does inclusive design relate to good design? Designing as a deliberative enterprise. *Design Studies, 34*(1), 93–110.

Higher Education Opportunity Act. (2008). Pub. L. No. 110-314, 122 Stat. 3078.

Hoff, D., Varney, E., Enein-Donovan, L., Thomas, C., & Fesko, S. (2009). Access for all customers: Universal strategies for one-stop career centers. *The Institute Brief No.* 26. Boston, MA: Institute for Community Inclusion.

Humayun, M. S., Dorn, J. D., da Cruz, L., Dagnelie, G., Sahel, J. A., Stanga, P. E., & Argus II Study Group (2012). Interim results from the international trial of Second Sight's visual prosthesis. *Ophthalmology, 119*(4), 779–788.

Mace, R. L. (1985). Universal design: Barrier free environments for everyone. *Designers West, 33*(1), 147–152.

Mackelprang, R. W., & Clute, M. A. (2009). Access for all: Universal design and the employment of people with disabilities. *Journal of Social Work in Disability & Rehabilitation, 8*(3/4), 205–221.

McGuire, J. M., & Scott, S. S. (2006). Universal design for instruction: Extending the universal design paradigm to college instruction. *Journal of Postsecondary Education and Disability, 19*(2), 124–134.

McGuire, J. M., Scott, S. S., & Shaw, S. F. (2003). Universal design for instruction: The paradigm, its principles, and products for enhancing instructional access. *Journal of Postsecondary Education and Disability, 17*(1), 10–20.

McGuire, J. M., Scott, S. S., & Shaw, S. F. (2006). Universal design and its applications in educational environments. *Remedial and Special Education, 27*(3), 166–175.

Mitra, S. (2006). The capability approach and disability. *Journal of Disability Policy Studies, 16*(4), 236–247.

National Institute on Deafness and other Communication Disorders (NIDCD). (2011). *NIDCD fact sheet: Assistive devices for people with hearing, voice, speech, or language disorders.* Retrieved from http://www.nidcd.nih.gov/staticresources/health/hearing/NIDCD-Assistive-Devices-FS.pdf

Pace, D., & Schwartz, D. (2008). Accessibility in post secondary education: Application of UDL to college curriculum. *US-China Education Review 5*(12), 20–26.

Rehabilitation Act of 1973. (amended in 1998). 29 U.S.C., Pub. L. No. 93-112 § 794 *et seq.*

Riemer-Reiss, M. L., & Wacker, R. R. (2000). Factors associated with assistive technology discontinuance among individuals with disabilities. *Journal of Rehabilitation, 66*(3), 44-50.

Riley-Huff, D. A. (2012). Web accessibility and universal design. *Library Technology Reports, 48*(7), 29–35.

Roberts, K. D., Park, H. J., Brown, S., & Cook, B. (2011). Universal design for instruction in postsecondary education: A systematic review of empirically based articles. *Journal of Postsecondary Education and Disability, 24*(1), 5–15.

Sanford, J. A. (2012). *Universal design as a rehabilitation strategy: Design for the ages.* New York, NY: Springer.

Sapp, W. (2007). Myschooldayonline: Applying universal design principles to the development of a fully accessible online scheduling tool for students with visual impairments. *Journal of Visual Impairment & Blindness, 101*(5), 301–307.

Scherer, M. J. (2007). *Living in the state of stuck: How assistive technology impacts the lives of people with disabilities.* Brookline, MA: Brookline.

Silver, P., Bourke, A., & Strehorn, K. C. (1998). Universal instruction design in higher education: An approach for inclusion. *Equity and Excellence in Education, 31*(2), 47–51.

Story, M. F., Mueller, J. L., & Mace, R. L. (1998). *The universal design file: Designing for people of all ages and abilities: Revised edition.* Raleigh, NC: North Carolina State University, Raleigh Center for Universal Design.

Wandke, H., Sengpiel, M., & Sönkse, M. (2012). Myths about older people's use of information and communication technology. *Gerontology, 58*(6), 564–570.

Wehmeyer, M. L., Palmer, S. B., Smith, S. J., Parent, W., Davies, D. K., & Stock, S. (2006). Technology use by people with intellectual and developmental disabilities to support employment activities: A single-subject design meta analysis. *Journal of Vocational Rehabilitation, 24*(2), 81–86.

Zolna, J. S., Sanford, J., Sabata, D., & Goldthwaite, J. (2007). Review of accommodation strategies in the workplace for persons with mobility and dexterity impairments: Application to criteria for universal design. *Technology & Disability, 19*(4), 189–198.

About the Authors

R. David Black, Ed.D., MPH, L.P.C., C.R.C., is a researcher in universal design in education and the workplace, assistive technology, and disability associated with chronic disease and public health. He provides lectures in these areas at California State University, Los Angeles (CSULA). Within the community, Dr. Black assists individuals with disabilities, survivors of trauma, adolescents, and veterans returning to higher education.

Martin G. Brodwin, Ph.D, C.R.C., is Professor and Coordinator of the graduate Rehabilitation Counselor Education Program at CSULA. As a vocational expert for the Office of Disability Adjudication and Review, Social Security Administration, he provides testimony on disability-related issues. Dr. Brodwin has published over 100 refereed journal articles, book chapters, and books on the subjects of medical aspects of disability, counseling, disability, rehabilitation, and accommodation.

Chapter 32

SICKLE CELL DISEASE AND HEMOPHILIA

John J. Howard, M.D., M.P.H.

Introduction

Hematology is the study of blood, blood-forming organs like bone marrow, and blood diseases. Blood is composed of cellular and fluid components. The cellular components are formed from stem cells in the bone marrow and are of three major types: red blood cells (RBCs), white blood cells (WBCs), and platelets. The fluid component of blood is called plasma. Plasma is composed mainly of water, but also contains proteins responsible for clotting (coagulation) to prevent uncontrolled bleeding and fight infection (antibodies). The plasma also serves as the main fluid transport system of the body, delivering molecules such as glucose, cholesterol, triglycerides, fatty acids, and electrolytes, like sodium and potassium, throughout the body.

RBCs are the most numerous of the cellular components circulating in the blood. Each RBC contains molecules of hemoglobin, an iron-containing protein that is responsible for transporting oxygen from the lungs to the rest of the body. Diseases affecting hemoglobin are numerous; this chapter concentrates on one—sickle cell disease.

There is a cascade of plasma proteins responsible for blood coagulation. The protein coagulation cascade serves as one of the body's most important methods of self-repair after trauma (Hoffman et al., 2013). Disorders affecting coagulation are numerous. Sickle cell disease and hemophilia are the two most common conditions that a rehabilitation counselor is likely to encounter when providing services to people with blood disorders.

Sickle Cell Disease

Sickle cell disease (SCD) is caused by the production of abnormal hemoglobin, called hemoglobin S (HbS). Presence of HbS leads to chronic anemia and acute and chronic tissue damage secondary to blockage of blood flow produced by abnormally shaped RBCs. SCD occurs most commonly in persons of African ancestry, but also affects persons of Mediterranean, Caribbean, South and Central American, Arab, and East Indian ancestry. An advantage of the sickle cell carrier is that it confers partial protection against malaria caused by *Plasmodium falciparum* (Bunn, 1997).

Genetics

The single amino acid change in the β globin chain of the hemoglobin molecule—valine for glutamic acid in the 6th residue—produces HbS. SCD is inherited from both parents. If an individual inherits the sickle cell gene from only one parent, the person is said to have the *sickle cell trait*. Individuals with sickle cell trait do not exhibit any symptoms of SCD. If an individual inherits the sickle cell gene from both parents, he or she has *sickle cell disease*. In the United States, about 8% of African Americans carry the sickle cell trait, and approximately 1 in 375 African American newborns are born with both genes and have sickle cell disease (Serjeant & Serjeant, 2001).

Clinical Manifestations

HbS is a hemoglobin molecule of reduced solubility; when deoxygenated (lacking oxygen), it becomes rigidly polymerized. Polymerization of HbS inside the RBC converts the RBC from its normal biconcave shape to a crescent- or sickle-shape. RBC flexibility is reduced by polymerization. As a result, the blood as a fluid under flow conditions becomes more viscous (thicker). Sickled RBCs block small blood vessels and sometimes large ones, causing damage to them and eventually death to the cells supplied by the affected blood vessels. The sickled RBCs are responsible for producing all the clinical manifestations of disease in people who have SCD.

Acute pain is the first symptom in most individuals and is the hallmark of SCD. Acute blockage of blood vessels (vaso-occlusion) by sickled RBCs accounts for most of the severe complications and can present as acute episodes causing pain in the chest, back, abdomen, and extremities. A painful vaso-occlusive crisis has a sudden onset, usually lasting five to six days, and may be localized in one area of the body or generalized. One type of vaso-occlusive crisis, acute chest syndrome, is the leading cause of death and hospitalization in SCD (Golden, Styles, & Vinchinsky, 1998). Acute chest syndrome is commonly understood as being caused by simultaneous vaso-occlusion and infection, and can progress to respiratory failure if not treated aggressively with antibiotics, transfusions, and bronchodilators to improve oxygenation (Castro, Brambilia, & Thorington, 1994).

Other organs of the body can be affected by vaso-occlusive complications. For example, leg ulcers occur due to cell death in the skin around the ankles. Prolonged standing in one position makes these ulcers worse. Vaso-occlusion involving the joints can be physically limiting. Bone infarcts (aseptic necrosis) in the lower extremities and the vertebrae of the spinal cord precipitate collapse of the involved bone and lead to degenerative osteoarthritis in older individuals. Occlusion of the arteries supplying the brain causes thrombosis and can result in a cerebrovascular accident (stroke). Both intellectual and physical disabilities may result from central nervous system complications in childhood, leading to limitations in adulthood.

Treatment

Management of SCD is primarily supportive, and includes monitoring the severity of the anemia, transfusing blood only when necessary, providing immunizations, treating infections early with antibiotics, and avoidance of dehydration. In addition to supportive treatment, the drug *hydroxyurea* is used to shift hemoglobin production from HbS to fetal hemoglobin, which does not sickle as readily (Platt, 2008). Gene therapy for SCD is also a possibility for future treatment (Pace, 2007). Gene therapy to correct the sickle cell mutation has already proved successful in mouse models (Chang, Ye, & Kan, 2006).

Functional Limitations

As in other chronic diseases with onset in childhood, an individual with SCD has physical as well as psychosocial issues that play a role in the potential for vocational rehabilitation. A full range of medical, psychiatric, and social services are needed to maximize overall functioning for successful rehabilitation.

Physical Limitations

Physical limitations are primarily the result of the decreased energy level associated with the chronic anemia of SCD, and the pain associated with sickle cell crises (Raphael, 2011).

Chronic anemia. Chronic hemolytic anemia is a hallmark of SCD. Sickled RBCs are destroyed randomly throughout the body, including in the spleen and liver, resulting in an average RBC lifespan of only 17 days compared to 120 days for a RBC in a non-affected individual. Chronic anemia can decrease an individual's energy level and make activities requiring physical exertion difficult.

Pain crisis. Although variable by individual, painful sickle cell crises typically occur on an average of twice a year (Platt et al., 1991). The crisis usually resolves within a week, but there may be an additional five to ten days during which the individual has residual symptoms. Some maintain work activity throughout a pain crisis, but others need to take time off work—from one to several days and up to two weeks, depending on the energy level needed for an employee's work. Counselors need to consider the level of work when providing vocational rehabilitation (Brodwin, Parker, & DeLaGarza, 2010). Employees with sedentary or light jobs are able to continue working through sickle cell crises more often than persons who have physically demanding jobs.

Pulmonary complications. In the presence of lung disease, shortness of breath becomes the limiting factor for work requiring exertion (Greer et al., 2013). Analysis of the physical demands of the job is helpful. Job restructuring or accommodation is useful when a position even has occasional physical demands beyond the person's capacity.

Neurologic complications. Seizures (especially in childhood SCD), spinal cord compression, central nervous system infections, vestibular dysfunction, and hearing loss are neurologic complications of sickle cell disease. The most serious of the neurologic complications is the occurrence of a stroke. Approximately 11% of individuals with SCD have clinically apparent strokes—overt or silent—before the age of 20 years; that risk increases to 24% by the age of 45 years (Ohene-Frempong et al., 1998). The residual effects of strokes can include mild muscle weakness and sensory impairment.

Eye complications. In SCD, visual field defects and visual loss in one or both eyes can occur because the retinal artery is vulnerable to vaso-occlusion. Functional limitation is dependent on extent of visual loss; improvement in function can occur with use of visual aids.

Skin complications. Leg ulcers produce pain and limitations of motion in the affected extremity. This interferes with activities such as standing, walking, climbing, and balancing. Prolonged standing is one possible cause of these ulcers (Falvo, 2014).

Bone and joint complications. Bone and joint disease interfere with physical activity because of pain, deformity, and loss of strength. Walking, standing, bending, climbing, and balancing may be affected. Some limitations are overcome by learning new techniques for physical activities through physical therapy. Prosthetic implant surgery has been a successful technique in this area.

Environmental Factors

Several environmental conditions exacerbate symptoms. Jobs involving exposure to cold and damp conditions need to be avoided since these environmental factors precipitate RBC sickling. Exposure to employment environments with noxious fumes, high levels of dust, and poor ventilation are not tolerated well, especially for individuals with pulmonary problems. Hot and humid conditions add stress on the heart and precipitate dehydration. On all jobs, persons with SCD need easy availability of water and other fluids to prevent potential dehydration (Francis & Johnson, 1991).

Psychosocial Issues

Emotional stress can exacerbate symptoms and make management of SCD difficult. An inability to predict or control symptoms leads to heightened anxiety and increased frustration. Recurrent painful episodes of sickle cell crises add to emotional distress. Depression is the major psychological factor associated with this disease; it affects ability to cope with the variable nature of the disease (Brodwin et al., 2010). Consequently, psychological consultation may be helpful when preparing a client for vocational rehabilitation.

Rehabilitation Potential

Most individuals with SCD will not need vocational rehabilitation services, but individuals with recurrent sickle cell crises that interrupt their work lives, and those individuals with chronic complications may benefit from rehabilitation services. Counselors need to explain to employers what SCD is and its symptoms.

An employee with an otherwise good employment record may be able to use accumulated sick leave for occasional sickle cell crises. Reasonable accommodation can facilitate a successful return to work for someone with moderate to severe sickle cell symptoms (Brodwin et al., 2010). An example of reasonable accommodation for an employee with SCD is an agreement with the employer that the individual will work through minor illnesses and save or accumulate sick days to be used for occasional sickle cell crises. Another accommodation is to have the worker put in non-paid overtime between crises to be used when work is missed during a crisis.

Onsite observation of the job helps the counselor modify physical aspects of the position. When a worker is having difficulty with physical exertion, the counselor can assist the client and employer in modifying the amount of lifting and carrying required (Falvo, 2014). One may be able to break down the amount lifted and carried into lighter loads; if this is not possible, the counselor may want to recommend job restructuring.

Mental stress present on the job and its effect on potential development of sickle cell crisis needs careful assessment. Modification of emotional stressors is more difficult than alteration of physical activities. Often, it is impossible to change emotional stress factors. At times, positive facilitation by the counselor is effective and results in decreasing emotionally stressful aspects of the job. Employer education creates a more thorough understanding of SCD, helping diminish work-related stressors.

When determining rehabilitation potential, the counselor should evaluate any physical complications the individual has and whether time off from work may be necessary when sickle cell crises occur. With this information, in conjunction with appropriate medical consultation and an understanding of the provisions of the Americans with Disabilities Act (42 United States Code Section 12101), the rehabilitation counselor is equipped to provide rehabilitation for persons who have SCD.

Hemophilia

Hemophilia refers to a collection of hereditary bleeding disorders which arise as a result of deficiencies in the plasma proteins which control blood coagulation. Blood coagulation is necessary to prevent hemorrhage (severe bleeding). Severe hemophilia causes lifelong recurrent bleeding into soft tissues, muscles, and most importantly, joints.

There are three main types of hemophilia: (1) deficiency of factor VIII results in the coagulation disorder known as *hemophilia A* (classic hemophilia); (2) deficiency of factor IX results in *hemophilia B* (Christmas disease); and (3) deficiency of factor XI results in *hemophilia C* (Rosenthal Syndrome). Hemophilia occurs in 1 in 10,000 male births in the United States—85% are deficient in factor VIII, 14% are deficient in factor IX, and only 1% are deficient in factor XI, or one of the other coagulation factors (Greer et al., 2013). Survival beyond young adulthood of people with severe hemophilia was uncommon before 1960. Since then, timely treatment of bleeding and the preventive (prophylactic) use of clotting factors have decreased the disability associated with hemophilia and normalized the lifespan of persons with hemophilia (Soucie et al., 2000).

Genetics

The genetic defects accounting for deficiency of factors VIII and IX both occur on the X chromosome. Males have one X and one Y chromosome (XY), whereas females have two X chromosomes (XX). A mother carrying the genetic defect causing hemophilia (X^h) on one of her X chromosomes (X^hX) may transmit hemophilia to her son (X^hY), or pass the defect to a daughter (X^hX), who then becomes a carrier for hemophilia. The mother may transmit her normal X chromosome to her son (XY) or daughter (XX), and no genetic transmission of the mutated gene takes place. Sons of a carrier mother and a normal father have a 50% chance of having hemophilia; daughters have a 50% chance of being carriers. Since a father with hemophilia (X^hY) contributes only his Y chromosome to his sons, none of his sons will have hemophilia, but all his daughters will receive his X^h chromosome and will be carriers (X^hX). This explains why hemophilia is almost exclusively a disease among males. Usually, a male inherits his mutant gene (X^h) from his carrier mother (X^hX), but in about 30% of cases of hemophilia, there is no family history and hemophilia is believed to arise from a spontaneous mutation (Mannucci & Tuddenham, 2001).

Hemophilia C is a mild form of hemophilia and is uncommon. Unlike hemophilia A and B, the inheritance of hemophilia C follows an autosomal recessive pattern. The gene that causes deficiency of factor XI is not present on a sex chromosome (X or Y)—rather on chromosome number 4. Therefore, hemophilia C affects both genders equally.

Disease Severity

There is a close relationship between disease severity and the activity level of the coagulation factor. Individuals without hemophilia have from 50% to 170% activity of any coagulation factor. Individuals with less than 1% activity have severe hemophilia with frequent, life-threatening bleeding. Individuals with 1% to 5% activity have moderate hemophilia with bleeding episodes weekly or monthly. Patients with greater than 5% activity have mild hemophilia with infrequent bleeding (Greer et al., 2013). However, the bleeding risk for hemophilia C is not always influenced by the severity of the deficiency of factor XI.

Clinical Manifestations

The major clinical manifestations of hemophilia are bleeding into a joint (hemarthrosis), a muscle, or other soft tissue (hematoma). Hemarthroses occur primarily within the knees, but can occur in the elbows, ankles, shoulders, hips, and wrists, and cause pain, swelling, and limitation of joint motion. The frequency of hemarthrosis varies widely from patient to patient despite similar levels of coagulation factor activity.

Bleeding into the joint initiates the development of hemophilic arthropathy, a disabling chronic joint disease. During a joint bleed, various blood components cause inflammation of the lining of a joint, resulting in synovitis. The joint responds to repetitive bleeds by producing a fibrous, highly vascular tissue, replacing the normal joint lining tissue. This vicious cycle leads to progressive degeneration of cartilage, destruction of bone, and replacement of joint space with fibrous (scar) tissue. Bones may fuse (ankylosis) resulting in deformity and severely impaired range of motion in the affected joint (Rosendaal et al., 1998). The early stage of synovial proliferation and joint destruction resembles the disease process of rheumatoid arthritis, whereas end-stage hemophilic arthropathy is similar to severe osteoarthritis (Papadakis, McPhee, & Rabow, 2013).

Diagnosis

Genetic testing for hemophilia is recommended to determine carrier status when there is a known family history of hemophilia on the maternal side of a family (Greer et al., 2013). At birth, a diagnosis of hemophilia can be made by analysis of umbilical cord blood. When there is no family history of hemophilia, any episode of prolonged bleeding suggests the presence of hemophilia. The diagnosis of hemophilia is then made by laboratory testing to establish the type of hemophilia (deficiency of factor VIII, IX, or XI), and level of factor activity.

Treatment

Effective care of a person with hemophilia requires a multidisciplinary health care team. The team concept gave rise to a comprehensive network of hemophilia treatment centers (HTCs) throughout the nation and in many parts of the world (Hoots, 2003). Persons with hemophilia who receive care in HTCs have a 60% reduction in mortality compared to those not seen at HTCs (Soucie et al., 2000).

The mainstay of treatment for hemophilia A and B is periodic replacement of the deficient factor with human blood products (factor concentrates). Factor concentrates were first extracted from pooled or multiple donor plasma, but substantial numbers of men with hemophilia developed antibodies to the human immunodeficiency virus (HIV), and many developed the acquired immunodeficiency syndrome (AIDS) (Mannucci & Tuddenham, 2001). Now, factor concentrates are synthesized by newer and safer recombinant technology and do not carry HIV.

Self-administered factor concentrates have led to prompt control of bleeding, reduced joint and muscle damage, and a longer lifespan. Studies have shown that a home-based program for self-infusion significantly reduces bleeding complications and absences from school or work (Soucie et al., 2001). Furthermore, prophylaxis (providing concentrate in anticipation of trauma, as opposed to treatment when a bleed occurs) reduces medical costs and minimizes loss of productivity (Papadakis et al., 2013). Medical advances in the treatment of hemophilia have resulted in a greater number of individuals being employed (Serjeant & Sergeant, 2001). Although bleeding in individuals with hemophilia A can generally be controlled with infusion of factor concentrates, 30% of individuals with hemophilia A develop an inhibitor to factor VIII which places them at increased risk for uncontrolled bleeding. Some types of anti-inhibitor therapy are successful at decreasing the number of bleeding episodes (Leissinger et al., 2011).

The annual costs for an adult for clotting factors for hemophilia are approximately $150,000 for on-demand therapy and $300,000 for prophylaxis (Manco-Johnson et al., 2007). This has led to a search for treatments that reduce the frequency of infusions. One method that has shown promise is gene therapy for hemophilia B. In a landmark study, long-term expression of factor IX at therapeutically relevant levels was achieved (Nathwani et al., 2011).

Functional Limitations

The rehabilitation counselor can expect to encounter widely different degrees of functional limitations among individuals with hemophilia. The extent of limitation usually correlates inversely with the individual's factor activity level. Those with severe disease who have not had the benefits of modern treatment have severe, generalized arthropathy. These individuals need to use wheelchairs for ambulation if they have not had surgical correction or insertion of endo-prostheses to restore function (Logan, 1995). Individuals with hemophilia who grew up during the era of modern treatment have few vocational limitations. Counselors should concentrate on surmounting any erroneous notions surrounding individuals with hemophilia. These incorrect notions include beliefs that people with hemophilia: (1) necessarily require sedentary jobs; (2) must be in protected environments; (3) cannot perform manual labor jobs; (4) and frequently miss work because of the disease. Many individuals work successfully in physically demanding jobs and also in light and sedentary white-collar and blue-collar vocations. However, persons with severe hemophilia, especially those who bleed more frequently despite maximal therapy, need counseling regarding jobs that require maneuvers that are potentially traumatic to joints or require maximal joint motion. Since an individual with hemophilia can normalize coagulation within minutes by injection of a factor concentrate, many potentially hazardous jobs have little risk.

Intellectual Functioning

Persons with hemophilia do not display any inherent intellectual limitations. Lower scores on intelligence tests and achievement tests in the 1960s are generally attributable to disrupted school attendance. Within two decades following the advent and implementation of factor replacement and self-supervised treatment, individuals with hemophilia were attaining educational levels at least equivalent to age-matched, unaffected men (Colegrove & Hurtzinger, 1994; Hoffman et al., 2013).

Psychosocial Factors

Psychosocial dynamics in men with hemophilia have provided focus for considerable investigation. As a group, these individuals display the same range of psychological variation present in non-affected persons. There is no general personality pattern for persons with hemophilia. Repeatedly, it is noted that many men with hemophilia are optimistic and exhibit strong ego strength. These men believe that coping with their disease has given them a *hardihood* they would not otherwise have developed. Despite these observations, the rehabilitation counselor needs to be aware of specific psychological limitations that sometimes occur (Falvo, 2014).

Particularly in previous years, when a boy with hemophilia was born, the mother frequently experienced varying degrees of guilt because of what she perceived as her *genetic responsibility*. Commonly, these mothers became inappropriately anxious and overprotective. Severe curtailment of her son's activities coupled with excessive attention and indulgence sometimes led to development of an overly dependent, passive, anxious person who experiences feelings of hopelessness, pessimism, and social isolation. By contrast the boy sometimes responded with denial leading to reckless, *daredevil* activities and pathologic risk taking. Hemophilia treatment centers have been able to do much to provide families with counseling and education. Better understanding of the disease and awareness of the dramatic effects of modern medical treatment have helped mitigate unhealthy parental concerns.

Employment remains a concern for people with hemophilia. Clearly, unemployment diminishes self-esteem and fosters passivity, pessimism, and depression (Raphael, 2011). A client's self-concept as being *unemployable* may be a key reason for reluctance to seek a job and failure to present oneself in the most positive light when seeking employment. Failure to find a job often reinforces initial self-doubts. If the rehabilitation counselor can help the client surmount reticence and negativism regarding employability, the client will be able to take a significant step forward.

Specific Functional Limitations

Physical limitations vary with each person. Arthropathy of a lower extremity weight-bearing joint is most likely to be physically limiting. For some individuals, elbow or shoulder joint disease may pose the greatest limitation. The client can provide reliable information about which joints are disabling and in what manner. For example, a person with a knee with almost no range of motion due to severe arthropathy, but who has only rare hemarthroses is less disabled for work than is a person with severe chronic synovitis and frequent hemarthoses involving the dominant upper extremity.

Occupational Limitations

Occupational limitations correlate closely with severity of hemophilia. There is also a close correlation between successful self-management of the disease and ability to function in the workplace. Clients with severe hemophilia who are on self-supervised treatment are best able to manage the effects of a job injury that causes a bleed. A 15-minute break is generally sufficient for an individual to self-infuse a factor concentrate (Raphael, 2011). Most clients with mild to moderate disease have few vocational limitations. A characteristic feature of severe hemophilia is unpredictability. Therefore, persons with severe hemophilia may not always optimally perform certain tasks out of their routine or familiarity.

The rehabilitation counselor must evaluate the client's vocational limitations individually (Brodwin et al., 2010). Members of the comprehensive hemophilia treatment team can provide precise assessment of functionality. Most employees with hemophilia can perform equal to their peers who do not have hemophilia in a variety of jobs and professions. Inaccurately perceived limitations by prospective employers outweigh actual functional limitations of the individual with hemophilia.

Rehabilitation Potential

Rehabilitation potential for people with hemophilia is excellent. Effective treatment of bleeding episodes, prevention or minimization of the disabling complications of joint bleeds, and the ability to correct deformities through surgery has greatly enhanced employability. Because of modern treatment modalities, many persons have completed high school, and increasingly, pursue higher education.

Rehabilitation counselors need to educate employers to maximize potential employment opportunities for these clients (Brodwin et al., 2010; Falvo, 2014). Most employers are unfamiliar with self-supervised infusion that allows persons with hemophilia to live near-normal lives. Contrary to popular misconception, persons with hemophilia are not fragile individuals only suitable for very specialized jobs located in protected environments. Often called "bleeders," many people erroneously believe individuals with hemophilia are vulnerable to rapid blood loss upon exposure to the slightest trauma. Actually, individuals with hemophilia bleed no more rapidly or excessively from minor cuts and superficial abrasions than do persons who do not have this condition.

Appropriate medical treatment can prevent further progression of existing disabilities and help avoid additional complications. The rehabilitation counselor may consider the initial status upon first seeing the client as being relatively stable and jointly work toward selecting a vocation in which the disability will not adversely affect functioning on the job. For clients who bleed frequently, the opportunity to self-infuse at the worksite effectively reduces morbidity and lost work time. Capacity to store concentrate and necessary accessories (needles, syringes, and gauze pads) is needed.

Individuals self-infuse in their offices or in restrooms. Some self-infuse at a nearby gasoline station or restaurant to conceal their hemophilia. Many employers have a first aid room where employees can self-infuse at the worksite. Persons with hemophilia frequently learn to compensate for their limitations and, therefore, often have fewer injuries than other workers in similar jobs. In many respects, people with hemophilia may be optimal clients for vocational rehabilitation because the disease itself can be effectively controlled (Brodwin et al., 2010).

Case Study

Mr. Leo Jones is a 53 year-old college-educated, self-employed machinist, with sickle cell disease. He is married and has two young children (ages 7 and 10). Mr. Jones developed bacterial septicemia (infection in the blood) and multiple complications of sickle cell disease requiring intermittent hospitalization over several months time. Both his marriage and business failed. Mr. Jones' wife is Chinese and bicultural, maintaining some of the beliefs of traditional Chinese culture. Her parents always wanted her to marry within their ethnicity and maintain a traditional Chinese home. This has caused emotional issues, especially when it comes to raising their children. His wife left him and moved to another state, taking their two children with her and moving in with her elderly parents.

Marriage problems and the failed business contributed to Mr. Jones' anxiety and depression. Dr. Carla Williams, his treating physician, noted that Leo had severe depression and referred him for psychological counseling. As a result of his condition, Mr. Jones developed a fatalistic attitude and did not complete the recommended course of counseling. Consequently, his depression deepened. Dr. Williams restricted Mr. Jones to light work. There are some limitations in the areas of standing and walking.

The daily work activities of a machinist (National Center for O*Net Development [2012], #51-4041.00 Machinists. See http://www.onetonline.org/link/summary/51-4041.00) include setting-up and operating machine tools and fitting and assembling parts to make or repair metal parts, mechanisms, tools, and equipment. One reads blueprints, diagrams, and mechanical drawings, uses precision-measuring tools, and understands a variety of machining procedures. Machinists use hand tools and power tools throughout the work shift. Mr. Jones had been self-employed for 30 years in this line of work.

Due to physical limitations related to bone destruction (avascular necrosis) in both hips, Mr. Jones was unable to return to his machinist business, which often required ten-hour days, six days a week. Besides him, he had two helpers in the business that did general machining. Work in the machine shop involved occasional lifting up to 80 pounds when shipment orders arrived, and regular lifting of 45 pounds, with repetitive lifting of 20-25 pounds. Mr. Jones stood or walked 50% of the workday.

After the business failed and for the next ten years, Leo filled his days with a variety of activities related to his church and various social clubs. By assuming a demanding schedule of responsibilities associated with these activities, he kept busy. During this period, Dr. Williams needed to hospitalize him as often as six times a year for acute pain crises and recurrent bone infections (osteomyelitis). Eventually, Mr. Jones was reunited with his children when they returned to the city to attend college. With these new family responsibilities, he gave up many of his outside activities and concentrated on assisting his children with their studies and making a home for them. Within a few months, Leo noticed a remarkable decrease in the frequency of hospital admissions, which he related to improved self-care. Proper rest, careful attention to fluid intake, and monitoring of physical activities contributed to the improved clinical course of the disease.

Mr. Jones' depression cleared. Subsequently, he felt the need for a higher income and sought vocational rehabilitation services. A counselor from the state department of rehabilitation provided counseling, guidance, and job placement. These services were successful and Leo was placed as a reader and driver for people with visual impairments.

Questions

1. Discuss physical, environmental, and psychosocial aspects of sickle cell disease.
2. Outline a vocational profile for Mr. Leo Jones including age category, educational level, work history (exertion and skill levels), occupationally significant characteristics, and transferable skills.
3. If Leo had decided to make further attempts to make his machinist business succeed, how would you as his rehabilitation counselor approach this decision? Provide supporting arguments.
4. Would you recommend use of transferable skills as a viable vocational rehabilitation option for Mr. Jones? If so, describe what skills are transferable to other skilled and semiskilled jobs.
5. Discuss the rehabilitation goal pursued in this case and explain why the counselor may have recommended it. Do you agree with this rehabilitation plan?

6. Speculate on how Mr. Jones was able to achieve his vocational goal.
7. Evaluate this case from a multicultural perspective.

References

Americans with Disabilities Act (ADA) of 1990, Pub.L. 101-336, 104 Stat 327, codified at Title 42, United States Code Section 12101. Retrieved from http://www.ada.gov/

Brodwin, M.G., Parker, R. M., & DeLaGarza, D. (2010). Disability and reasonable accommodation. In E. M. Szymanski & R. M. Parker (Eds.), *Work and disability: Issues, contexts, and strategies for enhancing employment outcomes for people with disabilities* (3rd ed., pp. 281–323). Austin, TX: Pro-ed.

Bunn, H. F. (1997). Pathogenesis and treatment of sickle cell disease. *New England Journal of Medicine, 337*(11), 762–769.

Castro O., Brambilia D. J., & Thorington B. (1994). The acute chest syndrome in sickle cell disease: Incidence and risk factors: The Cooperative Study of Sickle Cell Disease. *Blood, 84,* 643–649.

Chang J. C., & Ye L., & Kan, Y. W. (2006). Correction of the sickle mutation in embryonic stem cells. *Proceedings of the National Academy of Sciences, 103*(4), 1036–1040.

Colegrove, R., & Hurtzinger, R. (1994). Academic, behavioral, and social adaptation of boys with hemophilia/HIV disease. *Journal of Pediatric Psychology, 19*(4), 457–473.

Falvo, D. R. (2014). *Medical and psychosocial aspects of chronic illness and disability* (5th ed.). Sudbury, MA: Jones and Bartlett Learning.

Francis, R. B., & Johnson, C. S. (1991). Vaso-occlusion in sickle cell disease: Current concepts and unanswered questions. *Blood, 77,* 1405–1414.

Golden, C., Styles, L., & Vinchinsky, E. (1998). Acute chest syndrome and sickle cell disease. *Current Opinion in Hematology, 5,* 89–92.

Greer, J. P., Arber, D. A., Glader, B., List, A. F., Means, R. T., Paraskevas, F., . . . Foerster, J. (Eds.). (2013). *Wintrobe's clinical hematology* (13th ed.). Baltimore, MD: Lippincott Williams and Wilkins.

Hoffman, R., Benz, E. J., Silberstein, L., Heslop, H., Weitz, J., & Anastasi, J. (Eds). (2013). *Hematology: Basic principles and practice* (6th ed.). Philadelphia, PA: Elsevier Saunders.

Hoots, W. K. (2003). Comprehensive care for hemophilia and related inherited bleeding disorders: Why it matters. *Current Hematology Reports, 2,* 395–401.

Leissinger C., Gringeri A., Antmen B., Berntorp, E., Biasoli, C., Carpenter, S., . . . Mantovani, L. (2011). Anti-inhibitor coagulant complex prophylaxis in hemophilia with inhibitors. *New England Journal of Medicine, 365*(18), 1684–1692.

Logan, L. J. (1995). Hemostasis: Hemorrhagic and thrombotic disorders. In J. J. Mazza (Ed.), *Manual of Clinical Hematology* (2nd ed., pp. 349–379). Boston, MA: Little Brown.

Manco-Johnson, M. J., Abshire T. C., Shapiro A. D., Riske, B., Hacker, M. R., Kilcoyne, R., . . . Evatt, B. L. (2007) Prophylaxis versus episodic treatment to prevent joint disease in boys with severe hemophilia. *New England Journal of Medicine, 357*(6), 535–544.

Mannucci, P. M., & Tuddenham, E. G. D. (2001). The hemophilias: From royal genes to gene therapy. *New England Journal of Medicine, 344*(23), 1773–1779.

Nathwani A.C., Tuddenham E.G.D., Rangarajan S, Rosales, C., McIntosh, J., Linch, D. C., . . . Davidoff, A. M. (2011). Adenovirus-associated virus vector-mediated gene transfer in hemophilia B. *New England Journal of Medicine, 365,* 2357–2365.

National Center for O*Net Development. *Occupational Information Network (ONet).* Retrieved from http://www.onetonline.org/

Ohene-Frempong K., Weiner S. J., Sleeper L. A., Miller, S. T., Embury, J. W., Moohr, J. W., . . . Gill, F. M. (1998). Cerebrovascular accidents in sickle cell disease: Rates and risk factors. *Blood, 91*(1), 288–294.

Pace, B. S. (Ed). (2007). *Renaissance of sickle cell disease research in the Genomic Era.* London, England: Imperial College.

Papadakis, M. A., McPhee, S. J., & Rabow, M. W. (Eds.). (2013). *Current medical diagnosis and treatment* (43rd ed.). New York, NY: McGraw-Hill Lange.

Platt, O. S. (2008). Hydroxyurea for the treatment of sickle cell anemia. *New England Journal of Medicine, 358*(13), 1362–1369.

Platt, O. S., Thorington, B. D., Brambilla, D. J., Milner, P. F., Rosse, W. F., Vichinsky, E., & Kinney, T. R. (1991). Pain in sickle cell disease. *New England Journal of Medicine, 325*, 11–16.

Raphael, B. G. (2011). Hematological disorders. In S. R. Flanagan, H. H. Zaretsky, & A. Moroz (Eds.), *Medical aspects of disability: A handbook for the rehabilitation professional* (4th ed., pp. 223–236). New York, NY: Springer.

Rosendaal, G., Vianen, M. E., Wenting, J. G., van Rinsum, A. C., van den Berg, H. M., Hafeber, F. P., & Bijlsma, W. J. (1998). Iron deposits and catabolic properties of synovial tissue from patients with haemophilia. *Journal of Bone and Joint Surgery, 80-B*(3), 540–545.

Serjeant, G. R., & Serjeant, B. E. (2001). *Sickle cell disease* (3rd ed.). Oxford, England: Oxford University.

Soucie, J. M., Huss, R., Eratt, B., Abdelhak, A., Cowan, L., Hill, A., . . . Wilbur, N. (2000). Mortality among males with hemophilia: Relations with source of medical care. *Blood, 96*(2), 437–442.

Soucie, J. M., Symons II, J., Evatt, B., Brettler, D. Haszti, M., & Linden, J. (2001). Home-based factor infusion therapy and hospitalization for bleeding complications among males with hemophilia. *Hemophilia, 7*, 198–206.

About the Author

John J. Howard, M.D., M.P.H., J.D. is Professorial Lecturer in Environmental and Occupational Health, School of Public Health and Health Services, The George Washington University, Washington, D.C. Dr. Howard is board-certified in internal medicine and occupational medicine. He is admitted to the practice of medicine and law in California and the District of Columbia.

Chapter 33

GENETIC TESTING, DISCRIMINATION, AND COUNSELING

John J. Howard, M.D., M.P.H.

Introduction

The initial sequencing and analysis of the human genome was published in 2001 (International Human Genome Sequencing Consortium, 2001). Since then, genetic tests have been developed for more than 2,200 diseases, of which about 2,000 tests are currently available for use in clinical settings (Centers for Disease Control and Prevention [CDC], 2012). A genetic test involves "the analysis of human DNA, RNA chromosomes, proteins, and certain metabolites in order to detect heritable disease-related genotypes, mutations, phenotypes, or karyotypes for clinical purposes" (Holzman & Watson, 1999).

Genetic testing can be used for many reasons (Burke, 2002). Genetic tests can be used to screen carriers of gene mutations. These tests aim to identify unaffected individuals who carry one copy of a gene for a condition (like sickle cell disease) that requires two copies to be present to develop the symptomatic form of the genetic disease. Genetic tests can also be used for prenatal and newborn screening, predicting the probability of developing a neurological disease or a type of cancer, predicting whether an individual will respond to particular types of chemotherapy, or for forensic identification purposes (Hartl, 1999).

Genetic testing raises concerns that results of the test may be used in discrimination in employment and insurance. For example, individuals who test positive for a genetic test relating to a particular disease may be perceived by an employer or an insurer as actually having the disorder. In 2008, this concern led to enactment of a new federal anti-discrimination law called the Genetic Information Nondiscrimination Act of 2008 (GINA, 2008). This act serves to prevent discrimination in employment and insurance based on one's genetic makeup.

Since genetic testing may cause legal, ethical, and psychological concerns, genetic testing should be, and often is, accompanied by counseling. Genetic counseling is the process of helping people understand and adapt to the medical, psychological, and familial implications of genetic contributions to disease. This process integrates: (1) interpretation of family and medical histories to assess the chance of disease occurrence or recurrence; (2) education about inheritance, testing, management, prevention, resources, and research; and (3) counseling to promote informed choices and adaptation to the risk or condition (National Society of Genetic Counselors, 2005).

This chapter briefly reviews genetic testing, genetic discrimination, genetic counseling, and the role of the rehabilitation counselor. Three brief case studies conclude the chapter.

Genetic Testing

The three major types of genetic tests include: (1) gene tests (e.g., individual genes or relatively short lengths of DNA or RNA are tested); (2) chromosomal tests (e.g., whole chromosomes or very long lengths of DNA are tested); and (3) biochemical tests (e.g., protein levels or enzyme activities are tested) (Burke, 2002). Most genetic tests look at single genes and are used to diagnose rare genetic disorders, but a growing number of tests are being developed to look at multiple genes that may increase or decrease a person's risk of common diseases, such as cancer or diabetes (CDC, 2012).

Genetic tests have the potential to improve individual health, but many genetic tests are based on limited scientific information and may not yet provide valid or useful results. For example, genetic testing does not establish the onset date, nature, severity, course of a disease, or ensure the efficacy of treatment for a genetic disorder. All we know definitely is that "significant scientific uncertainty surrounds much genetic testing" (Gostin, 1991).

Individuals need not utilize a physician to gain access to genetic testing. Direct-to-consumer marketing for genetic testing occurs through the Internet, television, and other media. This has prompted concerns that such testing does not provide appropriate counseling, and will create the potential for physical or psychological harm to individuals (Wolfberg, 2006).

Most members of both the general public and at-risk groups express favorable attitudes toward, and interest in, being tested (Croyle & Lerman, 1995). Likewise, persons with disabilities who seek genetic counseling are generally favorable to the service (Chen & Schiffman, 2000).

Genetic Discrimination

The history of genetic discrimination started in the early 19th century during the eugenics movement. Eugenics advocated various practices designed to improve the genetic composition of the human population. This negative and discriminatory practice was evident during the late 19th and early 20th centuries in Germany where the term *eugenics* originated. Eugenics was also evident in the United States. By 1937, 32 states had passed sterilization laws aimed at preventing people with disabilities, especially those with intellectual disabilities, from having offspring (Houser & Lash, 1996).

The current genetic testing industry—a multi-billion dollar business—is growing by 25% annually (Pollack, 2006). As genetic testing increases, so does the potential of an employer, a health or disability insurer, or other entity to discriminate against an individual based on the results of his or her genetic test. The potential for discrimination exists because the increasing costs of health, life, and disability-related insurance, may encourage employers and insurers to use genetic tests to exclude those with the potential to incur expensive medical or disability claims. Genetic information could become available to employers, insurers, educators, law enforcement, and others who might not have the skill to understand or correctly serve individuals with a propensity for disability (whether perceived or actual) (Hudson, 2011). In sum, genetic testing can have serious negative implications for the individual tested. It has been noted that "prejudice, alienation, and exclusion often accompany genetic disorders, even though the conditions are neither the result of willful behavior nor subject to the person's control" (Gostin, 1991).

To date, there have been very few cases of genetic discrimination in health insurance and employment, but the fear of such discrimination prompted passage of federal legislation to protect genetic information (Hudson, Holohan, & Collins, 2008). On May 21, 2008, the GINA was signed into law by President George W. Bush.

GINA defines *genetic information* as including a person's genetic tests, genetic tests of a person's family members (up to and including fourth-relatives), any manifestation of a disease or disorder in a family member, and participation of a person or family member in research that includes genetic testing, counseling, or education (GINA, 2008). Genetic services are defined as testing, counseling, and education. Examples of protected tests include: (1) tests for BRCA1/BRCA2 (breast cancer) or HNPCC (colon cancer) mutations; (2) classifications of genetic properties of an existing tumor to help determine therapy; (3) tests for Huntington's disease mutations; and (4) carrier screening for disorders such as cystic fibrosis, sickle cell disease, spinal muscular atrophy, and fragile X syndrome (GINA, 2008).

GINA prohibits genetic discrimination in employment and health insurance. However, GINA does not apply to life insurance, disability insurance, long-term care insurance, or other potential uses of genetic information, so it is not entirely clear that "its limited protections will be sufficient to allay the fears of individuals currently dissuaded from undergoing genetic testing" (Rothstein, 2008). Nor does GINA prohibit an employer (as provided by the Americans with Disabilities Act of 1990 [ADA, 1990]), after making a conditional offer of employment to an individual, to require that person to sign an authorization to disclose all of his or her health records to the employer (Rothstein, 2008). This could result in the employer gaining access to genetic information about the individual.

Genetic Counseling

Genetic counseling is "a communication process which deals with the human problems associated with the occurrence or risk of occurrence, of a genetic disorder in a family" (Fletcher & Evans, 1994). Physicians who specialize in genetic disorders (medical geneticists), and non-physicians who have an academic background in genetics and training in counseling, do genetic counseling. Genetic counseling is a new field that began in 1959 with the first application of educating about human genetics (Gardner, McKinley, Sutherland, & Shaffer, 2012).

Genetic counselors apply what is known about human genetics in providing advice to: (1) those concerned about the possibility of having a genetic disease themselves (genetic diagnosis); (2) those family members concerned about having the same genetic disease as an affected family member (familial risk); and (3) those concerned about passing a genetic mutation to their offspring (prenatal genetic testing).

Genetic counselors assist the client in understanding the medical facts including diagnosis, probable cause, and management of the genetic disorder. They also provide an understanding of how heredity contributes to the disorder and the risks for family members. Counselors assist the client in selecting the most appropriate course of action after considering the risks, resources, and long-term family goals. Counselors also assist the client in making the best possible adjustments to a disorder in an affected family member or in dealing with the risks of recurrence of the disorder (Shiloh, 1996a, 1996b).

Before genetic testing is performed, counselors can advise a client about what would happen if genetic test results should become available to other parties, particularly potential or current employers and insurers; whether genetic disorders would make it impossible for applicants to obtain health, life, or disability coverage; and whether insurance companies would decrease benefits for certain conditions (Resta, 2007). Genetic counseling addresses the medical, employment, insurance, and psychological problems associated with the risk of a genetic disorder, not with the medical management of the disorder itself (Godard et al., 2003). Goals of genetic counseling include helping clients learn, understand, choose, cope, and adjust to unexpected circumstances (Veach, Le Roy, & Bartels, 2003).

Role for Rehabilitation Counselors

Counselors—whether they are rehabilitation counselors or genetic counselors—share much in common. Several additional roles for rehabilitation counselors related to genetic counseling have been identified. These include education, support, advocacy, and technical assistance (Bennett, Pettersen, Niendorf, & Anderson, 2003; Evans & Biesecker, 2006).

Education has been identified as a prerequisite for providing genetic services for both the public and professionals (Le Roy, Veach, & Bartels, 2010). Counselors need to be well versed and current in human genetics and possess sensitivity in working with clients. In regard to client education, rehabilitation counselors can assist in several activities. Counselors need to provide information concerning genetic processes and explain potential procedures and results in ways that are understandable and meaningful to clients.

In the supportive role, rehabilitation counselors perform a variety of services. These include assisting families to identify and address underlying psychosocial and cultural issues related to genetic concerns and provide referral to support groups when beneficial to persons and their loved ones. Counselors assist clients while making decisions and providing supportive follow-ups. They help clients understand and cope with the reactions of family members. Counselors may also mediate peer counseling.

In the role of advocate, rehabilitation counselors discuss issues concerning employment, insurance, and other types of social discrimination against clients (Biesecker, Schwartz, & Marteau, 2013). Potential counseling interventions include informing employers and insurers about the legal protections afforded persons with disabilities, potential accommodations for those persons in the workplace, and providing information to clients about their legal rights.

In addition, rehabilitation counselors can assist clients by providing technical assistance. This type of technical assistance may involve construction of a life care plan for the individual and the family (Blackwell, Weed, & Powers, 1994). The life care plan can identify potential services and costs that may be required for the family and child, as well as resources to secure such services. The use of life care plans is a practical means by which to inform the client of future responsibilities engendered by an adult and child with a disability. It can serve as a basis for planning future life care services and avoiding lapses in the provision of services for the foreseeable future.

Case Studies

Descriptions of three case scenarios adapted from Fletcher & Evans (1994) are provided to show the complexity and interaction of issues encountered during genetic counseling. Analysis of these cases will help the counselor understand genetic counseling. These cases illustrate the need for counselors to have a firm understanding of their own beliefs. It is essential to provide meaningful discussions with the client and others involved, to carefully examine their own personal beliefs, without actually giving advice about what choice to make.

Case 1. A 42 year-old woman is considering prenatal diagnosis for possible Down Syndrome. Down Syndrome, or trisomy 21, is a chromosomal condition caused by the presence of all or part of a third copy of chromosome 21. Down Syndrome is the most common chromosome abnormality in humans and causes moderate to severe congenital intellectual disability. She and her husband have a child with this condition. They tell the counselor that abortion is not an option and that she plans to carry the fetus to full term despite the results of genetic testing. The family's reason for seeking the diagnosis is to provide more time for preparation if this child has Down Syndrome. They ask for the counselor's advice. How should the counselor proceed? Discuss various options.

Case 2. A 25 year-old woman with no history of genetic disorders in her family is considering prenatal diagnosis. This client has a problem with alcohol but is in denial, believing she is only a social drinker. She is a client because she acquired a below elbow upper extremity amputation as a result of an automobile accident. Although she did not have any abnormal sequelae, at the time of the amputation she received several blood transfusions and is concerned she may have contracted hepatitis or AIDS. The client appears very anxious about the normalcy of the fetus, even after being told that, in her case, the potential medical risks of the genetic procedure (including possible miscarriage) are greater than the likelihood of diagnosing an abnormality. She asks for the counselor's advice. As her counselor, describe what approach you might take.

Case 3. A couple in their late twenties requests prenatal diagnosis to determine the sex of their fetus. The father is a client of yours due to a recent back injury. They already have four girls and feel desperate to have a son. They stated that if it is a girl, they plan to abort the fetus and keep trying to have a boy. If they cannot have testing, they will abort the fetus rather than face the possibility of having another girl. They have requested your advice. Discuss the ramifications of this case.

References

Americans with Disabilities Act of 1990 (ADA), 42 U.S.C. §12101 *et seq.*

Bennett, R. L., Pettersen, B. J., Niendorf, K. B., & Anderson, R. R. (2003). Developing standard recommendations (guidelines) for genetic counseling practice: A process of the National Society of Genetic Factors. *Journal of Genetic Counseling, 12*(4), 287–295.

Biesecker, B. B., Schwartz, M. D., & Marteau, T. M. (2013). Enhancing informed choice to undergo health screening: A systematic review. *American Journal of Health Behavior, 37*, 351–359.

Blackwell, T. L., Weed, R. O., & Powers, A. A. (1994). *Life care planning for spinal cord injury: A resource manual for case managers.* Athens, GA: Elliott and Fitzpatrick.

Burke, W. (2002). Genetic testing. *New England Journal of Medicine, 347*(23), 1867–1875.

Centers for Disease Control and Prevention (CDC). (2012). *Genetic testing*. Retrieved from http://www.cdc.gov/genomics/gtesting/index.htm

Chen, E. A., & Schiffman, J. F. (2000). Attitudes toward genetic counseling and prenatal diagnosis among a group of individuals with disabilities. *Journal of Genetic Counseling, 9*(2), 137–152.

Croyle, R. T., & Lerman, C. (1995). Psychological impact of genetic testing. In R. T. Croyle (Ed.), *Psychosocial effects of screening for disease prevention and detection* (pp. 11–38). New York, NY: Oxford University.

Evans, C., & Biesecker, B. B. (2006). *Genetic counseling: A psychological approach*. New York, NY: Cambridge University.

Fletcher, J. C., & Evans, M. E. (1994). Ethics in reproductive genetics. In J. F. Monagle & D. C. Thomasma (Eds.), *Health care ethics: Critical issues* (pp. 24–42). Gaithersburg, MD: Aspen.

Gardner, R. J., McKinley, L. M., Sutherland G. R., & Shaffer L. G. (2012). Chromosome abnormalities and genetic counseling. *Oxford Monographs on Medical Genetics No. 61*. New York, NY: Oxford University.

Genetic Information Nondiscrimination Act of 2008 (GINA). Public Law 110-233, 122 Stat. 881. Retrieved from http://www.eeoc.gov/laws/statutes/gina.cfm

Godard, B., Raeburn, S., Pembrey, M., Bobrow, M., Farndon, P., & Aymé, S. (2003). Genetic information and testing in insurance and employment: Technical, social, and ethical issues. *European Journal of Human Genetics, 11*, 11–12. London, Great Britain: Nature.

Gostin, L. (1991). Genetic discrimination: The use of genetically based diagnostic and prognostic tests by employers and insurers. *American Journal of Law and Medicine, 17*, 109–144.

Hartl, D. L., & Jones, E. W. (2012). *Essential genetics* (6th ed.). Sudbury, MA: Jones and Bartlett.

Holzman, N. A., & Watson, M. S. (Eds.). (1999). *Promoting safe and effective genetic testing in the United States: Final report of the Task Force on Genetic Testing*. Baltimore, MD: Johns Hopkins University.

Houser, R., & Lash, M. (1996). Implications of research from the Human Genome Project for rehabilitation counselors. *Journal of Applied Rehabilitation Counseling, 27*, 3–7.

Hudson K. L. (2011). Genomics, health care, and society. *New England Journal of Medicine, 365*(11), 1033–1041.

Hudson, K. L., Holohan, M. K., & Collins, F. S. (2008). Keeping pace with the times – The Genetic Information Nondiscrimination Act of 2008. *New England Journal of Medicine, 358*(25), 2661–2663.

International Human Genome Sequencing Consortium. (2001). Initial sequencing and analysis of the human genome. *Nature, 409*, 860–921.

Le Roy, B. S., Veach, P. M., & Bartels, R. M. (2010). *Genetic counseling practice: Advanced concepts and skills*. Hoboken, NJ: John Wiley and Sons.

National Society of Genetic Counselors. (2005). *Genetic counseling as a profession*. Retrieved from http://www.nsgc.org/About/FAQsDefinitions/tabid/97/Default.aspx

Pollack, A. (2006, April 13). A crystal ball submerged in a test tube: Genetic technology reshapes the diagnostics business. *New York Times,* Business/Financial.

Resta, R. G. (2007). *Genetic counseling: Coping with the human impact of genetic disease*. Retrieved from http://www.accessexcellence.org/AE/AEC/CC/counseling_background.html

Rothstein, M. A. (2008). GINA, the ADA, and genetic discrimination in employment. *Journal of Law, Medicine, and Ethics, 36*(4), 837–840.

Shiloh, S. (1996a). Decision-making in the context of genetic risk. In T. Marteau & M. Richards (Eds.), *The troubled helix: Social and psychological implications of the new human genetics* (pp. 82–103). Cambridge, Great Britain: Cambridge University.

Shiloh, S. (1996b). Genetic counseling: A developing area of interest for psychologists. *Professional Psychology: Research and Practice, 27*, 475–486.

Veach, P. M., Le Roy, B. S., & Bartels, D. M. (2003). *Facilitating the genetic counseling process: A practice manual*. New York, NY: Springer-Verlag.

Wolfberg, A. J. (2006). Genes on the Web – Direct-to-consumer marketing of genetic testing. *New England Journal of Medicine, 355*(6), 543–544.

About the Author

John Howard, M.D., M.P.H., J.D. is Professorial Lecturer in Environmental and Occupational Health, School of Public Health and Health Services, The George Washington University, Washington, D.C. Dr. Howard is board-certified in internal medicine and occupational medicine. He is admitted to the practice of medicine and law in the State of California and the District of Columbia.

Acknowledgement

The author would like to acknowledge the work of Joseph Havranek, Ph.D., the author of the original chapter on Genetic Counseling, for his lifetime of contributions to the field of rehabilitation counseling.

Chapter 34

REGENERATIVE MEDICINE AND DISABILITY

John J. Howard, M.D., M.P.H.

Introduction

Prometheus, a Greek Titan, was punished by Zeus for giving fire to mankind. Zeus had him chained to a rock and sent an eagle to eat his liver each day, but Prometheus' liver regenerated each night. Like Zeus, medical science is now creating new tissues to replace or repair organs lost to congenital defects, age, disease, or trauma. These newer scientific technologies involve growing tissues and organs in the laboratory and then implanting them into the body when the body's own healing responses fail to restore function (Atala, Lanza, Thomson, & Nerem, 2010). The term *regenerative medicine* was first used in 1992 to describe futuristic medical technologies (Kaiser, 1992), and the field has progressed since then thanks to advances in cell and developmental biology, biomaterials science, and biomedical engineering (National Institutes of Health, 2006).

The human body has the ability to replenish some cells and tissues, but that ability is limited to blood, skin, and intestinal lining cells. Humans cannot grow another limb like a newt, grow new heart muscle cells after a heart attack, or grow new nerves after a spinal cord injury. A human embryo's cells differentiate into specialized cell types after only a few divisions following conception. After that, they go into a type of cellular *lock down* when cellular differentiation ceases and cells are committed to their genetic fate (DeWitt, 2008).

Regenerative medicine has taken medical science beyond living donor or cadaveric transplants, first introduced in the early 20th century. By 1954, the first human kidney transplant had been performed. Currently, donor organ transplant surgery involves many different organs. The most common are bone marrow, heart, kidney, and lung transplants. Organ transplantation has become so successful that there is a shortage of donor organs; people needing organs remain on waiting lists for extended periods. Regenerative medicine has the potential to alleviate this organ shortage problem by providing a laboratory-grown source for replacement organs.

There is a wide array of unmet medical needs affecting tens of millions of people which could be addressed by regenerative medicine. Among these needs are spinal cord injuries, heart diseases, Parkinson's disease, Alzheimer's disease, birth defects, diabetes mellitus, severe burns, and bone and muscle diseases (Committee on the Biological and Medical Applications of Stem Cell Research, 2002). Over the past twenty years, several therapeutic applications of regenerative medicine have been introduced into everyday medical practice, or are in animal or human trials to test their safety and efficacy.

Research investments in cell-based therapies that characterize advanced regenerative medicine have come primarily from private industry. Government funding has been problematic because the source of some of the cells used to grow tissues and organs in the laboratory—cells harvested from human embryos—is controversial. Financial investment by the government is increasing, though, as other non-embryonic cell sources are identified. For example, the *Armed Forces Institute for Regenerative Medicine* (AFIRM) is a multi-institutional, inter-disciplinary network funded by the U.S. Army. AFIRM is working to develop treatment options using multiple different cell sources for severely wounded servicemen and women in six areas: (1) limb and digit salvage; (2) craniofacial reconstruction; (3) scarless wound healing; (4) burn repair; and (5) compartment injuries arising from blast injuries (AFIRM, 2013).

This chapter presents a brief introduction to the emerging field of regenerative medicine. Although the present practice of rehabilitation counseling has not been affected as yet, regenerative medicine is a field of therapeutics that has the potential to greatly improve the lives of people with disabilities and significantly affect the practice of rehabilitation counseling.

Basics of Regenerative Medicine

Cell-based regenerative medicine therapies involve three steps. First, a cell must be obtained that ideally possesses the twin traits of self-renewal and pluripotency. Self-renewal means that the cell can go through numerous cell divisions but still remain in a relatively undifferentiated state. Potency means that the cell has the capacity to differentiate into many different specialized cell types when stimulated in the laboratory. The cells that are the starting point in developing many regenerative medicine applications are known as stem cells. Second, techniques are used to produce the desired cell type from the source cell by modulating the source cell's microenvironment in the laboratory. Third, the specialized cells produced from source cell are then embedded into a tissue matrix structure or scaffold by means of *tissue engineering* and transplanted into the body to replace damaged cells (Khang, 2012).

Types of Stem Cells

Stem cells are generally divided into three categories depending on their origin: (1) embryonic stem cells; (2) fetal stem cells; and (3) adult stem cells. Embryonic stem cells—derived from inner cell mass of the blastocyst phase of an early human embryo—are capable of infinite self-renewal and are broadly *pluripotent*, meaning they can differentiate into all cell lines—ectoderm, mesoderm, and endoderm. Obtaining human embryonic stem cells requires the destruction of early human embryos which makes obtaining this type of stem cell ethically very controversial. Because of the controversial nature of stem cells, the authority of the Federal government to fund and conduct embryonic stem cell research was restricted in 2007 by President George W. Bush (Bush, 2007). In 2009, President Barach Obama removed the restrictions and expanded support of human stem cell research (Obama, 2009). However, regenerative medical research involving human embryonic stem cells remains controversial.

Fetal stem cells are derived from the placenta, amniotic fluid, or from umbilical cord blood. Harvesting fetal stem cells does not require destruction of the fetus. Adult stem cells, also known as *somatic* stem cells, are found throughout the body but in very small numbers. As a source of stem cells, adult stem cells are not considered controversial as they are derived from adult tissue samples through biopsy or organ donation rather than from destroyed human embryos (Atala et al., 2010). However, fetal and adult stem cells lack the same power of self-renewal and pluripotency as do embryonic stem cells; they need more coaxing in a laboratory to express those traits. But these types of stem cells are becoming an important source for regenerative medicine.

Laboratory Modulation of Stem Cells

All cells are influenced by their microenvironments. Stem-cell modulation technologies are a complex area of laboratory science that involves manipulating the stem cell into desired specialized cell types. A full description of these techniques is beyond this chapter, but suffice it to say that stem cells can now be grown and coaxed into differentiating into stable cell lines of various tissues such as heart muscle cells, nerve cells, and muscle cells, by means of advanced cell culture techniques and stem-cell technologies.

Tissue Engineering

The procedure of replacing damaged tissue with new cells is called tissue engineering (Berthiaume, Maguire, & Yarmush, 2011). Tissue engineering uses laboratory-grown source cells embedded in a biomaterial-derived matrix structure that has the capability of functioning in three dimensions (Liu, Hui, Bhatia, & Chen, 2009). Engineered scaffolds derived from porcine intestines are used to provide a matrix for embedding regenerated cells. The cell-matrix is incubated in the laboratory to promote cell adhesion and organ formation and then transplanted into the body (Viola, Lal, & Grad, 2003). Advanced tissue engineering envisions a technology for 3D organ printing which would dramatically accelerate and optimize tissue and organ assembly (Mironov, Boland, Trusk, Forgacs, & Markwald, 2003). Through tissue engineering techniques, regenerative medicine is moving closer to developing therapeutic applications for damaged organs that would significantly expand what rehabilitation medicine can offer people with disabilities (Khademhosseini, Langer, Borenstein, & Vacanti, 2005).

Therapeutic Applications

Although few medical therapies using stem cells are in clinical practice at this time, regenerative medicine holds great promise for people who have severe burns, are disabled by a spinal cord injury, who sustain a heart attack and lose heart muscle cells, or who undergo cartilage loss. Regenerative medicine research is leading to solutions to these conditions and many others (Committee on the Biological and Medical Application of Stem Cell Research, 2002). The following four examples illustrate the potential future impact of regenerative medicine for people with disabilities (Badylack & Nerem, 2010).

Burns

Mortality from full-thickness burns is high due to the slow pace of wound healing. Approaches to the treatment of severe burns involve skin auto-grafting, but this technique is limited in extensively burned individuals because such individuals have so little healthy skin available for auto-transplantation. Transplanting skin from healthy donors to the burned individual is another approach, but transplant rejection often occurs (Gerlach, Wolf, Johnen, & Hartman, 2010). Newer cell-based regenerative medical therapies are also being investigated. A very small population of the burned individual's skin cells (*keratinocytes*) are harvested and rapidly reproduced in the laboratory. The new keratinocytes are applied to the burned area, either by embedding them in a tissue scaffold or by spraying them on the burned area. Fetal skin-derived cells can also serve as a source of keratinocytes in burn therapy (Hohlfeld et al., 2005).

Spinal Cord Injury

One of the first studies using a human embryonic stem cell involved individuals with neurologically complete traumatic spinal cord injuries. Currently, cell-based regenerative medical research into spinal cord regeneration is focused on determining which stem cell would best restore spinal nerve function.

An obstacle to nerve cell regeneration is the tendency of scar tissue to form at the site of the spinal cord injury. Scar formation can block the growth of any transplanted cells, rendering cell-based regenerative medicine solutions to spinal cord injury ineffective. Scarring is promoted by axon growth inhibitors (Kingwell, 2011). In animal studies where these axon growth inhibitors are blocked, some axon *sprouting* and functional recovery has been seen (Lee, McKeon, & Bellamkonda, 2010). Other studies have shown that stabilization of the axonal microtubule with paclitaxel (a cancer drug) promotes axon growth in animals (Hellal et al., 2011).

Heart Disease

Heart failure following a heart attack is a leading cause of death worldwide (World Health Organization [WHO], 2011). After cardiac muscle cells (cardiomyocytes) die from a lack of oxygen (ischemia) during a heart attack, they are replaced by fibrotic scar tissue, not by new heart muscle cells. Scar tissue does not contract like normal cardiomyocytes. The pumping function of the heart is impaired and heart failure may result. Heart failure treatment is limited, as are donor hearts for replacement. These factors have spurred the development of approaches to replace damaged cardiomyocytes through cell-based therapies (Laflamme & Murray, 2011). Studies with human adult stem cells or with human embryonic stem cells have shown promise in achieving cardiomyocyte regeneration and restoration of cardiac function (Passier, van Laake, & Mummery, 2008). Clinical trials using adult stem cells in post-heart attack therapy are among the most advanced regenerative medicine applications of stem cells to date (Ahsan, Doyle, & Nerem, 2010).

Cartilage

Adults lack the regenerative ability to repair cartilage that becomes damaged by osteoarthritis, traumatic injury, or joint disorders like rheumatoid arthritis. Currently, chrondrocytes (cells which make cartilage) can be harvested from an individual with damaged cartilage, multiplied in the laboratory, and surgically transplanted back into the individual. Although effective, this process involves a complex surgical procedure. A search for cell-based regenerative therapies has begun. Cell-based therapies using a type of adult stem cells, such as mesenchymal stem cells (MSCs), and a scaffold of self-assembling biofibers, have shown promise in animal models of cartilage regeneration (Shah et al., 2010). Also, a simple intra-articular injection of a chemical called kartogenin into the joint stimulates endogenous MSCs to differentiate into cartilage-producing chondrocytes (Johnson et al., 2012). Stimulating an individual's own MSCs to differentiate and populate the joint surface with mature cartilage by an injectable chemical would be more effective than what is currently available (Marini & Forlino, 2012).

Risks

No medical therapy is free of risk. Three risks associated with cell-based regenerative medicine are important to mention.

Neoplasms

Differentiation of a source cell into a particular cell type so that only cells of the desired cell type grow in the recipient is the aim of regenerative medical therapies. However, cells can differentiate into unwanted cell types after being transplanted. If this occurs, a tumor mass of unwanted cells, usually of different cell types occurs. This is called a *teratoma*. For example, transplanted heart muscle cells could continue to differentiate after being transplanted into a person's heart, forming a neoplasm of cartilage, neural cells, teeth, bone, or other cell types. Development of a teratoma defeats the purpose of the cell therapy and can further impair the function of an already damaged heart.

Immune Rejection

A second risk is rejection of the transplanted cells by the person's immune system. Source cells obtained from the same individual into whom they will be re-implanted, called *autologous* cells, have little risk of rejection. If autologous cells cannot be obtained, cells which come from a donor of the same species, called allogeneic cells, can be used as source cell. Allogeneic cells and xenogenic cells (cells from another species) can also be used as source cells, but increase the risk of rejection.

Zoonosis

Zoonosis refers to the transmission of animal diseases to humans. Scaffolds that are used to form the structural support for source cells used as replacement tissues are produced from animals, most commonly pigs. Although the scaffold is washed clean of animal cells leaving only the connective tissue scaffold, the risk of contamination with animal viruses still exists (Khang, 2012).

A Word about Cloning

In 1962, Sir John Gurdon of Great Britain found that the specialization of adult somatic cells is reversible. Gurdon replaced the nucleus of a frog egg cell with a mature frog intestinal cell nucleus. The modified egg cell grew into a normal tadpole. He proved that the nucleus of the mature frog intestinal cell, which many thought up to that time had lost the ability to direct new life, still contained the ability needed to grow all the cells of a frog. The reprogramming of somatic nuclei to direct the differentiation of enucleated eggs is known as somatic cell nuclear transfer (SCNT). In 2012, Gurdon shared the Nobel Prize in Medicine with Shinya Yamanaka of Japan for the discovery that mature cells can be reprogrammed to become pluripotent. Their research showed that somatic cells that normally cannot regenerate other cell lines, because they are already specialized to perform specific functions in the body, can be stimulated to do so under certain circumstances. This is the basis of reproductive and therapeutic cloning.

Reproductive Cloning

The most controversial aspect of SCNT involves cloning of an entire individual. In 1996, Dolly, a female domestic sheep, was the first mammal to be cloned by SCNT (Wilmut, Schnieke, McWhir, Kind, & Campbell, 1997). A mammary gland cell nucleus was used. The production of a healthy cloned sheep proved that a highly specialized cell like a mammary gland cell could be made to recreate a whole individual. Reproductive cloning that creates a genetically identical copy of an existing, or previously existing, human being is very controversial. In fact, 15 states have passed laws prohibiting reproductive human cloning (National Conference of State Legislatures, 2008).

Therapeutic Cloning

Only slightly less controversial is therapeutic cloning. SCNT is used to implant a somatic cell nucleus into an enucleated human egg; the egg is then stimulated to divide into a blastocyst. The inner cells of the blastocyst are isolated and used to create embryonic stem cells for regenerative medical purposes. In addition to the advantages of embryonic stem cells, self-renewal and pluripotency, another advantage is that the risk of immune rejection is less because the individual who will benefit from the transplanted source cells is the source of the DNA used in SCNT. Since therapeutic cloning results in destruction of an embryo, it is as controversial as reproductive cloning.

Future

There is no doubt that regenerative medicine has the potential to improve the lives of people with disabilities. Many scientific and ethical hurdles remain before that potential can be fully achieved, but already counseling is undergoing change as a result of the advances that regenerative medicine is bringing to the practice of rehabilitation. Rehabilitation specialists are now working with regenerative scientists to guide the development of clinical protocols for individuals with disabilities who are undergoing regenerative medical procedures (Ambrosio, Wolf, & Delitto, 2010). The practice of rehabilitation counseling will expand in the future to include not only traditional whole body, physiological and mechanical approaches, but also cellular and molecular regenerative medicine approaches (Ambrosio & Russell, 2010).

References

Ahsan, T., Doyle, A. M., & Nerem, R. M. (2010). Stem cell research. In A. Atala, R. Lanza, J. Thomson, & R. Nerem (Eds.), *Foundations of regenerative medicine* (pp. 28–47). New York, NY: Elsevier.

Ambrosio, F., Wolf, S. L., Delitto, A., Fitzgerald, G. K., Badylak, S. F., Boninger, M. L., & Russell, A. J. (2010). The emerging relationship between regenerative medicine and physical therapeutics. *Journal of the American Physical Therapy Association, 90*(12), 1807–1814.

Ambrosio, F., & Russell, A. (2010). Regenerative rehabilitation: A call to action. *Journal of Rehabilitation Research and Development, 47*(3), xi–xv.

Armed Forces Institute for Regenerative Medicine (AFIRM). (2013). Retrieved from http://www.afirm.mil/

Atala, A., Lanza, R., Thomson, J., & Nerem, R. (2010). *Foundations of regenerative medicine.* New York, NY: Elsevier.

Badylak, S. F., & Nerem, R. M. (2010). Progress in tissue engineering and regenerative medicine. *Proceedings of the National Academy of Sciences, 107*(8), 3285–3286.

Berthiaume, F., Maguire T. J., & Yarmush, M. L. (2011). Tissue engineering and regenerative medicine: History, progress, and challenges. *Annual Review of Chemical and Biomolecular Engineering, 2*, 403–430.

Bush, G. W. (2007). *Expanding approved stem cell lines in ethically responsible ways.* Executive Order 13435 (June 20, 2007). Retrieved from http://georgewbushwhitehouse.archives.gov/news/releases/2007/06/20070620-6.html

Committee on the Biological and Medical Applications of Stem Cell Research. (2002). *Stem cells and the future of regenerative medicine.* Washington, DC: National Academy. Retrieved from http://www.nap.edu/openbook.php?record_id=10195&page=R1

DeWitt, N. (2008). Regenerative medicine. *Nature, 453*(7193), 301–302.

Gerlach, J. C., Wolf, S. E., Johnen, C., & Hartman B. (2010). Innovative regenerative medicine approaches to skin cell-based therapy for patients with burn injuries. In A. Atala, R. Lanza, J. Thomson, & R. Nerem (Eds.), *Foundations of regenerative medicine* (pp. 688–711). New York, NY: Elsevier.

Hellal, F., Hurtado, A., Ruschel J., Flynn, K. C., Laskowski, C. J., Umlauf, M., . . . Bradke, F. (2011). Microtubule stabilization reduces scarring and causes axon regeneration after spinal cord injury. *Science, 331*(6019), 928–921.

Hohlfeld, J., de Buys Roessingh, A., Hirt-Burri, N., Chaubert, p., Gerper, S., Scaletta, C., . . . Applegate, L. A. (2005). Tissue engineered fetal skin constructs for pediatric burns. *Lancet, 366,* 840–842.

Johnson, K. Zhu, S., Tremblay, M. S., Payette, J. N., Wang, J., Bouchez, L. C., Meeusen, S., Schultz, P. G. (2012). A stem cell-based approach to cartilage repair. *Science, 336*(6082), 717–721.

Kaiser, L. (1992). The future of multihospital systems. *Top Healthcare Financing, 18,* 32–38.

Khademhosseini, A., Langer, R., Borenstein, J., & Vacanti, J. (2005). Microscale technologies for tissue engineering and biology. *Proceedings of the National Academy of Sciences, 103*(8), 2480–2487.

Khang, G. (Ed). (2012). *Handbook of intelligent scaffold for tissue engineering and regenerative medicine.* Singapore: Pan Stanford.

Kingwell, K. (2011). Regeneration: A regenerative medicine. *Nature Reviews Neuroscience, 12,* 123.

Laflamme, M. A., & Murray, C. E. (2011). Heart regeneration. *Nature, 473,* 326–335.

Lee, H., McKeon R. J., & Bellamkonda R. V. (2010). Sustained delivery of thermostablized chABC enhances axonal sprouting and function recovery after spinal cord injury. *Proceedings of the National Academy of Sciences, 107*(8), 3340–3345.

Liu, W. F., Hui, E. E., Bhatia, S. N., & Chen, C. S. (2010). Engineering cellular environments. In A. Atala, R. Lanza, J. Thomson, & R. Nerem (Eds.), *Foundations of regenerative medicine.* New York, NY: Elsevier.

Marini, J. C., & Forlino A. (2012). Replenishing cartilage from endogenous stem cells. *New England Journal of Medicine, 366*(26), 2522–2524.

Mironov, V., Boland, T., Trusk, T., Forgacs, G., & Markwald, R. R. (2003). Organ printing: Computer-aided jet-based 3D tissue engineering. *Trends in Biotechnology, 21*(4), 157–161.

National Conference of State Legislatures (2008). *Human cloning laws.* Retrieved from http://www.ncsl.org/issues-research/health/human-cloning-laws.aspx

National Institutes of Health (NIH). (2006). *Regenerative medicine.* Retrieved from http://stemcells.nih.gov/staticresources/info/scireport/PDFs/Regenerative_Medicine_2006.pdf

Obama, B. (2009). *Removing barriers to responsible research involving human stem cells.* Executive Order 13505 (March 9, 2009). Retrieved from http://www.gpo.gov/fdsys/pkg/FR-2009-03-11/pdf/E9-5441.pdf

Passier, R., van Laake, L. W., & Mummery, C. L. (2008). Stem-cell-based therapy and lessons from the heart. *Nature, 453,* 322–329.

Shah, R. N., Shah, N. A., Del Rosario Lim, M. M., Hsieh, C., Nuber, G., & Strupp, S. I. (2010). Supramolecular design of self-assembling nanofibers for cartilage regeneration. *Proceedings of the National Academy of Sciences, 107*(8), 3293–3298.

Viola, J., Lal, B, & Grad, O. (2003). *The emergence of tissue engineering as a research field.* Cambridge, MA: Abt Associates. Retrieved from http://www.abtassociates.com/reports/emergence_tissue_engineering_research.pdf

Wilmut, I., Schnieke, A. E., McWhir, J., Kind, A. J., & Campbell, K. H. S. (1997). Viable offspring derived from fetal and mammalian cells. *Nature, 385,* 810–813.

World Health Organization (WHO). (2011). *Top ten causes of death.* Retrieved from http://www.who.int/mediacentre/factsheets/fs310/en/index.html

About the Author

John Howard, M.D., M.P.H., J.D. is Professorial Lecturer in Environmental and Occupational Health, School of Public Health and Health Services, The George Washington University, Washington, D.C. Dr. Howard is board-certified in internal medicine and occupational medicine. He is admitted to the practice of medicine and law in the State of California and the District of Columbia.

Appendix

MASTERING MEDICAL TERMINOLOGY

Prefixes

Word roots can be modified by prefixes that denote:

1. Position in time or space
   - ab - means **away from**

   abnormal – away from normal

   abduction – drawing away from the midline of the body by the arm or leg
   - circum – means **around**

   circumcision – a cutting around of the prepuce

   circumarticular – around a joint

2. Quantitative information
   - a or an – means **without**

   anorexia – without appetite

   anoxia – without enough oxygen
   - hemi – means **half**

   hemiplegia – paralysis of one lateral half of the body

   heminephrectomy – removal of a portion of a kidney
   - diplo – means **double**

   diplopia – double vision

   diploscope – an apparatus for study of binocular vision
   - quint – means **fifth**

   quintipara – a woman who has five pregnancies continued beyond the 20th week of gestation

   quintuplet – one of five offspring produced in one gestation period

3. Qualitative information
   - mal – means **bad** or **ill**

   malfunction – defective function

   malocclusion – faulty positioning of the upper or lower teeth in relation to the other
   - eu – means **good** or **healthy**

   euphoria – sense of well-being or condition of good health

   euthanasia – easy or painless death

4. Sameness and difference
   - hetero – means **different**

   heterogeneous – differing in kinds or nature

heterosexual – sexual orientation directed to the opposite sex
- homo – means **same**

homogeneous – of the same kind

homosexual – sexual orientation directed to the same sex

5. Physical attributes (size, shape, color)
    - micro – means **small**

microcephalia – abnormal smallness of the head

micromelia – abnormal smallness or shortness of the extremities
- brachy – means **short**

brachycephalia – having a short head

brachydactylia – having abnormally short fingers and toes
- oxy – means **pointed** or **sharp**

oxycephaly – having a high and pointed head
- albo – means **white**

albinism – absence of pigmentation

albinuria – passing of white or colorless urine

Suffixes

Suffixes and significant word endings characteristically function in compound words to:
1. Form adjectives
    - -al means **pertaining to**

peritone**al** – pertaining to the peritoneum

arteri**al** – pertaining to an artery
- -ible, or –able means **ability**

digest**ible** – capable of being digested

oper**able** – subject to being operated

2. Express diminutive size – a number of suffixes serve this purpose,
    - -cule, –icle, –ium, –ole, –ule, and variations

arteri**ole** means a small artery

gran**ule** means a small grain

3. Indicate a surgical procedure
    - -ectomy means **removal** of an organ or part

append**ectomy** – removal of the appendix
- -lysis means **loosening**, usually of adhesions

cardio**lysis** – freeing of the heart of pericardial adhesions
- -ostomy means an operation in which an **artificial opening** is formed between two hollow organs or between one or more such viscera and the abdominal wall for discharge of intestinal content or urine.

colo**stomy** – the surgical creation of an opening between the colon and the exterior of the body
- -pexy means **fixation**

nephro**pexy** – the surgical attachment of a floating kidney

- -plasty means **plastic surgery**

blepharo**plasty** – plastic surgery of the eyelids

- -rrhaphy means **suture** or **operative repair**

teno**rrhaphy** – the suturing of a tendon

- -scopy means **viewing** or **examining**, usually with an instrument

endo**scopy** – visual inspection of any body cavity by means of an endoscope

- -tomy means **cutting** or **incision**

laparo**tomy** – the surgical opening of the abdomen

- -tripsy means the **intentional surgical crushing** of a structure

litho**tripsy** – the disintegration of a kidney stone by a high-energy shockwave

4. Express conditions or changes related to pathological processes

- -mania means **excessive excitement** or **obsessive preoccupation**

pyro**mania** – an irrational compulsion to set fires

- -sis means an **action**, **process**, or **condition**

silico**sis** – a fibrotic disorder of the lungs following inhalation of dust containing silicone dioxide

thoracente**sis** – surgical puncture of the chest wall for removal of fluid

- -itis means **inflammation**

appendic**itis** – an inflammation of the appendix

Besides these loosely formulated classes of suffixes, there are a number of miscellaneous word endings, the most significant of which is included in the basic prefix/suffix vocabulary that follows. Rehabilitation counselors need to be familiar with this vocabulary.

Basic Prefix and Suffix Terms

The following list of prefix and suffix terms aid in understanding medical terminology. This list will familiarize the reader with the flexibility of nomenclature. As new terms are encountered, the counselor can more readily recognize the components from which they are made.

Prefix/Suffix	Definition	Example
-algia	pain	neur**algia**
angio-	blood vessel	**angio**gram
ante-	before	**ante**cubital
arth-	joint	**arth**roscopy
blephar-	eyelid	**blephar**ospasm
cardi-	heart	electro**cardi**ography
cele-	1) a swelling	varico**cele**
	2) a hernia	recto**cele**
cerebr-	cerebrum	**cerebr**al
chole-	gall or bile	**chole**cystectomy
chondr-	cartilage	**chondr**ocostal
contra-	opposed to	**contra**ception
cost-	rib	inter**cost**als

cyst-	bladder	**cyst**itis
-desis	fusion	arthro**desis**
derm-	skin	**derm**atology
dys-	difficult, abnormal	**dys**pnea
ect-	outside	**ect**omorph
-ectomy	removal	spen**ectomy**
-emia	condition of the blood	polycyth**emia**
enceph-	brain	**enceph**alitis
end-	within	**end**ocrine
enter-	intestine	**enter**ostomy
epi-	upon, above	**epi**thelium
genic-	giving rise to	psycho**genic**
glyco-	sugar	**glyco**suria
hemi-	half	**hemi**plegia
hepat-	liver	**hepat**itis
hyper-	in excess	**hyper**tension
hyster-	uterus	**hyster**ectomy
-iosis	a pathologic condition	ameb**iosis**
-itis	inflammation	tonsill**itis**
leuk-	white	**leuk**ocyte
lip-	fat	hyper**lip**emia
-lith	stone	nephro**lith**iasis
-megaly	a state of largeness	hepato**megaly**
myel-	1) bone marrow	**myel**ocyte
	2) spinal cord	polio**myel**itis
myo-	muscle	**myo**cardium
neph-	kidney	**neph**rosis
-oid	resembling	thyr**oid**
-oma	tumor or swelling	carcin**oma**
-oscopy	visual examination	lapar**oscopy**
-osis	disease process or condition	nec**rosis**
osteo-	bone	**osteo**arthritis
-ostomy	creation of an artificial opening in an organ	trache**ostomy**
-otomy	incision	crani**otomy**
para-	near, alongside, beyond, outside	**para**vertebral
-pathy	disease of	cardiomyo**pathy**
-penia	lack of	leuko**penia**
-plasty	reparative or reconstructive surgery	rhino**plasty**

pneumo-	air	**pneumo**thorax
pre-	before	**pre**cancerous
pro-	in front of, before	**pro**gnathism
proct-	rectum or anus	**proct**ology
-ptosis	lowering of an organ or part	nephro**ptosis**
pyel-	pelvis	**pyel**ogram
pyo-	pus	**pyo**rrhea
spondyl-	vertebra	**spondyl**olysis
sub-	under	**sub**mandibular
super-	above, excessive	**super**sensitivity
supra-	above	**supra**ventricular
syn-	together	**syn**arthrosis
trans-	across	**trans**urethral
tri-	three	**tri**ceps

Anatomical Landmarks

A rehabilitation counselor should be familiar not only with the names of anatomic structures and pathological conditions, but with the "landmark" terms that designate anatomic position and direction. These are described in relation to the patient who is standing in the erect position, looking forward, with arms to the side of the body, and hands with palms forward (see Figure 1). The most commonly used landmark terms are the following:

lateral	to the side (used in contradistinction to medial)
medial	to the center
superior	above (used in contradistinction to inferior)
inferior	below
anterior	before or in front (used in contradistinction to posterior)
posterior	behind or in back
proximal	nearest to the point of attachment or center of the body (used in contradistinction to distal)
distal	farthest from the center
prone	lying face downward (used in contradistinction to supine)
supine	lying face upward
volar	pertaining to the sole of the foot or the palm of the hand
dorsal	pertaining to the back (used in contradistinction to ventral)
ventral	pertaining to the front or abdominal surface
palmar	pertaining to the palm of the hand
plantar	pertaining to the sole of the foot

Body Areas

Specific sites of illness or injury are usually designated by terms derived from the adjacent anatomic structure. Among the commonly used terms to indicate body areas are the following:

abdominal	pertaining to the stomach and intestinal area
carpal	pertaining to the wrist

FIGURE 1
Anatomical Positon of the Human Body for Descriptive Purposes

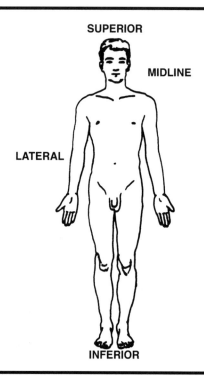

cervical	pertaining to the seven vertebrae in the neck, or the neck region
costal	pertaining to the ribs
cranial	pertaining to the skull
femoral	pertaining to the thigh
frontal	pertaining to the forehead
lumbar	pertaining to the five vertebrae in the lower portion of the back, or that region
pelvic	pertaining to the pelvic girdle
renal	pertaining to the kidney area
sacral	pertaining to the four vertebrae in the lowest portion of the back, or that region
sternal	pertaining to the sternum or breastbone
thoracic	pertaining to the twelve vertebrae in the upper portion of the back, or that region

Medical Abbreviations

Abbreviations denote instructions that are included in prescriptions for medications; some signify symptoms as reported by patients, and some refer to anatomic parts or body systems. Examples are noted:

a.c.	before meals (ante cibum)
b.i.d.	twice daily (bis in die)
B.P.	blood pressure
C-1 through C-7	cervical vertebrae by number
CBC	complete blood count
C.C.	chief complaint

C.N.	cranial nerve
C.N.S.	central nervous system
CPR	cardiopulmonary resuscitation
CT	computerized tomography
CVA	cerebrovascular accident
DB	decibel
DX	diagnosis
ESR	erythrocyte sedimentation rate
F.H.	family history
FX	fracture
GI	gastrointestinal
Hg	hemoglobin or mercury
GU	genitourinary
HBV	hepatitis B virus
HDL	high density lipoprotein
h.s.	at bedtime (hora somni)
H & P	history and physical examination
HX	history
L-1 through L-5	lumbar vertebrae by number
L.L.Q.	left lower quadrant
L.M.P.	last menstrual period
L.U.Q.	left upper quadrant
MRI	magnetic resonance imaging
OA	osteoarthritis
O.D.	right eye (oculus dexter)
O.S.	left eye (oculus sinister)
p.c.	after meals (post cibum)
P.H.	past history
P.I.	present illness
p.r.n.	as needed (pro re nata)
q.i.d.	four times daily (quater in die)
RA	rheumatoid arthritis
R.B.C.	red blood count
R.L.Q.	right lower quadrant
R/O	rule out
R.U.Q.	right upper quadrant
Rx	prescription
S-1 through S-5	sacral vertebrae by number
SOAP	subjective findings, objective findings, assessment, plan
T-1 through T-12	thoracic vertebrae by number

t.i.d.	three times daily (ter in die)
TX	treatment
W.B.C.	white blood count

The abbreviations cited are examples of the hundreds, perhaps thousands, in use. Unlike medical nomenclature, abbreviations cannot be divided logically into components, nor is it feasible to try to memorize a list of abbreviations. With experience, one becomes increasingly competent in interpreting this medical shorthand.

Index

A

AA – see Alcoholics Anonymous
abbreviations – see medical abbreviations
acquired brain injury – see traumatic brain injury
acquired immunodeficiency syndrome – see HIV/AIDS
acupuncture, 144-146
acute retroviral syndrome – see HIV/AIDS
acute stress disorder, 278
addiction, 295-308
age categories, 2
AIDS – see HIV/AIDS
ALANON, 312
albinism, 125
alcohol abuse, 309
Alcoholics Anonymous (AA), 311, 314-315
alcoholism, 310
alcohol-related disorders, 309-316
alternative medicine – see Integrative medicine
Americans with Disabilities Act, vii, 8, 47, 61, 81, 112, 189, 213, 228, 229, 304, 318, 322, 324, 335, 393, 410
amputation, 7, 51-53, 56, 357-361
aneurysm, 172
aneurysmal subarachnoid hemorrhage, 172
angina pectoris, 69-73, 80
ankylosing spondylitis, 264-265
anxiety disorders, 274-275
aphasia, 199-200
arterial sclerosis, 53
arterial venous malformation – see cerebral vascular malformation
arthritis – see rheumatic disease
Asperger's syndrome, 343, 344
assistive technology, 110-111, 123, 125, 127 162-163, 176-177, 226, 228-229, 323, 364, 385, 389-391
asthma, 77-83
AT – see assistive technology
atraumatic brain injury, 157
auditory system, 101-102
aural rehabilitation, 108-109
autism spectrum disorder, 343-351

B

biofeedback/neurofeedback, 137, 149-151
biologic therapy, 43
bipolar disorders, 277
blast injuries, 156-157

blood pressure – see hypertension
brain injury, 155-164
brain tumor, 172, 181
bronchitis, 77-78
burn injuries, 367-376, 417

C

cancer, 37-50
Cannabis – see marijuana
cardiac muscle, 18, 22, 68, 234, 417
cardiac transplantation, 72
cardiomyopathy, 65
cardiovascular disease, 53, 65-68
cardiovascular system, 25-28
carpal tunnel syndrome, 133, 202, 381, 383
case study analysis, 13-14
cataract, 125
central nervous system, 22
cerebral embolus, 171
cerebral hypertensive hemorrhage, 171
cerebral palsy, 219-232
cerebral thrombus, 171
cerebral vascular accident – see stroke
cerebral vascular malformation, 172
chemotherapy, 43-45, 48, 90
chiropractic, 147-149
chronic bronchitis – see bronchitis
chronic obstructive pulmonary disease, 77-85
chronic pain management, 131-141, 212, 382, 400
circulatory system, 26
cloning, 418-419
closed head injury, 156
cochlear implant, 108
complementary medicine – see integrative medicine
computerized tomography, 195
conductive hearing loss, 104-105
congenital heart disease, 66
congestive heart failure, 72
contracture, 211
COPD – see chronic obstructive pulmonary disease
coronary artery disease, 69-70
CVA – see stroke

D

Deaf, 104
Deafness – see hearing loss
deinstitutionalization, 281, 333-334
dementia, 198-199

431

depression, 276
dermatomyositis, 263-264
detoxification, 302, 304, 310-313
diabetes mellitus, 51-57
diabetic nephropathy, 53
diabetic retinopathy, 53, 123
dialysis, 59
digestive system, 31-32
drug use, 295-308
DSM – see autism spectrum and psychiatric diagnoses

E

echocardiogram, 71
educational categories, 3
electroencephalogram, 195
electromyography, 195
emotional lability, 158, 160, 300
emphysema, 77, 84
endocrine system, 34-35
epilepsy, 181-192
exertion/physical demand levels, 4-5

F

fibromyalgia, 133
functional limitations, 6-7

G

gene transformation, 38-39
generalized anxiety disorder, 275, 347
genetic counseling, 411-412
genetic discrimination, 410-411
genetic testing, 409-410
genetics, 399, 402, 409-412
genitourinary system, 32-34
glaucoma, 123

H

hallucinogens, 295, 296, 299
hand injuries – see upper extremity injuries
hard-of-hearing – see hearing loss
hearing aids, 107-108
hearing loss, 101-115
heart disease – see cardiovascular disease
heavy – see exertion/physical demands
hematological diseases, 399-408
hemiplegia (see stroke), 162, 173
hemophilia, 402-405
HIV/AIDS, 87-100
holistic rehabilitation, 1-2, 10-11, 237-239

homeopathy, 146-147
human immunodeficiency virus – see HIV/AIDS
Huntington's disease, 200
hypertension, 68-69, 175-176
hypertensive heart disease, 68-69

I

integrative medicine, 143-153
integumentary system, 28
intellectual developmental disorders, 329-342
internal medicine, 12
intracranial hemorrhagic stroke, 171-172
ischemic stroke, 171

J

JAN – see Job Accommodation Network
Job Accommodation Network, 10
job accommodation/modification, 8-9, 112, 189-190, 361, 364
job coaching, 164, 338
job modification, 8-10
job restructuring, 8-10, 112

K

kidney disease, 57-61
kidney transplantation, 59-60

L

LD – see learning disabilities
learning disabilities, 317-328
light – see exertion/physical demands
lower extremity impairment, 354-359
lungs – see chronic obstructive pulmonary disease
lymphatic system, 27

M

macular degeneration, 119, 124
magnetic resonance imaging, 195
major depressive disorder, 276-277
manual techniques, 135
marijuana, 295-300, 310
medical abbreviations, 428-430
medical specialties, 11-13
medical terminology, 423-430
Medicare functional levels, 363-364
medium – see exertion/physical demands
mitral valve prolapse, 67
mixed hearing loss, 104-105
mononeuropathy, 195, 202
mood disorders, 276-277

motor neuron disease, 194, 198, 200
multiple sclerosis, 243-253
muscular dystrophy, 200, 233-242
musculoskeletal system, 18-20
myocardial infarction, 53, 70, 80
myocardiopathy – see cardiomyopathy

N

neuromuscular disease, 233, 236-239
neuropathy, 201-202
nicotine, 70, 304
noise-induced hearing loss, 105
normalization, 333-335

O

occupational therapy, 224
occupationally significant characteristics, 5, 6, 123
open head injuries, 157
opiates, 135, 297
optic atrophy, 123
oral hypoglycemic agents, 54-55
organ level, 18
orthotics, 106, 353-357
osteoarthritis, 106, 260-261
otosclerosis, 106
ototoxicity, 106

P

pancreas, 31-34
panic disorders, 275
paralysis, 172-173
paraplegia, 206, 210, 214
paresis, 158, 173, 262
Parkinson's disease, 120, 159, 198, 200
peripheral nervous system, 22-23, 53
peripheral neuropathy, 51, 52, 53, 90
peripheral vascular insufficiency, 52, 53
peroneal neuropathy, 202
personality disorders, 279-280
phantom limb, 131, 364
phantom limb pain, 133, 359
physical exertion categories – see exertion/physical demands
physical therapy, 135, 224
polymyositis, 106, 263-264
positron emission tomography, 196
post-traumatic stress disorder, 277-278
presbycusis, 106
pressure sores, 211
prosthetics, 353-354, 359, 361-364
psychiatric diagnoses, 269-284

PTSD – see post-traumatic stress disorder
pure tone audiometry, 103

Q

quality of life, 229

R

radiation therapy, 42-43
reasonable accommodation, 8-9, 47, 189-190, 304, 321-324
regenerative medicine, 415-421
rehabilitation intervention, 1, 8-10
rehabilitation potential, 46, 56
renal failure – see kidney disease
residual functional capacity, 4
respiratory system, 29-30
retinal diseases, 53, 120, 121, 123
retinitis pigmentosa, 124
retinopathy of prematurity, 125
return-to-work, 214
rheumatic disease, 255-268
rheumatic heart disease, 67
rheumatoid arthritis, 133, 256-260

S

schizophrenia, 278-279
scleroderma, 262-263
sedentary – see exertion/physical demand
seizures, 181-192
semiskilled – see skill requirements
sensorineural hearing loss, 104-105
sensory system, 30-31
sexuality, 210-211, 285-293, 345, 372-374
sexuality and disability, 46, 239, 285-293, 345, 367, 370-374
sheltered workshops, 337, 348
sickle cell disease, 399-402
skeletal system, 3-4
skill requirements, 3-4
skilled – see skill requirements
skin – see integumentary system
somatic nervous system, 124
spasticity, 211
spinal cord injuries, 205-215, 391, 415, 417
Stargardt's disease, 120, 124
stem cell, 416-417
stroke, 169-180
substance abuse, 134, 158, 168
supported employment, 336-338
systemic lupus erythematosus, 261-262

T

TBI – see traumatic brain injury
tolerance, 310
transferability of skills, 5-6
transplantation, 42, 43, 59-60, 262, 415, 417
traumatic brain injury, 155-167

U

ulnar neuropathy, 202
universal design, 392-396
unskilled – see skill requirements
upper extremity impairment, 377-388

V

valvular heart disease, 65, 67
very heavy – see exertion/physical demands
vestibular disorders, 106-107
veterans, 213-214
vision aids, 121-122
vision enhancement, 127
vision substitution, 127
visual disabilities, 117-130
visual system, 120-121
vocational profile, 2-5, 13-14
vocational skills, 5-6

W

whole medical systems, 143-144